Accident and Emergency Medicine

Accident and Emergency Medicine

EDITED BY

William H. Rutherford
OBE MB BCh FRCS(Ed) FRCSE
Honorary Consultant in Accident & Emergency Medicine
Royal Victoria Hospital
Belfast
Emergency Planning Adviser
Department of Health and Social Services
Northern Ireland

Robin N. Illingworth MA BM BCh MRCP
Consultant in Accident & Emergency Medicine
St James' University Hospital
Leeds

Andrew K. Marsden MB ChB FRCS(Ed)
Consultant in Accident & Emergency Medicine
Pinderfields General Hospital
Wakefield

Peter G. Nelson MB BCh FRCP (Lond)
Consultant in Accident & Emergency Medicine
Royal Victoria Hospital
Belfast

Anthony D. Redmond MD MRCP FRCS
Consultant in Accident & Emergency Medicine
Wythenshire and Withington Hospitals
Manchester

David H. Wilson MB ChB FRCS(Ed) FRCS
DTM&H
Dean of Postgraduate Medical Education
Faculty of Medicine
University of Leeds
Leeds

SECOND EDITION

CHURCHILL LIVINGSTONE
EDINBURGH LONDON MELBOURNE AND NEW YORK 1989

CHURCHILL LIVINGSTONE
Medical Division of Longman Group UK Limited

Distributed in the United States of America by Churchill Livingstone Inc.,
1560 Broadway, New York, N.Y. 10036, and by associated companies, branches
and representatives throughout the world.

First published 1980
Second edition 1989

ISBN 0 443 038201

British Library Cataloguing in Publication Data

Accident and emergency medicine. — 2nd ed.
  1. Medicine. Emergency treatment — For hospital doctors
  I. Rutherford, William H.
  616'.025

Library of Congress Cataloging in Publication Data

Accident and emergency medicine/edited by William H. Rutherford ...
  [et al.]. — 2nd ed.
  Bibliography: p.
  Includes index.
  1. Emergency medicine. 2. Traumatology I. Rutherford, William Harford.
  [DNLM: 1. Accidents. 2. Emergency Medicine. 3. Emergency
Service, Hospital WX 215 A171]
RC86.7.A26 1989
616'.025 — dc19
DNLM/DLC
for Library of Congress

Printed in Great Britain
at the University Printing House, Oxford

Preface to the Second Edition

When the first edition of this book was written, the specialty of accident and emergency medicine was young. The main aim in writing then was to provide an authoritative textbook for those who had chosen to make a career in the specialty and were entering their senior registrar training.

In practice the book's use was not restricted to academic study nor to senior trainee grades. It was used not only by doctors of all grades but also by nurses, though in this case mainly by those who intended to work permanently in A & E departments and were studying for the certificate in A & E nursing. While this edition is a very thorough revision of the first, the general style and content are similar and hopefully it will again appeal to a wide spectrum of users.

Shortly after the first edition was written Mr Peter Weston left the A & E department of the University Hospital in Nottingham and went to a general surgical post in Mbeya, Tanzania. When a second edition was planned he asked to be excused. Dr Peter Nelson, Mr David Wilson and I who worked with him on the first edition are particularly aware of how much we owe him and how much that he wrote survives into the second edition. For this edition we have been joined by three new editors, Dr Robin Illingworth, Mr Andrew Marsden and Mr Tony Redmond. Unlike the original authors, these men have had the benefit of the senior registrar training scheme. Much of the improvement in this volume is due to their knowledge and enthusiasm.

In the first edition the identity of the author of the original draft of any chapter was not declared. The drafts were subjected to much mutual criticism and rewriting, and in the end we felt that the whole book and each of its chapters belonged to us all. In this edition we again followed the discipline of submitting every draft to all the editors, and again the criticism and rewriting have greatly improved the quality of the text. However in the end we felt it best that the responsibility for each chapter should be placed on a declared author. We hope that the very considerable consensus and the strong bonds of friendship between the six of us will again have helped to produce a book which reads almost as if it had been written by a single author.

The editors are all from the United Kingdom and the book necessarily reflects the conditions of the specialty in our own country. We have, however been in touch with colleagues, specialist associations and specialist colleges in other lands. We hope that this has influenced us as we write, and that our book may be of value to doctors working in the field of emergency medicine throughout the world.

Between the first and second editions, word processors have come into their own. We are deeply indebted to Julie Connolly, Kate McAteer, Maria McConvey and Christine McMillan in the Royal Victoria Hospital, Belfast, who prepared the disks from which the book was printed. We are also grateful to a host of other secretaries in all our hospitals. This edition also owes much to the wise planning and advice of Mr Peter Richardson and the careful editorial control of Mrs Elif Fincanci-Smith of Churchill Livingstone. It has been a pleasure to work with them.

Accident and emergency medicine is a specialty covering a very broad field, where decisions of importance often have to be made in conditions of stress. Our aim was to produce a practical book where doctors and nurses could find succinct and trustworthy advice. We hope that we have succeeded in that aim.

Belfast, 1989   W.H.R.

Preface to the First Edition

Ever since the first hospitals came into being, doctors have had to deal with patients arriving with a great variety of injuries and other acute medical complaints. This aspect of hospital medicine was usually dealt with by junior doctors, often working in the reception area for a few months of their training period.

During the past two decades, it has been realised that correct treatment in the first few minutes in hospital influences the mortality and morbidity of seriously ill patients as much or more than any subsequent treatment, and that to achieve high standards it is necessary to place accident and emergency departments in the hands of doctors who will make this subject their permanent interest and responsibility.

In the UK, the appointment of a few consultants as an experiment proved so successful that the demand for more appointments mushroomed at an alarming speed. As it became evident that these doctors would be a permanent part of the medical services, arrangements had to be made for the training of new consultants. The Royal Colleges of Physicians and Surgeons set up a Specialist Advisory Committee in 1975. It was this body which gave the specialty its name — accident and emergency medicine.

Many books have already been written about both medical emergencies and trauma. There are also a number of books for the guidance of junior staff working in accident and emergency departments. But no British book has been written specifically for those who are training to work permanently in this field. This book is intended to fill that gap.

Accident and emergency medicine is a field where good clinical practice is difficult to achieve unless there is a sound basis of good organisation. We have therefore devoted the first section of the book to aspects of organisation. The next three sections deal with clinical problems. The conditions have been separated into life-threatening, major (stretcher patients) and minor (walking patients), and a section devoted to each. Within each of the three sections, conditions have been classified according to the chief problem with which the patient presents. Problems and diseases are considered from those points of view relevant to decisions in the A & E department: salient points which should be elucidated in the history; clinical signs which should be sought; whether X-rays or other tests should be carried out in the department; what immediate treatment is necessary; and which patients should be admitted, discharged or referred to a specialist clinic.

The fifth section of the book is devoted to various specialties which are of particular relevance to accident and emergency work. Finally, some useful information is listed in a series of appendices.

It has been difficult to keep each section and topic in proportion. Some comparatively rare conditions have been described because if they are not correctly diagnosed and treated, the outcome is serious or fatal. Some topics should be so well known to all doctors that prior knowledge has been assumed. The number of patients with fractures treated in different A & E departments varies widely. There are many excellent books about the management of fractures, and we have restricted ourselves to their diagnosis and immediate treatment. The chapter on minor head injuries is disproportionately long, but the information needed by doctors in A & E departments is not readily available from other sources.

The higher specialist training for accident and emergency medicine differs from the training for many other specialties in that those embarking on it may come from a wide range of medical backgrounds. They may have a higher degree in medicine, surgery, anaesthetics or general practice. Each individual's training programme is tailored according to his previous experience. In view of the varied backgrounds, it has been necessary to cover a wide field of medicine. We have had to assume that some trainees will be unfamiliar with each subject. It is inevitable that some parts of the book will seem very simple to those already well versed in that subject.

Writing a major textbook on a new specialty has been a challenging experience. During the process our understanding of the subject developed. The result is a book which we hope will be valuable not only to senior registrar trainees but to all doctors — junior and senior — working in accident and emergency departments. Indeed, doctors in other disciplines whose work includes the management of acutely ill patients may also find its problem-orientated approach and its emphasis on decision-making both stimulating and useful.

W.H.R
1979

Acknowledgements

Permission to reproduce the figures and tables listed below has been obtained from those who hold the copyright. We are very grateful to all who have helped us in this way.

Fig. 6.1 Physio Control UK Ltd.

Fig. 6.4 John Murray Ltd.

Fig. 6.6 Professor Miles Irving. Department of Surgery, Manchester.

Fig. 7.1 The Press Association.

Figs. 7.2 A and B Associated Press.

Figs. 10.1, 10.2, 10.3, 10.5, 10.6, 10.11, 10.13, 10.16, 10.27 (from original drawings by Asmund Laerdal, Norway) The Resuscitation Council.

Figs. 10.7, 10.21, 10.22 (from Fisher J, Marsden AK, Rogers J 1986 Save a Life. An Instructor's Guide) BBC Publications Ltd.

Fig. 10.8 and Tables 10.1, 10.3, 10.4, 10.5 (from Evans T(ed) 1986 The ABC of Resuscitation) The British Medical Journal publications.

Fig. 10.20 (from article by Stephenson H E Jr 1984 51: 370–377) The Missouri Medical Journal.

Fig. 14.1 (from Boyd CR, Kilson MA, Copes WA 1987 Evaluating Trauma Care — the TRISS method. 24(iv): 370–378) The Journal of Trauma.

Fig. 14.2 (from Knas WA, Draper EA, Wagner DP, Zimmerman JE 1985 A severity of diseases system. 13: 818–829) Critical Care Medicine.

Figs. 14.32, 14.33 (from Settle JAD. Burns — the first 5 days) Smith and Nephew Pharmaceuticals Ltd.

Fig. 14.35 Crown copyright reserved. From Porton Down.

Figs. 14.49, 14.50 Miss Helen McIllhenry.

Fig. 16.3 (from article by Prescott L F in Drugs 1983 25: 297 (fig. 4) Adis Press, Auckland.

Table 17.1 (modified from Lance J W 1982 Management of headache, 4th edn.) Butterworths Scientific, London.

Figs. 18.5, 18.7–18.12 (from Bennett D 1985 Cardiac Arrhythmias, 2nd edn.) Butterworths Scientific, London.

P. 313 Broad guidelines of good practice for the discharge of elderly patients from an A & E Department — The British Geriatrics Society.

Figs. 38.2, 38.3 St. John's Ambulance.

Fig. 40.6 and Table 40.1 The Neurosurgical and A & E units, Pinderfields General Hospital, Wakefield.

Contributors

Ian D Adams MD
Consultant in Accident & Emergency Medicine, St James'
University Hospital, Leeds

Michael J Cinnamond MB BCh FRCS(Ed),
Professor of Otolaryngology, The Queen's University of Belfast;
Consultant Otolaryngologist, Royal Victoria Hospital, Belfast

William J Cunliffe MD FRCP
Consultant Dermatologist, The General Infirmary, Leeds

David Hutchinson BChD LDS D(Orth) FDSRCS(Eng)
Consultant Oral Surgeon, Pinderfields General Hospital, Wakefield

Karen A Illingworth MB ChB FFARCS
Consultant Anaesthetist, St James' University Hospital, Leeds

Robin N Illingworth MA BM BCh MRCP
Consultant in Accident & Emergency Medicine, St James'
University Hospital, Leeds

Stewart S Johnston MB BCh FRCS
Consultant Ophthalmic Surgeon, Royal Victoria Hospital,
Belfast

Alan G Kerr MB BCh FRCS(Ed) DObstRCOG
Consultant Otolaryngologist, Royal Victoria Hospital, Belfast

Andrew K Marsden MB BCh FRCS(Ed)
Consultant in Accident & Emergency Medicine, Pinderfields
General Hospital, Wakefield

J O Manton Mills MB BCh DRCOG DMRD FRCR
Consultant Radiologist, Royal Victoria Hospital, Belfast

Peter G Nelson MB BCh FRCP (Lond)
Consultant in Accident & Emergency Medicine, Royal Victoria
Hospital, Belfast

Anthony D Redmond MD MRCP FRCS
Consultant in Accident & Emergency Medicine, Wythenshire
and Withington Hospitals, Manchester

William H Rutherford OBE MB BCh FRCS(Ed) FRCS
Honorary Consultant in Accident & Emergency Medicine,
Royal Victoria Hospital, Belfast, Emergency Planning Advisor,
Department of Health & Social Services, Northern Ireland

David H Wilson MB BCh DTM & H FRCS(Ed) FRCS
Dean of Postgraduate Medical Education, The Faculty of
Medicine, University of Leeds

Contents

SECTION ONE

Organisation

INTRODUCTION

The main functions of doctors working in accident and emergency departments are making an accurate diagnosis, giving immediate treatment and arranging for the patient's further care. Good organisation, thereby enabling the doctors to concentrate wholly on this aspect of their work, is the responsibility of the consultant. Section I therefore deals with the most important aspects of this organisation.

The nature and scope of accident and emergency medicine are described in the first chapter. Also the functions of the department are outlined. This leads on naturally to the second chapter which is concerned with the design and planning of the department.

The A & E department is on the interface between the hospital and the community and therefore good communications and records are essential. Much thought should go into this aspect of

A & E work. One reason for the necessity for good records is their medicolegal importance. The consultant must have a grasp of the common legal problems because he has a special responsibility to guide his junior colleagues in these matters. Many of the problems which affect patients attending A & E departments are social as well as medical, and the A & E doctor must be able to assess not merely the medical issues but to give due weight to the social.

While the chief responsibility of A & E doctors is in their own departments, they are inevitably interested in methods of lowering mortality and morbidity in the prehospital phase of patient care. The staff of the department should be trained not only to cope with normal day-to-day conditions, but also with the unpredictable demands of a disaster. In the investigation of A & E patients, a high percentage will require radiological examination or some other form of imaging. A chapter is devoted to this aspect, and another to pain control and anaesthesia.

Accident and emergency medicine

EARLY DEVELOPMENTS

Accident and emergency medicine is one of the most recent specialties to emerge. It is now a fully organised and recognised specialty in at least six countries — the UK, the Republic of Ireland, the USA, Canada, Australia and New Zealand. There are a number of other countries where it exists at some stage of development and where associations of doctors interested in the problems and opportunties of this field have been established. Organisation of the specialty in Ireland, Canada and New Zealand was to some extent secondary to its development in Britain, America and Australia. The specialty started independently in these countries, and at first those doctors involved in one country were not aware of the existence of a similar group in another. It would appear that there were forces at work in the field of medicine which brought about this development, and that they were operating strongly in the 25 years between 1960 and 1985. What were these factors?

The origins of specialism in medicine go back for some hundreds

of years. The separation of doctors who operated (i.e. surgeons) into a special group is at least 400 years old. Some doctors also chose to devote themselves entirely to the care of women during childbirth. The crucial factors which define different specialties vary greatly in their nature. For example, surgery and medicine are defined on the basis of whether operative treatment is or is not appropriate. Ophthalmology and dermatology are defined by anatomy. Paediatrics and geriatrics are defined by age.

In the 20th century the tendency towards specialisation increased and still appears to be increasing. Different groups of doctors confined their interests to one small field within medicine and, within that field, developed a degree of expertise which was only possible because of the restriction of their field of interest.

While specialisation was not restricted to hospital medicine, it was in the hospital that it reached its most advanced form. Hospitals became centres with clinics and wards catering for a large number of specialities. However, there was a tradition in many countries that the medical emergencies arriving at the hospital should be dealt with by a succession of the most junior doctors. As a result emergency patients in the most critical condition arrived in a hospital where excellent specialists worked, but the standard of immediate care was poor because the initial assessment and resuscitation were performed by doctors too inexperienced to be able to treat well and too inhibited to summon a senior specialist in the correct field.

Dissatisfaction with standards in Casualty (as the emergency receiving room was called) was voiced in Britain in the 1960s from two different sources. Firstly, a government report into medical services for the victims of accidents (commonly called the Platt Report after the chairman of the reporting committee, Sir Harry Platt) was concerned that the severely injured patients' condition was in danger of deteriorating after arrival in hospital because of poor arrangements for their reception. Secondly, Dr Frank Pantridge investigated the time factor in the early hours after a patient sustained a myocardial infarct and was more forthright. He called the casualty department the death trap — a prime site of inexcusable delay.

The Platt Report's solution was that, for each casualty department, three orthopaedic consultants should be appointed and expected to spend a substantial part of their time supervising the department. Few if any orthopaedic surgeons were so appointed. At that time, as well as large numbers of very junior doctors, there were here and there senior doctors working in the casualty department. They did not have consultant status, as was usual for senior doctors working in recognised specialities, but were appointed as assistant to a consultant in orthopaedics or general surgery who was nominally in charge, but rarely seen in the department. As a consequence of the debate which ensued from the Platt report in 1967 these assistant doctors formed themselves into the Casualty Surgeons Association. Their aims were recognition for their speciality and the appointment of consultants. In 1973 their campaign achieved its aim and some 30 such consultants were appointed. Prior to this there were only three or four consultants in the whole of the UK appointed to work full-time in this field.

It was natural in the National Health Service in Britain that the arguments should be debated in the British Medical Association and negotiated with the Department of Health. In the USA prior to 1960 the general situation in emergency rooms (the American term for casualty departments) was very similar to Britain. These were usually staffed by rotating interns who were too inexperienced for the responsibilities they were given. However, under a system of private medicine, it is easier for doctors to take local initiatives. In Michigan in 1961 a group of physicians made arrangements by which there would always be one senior physician on duty in the emergency room during the whole 24 hours of each day. Apart from their responsibilities on the rota, the physicians otherwise continued their normal practice. About the same time in Alexandra, Virginia another group of physicians decided that they would join together and work solely in the emergency room.

Similar experiments started in other areas. The doctors involved banded themselves together and in 1968 formed the American College of Emergency Physicians. Within a very short time they had over 1000 members. They discovered that they were practising a new specialty which was not recognised. As well as the direct battle for recognition it was necessary to establish residency training schemes, a certification board with standards and procedures, a journal and an academic and research body. Very similar developments were taking place in Britain with the development of a senior registrar training scheme, a specialist examination, a journal and a research society.

Developments in Canada were influenced by the geographical features of the country, with its areas of dense population and large conurbations contrasting with much larger areas where the population is minimal and widely scattered. The problems of making good organisational arrangements to deal with medical emergencies in these situations were formidable. During the 1970s many doctors practising in emergency departments joined the American College of Emergency Physicians and in 1978 they formed their own association, the Canadian Association of Emergency Physicians. The formal steps to establish and recognise the specialty were taken by the Royal College of Physicians and Surgeons of Canada in the early 1980s. Arrangements were made for training programmes, accreditation and certification. Simultaneously, the College of Family Physicians of Canada

established a one-year training course, which was to be added to their normal two-year course for family physicians. Completion of this three-year course was rewarded by a Certificate of Special Competence in Emergency Medicine.

In Australia, as in many other countries, until the 1960s medical staffing of casualty departments had been almost entirely by a succession of junior staff. The first senior doctor was appointed to a prominent post as Casualty Director in Gaelong, Victoria, in 1967. By 1973 there were enough such appointments to allow the establishment of the Association of Casualty Supervisors of Victoria Hospitals. This was an association for both doctors and nurses working in a supervisory capacity. In 1977 the Victoria government set up a committee to examine the reception of road accident victims. This focused attention on the problems of providing staff with adequate experience and training at the reception areas of hospitals.

In 1978 the Western Australian Society for Emergency Medicine was founded and by 1980 this society and the association in Victoria were superseded by the Australian Society of Emergency Medicine. Various New Zealand doctors were involved in very similar problems and developments, and the new society was almost immediately transformed into the Australasian Society for Emergency Medicine. The geography and the medical organisation of Australia and New Zealand imposed their own distinctive effects on the evolvement of the specialty. As the doctors sought to lay the foundations of a new specialty, they were aware of developments in the UK and the USA and were able to consider how far the structures in those countries would meet their own needs. They decided that the best method would be to form a College, somewhat similar to the American model. Progess was remarkably rapid. By 1983 the inaugural meeting of the Australasian College for Emergency Medicine was held in Surfers Paradise, Queensland. In 1985 the first primary examination was held, 35 doctors sat it and 7 passed. The first fellowship examination followed in 1986.

THE NATURE OF THE SPECIALTY

The emergence of a specialty is often connected with raising standards of care for a certain group of patients, and usually recognition of the specialty has been followed by reorganisation of medical facilities to allow the application of the newly gained knowledge. Accident and emergency medicine is unusual in that its organisational separation preceded by many years both its recognition as a specialty, and any serious efforts to develop standards of excellence for the treatment of its patients.

Accident and emergency medicine is differentiated on the basis of a particular time and a particular place. The time is the phase of urgency or crisis and the place is the reception area of a hospital. It is in the interplay of the time and the place which gives accident and emergency medicine its special characteristics. There are many critical situations and emergencies in medicine which are not appropriate to the reception area of a hospital, e.g. emergency complications of anaesthesia, or an emergency for the public health services such as an epidemic of food poisoning. Equally, there are conditions quite suitable for investigation and treatment at hospital outpatient clinics which have no element of crisis or emergency, such as most patients with skin rashes and chronic low back pain.

The resuscitation of patients arriving at hospital in extremis from a wide variety of different conditions is one of the prime responsibilities of A & E medicine. By accurately differentiating between the patients who do and do not require admission to hospital and by directing patients to wards and clinics of the appropriate specialty or back to the care of their general practitioners, doctors in accident and emergency medicine can do much to see that the acute hospital services are used to their maximum efficiency. The proper diagnosis and treatment of minor injuries (especially of the head, hand and neck) and minor septic conditions are also a significant part of the work.
Accident and emergency medicine overlaps with many other specialties. The specialty training recommendations in accident and emergency medicine therefore include experience in many other specialties. To some it appears as if accident and emergency is vainly attempting to take within its ambit the wisdom of all other specialties. This is not so. In relation to other specialties, accident and emergency medicine is a cross-section and, like a slice, a cross-section is broad but not very deep. Accident and emergency medicine is concerned only with those parts of other specialties relevant to the emergency reception services in a hospital.

WHAT'S IN A NAME?

In Britain the old name for the accident and emergency department was the casualty department. This was in many ways an excellent term. Everyone knew that it referred to a particular department in the hospital. It carried some of the same overtones as the term casualty as applied to a person, as in battle casualty — the victim of a serious accident.
However, when in 1961 the Platt Committee came to investigate arrangements in hospitals for the reception and treatment of accidents, they found standards poor and morale low. They were concerned about the problems of 'casual' attenders. Wishing to give the public a clearer idea of what kind of work these departments were meant to do, they suggested that they should be renamed accident and emergency departments. The name was quickly accepted by those departments which were attempting to make improvements, so that it became associated with feelings of hope and aspirations towards excellence. The term casualty, so much more succinct and essentially meaning the same thing, became more and more associated with departments which had not changed with the times. When a specialist advisory committee was set up to devise a training programme for the newly emerging specialty, it gave its blessing to the term accident and emergency medicine. We have accepted this term throughout our book. For the shortness and simplicity we have often shortened 'accident and emergency' to 'A & E'.

There is no doubt that in some ways 'accident and emergency medicine' is a cumbersome phrase. In America the specialty has opted for the more succinct term 'emergency medicine'. However this also is not without difficulty. Emergencies in medicine cover a very wide field. Emergency situations may arise in all the different specialties not merely at the time of arrival at hospital, but at any point in the time scale of an illness. Emergency medicine and emergencies in medicine could easily be confused. The term accident and emergency medicine, though clumsy, is unlikely to be confused with any other entity.

As this is a British textbook, we will use this accepted British name for the specialty. We trust that it will cause little confusion even in countries where the term emergency medicine is more commonly used.

THE EFFECT OF OPEN ACCESS

One essential feature of any good emergency service must be ease of access. Some emergencies are life threatening. It is obviously inappropriate to have any elaborate screening of patients before arrival at the department, as the delay so caused may increase morbidity or mortality rates. In practice, A & E departments are open not merely to all medical practitioners for immediate referral of emergency cases, but also to patients in a crisis. The type of patients seen in any department is therefore dependent not only on the views of the A & E medical staff on its correct use, but also on the views of general practitioners and the expectations of the public. People who happen to live close to a hospital with an A & E department often choose to use it for any or every purpose merely because appointments are not required. Some general practitioners will use the department as an alternative to requesting an appointment at the appropriate specialty clinic, or occasionally just to get rid of a querulous patient.

Open access allows doctors and public to determine how the department is used, and A & E staff have no option but to see all patients who enter the department. However, individuals who attend inappropriately should be seen and advised where and how to seek help. It may be much less trouble merely to hand out some symptomatic treatment, but unless A & E doctors accept the burden of redirecting patients to appropriate services they are co-operating in the misuse of the department and must expect that misuse to increase. Local committees in hospital and in the community should be made aware of the problems so that informed discussion can take place about the correct referral for each type of patient.

PATIENTS ON THE A & E / GP INTERFACE

There are two groups of patients who find their way to A & E departments for whom, at least in theory, there are alternative sources of care.

1. The trivial injury or illness for which self-care at home would be quite adequate. The number of patients of this type is difficult to assess, but in a large urban A & E department roughly 5% of walking patients fall into this category.

2. Those with the less acute medical conditions who need the

help of a general practitioner, but present themselves at the A & E department, often because they have tried to contact their general practitioner but have been unable to do so. Some may have had to wait for an appointment with their family doctor. Such patients may think they will get more expert treatment at the hospital or that the GP will send them there anyway. Of the case load of a large urban hospital, 8% fall into this category.

These patients often receive scant attention and inadequate treatment from junior A & E doctors whose prime interests, training and skills lie in the treatment of the more serious acute illness and injury and who may not have time to enquire in sufficient depth into the physical or mental stresses which so often underlie presenting complaints. This problem could be tackled in four ways:

1. More effort could be made to educate the public in the proper use of the various branches of the health services. The staff of A & E departments must surely be involved in such schemes.

2. Some sorting by suitably trained nurses could be undertaken at the entrance to the A & E department. This would allow the patients with less acute problems, to be diverted either (a) to a different section of the department which would be staffed by doctors of a general practice background (either general practitioners, or vocational trainees), or (b) back to health centres in the community. This reverse referral to GPs would be much easier if there were health centres adjacent to, or integrated with, the hospital complex. This concept is already in existence where health centres and community hospitals have grown up together. For A & E departments such a policy would be a radical change and contrary to the present policy of the Casualty Surgeons Association which states that all patients should be seen by a doctor. However the exponential increase in attendances in A & E departments may require radical measures.

3. The hospital could be used (instead of general practitioners) as the source of primary care outside normal office hours. The majority of patients could be treated through a deputising service based within the hospital.

4. Efforts could be made to reverse the trend by operating a strictly limited number of health centres 24 hours a day and basing the deputising service in one of these centres.

Either the third or fourth of these solutions would require considerable readjustment of staffing and facilities, but either would be preferable to the present unhappy compromise which relies so heavily on the goodwill and patience of doctors and nurses in A & E departments.

A & E REGULARS

There are certain groups of patients for whom A & E departments have always accepted responsibility, for example, the drunks, the drug addicts, those diabetics and epileptics who cannot or will not take their medication regularly, the social misfits, psychiatric emergencies, those of no fixed abode and many patients whose problems are indicative of the social evils or ills of our time. It is desirable to have a register of 'regulars' so that a medical social worker (who is an essential member of the A & E team) and the

A & E doctor can periodically review them to ensure that appropriate action has been taken. There must also be a register of children who have sustained suspected or actual non-accidental injury.

Responsibility for 'regulars' and children with non-accidental injury is one way in which the medical social worker is involved in A & E medicine. This aspect is more fully dealt with in Chapters 4, 5 and 30. The police may also become involved in A & E work through the department's regulars.

GEOGRAPHICAL LOCATION

The appropriate use of an accident and emergency department will vary somewhat from place to place and from country to country. Large metropolitan cities are likely to have considerable numbers of tourists, temporary residents and commuters. When such patients fall ill with conditions which would normally be appropriate to general practice they may turn to the A & E department of a hospital. The hospital in a holiday resort town will find itself in a similar position during the tourist season. In these situations there is an area of overlap between accident and emergency medicine and general practice. The fact that almost any condition seen in general practice may also be seen in an A & E department does not mean that A & E medicine should be thought of as including the whole scope of general practice. The metropolitan and tourist centre A & E departments should be thought of as the exception rather than the rule.

The work in any particular A & E department will also be affected by the presence of other hospitals in the vicinity. Thus, a children's hospital, an eye hospital, an ear, nose and throat hospital in the vicinity may each have its own A & E department. The A & E department of a neighbouring general hospital may not then have to undertake supervision of patients in these specialties. However, A & E medicine as a whole must be thought of as including the emergency aspects of all these specialties.

ACCIDENT SERVICES

The move towards upgrading A & E departments in the UK historically emerged from the concern of some surgeons (mainly orthopaedic surgeons) about the inadequate arrangements for the reception of severely injured patients. Accidents are the fifth largest cause of death in all ages, and the most common cause of death for people aged under 40 years. If lives are to be saved and morbidity reduced, treatment of the severely injured in the first minutes after arrival in hospital must be of high quality. As accidents happen every day and at any time, organising such care is an important responsibility. A good A & E department should also provide high quality care for minor accidents and be involved in teaching and research relating to accidents.

The number of trauma patients, both major life-threatening cases and minor trauma and the proportion of trauma patients to non-trauma patients will vary somewhat from hospital to hospital.

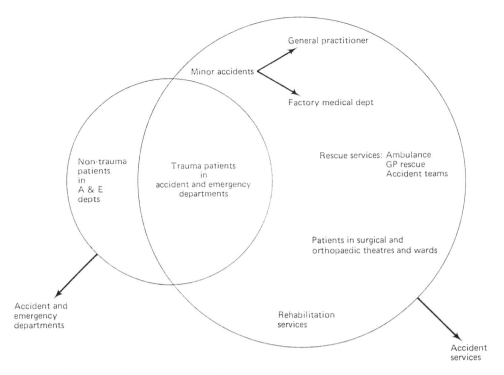

Fig. 1.1 The overlapping interests of A & E medicine and accident services.

However, it is obvious that accidents are an important part of the work of an A & E department. On the other hand, when A & E work is approached primarily from the aspect of accidents, it is all too easy to assume that everything going on in the department which is not accident work is of little importance or significance. From what has been written above, it can be seen that such a view is narrow and biased, and unlikely to lead to the development of good departments (Fig. 1.1). It is also dangerous.

ADMISSION POLICY

The work in different A & E departments will vary depending on the local hospital admission policies. In some hospitals this is arranged between the practitioner and the consultant in charge of the ward. In others all such cases are received in the A & E department and the final decisions about admissions are made there.

Although this will, to some extent, change the types of patients dealt with, it does not alter the nature of A & E medicine as a whole. Cases similar to those sent by general practitioners will still arrive either as self-referrals, or as patients received through the emergency and ambulance services responding to a 999 call.

A & E DESIGN AND FUNCTION

When considering how to plan and design a department (Ch. 2) we argue that good planning depends on understanding its proper function. It is also true that the design features which have come to characterise most A & E departments indicate the nature of the work.

The resuscitation room demonstrates the important place in A & E medicine of the resuscitation of patients with life-threatening emergencies. Some cubicles are usually designated for the treatment of major, though not life-threatening conditions. Decisions need to be made about whether these patients require hospital admission. Other cubicles are designated for patients with minor conditions, few of whom will need hospital admission. Usually a few cubicles will be reserved for the follow-up care of patients with appropriate conditions within the A & E department. A dressings room is a feature because some patients with wounds and minor burns will attend over a period of time for dressings. The operating theatre shows that A & E medicine also encompasses minor surgery. The x-ray rooms draw attention to the key place of radiology. Most departments have observation wards where patients whose conditions are on the borderline of needing hospital treatment may be held for 24 hours, and this responsibility is counted as part of the specialty.

THE CLINICAL DIMENSION

One of the features which characterise A & E medicine is that its care of patients is episodic rather than continuous. Patients present in hospital with a problem — vomiting, abdominal pain, collapse, road accident. The skills of this specialty are in knowing, for any particular problem what precise points need to be established in the medical history, which are the important aspects of the physical examination, whether radiological investigations are required and what other special tests are of value. A & E medicine is concerned with the criteria for admission to hospital and possible alternative management. It is concerned with such medical treatment as is likely to be needed while the patient is in the A & E department, with the criteria used for monitoring patients in the department or observation ward and with the conduct of review clinics.

THE ORGANISATIONAL DIMENSION

Good organisation is of paramount importance in an A & E department. It is not enough to be able to understand the clinical problems of patients. It is necessary to initiate and maintain good record systems, to make plans for disaster situations and to deal with complaints and legal problems. By its nature as a cross-section of many specialties, there are problems of relationships with many other hospital departments and, because this department is on the interface between the hospital and the community, relationships have to be maintained with people and institutions outside the hospital. It is essential that the A & E doctor knows how to work tactfully yet firmly with many other people, and how to act as a member of a team which includes all those who work within the department.

TIME

Every aspect of medicine has its characteristic tempo. The tempo of the A & E department is one of movement, not hectic movement, for the confidence and skill of the staff should impart a feeling of calm no matter how great the pressure. But it should be obvious to patients, to relatives and to the staff that the work is going forward.

The time a patient spends in the A & E department is sandwiched between the prehospital phase of his illness or accident and the definitive treatment in the ward or theatre. Some severely injured or seriously ill patients will undergo resuscitation as a result of which their condition may be much improved. This may affect the mortality and morbidity as much as anything done at a later stage. But the majority of patients are not undergoing resuscitation. They are being assessed. To spend up to an hour in assessing such patients, and thus making sure that the right patients are admitted to hospital and that they go to the most appropriate unit for treating their complaint, is time well spent. But it is not justifiable to keep patients with serious illnesses or injuries lying on trolleys in an A & E department for two, three or four hours.

Similarly, many patients with minor injuries — wounds, sprains, small burns, fractures of the hand or arm — should be examined and treated within 20 minutes. Some may take up to an hour, as there will be times when patients with minor injuries must allow the doctors and nurses to deal first with patients with more serious complaints. Nonetheless, an hour is a reasonable target time for both major and minor patients. When decisions are being made, treatments given and few, if any, patients waiting beyond an hour, the whole department enjoys a sense of work being well done.

By contrast, when delays of three or four hours build up, the patients and relatives become irritated. Usually they communicate their irritation, first to the receptionists and somewhat later to the nurses. Only after a considerable interval do patients complain to doctors.

No department can totally avoid times of long delay, but 80–90% of patients should be seen and decisions made within an hour. Where there are repeated delays, either the staff does not understand how to do its work well, or the allocation of staff is insufficient for the workload.

TEACHING

Wherever good medicine is practised, it should be taught. In departments which have been approved by the Specialist Advisory Committee for higher training in A & E medicine, the most senior trainee will be a senior registrar who intends to practise the speciality. The senior staff will arrange for secondment of this senior registrar to the many other specialist departments where he or she needs to acquire experience.

A & E departments play their part in the education of young surgeons, such experience being a compulsory requirement for the FRCS examination and recognised as acceptable in preparation for the MRCP examination. The departments are also used in the hospital training of general practitioners.

For junior doctors, the departments have the great advantage that, when the doctor has examined a patient, he can make his own decision if he feels the matter within his competence. Decision making is an educative experience more accessible to the young doctor in the A & E department than in almost any other hospital specialty. It is, of course, important that he always has access to senior colleagues, so that he is not forced into responsibility beyond his competence. Some A & E departments have introduced case reviews and self-monitoring, and this has been found to be very helpful in raising standards. Once- or twice-weekly case conferences or other teaching sessions should be carried out in all the larger departments.

For medical students the departments are of value both in giving experience in the management of serious emergencies and also for teaching about some of the minor conditions which it is assumed that every doctor knows, yet which so rarely are formally taught.

A & E departments should also form part of the experience of nurses during their training. If possible, tutorial sessions should be fitted in at times when the department is not too busy. The skills of bandaging, strapping and splinting should be taught to doctors, nurses and medical students.

RESEARCH

Because of the large number of patients seen, A & E departments are especially suitable for small programmes of clinical research which can be completed in the 6 or 12 months during which a young doctor is attached to the department. The specialty also provides material suitable for more long-term studies by senior members of staff, and some valuable contributions have already been made, including a multicentre study on the effectiveness of seat belt legislation in the UK.

TRAINING

Training to enter the specialty

When opening a new school, it is customary to start with an intake of the most junior form, and year by year allow this group of students to progress into a higher form, adding a new bottom class until there is a full set of classes from senior to junior. Historically, A & E medicine has set this process on its head, firstly appointing consultants, then arranging for senior registrar training and only recently devoting attention to the earlier phases of training.

Having decided, in 1973, to appoint consultants, the original appointees were either drawn from subconsultant grades where the candidates had worked for some years in A & E departments and gained experience, or from doctors whose backgrounds had given them a particularly wide experience, for example from service in the Third World or the armed services. In order to provide replacements as these men retired and to fill newly created posts, it was necessary to create a cadre of senior registrars. The first step was to establish a Specialist Advisory Committee for the accreditation of departments suitable for supervising senior registrar training and to lay down guidelines for the training. Because the sphere of work did not fall entirely within the remit of either the Royal College of Surgeons or the Royal College of Physicians, a joint working party was established. This joint committee laid down the rules and policies. After these were agreed, for ease of administration the Specialist Advisory Committee was appointed by the Royal College of Physicians. The membership of the committee continued to be drawn from both surgeons and physicians alongside a number of doctors already working in A & E departments.

A higher degree was deemed an essential qualification and it was agreed that this might be in medicine (MRCP), surgery (FRCS) or anaesthetics (FFARCS). Some years later the Royal College of Surgeons of Edinburgh felt that there should be a special higher examination designed to meet the needs of the new specialty. Although administered by a surgical college, the examination is set and examined by general surgeons, general physicians and A & E specialists. The resulting qualification is known as FRCS(A & E). This has also been accepted as a suitable entrance qualification for senior registrar training.

Because A & E medicine covered such a wide spectrum of diseases, the senior registrar training consisted to a large extent of secondments to other departments. The initial requirements for each trainee were drawn up to complement his previous experience. Surgeons were required to spend time in medical and cardiology wards as well as anaesthetics. Physicians were given a surgically based programme.

Although these programmes have worked reasonably well, they have had their problems. The trainee at senior registrar level finds himself repeatedly having to work in a very junior capacity during his secondments to various wards and units. In these units the training programmes are designed mainly to produce specialists in the discipline of that unit. The senior registrar seconded from the A & E department may find that he is being involved in many things which have no direct relevance to A & E medicine.

As the consultants in A & E departments become more and more expert over the whole of their specialty it would seem that they will gradually take over the training of those entering the speciality. In time the cardiology or orthopaedics appropriate for an A & E senior registrar may be better taught in the A & E department than in the cardiology or fracture wards and the need for secondments may disappear.

Competition to get into senior registrar posts has been intense. This has not infrequently resulted in trainees having two or three higher degrees. In acquiring these degrees and the related experience at an earlier stage of their careers, young doctors have already secured junior posts in a wide variety of specialties. This is altering the type of programme that is necessary in the senior registrar phase.

During senior registrar training, doctors are encouraged to undertake research. The senior registrars club has been a forum for early discussion of research topics, for the presentation of papers and for discussing the problems of the specialty in general and training requirements in particular. Most senior registrars have travelled at least within their own country. Crossing the Atlantic to work in the very different environment of emergency medicine in the USA has been particularly stimulating for those who have found ways of overcoming the conflicting requirements of registration in the different countries. The specialty of A & E medicine is still in a formative phase and as developments take place, adjustments have to be made in training. The Specialist Advisory Committee is responsible for making these adjustments.

The position is much more fluid in the earlier stages of training. There was a time when many entrants to the specialty had originally commenced training in some other medical or surgical branch and, finding advancement blocked, they transferred to A & E medicine as a second choice. As the specialty has become established a high percentage enter this training as their specialty of first choice. The stage at which doctors select A & E medicine as their chosen career has moved backwards to registrar, senior house officer, junior house officer and sometimes even medical student level. These early entrants have sought advice on how to plan their careers.

When senior registrar training was first established aspirants were advised to go into a training scheme for surgery, medicine or anaesthetics and to stay in that discipline until obtaining a higher degree. At this point the trainee needed to find a job in an A & E department for 6–12 months, followed by a training post in a discipline complementary to that originally studied. This has resulted in a number of trainees acquiring both FRCS and MRCP degrees. People thus qualified were ideally placed to sit the FRCS(A & E) examination and with this collection of degrees were in a very strong position to compete for senior registrar posts. Whilst this is still an acceptable path, there is much to be said in favour of making the FRCS(A & E) examination the primary objective of the early years. The obligatory requirements required for sitting the examination include one year of A & E medicine, one year of general surgery and one year of general medicine. Those who are successful in passing the FRCS(A & E) examination and cannot immediately obtain to an A & E senior registrar post may then consider doing an extra period in medicine, surgery or, maybe most valuable of all, anaesthetics including intensive care. It will be sad if it should always prove necessary to enhance one's chances of securing good senior posts by taking a multiplicity of higher degrees.

The early stages of training for A & E medicine are in a fluid state at present. It is becoming increasingly important to balance the numbers of senior registrar and registrar posts. The position is complicated in that some registrar posts in A & E departments are training posts for fracture and orthopaedic work, and not true A & E registrar posts.

PREVENTION OF ACCIDENTS

The A & E doctor sees the suffering of patients in a personal and dramatic way. He can also see the difficulties in the organisation of accident services and the limited success of treatment. He should therefore be motivated to play his part in the community to try to prevent unnecessary injury. This he may do by studies of the situation, external cause and nature of injuries. This may draw attention to the danger of particular industrial processes, dangers in particular sports and the injuries of road traffic accidents. While the incidence of various conditions in any particular A & E department is not necessarily proportional to the incidence in the community as a whole, epidemiological analysis may serve to draw attention to factors which can be modified to prevent accidents. How this can be done and how A & E records can be linked to other records for such research is discussed more fully in Chapter 3.

As well as helping prevention by such statistical research, A & E doctors can involve themselves with associations such as the Royal Society for the Prevention of Accidents and the Medical Commission for the Prevention of Accidents. Accident prevention often requires legislation, and this type of legislation often gets low priority unless the community is made aware of its importance. The A & E doctor should play his part in this work. Like other doctors he also has a responsibility to help in campaigns for the prevention of medical conditions such as heart disease, alcoholism, smoking related diseases etc.

HUMANE MEDICINE

The episodic nature of A & E medicine has been referred to already. In this it is very different from general practice, where a doctor cares for the same people over a long period — sometimes for a person's whole life. The A & E doctor each day faces large numbers of new patients, most of whom he will never see again. The short contact and the high turnover rate makes this medical work similar in shopping terms to a supermarket. There is a very real danger that daily work under these conditions will lead to the practice of a brand of supermarket medicine. Any doctor who has been the victim of supermarket medicine will know the importance of deliberately striving to cultivate a true humanity. Every patient is a person and wants to be treated as such. What is humdrum and minor to the doctor may be a matter of great anxiety to the patient. Not everybody's problem can be diagnosed, not everybody's sufferings can be relieved, but to some extent everybody's feelings can be appreciated and shared.

While this is true for all patients, it is of particular importance for the nervous, the elderly and children. Too often the term 'social problem' is introduced at an early stage of an encounter with an elderly patient. It then acts as a mental block, preventing true understanding. A real effort needs to be made to understand how children feel when, in the middle of an experience of anxiety and suffering, they are confronted with the strange world of the hospital. Much thought should be given to eliminating for them unnecessary encounters with other patients' sufferings.

The anxiety and suffering is not confined to patients. Often relatives will have come to the department with the patient. The A & E doctor should ask about them. He should also be prepared to explain as much as he can, simply and sympathetically. His hardest task in this field is when he has to inform them that the patient has died. There is no easy way of doing this, but it does make a difference to the relatives if the doctor is prepared to spend time with them. The value of having proper accommodation where this can be done is stressed in Chapter 2.

CONCLUSION

We have tried within the limits of a chapter to state in outline our concept of A & E medicine. The chapter is an introduction to the book, and the whole book is to be understood as a fuller statement about the specialty as it exists today. We believe that the development of this specialty offers the best opportunity for improving the care of patients with accidents and emergencies on their arrival at hospital.

FURTHER READING

Casualty services and their setting 1960 Nuffield Provincial Hospital Trust, London

Report of the Sub Committee on Accident and Emergency Services (The Platt Report) 1962 Standing Medical Advisory Committee of Central Health Services Council, Ministry of Health, HMSO, London

Report of the Working Committee on Accident Services 1970 Review Committee of Great Britain and Ireland; Chairman, Sir Henry Osmond-Clarke. British Medical Association, London

An integrated emergency service 1973 The Casualty Surgeons Association: c/o Royal College of Surgeons, London

Report on Medical Staffing of Accident and Emergency Services (The Lewin Report) 1978 British Medical Association, London

The accident and emergency department — design and planning

INTRODUCTION

An A & E department must be an integral part of a general hospital. It should be centrally located within the hospital complex and have easy access to all the other clinical departments. Ideally it should be possible to manage all types of emergency patients within the one hospital. Transporting sick children, acutely ill medical patients, or the recently injured from the A & E department to another hospital is detrimental to good medical care and occasionally may prove to be disastrous.

The A & E department depends day and night on certain support services (e.g. the blood bank and various laboratories) and these should be within or close to the department.

For most patients admitted to the hospital the A & E department is their way into the hospital, and for many patients the A & E department is the only section of the hospital they visit. The public image and esteem of the hospital can be made or marred by this one department. Because the A & E department is open to the public continuously, the demand for cleaning, maintenance, repairs, painting and general support from the hospital administration is of a much greater order than any other section of the hospital.

ACCESS TO THE DEPARTMENT

There must be rapid, unhindered access for emergency ambulances to reach the department and they should be able to unload their patients in a sheltered, protected, illuminated area, free from public

gaze and adjacent to the resuscitation room (Fig. 2.1). The vehicle should then be able to move off to a nearby ambulance park. The professional ambulance team will ensure that this arrangement works smoothly. Problems arise when a private car driver brings a friend or relative who has suddenly been taken ill. They may park their car as near as possible to the entrance to the department and leave it there so that they can stay with the patient. Sympathetic firmness is required by a member of staff designated with the responsibility of controlling the access area. It is essential that there are car parking spaces nearby which are reserved for this recurring problem.

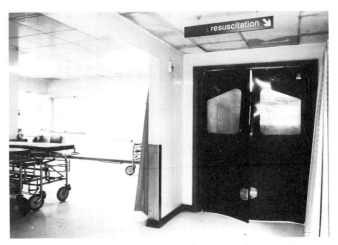

Fig. 2.1 Ambulance bay and trolley patients' entrance adjacent to the resuscitation room.

The hospital administration must ensure that vehicular movement in the access area is not impeded by hospital service vehicles or visitors' private cars at any time of day or night.

RECEPTION OF PATIENTS

Patients brought by ambulance will be taken directly to an appropriate area by the ambulance crew and either an ambulance man or a relative will give the patient's details to the receptionist.

Porters, reception staff and nurses must constantly be alert to the needs of a seriously ill patient who arrives in a private car. Emergency trolleys must always be ready for such patients and simple arrangements be available for their registration.

In planning the department it is necessary to allocate space for the storage of trolleys and wheelchairs. Emergency equipment which can be taken to the scene of an accident must also be stored near the entrance.

Clear signposting is essential for guiding walking patients to the reception desk. The receptionists must work in close liaison with the nursing staff so that seriously ill or injured patients are not kept waiting. Ideally the waiting area should be adjacent to the reception desk so that if there is a rush of new patients they can sit down under the supervision of the triage nurse until the receptionist is available to register them, rather than having to form a queue in which they may overhear preceding patients give their personal details to the receptionist.

During daytime hours the reception desk can be open so that patient and receptionist can have a face to face interview. Unfortunately, at night-time the unruly behaviour of some patients or their friends make it necessary to give some physical protection to the receptionist, e.g. by a plastic louvered window. There must always be adequate space for the storage of records and in future the reception desk must be large enough to accommodate computer hardware (Fig. 2.2).

Once the patient's record card has been prepared it is the responsibility of the triage nurse to decide on the priority of patients to be seen and treated by the doctor. If children cannot be attended to immediately they should be able to wait in a suitably furnished children's waiting room, but still under the close supervision of the triage nurse.

FRIENDS AND RELATIVES

The nurse must also be aware of the needs of any relatives or friends who have accompanied the patient.

Relatives who do not accompany an adult patient when they go to be examined should be told how long the patient is likely to be in the department. A canteen during the day and drinks dispenser at night should be provided for patients' relatives and friends. Patients should not have anything to eat or drink before seeing the doctor in case they require a general anaesthetic. If a mother has brought other children with her, apart from the patient, they should be accommodated in a play area until the whole family is ready to leave the department.

Relatives of a patient who has suffered a catastrophic injury or illness and whose life is in danger should be able to wait in a separate 'relatives room' where they can be given details at regular intervals of the patients' progress. Should there be a fatal outcome, the senior doctor and nurse who have been involved with the patient can then use this room to inform the relatives and console them in their distress (Fig. 2.3). The room should be pleasantly furnished with a hand basin and mirror and a telephone so that contact can be made with those who can give continuing support to the family.

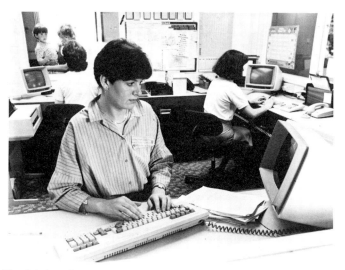

Fig. 2.2 A modern reception area designed to accommodate a computer-based accident and emergency record system.

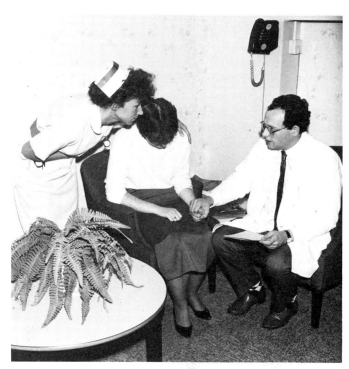

Fig. 2.3 The relatives room. Consoling a widow is the responsibility of the senior doctor and nurse who were involved in the attempted resuscitation of her husband.

FACILITIES FOR THE EXAMINATION OF PATIENTS

Patients may be divided into eight categories:

A. Walking patients
1. Do not need to be undressed
2. Need to be undressed for examination
3. Eye, ENT and dental patients
B. Trolley patients
4. Do not require resuscitation
5. Require, or may require, resuscitation
6. Patients found dead on arrival
C. Other Patients
7. Require immediate isolation
8. Patients making return visits

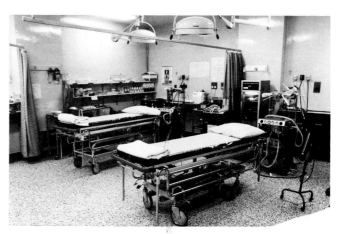

Fig. 2.4 The resuscitation room must have space, privacy and equipment in good working order. Good communication with other sections of the A & E department and the hospital are essential.

1. Walking patients who do not need to be undressed can be seen by a doctor sitting at a consultation desk adjacent to the waiting room. Many of these patients only require treatment for a minor wound and this can be conveniently given in an adjoining cubicle so that the patient can leave the department immediately after treatment.

2. Patients who require to be partially undressed for their physical examination can walk to clearly numbered cubicles reserved for this purpose. It is useful to have an indicator light outside each cubicle to show when a patient is ready for examination by a doctor.

3. Examination and treatment of patients with eye, ear, nose and throat, or dental problems require special lighting and equipment which can be provided in a cubicle specifically designed and equipped for this purpose.

4. A patient with a serious, but not life-threatening condition can be conveniently examined on a trolley. The nurse who receives the patient into the cubicle will record the basic history and vital signs, whilst preparing them for the doctor's examination.

All the examination and treatment cubicles mentioned above require privacy, good lighting and easy access to the remainder of the department. Wall mounted fittings will include oxygen and suction, a hand-basin, a writing surface and stationery rack. A mobile lamp on an extension bracket, a viewing screen for radiographs, electric sockets, a sphygmomanometer and shelves for dressing materials.

5. Patients requiring resuscitation and patients with central chest pain who may suffer a cardiac arrest, should be taken directly to the resuscitation room (Fig. 2.4). This room should be adjacent to the ambulance arrival bay. It must have adequate floor space (25 square metres per patient to be treated), privacy, warmth (25°C) and all equipment must be clearly labelled and in good working order. It should be checked every day and disposable items replenished immediately after use.

6. Patients found to be dead on arrival at hospital should be accommodated in a room set aside for this purpose adjacent to the ambulance bay. Police or relatives may wish to view the body. It is important that forensic evidence should be noted and the coroner or his officer can be contacted if necessary. Precise

identification of the deceased person is essential before information is given to relatives.

For the eventual discharge of the body, the A & E department must have an agreed policy which has been worked out with the coroner, the police, the public mortuary and local undertakers.

7. Patients requiring immediate isolation may have been victims of radiation or may be suffering from exotic diseases, such as Lassa fever. The former are discussed in Ch. 27 and the latter in Ch. 25. A room must be designated for the reception and assessment of these patients. It must be located away from the main part of the department so that as few staff as possible and no other patients are put at risk, and it must have shower facilities and a telephone. The shower may also be useful for a patient with chemical burns. A flea infested patient can also be managed in this room.

8. Patients making return visits. Follow-up clinics organised within the A & E department require separate accommodation so that there is no competition for its use between new and old patients — except in the event of a major disaster, when the follow-up clinic area will be used to increase the resources of the department. Follow-up clinics should be conducted by the senior staff of the department to check the appropriateness of patients' management and ensure that no injuries have been missed.

This suite of cubicles may also be used for specific clinics, for instance redressing of burns, a hand injury clinic, or a sports injury clinic, depending on agreed local policy.

PATIENT INVESTIGATION

An acute measurements laboratory for blood gases, electrolytes, glucose and alcohol estimations should be situated near to the resuscitation room (Fig. 2.5). Some departments are now also equipped with computer-aided diagnostic facilities.

The radiology department is the most used and the most expensive investigational service. Radiographers must provide a 24-hour service. Ideally two rooms are required, both capable of routine work, but one of them should also be equipped for skull

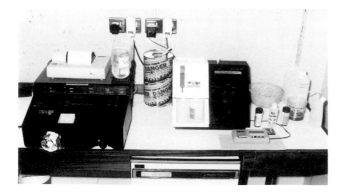

Fig. 2.5 An acute measurements laboratory adjacent to the resuscitation room.

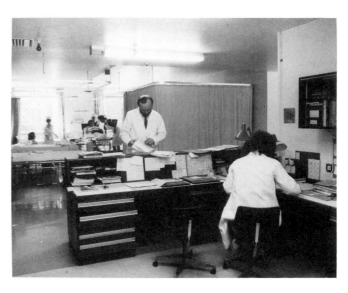

Fig. 2.6 The observation ward is an integral part of the A & E department.

and facial bone radiography. There must also be provision for radiography in the resuscitation room. Image intensification equipment is valuable for the rapid assessment of an unconscious injured patient, or for the insertion of a cardiac pacemaker.

Computerised tomography is now an essential service for a hospital with a major accident department. Some A & E departments use an ultrasound mid-liner as a preliminary investigation of a head injury patient.

Finally there should be radiological facilities in the plaster room to check accuracy of reduction of fractures and dislocations before the anaesthetic is terminated. A rest-room for the radiographers and a reporting room for the radiologist should be provided. The detailed use of radiology and imaging for emergency patients is discussed in Ch. 8.

is approximately 1 per 30 000 population in the catchment area. It is convenient to have a sound attenuated room with plastic windows adjacent to the nursing station for the observation of drunk or psychiatrically disturbed patients. Another very valuable asset is an interview room, which can be shared by the various doctors and paramedical personnel involved in patients' management.

The observation ward should be regarded as an integral part of the A & E department.

PATIENT TREATMENT

Much of the routine treatment of dressing wounds, bandaging, strapping and injections can be carried out in the examination cubicles. For more serious conditions two operating theatres are required with an associated anaesthetic room, a recovery room and utility room. Clean wounds will be explored and sutured in one of the theatres, the other being used for the treatment of infected wounds and abscesses and for the manipulation of closed fractures or dislocations. It is preferable to have a separate plaster room for the application and removal of casts and, like the two theatres, this room should be equipped for administration of general anaesthetics and for resuscitation.

OBSERVATION WARD

The provision of this facility is essential for the good and safe management of patients and is an economic way of avoiding unnecessary, disruptive and expensive admission of a patient to a general hospital ward (Fig. 2.6). The number of beds required

HOUSEKEEPING

For the efficient, smooth running of the department there must be an adequate storage space for the delivery and reception of supplies, a clean utility room for preparation and a dirty utility room for the disposal of waste. Adequate space must also be allocated for cleaning materials and equipment.

NURSING STATION/DEPARTMENTAL CONTROL BASE

Co-ordinated supervision of the whole department is essential for its effective function. The control point should be centrally situated. It should give nurses and doctors sufficient privacy to discuss patients and to make telephone calls without being overheard by patients or their relatives. The drugs cupboard and a small safe for patients' valuables can also be located here. Departmental information such as duty rotas, drug and treatment policies and the major accident plan should be kept here. It must be maintained as a work area and is not the appropriate location for reading the newspaper or drinking coffee. If closed-circuit television is used for surveillance of the department at night then the monitor screen should be in the nursing station.

EDUCATION FACILITIES

The range of work in an A & E Department is so wide that nobody can know everything. There is a constant need for learning and keeping up to date. Junior medical and nursing staff change so frequently that an active teaching programme is essential to maintain standards and to impart the full potential of the academic and practical components of the specialty.

Every department must have its own library where books are always available for reference or study (Fig. 2.7). In smaller departments the library may also serve as a teaching room. In larger departments, especially those which are responsible for teaching medical students, a separate seminar room is required (Fig. 2.8). The library may also serve as the centre for departmental research and accident prevention studies. Prepared programmes of teaching for the medical staff, nurses and medical students can be reinforced by open access to tape-slide or video teaching material. The equipment for this must be maintained in good order and the teaching material appropriate and up-to-date (Fig. 2.9). This requires an allocation of funds which should not be less than one penny per new patient each year.

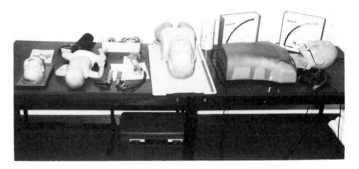

Fig. 2.9 Resuscitation manikins are useful for demonstrating, practising and testing practical skills.

STAFF FACILITIES

Offices are required for the senior nursing and the consultant staff, with associated secretarial space. The administrator responsible for the department will also require an office. Associated staff, such as paediatric health visitors, medical social workers and community psychiatric nurses, will be able to give a much more complete service if they have a base within the department.

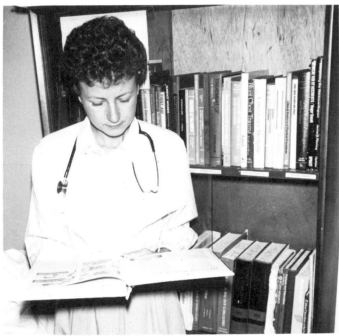
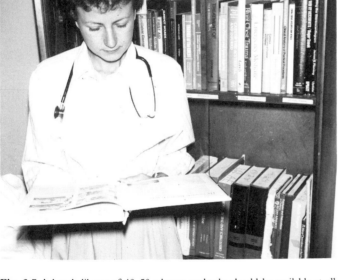

Fig. 2.7 A bench library of 40–50 relevant textbooks should be available at all hours within the A & E department.

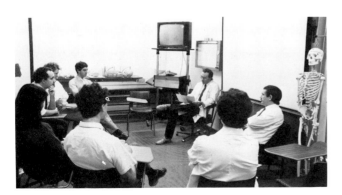

Fig. 2.8 The departmental seminar room is used for postgraduate training, undergraduate teaching and self-access learning.

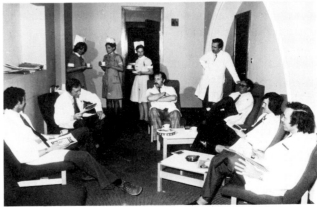

Fig. 2.10 The departmental sitting room is the hub of the department and provides resuscitation for the staff.

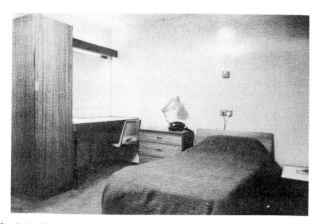

Fig. 2.11 The night-duty doctor's bedroom: it may sometimes be possible to have a few hours sleep.

It is also essential for the porters to have a room adjacent to the ambulance bay.

The most important staff facility is the 'sitting room' (Fig. 2.10). Much of the work in an A & E department is stressful and it is essential that all members of staff can sit down together and 'unwind' over a cup of tea or coffee. The sitting room is the place where harmony and unity of purpose is achieved among the staff.

Finally, for those departments where the caseload allows it, or the structure of the duty rota makes it necessary, a bedroom for the overnight doctor is required (Fig. 2.11).

Communication and records

In A & E departments large numbers of patients pass through in a short time and most of them do not return. During this brief visit important decisions are made which are of concern both to the patient and also to other interested people and organisations. These include other doctors and departments within the hospital, general practitioners and possibly social workers, rescue services outside the hospital, or national bodies concerned with the public's health and protection. A & E doctors themselves need to know what is going on in their own department in order that they may assess the work of the department and the part which they play in it.

COMMUNICATION

This chapter outlines some of the ways in which good communications may be maintained. The problem will be considered from the point of view of the care of individual patients and also from a general aspect, concerned with the wider organisation of the department.

Communication within the department

About the patient

Good personal communication with patients is essential. This requires time to listen, even though the patient may not be a good communicator. The feelings and worries of anxious relatives are equally important and they, too, require time spent in conversation.

We must not lose sight of why we are there. Patients bring their troubles to the A & E department because they perceive that this is the correct place to come. A medical training irrevocably changes your own perception of what constitutes an emergency. Even when patients have attended inappropriately it is no cost to be polite and courteous.

Explain clearly and without jargon any procedure or conclusion. It is well known that patients comprehend only a part of what the doctor tells them. A nurse may later amplify and reinforce what the doctor has said, but the doctor must be prepared to repeat the interview.

Sometimes the doctor may not be able to speak or understand the patient's language. A list should be available of hospital staff who speak foreign languages, and of local sources of interpreters. Multilingual lists, with standard questions and answers relevant to an accident or emergency (such as those produced by the British Red Cross), are very useful. Deaf patients may be a problem. A simple electrical device which magnifies sound into earphones may be of value and a friend or relative may be able to help. The deaf and dumb 'finger language' is easy to learn and may be the only way of communicating.

General communication

Administrative communication within an A & E department is important — but difficult. Because staff work in shifts throughout the 24 hours and on weekends and holidays, the whole staff is never together in the department at any one time, yet each member must know about changes in departmental instructions and policy. Administrative consultation and communication is important between the various levels of staffing, including porters, clerks, nurses of all grades, radiographers, social workers, administrators and doctors.

Formal structures for communication may be set up. Meetings are useful in sorting out problems, sharing view points and in disseminating information. If there is no official structure, interstaff communication on an informal basis is doubly important.

Communication within the hospital

About the patient

In handing over patients to other doctors in the wards, in the fracture clinic or other outpatient clinic, the A & E doctor should aim to speak personally to his counterpart, either face to face or by telephone as often as this is possible.

It is within the nature of A & E work that our relationship with our patients is usually transitory. Definitive in-hospital care is usually provided by another specialty. The speed with which the patient is referred to the appropriate specialty often determines the outcome. Referral can usually be facilitated if the referring doctor knows beforehand the information the receiving doctor will require. For example, before discussing a case with a neurosurgeon it is essential to have recorded the full neurological status of the patient and be able to convey this in a way that has meaning.

There is a skill in referring a patient. The receiving doctor will need to know personal details of the patient and will appreciate a clear and concise account of why he has come to hospital. Outline the relevant clinical findings. Have the completed notes in front of you and the results of any tests. When asked for further details they will be immediately to hand. You should plan what you are going to say and be polite. Introduce yourself and establish to whom you are speaking and ensure that the grade of each correspondent is known to the other. State what you want from the specialist (advice, admission) and why you would like it. Avoid accepting a diagnosis over the phone if this means the patient will go home on the strength of it. It is better to ask the doctor to come and examine the patient and commit his opinion to the patient's notes. Whenever you feel unhappy or unsure about the advice that is being offered state your reservations. If necessary, discuss the case with the senior doctor of the A & E department.

Similarly, when doctors in the A & E department are changing over at the end of a shift, they should hand over patients by speaking personally to each other.

Contact with other disciplines in the hospital should be fostered and maintained by encouraging medical staff to attend clinical teaching sessions and, conversely, encouraging doctors from other disciplines to participate in the teaching sessions within the A & E department. Such contacts will serve to facilitate subsequent interdepartmental discussions about individual patients.

A & E departments are, by their very nature, informal. There is a sharing of duties and many professions overlap. Patients will only gain the optimum treatment when interdisciplinary boundaries are easily crossed and staff communicate freely. For example, a senior nurse will have more experience in emergency care than a newly qualified doctor. The atmosphere in the department must encourage the sharing of this experience without of course undermining an individual's professional role.

General communication

Both A & E nursing and medical staff should be represented in the hospital management structure, otherwise the department will be represented (or misrepresented) at second hand. The volume of patients seen in A & E departments, the importance of relationships with patients and public and the close inter-relations with all other departments of the hospital are clearly sufficient to justify this direct representation.

Communication outside the hospital

About the patient

Communication with general practitioners may be at two levels. For those patients whose condition will need no further immediate help from the general practitioner, brief details of the patient's visit to the department can be sent in a letter through the post (Fig. 3.1). Telephone discussion between A & E staff and general practitioners can often prevent inappropriate referral and ease the discharge of a patient from the A & E department.

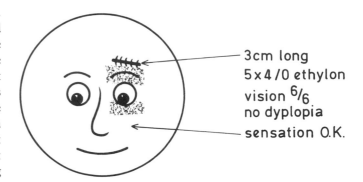

Fig. 3.1 This simple drawing shows the location of a wound and the type and number of sutures used. It also shows that there was no clinical evidence of a fracture of floor of the orbit.

Secondly, more direct communication is required about patients who are seriously ill. They may have been referred by the general practitioner or arrived unannounced. If they are to be sent home and will require further care from the general practitioner they should carry a letter with them giving a presumptive diagnosis, details of the history, physical examination, investigations and any treatment carried out. Suggestions for the continuing care of the patient and details of arrangements for any subsequent visit to hospital must also be included. In many cases attempts should also be made to contact the general practitioner on the telephone. This may be necessary to obtain information about a previous illness or current medication in a patient brought in following injury or the sudden onset of an illness.

Ambulance personnel have a sphere of expertise different from the A & E staff. A & E doctors can give advice when it is asked for but it is a serious mistake to think that experience gained in the resuscitation area and theatre of a large hospital can be immediately transferred to the streets and ambulances. Work *with* the ambulance service not over it.

The paths of *police officers* and A & E doctors often cross. There are times when the duties of each may be in conflict, but this is rare. Close co-operation and mutual understanding will help the individual patient and substantially helps the community at large.

Social workers have an independent professional status and will be aggrieved when their assessment of a patient is ignored. Furthermore, many 'social problems' are a complex mixture and have usually not happened overnight. Foresight in the management of at-risk patients will often prevent the development of a 'social problem' and certainly prevent the 'dumping' of these cases on the hapless social worker. By identifying patients as socially 'at risk' they can be referred to social services at a remedial point in their history. The primary care team can be mobilised and problems averted. Clearly the circumstances which increase risk are many but certain ones are common and are outlined in Ch. 5.

General communication

A senior member of the A & E staff should have administrative contact with one of the general practitioner committees, especially one which, in a large city, is concerned with the deputising services.

Similarly the department must be fully represented on the joint rescue services committee. It may only meet infrequently, but it can help to cross the boundaries of police, fire service, ambulance service, local authority and hospital. It should promote agreed plans for first-aid training, accident prevention, health education and major disaster organisation. It should also seek to evaluate the effectiveness of these co-operative ventures.

Regular good communication will lead to effective co-operation on a day-to-day basis and in a crisis (Fig. 3.2). Its absence is almost certainly a harbinger of disaster and chaos.

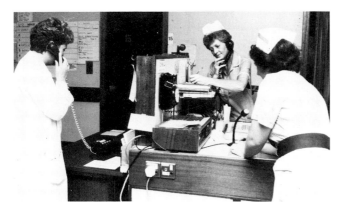

Fig. 3.2 Shows short-wave radio communication with an ambulance, reception of a phone call from outside the hospital and communication within the hospital all occurring simultaneously.

RECORDS

The introduction of computing into medical records is creating a revolution. For well over a century the only progress was the replacement of the quill pen by a fountain pen, which was then supplanted by the ballpoint pen. These minor modifications pale into insignificance in the face of current changes in record-keeping. Nevertheless, at the time of writing, the majority of A & E departments in the UK are still relying on hand-written records.

Whilst verbal communication is always necessary when the co-operation of another person or department is needed immediately, the advantage of written communication is that there is a permanent record. Neither the immediate nor the long-term value of a written record will be achieved unless it is legible. Those who are choosing A & E medicine as a specialty would do well to reflect on the quality of their handwriting and, if necessary, spend considerable effort in increasing its legibility.

The need for good records

The importance of the record for communication has already been stressed, but good records are also needed for the following reasons:

1. Patient care. Many people may share in the care of a patient. The correct understanding of the complaint and proper co-operation in administering treatment are only possible when an accurate record is made of everything that has been learned about and done to the patient.

2. As a defence against unjust complaints. The A & E department is an area where decisions often have to be made under pressure. Several urgent cases may arrive together. Admission to hospital may seem advisable, but beds may not be available. It is unfortunately inevitable that occasional mistakes will be made. Yet many complaints which are made are either unfounded or greatly exaggerated. A careful, legible record is the foundation of a good defence. Without it a doctor is open to blame beyond anything justified by his actions or omissions.

3. The A & E record may be the only record. This is so when the patient dies in the A & E department or when, in a case of extreme urgency, the patient is taken immediately to the operating theatre. The only preoperative record then will be the one made in the emergency department.

4. The record may subsequently be required for medicolegal purposes. This may not arise for months or years later and an accurate, legible record is essential for the preparation of a medicolegal report or the presentation of evidence in court. An illustration of the injury is particularly valuable.

5. For research work. The importance of a record for research purposes may only be realised at a later date. An incomplete, inaccurate or illegible record may then mislead the research or detract from the quality of the research work.

6. Doctors involved in A & E medicine must have a concern for accident prevention. Epidemiological studies rely on good records and this is essential to achieve a sound policy for prevention.

7. *Never write anything in the record which could embarass you if it were read by the patient, the relatives or a solicitor.*

The format of the basic clinical record

There are two important aspects to the patient's record (Fig. 3.3). It has a clinical function and a statistical function. The former is the more important but the latter is frequently ignored. The format of the record will depend on whether the records are being created by pen on paper, or being generated by a computer-based system.

Manual records

In both methods certain basic information must be recorded. At the reception of the patient this includes name, age, sex and address of the patient, the date and time of registration, the name and address of the patient's general practitioner, the cause of an accident and the patient's complaint.

The patient's record then passes from the receptionist to the triage nurse, who may record basic physical signs and social details.

The doctor who examines the patient must then create a structured clinical record, passing consecutively from History to Physical Examination, to Investigations, to Treatment and finally Disposal. In practice, for instance, for an unconscious patient with multiple injuries, the information is often only available in a

SURNAME   A & E No.
FORENAMES   REG. DATE
LOCAL ADDRESS   REG. TIME

                                                 SEX
                                                 D O B
TEL. No.   POST CODE   AGE

FAMILY GP   REVISITS 1/2/3/4/5/6/7/8/8+
                                   NO PREVIOUS EPISODES
                                   PREV. A/E NUMBER
OCCUPATION   HOSPITAL NUMBER

TYPE OF INCIDENT   LOCATION OF INCIDENT

INITIATOR OF REFERRAL   MODE OF ARRIVAL

INITIAL COMPLAINT

Seen by Dr.   CODE   NAME   at   HRS.
DIAGNOSIS   Patient Group   Diag   Anat Site
                1   1   1
                2   2   2
                3   3   3
         Amendments 1/2/3
Description of MAJOR DIAGNOSIS   Further Diagnosis Yes No

INVESTIGATIONS

         X RAY □ ECG □ Urine □ B/Bank □ Haematology □ Chem Path □ Bact □
TREATMENT

Dressing □   POP □   Manip □   Advice □
Injection □   Suture □   GA □   Obs Ward □
Prescription □   Incision □   Rehab □   Ref Trtmnt □

DEPARTURE DETAILS
TIME OF DEPARTURE
WARD No. (If admitted)

Fig. 3.3 The front of a record card prepared for the patient's details to be printed in the upper half by the computer at the reception desk. The information in the lower half of the card will be entered into the computer file when the patient leaves the department.

disjointed manner, but before the patient leaves the emergency department it is helpful to other medical staff if the A & E doctor makes a sequential summary of the information available to him. He must also sign the record and indicate the time at which he became involved with the patient.

Computer-based records

In the past decade pioneering work on computerised record systems has followed two paths. The one has seen its prime function to ensure the efficient use of the department's resources, to be able to locate any patient within the department and to facilitate and record their passage through the department. The other has placed its main emphasis on statistical analysis of data to provide information for the management of the department, audit of the medical activity, the epidemiological study of accidents and acute illness and to provide data for accident prevention work. Both these emphases are clearly beneficial to the A & E department and eventually the strong points from both systems will coalesce. Despite this current divergence, both systems impart outstanding advantages over a manual system. The patient has a printed record, there is an on-line enquiry system, a daily register is generated, reply letters for the patient's general practitioner can be printed and labels can be produced for specimen identification. Subsequent analysis and use of the information held on the computer will depend on the initiative and interest of the clinicians within the department. At all times the use of the information is controlled by the Data Protection Act of 1984, and the same principles apply regarding the confidentiality of medical information, regardless of the method of its recording. Irrespective of whether it is created manually or by computer, *the record card must never leave the A & E department*. An NCR copy or photostat of the card should accompany a patient who is transferred to another part of the hospital.

Recording of data and statistical reports

For many years each hospital has been required to report annually on the work of its A & E department, indicating the total number of patient visits and how many of these were 'first visits'.

Whether these patients were young or old, male or female, seriously ill or with only minor injuries, whether they were admitted to hospital, even whether they lived or died is not recorded in the official, annual SH3 statement.

In 1980 the NHS/DHSS Steering Group on Health Service Information was appointed, under the chairmanship of Mrs Edith Korner to review and improve all aspects of information in the Health Service.

For A & E departments still using a manual record system the Korner report has virtually no suggestions for improvements. For departments with computerised systems there is very detailed advice about information which should be captured for all patients with definitions of the groups and subgroups of the various categories. This part of the report is reproduced at the end of this chapter.

There are now a number of systems used for operating computers for A & E records and all of them should meet the requirements set out in the Korner report. CAER (the Computerisation of Accident and Emergency Records), the system which is most widely used in the UK, also allows the recording of up to three diagnoses, and an amended diagnosis, all of which can be cross tabulated with the anatomical site of the injury or illness.

Ideally the classification of acute injury or illness should follow the coding in the 9th edition of the International Classification of Diseases (ICD) and it is possible to recategorise the CAER-coded diagnoses in ICD terms. However, using the present edition of ICD either for the diagnosis or for the cause of injury (the E codes), is extremely time consuming, and A & E departments are not allocated the necessary staff for this. It is hoped that when the 10th edition of the ICD is introduced in 1992 the sections on injuries and their causes will relate more closely to the pattern of work which is seen in A & E departments.

Computer linkage

This description and discussion has been limited to activity and information within the A & E department. As computerisation progresses in other parts of the hospital, it will be possible to create links for the transfer of information. In some hospitals the A & E system is an integral part of the Patient Administration System (PAS). Other A & E departments have a stand-alone system which is independent of the PAS but can be linked to it. The reason for this latter arrangement is that the A & E department works 24 hours every day, including all public holidays and can ill-afford any down time on the computer. Having a stand-alone system with a rapid call-out contract for maintenance releases the A & E department from the inconvenience of problems on the more complex PAS computer.

The transfer of patient information between the A & E department and the hospital PAS can be complemented by linkages with computerised information systems in radiology, pathology, haemotology, microbiology and chemical pathology. By the use of a modem, it is already possible to interrogate the bank of information on toxic substances maintained by Scottish Poisons Information Bureau in the Royal Infirmary, Edinburgh.

Further development in A & E computing will include computerised communication with general practitioners and the community health services. This revolution in A & E records is gaining momentum and will have far reaching effects in enhancing many aspects of emergency care. Within the next 5 – 10 years all departments should have moved forward to using a computer-based record system.

CATEGORISATION OF DATA TO BE CAPTURED BY COMPUTERISED A & E SYSTEMS AS SET OUT IN THE KORNER REPORT

We recommend that a minimum set of data be available to allow each department to compare its workload with others and that the following data items be collected for each patient:

a. Accident and emergency department number
b. New or follow-up patient
c. Time and date of arrival
d. Date of birth
e. Sex
f. Area of residence code
g. Code of general practitioner
h. Initiator of referral
i. Mode of arrival
j. Patient group
k. Type of incident (if an accident or trauma case)
l. Method of departure

We recommend that the initiator of the attendance be classified as follows:

a. A written or telephoned request from a general practitioner
b. The patient sent by others (e.g. by foreman, schoolteacher)
c. The patient referring himself, and making his own arrangements for attendance
d. The patient being brought in by others, usually as a result of an emergency call to the ambulance service
e. Staff of the accident and emergency department

We recommend that the mode of arrival be classified as:

a. Walked to the department
b. Arrived by public transport, other than the ambulance service
c. Arrived by private transport
d. Brought in by ambulance

Nationally about 70% of new attendances at accident and emergency departments are due to accident or trauma, including poisonings. We thus recommend that the classification of patients into broad groups be as follows and that these data be input after the patient has been seen by a doctor:

a. Accidents
b. Deliberate self-harm
c. Assaults
d. Stings and bites
e. Conditions not due to trauma or an accident
f. Patients who had no abnormality detected
g. Patient dead

For trauma and accident cases (items a–d in the preceding paragraph) it is important to record the type of the incident. We recommend that this be classified as:

a. Accident or trauma at home (home being defined as for the Home Accident Surveillance System)
b. Road traffic accident
c. Injury due to sport
d. Accident or trauma at work
e. Accident or trauma in an educational establishment
f. Accident or trauma in a public place
g. Other types

We recommend that the method of departure be classified as:

a. Left the department before being treated
b. Left the department having refused treatment
c. Allowed home with or without an appointment at the department or at an outpatient clinic
d. Admitted to a bed associated with the department
e. Admitted to a hospital bed other than one associated with the department
f. Died in the department.

Additional items that might be collected in individual departments for internal management purposes include:

a. Name of the doctor seeing the patient
b. Time that patient was seen by a doctor
c. Time the patient left the department
d. Investigations ordered for the patient
e. Procedures ordered for the patient.

FURTHUR READING

Current perspectives in health computing Kostrewski Barbara (ed) 1984 Cambridge University Press

Legal aspects

The application of the processes of law to medical practice is the same whatever the field of medicine. The same expectations of competence and conduct should apply equally across the profession. Nevertheless, a doctor may suffer a greater degree of exposure to the offices and officers of the law in six months spent working as a junior doctor in an A & E department than at any other time in his/her professional career. Medicolegal problems are inclined to be particularly common and difficult in this area 'at the sharp end' of medicine.

The reasons for this are not difficult to perceive:

The type of work

The spectrum of clinical cases covers the whole field of medicine in its broadest sense, extending to cover many social emergencies as well. Many patients attend an A & E department as the result of violent injury either inflicted accidentally or deliberately. Cases of assault, child abuse and industrial or traffic accidents often result in requests for police statements or legal reports. The relationships between alcohol, drugs and accidents may be reasons for frequent professional contact with police officers. Episodes of self-harm may lead to conflict with family and employers raising issues of clinical confidentiality. Patients brought in dead or dying in the A & E department result in regular contacts with the coroner and his officers.

Mode of presentation

Most of the patients arrive unheralded and the pressures to make an instant diagnosis and to provide immediate treatment may be overwhelming. Under these circumstances the examination may be incomplete, complications may not be foreseen and the real reason for the patient's attendance may be overlooked.

Much of the work is undertaken at night, at weekends and during public holidays. At these times A & E department staffing levels may be poor and the back-up services in the hospital and in the community may also be reduced. In a large A & E department at least half of the patients will attend outside the normal working hours. A & E departments are often busy and noisy so doctors are often tired and interrupted: an ideal situation for making mistakes.

Patient expectations and demands

Attendances at A & E departments throughout the United Kingdom have been rising steadily in recent years. This has been accompanied not only by an increase in the number of investigations performed (such as radiological examinations), but also by an extension of the scope of work practised. It is not uncommon for a patient and A & E staff to disagree about the appropriateness of attendance for a particular condition at a particular time.

The patient who appears to be 'overanxious' or seems unnecessarily 'demanding' may have a real medical, social or psychiatric problem for which time and patience are required. In a busy department, such patients may provoke feelings of frustation which may interfere with clinical judgement and compassionate care.

In this increasingly litigious climate there are considerable pressures on staff to practise so-called 'defensive medicine' — a process which leads to practice by rote, removing logical thought and resulting in a sterile, non-trusting doctor–patient relationship. Defensive practices waste expensive resources.

External demands

There are often pressures not to admit patients to hospital unless they are obviously gravely ill. Experience is needed to withstand aggressive interrogation of a member of the receiving team anxious to project his beds.

Stresses in the hospital will be mirrored in the service outside the hospital if communications between A & E department staff and the general practitioner are poor. Good communications are important between doctor and patient. Explanations should be given to the patient in such a way that it is difficult for the patient to believe that treatment has been withheld by an unsympathetic doctor.

It is not possible to define rigidly what constitutes an emergency. A doctor should see all patients who attend an A & E department, but need only investigate and treat those for whom he thinks this is appropriate. If he decides that the patient might be more appropriately seen by his general practioner, or might need no medical attention at all, then the doctor should politely inform the patient of this. If necessary, advice should be given as to how and where the patient might best seek further help. Where there is a serious conflict of opinion it is wise for the doctor to seek the advice of a senior colleague. The threat of subsequent legal action should not influence the doctor's decision to investigate or treat the patient when management is not indicated on clinical grounds.

This attitude is particularly relevant to the question of radiographic examinations. Radiographs should be taken if they will help in the diagnosis and management of patients and not for 'medicolegal' reasons alone.

COMPETENCE

The threat of malpractice claims is a common anxiety amongst young doctors starting work as casualty officers. The number of civil claims for medical negligence is on the increase and the cost of settlement of such claims has led to considerable rises in the subscription fees to the medical defence societies. Negligence is a civil misdemeanour, known as a *tort*. For negligence to be proved it must be demonstrated that:

1. The doctor owed a duty of care to the patient.
2. The doctor was in breach of that duty.
3. The patient suffered damage as a result.

The actual law on medical negligence remains unaltered since 1957 when the High Court laid down the principle referred to as the *Bolam test:*

'A practitioner is not guilty of negligence if he has acted in accordance with a practice accepted as proper by a responsible body of medical men skilled in that particular art, even though a body of adverse opinion also exists among medical men.' [Furthermore] ' ... where you get a situation which involves the use of some special skill or competence the test is the standard of the ordinary skilled man exercising and professing to have that special skill.'

In other words, for the newly appointed A & E doctor, the level of knowledge and skill is that which would be reasonably expected from someone who has just completed the preregistration year; a doctor who has spent time in other disciplines would be expected to bring knowledge and experience gained in those other disciplines to bear on the work in the A & E department.

This test does not provide the young doctor with an excuse for sloppy work on the grounds of ignorance. Neither does it absolve the doctor from the 'duty of care' once assumed — either by virtue of the patient presenting or through referral from another doctor. Rather it gives the substance for some words of advice to guide the new doctor through the seemingly alien world of the A & E department.

Be aware of your own limitations

Don't 'bite off more than you can chew'. The A & E department is not the place for aspiring surgeons to practise their techniques unsupervised nor is it the place for doctors to attempt to learn new skills with no more than an instruction manual for guidance.

Follow the advice laid down

All good A & E dpeartments will have guidance notes for their medical staff reflecting local policies and codes of practice applicable to the department.

Don't be afraid to ask for help when you need it

Senior staff are appointed to take responsibility for the action of their juniors — use them! Consultants would far rather offer advice which may prevent a tragedy occuring than be held to account for the consequences that might follow.

Tackle one problem at a time

This may seem counsel of perfection during a particularly busy and demanding shift. Success in priority sorting ('triage') comes only with experience. Mistakes often occur, though, when the staff are under pressure and it is safest to see each case through properly even if it means that other patients might have to wait a little longer.

Take great care when handing over

Frequently problems arise when transferring responsibility to another A & E doctor or to the inpatient medical team. Before going off duty ensure that you have informed your colleague about remaining patients, especially those waiting for radiographs or other investigations; that adequate arrangements are made for follow-up or that appropriate communication has been made to the general practitioner. You should make it clear whether you are requesting admission of a patient, a 'second opinion' from a more experienced doctor, or merely advice or reassurance over the telephone. To request a second opinion and accept a diagnosis made by telephone may be a recipe for disaster.

Make good notes

The importance of the Accident Record Card has been stressed in the last chapter. The casualty record has to be clear, precise and succinct. It must show the relevant recent history without being discursive; the salient clinical findings (and, here, a sketch of the injury is invaluable for refreshing your memory when reviewing or re-examining the patient later) and, above all, your management decisions. It is the vehicle for formal communications between doctor and nurse and between departments. Its contents are frequently used as evidence during the judicial process. Don't write anything that you might be ashamed of later. Take care in recording LEFT and RIGHT and describe fingers by name rather than by number. Sign and date your notes and initial any treatments that you might order or administer.

All doctors, however junior, should try to keep abreast of developments, especially therapeutic advances, in their subject, for a situation which might not have been judged to be negligent some years ago might fall later into that category in the light of new knowledge.

There are a number of well known 'pitfalls' and danger spots in A & E work (see Guly 1984). These are regularly referred to in the annual reports of the medical defence societies. Table 4.1 is a list of common errors which may give rise to claims of medical negligence. Table 4.2 is a list of frequent radiographic traps. The application of radiology and imaging to emergency work is discussed in Ch. 8.

Table 4.1 Common errors in accident and emergency work

A. *Missed diagnoses*
1. Retained foreign bodies
   a. Glass anywhere
   b. Metal in eye
2. Injury to distal nerve, vessel or tendon in limb injuries
3. Proximal fracture or dislocation with distal limb injury
   a. Hip dislocation with fractured thigh or knee
   b. Axial compression injury with fractured os calcis
4. Soft tissue and tendon injury
   a. Achilles tendon rupture
   b. Quadriceps tendon rupture
5. Damage to heart or great vessels in blunt chest trauma
6. Neck trauma with head, face or jaw injury
7. Carpal fractures and dislocations
B. *Misdiagnoses*
1. The head injury as 'drunk' or 'CVA'
2. The testicular torsion as orchitis or appendicitis
3. The leaking abdominal aortic aneurysm as lumbar disc pain
C. *Incomplete diagnoses*
1. Extent of blood loss in blunt chest and pelvic injuries
2. Occult injury with blunt abdominal trauma
3. A small pneumothorax in a patient who needs ventilating
4. The Monteggia or Galeazzi fracture-dislocation
5. Injuries apparent on turning the patient over
6. Failure to record visual acuity after injury of eyes
D. *Mismanagement*
1. Failure to admit;
   a. The infant with abdominal pain
   b. The child with bone pain and fever
   c. The bronchitic with fractured ribs
   d. The chest pain with a heart attack
   e. The patient who cannot walk after injury
   f. The depressed overdose
   g. The limb grossly swollen after injury
   h. The near-drowning or smoke inhalation injury
2. Failure to arrange wound excision in compound fracture or joint injury
3. Failure to take care with plaster slabs, splints and tourniquets
4. Failure to stabilise a suspected cervical spine injury
5. Failure to delay the closure of a gunshot wound or animal bite

Table 4.2 Radiographic traps in A & E work

Inadequacy of examination
1. The odontoid peg
2. The cervicothoracic vertebral junction
3. The dorsolumbar vertebral junction
4. Spiral fractures which only show on one limb view
5. The injured joint above or below a fracture
6. Soft tissue views of the right density for glass foreign bodies

Failure to repeat the examination
1. Scaphoid fracture
2. March fracture
3. Elbow injuries with a positive fat pad

Unfamiliarity with the appearance
1. Linear skull fractures
2. Depressed skull fractures
3. Posterior dislocation of shoulder
4. Fracture of orbit or zygoma
5. Talar tilt with ankle ligament injuries
6. High patella with quadriceps ligament injuries
7. Compressed greenstick fracture in children
8. Fractured os calcis
9. Injury of subtalar or midtarsal articulation
10. Apical pneumothorax
11. Mediastinal haematoma
12. Collapse left lower lobe

Some examples

1. A patient may present with a history of pain in the eye which developed suddenly whilst using a hammer. If blindness or loss of the eye followed, failure to have taken a radiograph for an intraocular foreign body would be deemed negligent.

2. The patient who may reasonably be suspected of having sustained a fracture of the carpal scaphoid bone, but whose initial radiograph does not demonstrate a fracture, may be told to return if the pain persists. This type of advice may be misinterpreted by many patients and is inappropriate. Such patients should be clearly instructed to return after two weeks for a check radiograph and in the meantime the limb should be immobilised in a plaster cast pending review (see Ch. 35).

3. If a patient with chronic chest disease (especially an elderly patient) sustains fractures of the ribs, failure to admit him to hospital may be regarded as negligent. It is quite possible for such a patient to die. Even severe bruising of the chest wall may be sufficient to cause a bronchopneumonia in such a patient.

4. Abdominal pain in young children may pose diagnostic difficulties for even the most experienced paediatrician. Failure to request a more experienced second opinion before discharging such a patient from the department may be judged negligent if the child subsequently is shown to have a torsion of the testis or other serious intra-abdominal complication.

CONFIDENTIALITY

'It is a doctor's duty to his patient strictly to observe the rule of professional secrecy by refraining from disclosing voluntarily to any third party information which he has learned directly or indirectly in his professional relationship with his patient.'

General Medical Council 1983

This ethical guideline forms the basis of one of the most difficult and ill-understood areas in the practice of A & E medicine. It is the principle which, most frequently, brings the A & E doctor into conflict with the police and lawyers. Although, in English law, there is no strict legal obligation to preserve professional secrecy, it is generally understood that confidentiality is an implied term of the contract between a doctor and his patient and that unauthorised disclosure could give grounds for civil proceedings against the doctor. It is often unwitting rather than deliberate disclosure which serves as the doctor's pitfall.

The exceptions:

Where the patient gives consent

'If the patient or his legal adviser gives written and valid consent, information to which the consent refers may be disclosed'.

A discussion of the meaning of consent is given in the next section. In cases where it seems obvious that disclosure of information to a third party would be requested, then steps should be taken to ensure that the consent is informed and in writing. The responsibility for obtaining consent rests with the party requiring the information, not with the holder of the information. However, in straightforward accident or assault cases, it would seem a sensible precaution for the doctor to obtain the patient's written consent at the time of examination to prevent time and unnecessary effort being expended later. A simple declaration on the case record ('I consent to the disclosure of information about my injuries to the police if requested') would appear to suffice. Innocent victims of assault rarely refuse to give consent.

When a solicitor seeks information about a patient and states that he is acting for that patient then it can be assumed that he holds the patient's consent. However he does not, necessarily, hold the consent for disclosure of information about a relative of that patient. Doctors should be particularly aware of hazards of divulging information about domestic assault cases to solicitors involved with divorce proceedings.

Colleagues

Information about a patient may be shared with other doctors who assist with clinical management and also with other professional persons who are properly concerned with the patient's health (e.g. dentists, nurses, clerical staff and professions supplementary to medicine).

> It is the doctor's duty to ensure that those with whom information is being shared appreciate the rule of professional secrecy.

This principle should extend to personal health data held on computerised systems and subject to the regulations of the Data Protection Act (1986).

Under this heading can be included information about adverse drug reactions required by the Committee on the Safety of Medicines (see Ch. 16).

Statutory duty

> Information may be disclosed to the appropriate authority in order to satisfy a specific statutory requirement.

Examples of this include:

1. Notification of infectious diseases. If a doctor becomes aware or suspects that a person whom he is attending is suffering from a notifiable infectious disease he must send a certificate to the Medical Officer of Environmental Health of the local authority (see Ch. 25 on Infectious Diseases).

2. Notifications of births and deaths (Section 124 of the National Health Service Act 1977).

3. Notifications under the provision of the Abortion Act (1967).

4. Notifications of drug addicts under the provision of the Misuse of Drugs Act (1971). Any doctor who attends a person who he considers to be, or has reasonable grounds to suspect, is addicted to any drug controlled by the regulations shall, within 7 days of the attendance, furnish in writing to (in Britain):

The Chief Medical Officer at the Home Office, Queen Anne's Gate, London SW1H 9AT

the name, address, sex, date of birth and NHS number of the person, the date of attendance, and the name of the drug(s) concerned. Special forms are available.

5. Notification of occupational diseases and poisonings. RIDDOR (Reporting of Injuries, Diseases and Dangerous Occurrences Regulations 1985) replace the notification laws in the 1961 Factories Act, now placing responsibility for reporting poisonings and diseases on the employer.

6. Notification required by the Road Traffic Acts.

Under section 168 of the Road Traffic Act 1972, an A & E doctor might be compelled by the police to 'pass on such information which he has in his possession which may lead to the identification of the driver of a vehicle alleged to have committed the offence of driving a motor vehicle, knowing it to be stolen'. This unusual, but anomalous, piece of legislation has given rise to conflict in the past.

Information required by process of law

Unlike the privileges accorded to members of the legal profession, confidential medical information is not privileged from disclosure.

> If the doctor is directed to disclose information by a judge or other presiding officer of a court before whom he is appearing to give evidence, information may at that stage be disclosed.

Similarly,

> If, in the course of legal proceedings, a court requires knowledge about a patient's medical details, an order can be made which compels the doctor to reveal the details — or face proceedings for contempt of court.

However, where litigation is in prospect, unless the patient has consented to disclosure, or a court order has been served on the doctor, information should not be disclosed merely in response to demands from other persons, such as another party's solicitor or an official of the court.

Research

It is ethical to disclose information for the purpose of a proper medical research project for which approval has been given by a recognised ethical committee. The patients' identities should be concealed, if possible, by the use of reference numbers rather than names.

Where disclosure is required in the public interest

> Rarely, disclosure may be justified on the grounds that it is in the public interest which, in certain circumstances, might over-ride the doctor's duty to maintain his patient's confidence.

For example, the disclosure of medical information may exceptionally be justified if it can help to prevent or detect the commission of a serious crime or bring the perpetrator of such a crime to justice.

This is the most contentious exception to the general rule. The doctor may find his professional ethics in conflict with this public duty as a citizen in the country in which he practices. Department of Health guidelines advise that, before a disclosure is made, the following conditions must be satisfied:

1. The crime must be sufficiently serious for the public interest to prevail (see Section 109 of the Police and Criminal Evidence Act 1984 for a definition of 'serious crime')

2. It must be established that, without the disclosure, the task of preventing or detecting the crime would be seriously prejudiced or delayed.

3. Satisfactory undertakings must be obtained that the personal health data disclosed will not be used for any other purpose and will be destroyed if the subject is not prosecuted, or is discharged, or acquitted.

When faced with such a dilemma a junior doctor should ask his consultant who may consult with colleagues and his medical defence society. Rarely are matters so urgent that the doctor cannot reasonably ask for time in which to consider the request for information and seek advice.

> Whatever the circumstances a doctor must always be prepared to justify his action if he has disclosed confidential information.

Problem areas

Employers. It is better to hold firmly to the rule that no information may be divulged without the patient's consent. Where a factory medical unit refers a patient, A & E department staff are under a professional obligation to reply.

Relatives. Traditionally the doctor has been willing to discuss patient's illnesses with relatives to a greater or lesser extent. Where it is undesirable *on medical grounds* to seek the patient's consent the doctor may give information, in confidence, to a relative or other appropriate person. There may be times when the patient objects even to members of the family being told about the patient's presence in the A & E department. Take special care before giving information about drug or alcohol abuse, pregnancy or miscarriage and venereal disease. For example, it may be unwise to divulge to a parent the fact that a daughter is taking the contraceptive pill.

The police. There are no clear guidelines as to when legal obligations should be given precedence over the duty to patient confidentiality. In specific cases the doctor is left to use his commonsense and act according to his conscience (see above). For example, it is unlikely that a claim for breach of confidentiality would succeed against a doctor who informed the police that a patient had been brought to his department with obvious gunshot wounds — even if that patient were to refuse to given permission for such information to be divulged. Neither would there be problems in disclosing confidential information in relation to the investigations of murder, rape, armed robbery or offences against the State. However, other areas are not so clear cut. When there is good reason to believe that the driver of a car involved in an accident was under the influence of drugs, or was a diabetic suffering from an insulin overdose, or an epileptic who had had a fit, such information should only be given to the police if the patient gives his full permission. It is best to discuss these matters with one's medical defence society when in doubt, for it is as important to prevent a recurrence of a road accident as to deal with the effects of the present accident.

Many enquiries from the police relate to minor assault. If the police ask for the name and address of a patient who has been involved in a fight and is now in the department, this information could be given. It is, however, wrong to allow the police access to the A & E department patient register. Any further information should be given only after obtaining the patient's consent in writing. This is particularly important when a patient claims to have been assaulted by the police.

Traffic police officers — as part of their investigation into a Road Traffic Accident involving personal injury — are, in the UK, required to complete a statistical return (the 'Stats 19'). Such an officer can be told, in response to his request, the name, address and age of the patient; the general description of his injury ('head injury', 'leg injury' etc); the severity of his condition (critical, serious, minor) and his disposal (admitted to hospital, transferred for special care, home after treatment).

The news media.   The temptation for junior doctors and nurses to speak to the media about individual patients or incidents should be resisted. There should be a clearly defined policy in the hospital to deal with such situations. Guidelines for hospital administrators for dealing with the press are contained in the DHSS Health Memorandum (56)58. No personal details or clinical information should be divulged without the valid consent of the patient.

CONSENT

The examination and treatment of patients cannot be carried out without physical contact. Where physical contact takes place without the agreement of the patient, an assault may be said to have occurred. This may be a civil or a criminal offence or both. As a precaution against legal proceedings, therefore, the doctor should be sure that he has the patient's consent before any examination, procedure or treatment is commenced.

Consent itself is not always understood. There is more to it than the demonstration of a signature on a piece of paper. Even when not *expressed* it can be *implied*. For example the patient's presenting himself to an A & E department implies at least some degree of consent to treatment. If the patient undresses and lies upon the examination couch when the doctor indicates a wish to examine him then agreement to that procedure is implied. Express consent is said to be given when a patient states agreement to a request in clear terms, orally or in writing.

Whatever the form of consent, certain other criteria must exist for that consent to be valid:

1. The patient must be informed of the true nature of the procedure and any inherent risks. The meaning of informed consent has been fully debated recently in English law. There is no requirement, as in some United States federal laws, that every possible complication and side effect should be explained to the patient as a prerequisite to treatment. In the *Sidaway Case* in 1975, it was affirmed in the House of Lords that a decision about what degree of disclosure of risks of treatment to a particular patient must primarily be a matter of clinical judgement. The responsibility for resolving any conflict between medical expert opinion in a particular case would rest with the trial judge.

2. The patient must be competent to understand the nature of the procedure.

> In England any person of sound mind who has attained the age of 16 years may give a legally valid consent to surgical, medical or dental treatment or procedures (s8, Family Law Reform Act, 1969).

Below the age of 16 the situation is unclear — the law does not state that a person below the age of 16 years may not give consent! The preferred view is that the consent is valid so long as the child is competent to understand the nature and purpose of the treatment. Commonsense should prevail. Clearly, if there is doubt and the treatment can wait — then wait. If the treatment is urgent then common law and commonsense should be followed. Sufficient treatment should be administered to resolve the emergency but no more until consent can be obtained.

3. The consent must be clearly *voluntary*. Any degree of duress, fraud or deceit will invalidate the consent — implied or expressed.

Consent in an emergency

Treatment may be administered without consent under common law when there is 'urgent necessity'. This is not clearly defined in law but is usually meant to describe circumstances when 'life-saving' treatment is given. It also includes any 'emergency' which, in these circumstances is understood:

> when immediate action is necessary to preserve life or to prevent a serious and immediate danger to the patient or other people.

Any treatment or physical restraint employed in these circumstances must be 'reasonable' and sufficient only for the purpose of bringing the emergency, not necessarily the underlying condition, to an end.

'The principle to guide the practitioner is to act in good faith and in the immediate interests of the patient's health and safety. If there is any element of doubt there should be no hesitation in seeking the opinion and advice of one or more colleagues.'

Consent and evidence

In cases involving the police it is wise to ensure that any consent for forensic examination, for the taking of specimens for forensic analysis and for the provision of a written statement to the police based on the doctor's findings at that examination, should be fully informed and expressed in writing. The purpose of the examination should be explained to the subject, preferably in the doctor's presence, by the police officer in the case, explanation of the nature and extent of the examination are clearly the responsibility of the doctor. Special consent forms held by the police may be available.

This principle is particularly important in the execution of an *intimate body search*, which may be requested, for example, when a patient has concealed drugs, loot or contraband within a bodily cavity in order to escape detection and surgical instrumentation is required for its removal. An A & E doctor should not perform examinations of this nature but should advise the police to obtain help from a police surgeon. The issue of intimate body searches is covered within the regulations of the Police and Criminal Evidence Act 1984.

Consent and Jehovah's Witnesses

The refusal of blood transfusions by Jehovah's Witnesses or other religious sects occasionally presents difficulties for the staff of the A & E department. No doctor can force blood into an unwilling patient without violating the laws of consent already discussed. In an emergency it is not appropriate for the doctor to refuse to undertake treatment and he may be compelled by common law to accede to the patient's wishes and withhold blood, even though he is of the opinion that blood may be essential for the preservation of life. When the patient is volitional and the doctor is willing to undertake treatment then the full nature of the patient's condition should be explained to him together with the need for blood and the consequences of not giving it. This explanation should be given by a senior doctor and witnessed by a colleague. The patient should be asked to sign a written declaration of his refusal. When the patient is unconscious, the person from whom consent (or refusal!) is sought should be the nearest relative.

The main problem arises over the children of Jehovah's Witnesses for it is difficult to accept that a person who has not reached the legal age of consent can become sufficiently informed as to appreciate all the personal consequences of refusing a transfusion.

> Furthermore, the Children and Young Persons Act 1933 makes it a criminal offence for anyone over 16 who has the custody, charge or care of a child under 16 wilfully to ill-treat, neglect or abandon that child or expose him to unnecessary suffering or injury to health.

Should the child die as a result of such neglect a charge of manslaughter could ensue. The principle which should be followed is for the doctor in charge of the case to do what is genuinely believed to be best for the child. After all, it is the child who is the patient, not the parents. Before making such a difficult decision which will clearly over-ride the parental wishes, the doctor must take into account all relevant considerations, including the views of medical and nursing colleagues and the possible use of plasma substitutes. When time permits, the advice of a defence society should be sought.

Refusal of treatment

A small number of patients, not all of whom are psychiatrically disturbed, will refuse medical advice, however courteously and clearly this may be offered. The doctor can only give his considered advice. If the patient declines to accept this, he should be recommended to seek medical advice elsewhere. He should be discharged from the department after first having been asked to sign the 'refusal' document. Should the patient refuse to sign such a document, the doctor must repeat his advice to the patient in the presence of another doctor or a senior nurse. He must then record in his notes what he has done and ask the nurse to witness his account. The unsigned form should be filed with the doctor's notes.

The patient may then decline to leave and may request further examination. At this stage a decision should be made whether a psychiatric opinion is required or whether the police should be asked to remove the patient from the department. Such patients may waste much time and disrupt the work of the department. This is disturbing, not only for nursing and medical staff, but also for other patients in the department. Eviction should be implemented as quietly and efficiently as possible and with a minimum of force. Appropriate explanations should be made to the other patients or members of the public who may have witnessed the incident. It may be helpful to have a member of the hospital administration present so that any accusations of physical violence can be promptly answered. Full clinical notes must be made in the hospital records at the time of the incident.

THE LEGAL REPORT

A & E doctors are often asked for written reports of patients' injuries and/or treatment, for example:

1. An attendance certificate for school or employer
2. A 'medical certificate' for insurance company
3. A police statement
4. A medical report to a solicitor, trade union or insurance company used as the basis of a civil claim for damages
5. A report to HM Coroner in the event of a death which is the subject of a Coroner's Inquiry
6. A report to the health authority in the event of an untoward incident occurring to a patient
7. A report to a medical defence society.

Great care should be taken before putting anything on paper. Before acceding to a request for any sort of statement or report the doctor should satisfy himself for whom he is acting and that, where appropriate, the patient has given consent to disclosure. The content of the report should be in accordance with the instructions of the party requesting it — the doctor should confine himself to the relevant facts and not venture an opinion unless one is asked for. Where an opinion is expressed it should be fair and impartial and reflect the experience and expertise of the writer — if a doctor does not know the answer to a question asked he should say so. Most accident reports will be requested of and prepared by a senior doctor — usually the consultant in charge of the case. Any junior doctor faced with a request for a legal report, perhaps for the first time and who is not unnaturally apprehensive and perhaps ignorant of procedure should seek advice from his consultant.

The provision of most types of medical reports commands a fee. Many fees are fixed, e.g. the fee for preparation of a police statement or a report to the Criminal Injuries Compensation Board. Others will be charged in proportion to the work involved and the standing and expertise of the examiner. The work involved in submitting such reports is not private work — provision is made for it under Category 2 of the terms and conditions of service under the National Health Service Act — but when technical services such as radiology and pathology are used in connection with a clinical examination for a report charges will be due to the health authority. Monies gained from Category 2 work are subject to income tax and must be declared.

Police statements

Statements to the police should be set out on witness forms in a standard manner to the requirements of the Criminal Justice Act 1967, s9. It is useful to have an agreed departmental policy whereby the statement is prepared in private in the doctor's own time, usually by dictation to the secretary, and then submitted, in approved form, to the police administrative liaison officer. In this way the doctor will not feel under any pressure to rush his statement and say things that he did not intend to say. He will have the opportunity of modelling the layout upon a specimen statement produced by a senior colleague and will be able to ensure that hearsay, conjecture and bias are eliminated from the statement. The typography will be tidy, the spelling checked and a copy of the statement, record card and fee note retained by the doctor and within the department master file.

The accident report

Accident reports are of two main types: the factual report from the case notes outlines the circumstances of the attendance, the injuries noted and the treatment and disposal arranged; a 'comprehensive medical report' sets out details of the accident and the disability ensuing, the outcome, the findings at follow-up examination and an opinion relating to the cause and the prognosis. Clearly the latter should be undertaken only by a senior, experienced doctor.

Table 4.3 sets out the main headings of a full accident report and may serve as a useful aide-memoire.

THE MEDICAL WITNESS

In the English legal system, now that increasing reliance is being placed upon the written word of the police statement as deposition of evidence in committal proceedings, the number of occasions upon which an individual A & E doctor might be called upon to testify in a court of law is, fortunately, fairly small. The thought of having to appear in the unfamiliar surroundings of a court does, nevertheless, cause considerable anxieties for even the most experienced doctor. Although court procedure is beyond the scope of this review, a doctor who receives a witness summons or court warning would do well to consult the relevant section of a standard textbook on legal medicine for the purpose of familiarisation with form and protocol. There is a significant difference between criminal courts and the Coroner's inquest. Whilst the latter use the form of an enquiry in which all interested parties have a right to put questions to a witness, the former relies on the traditional adversarial system of examination-in-chief, cross-examination and re-examination.

Table 4.3 Aide-memoire for an accident medical report

Examiner: name, address, qualifications	
Subject: name, address, date of birth, reference no.	
Date of accident	
Date and place of examination	
Date of report	
HISTORY	History of current event
	Previous history relevant to current event
EXAMINATION AND TREATMENT IN IN HOSPITAL	Examination in A & E department. Injuries noted
	Investigations including radiographs
	Arrangements for subsequent treatment, surgery, rehabilitation
FOLLOW UP AND MEDICAL OUTCOME	
SUBSEQUENT PROGRESS SINCE HOSPITAL DISCHARGE	Activities of daily living
	Household activity
	Work: Period of total occupational disability
	Partial occupational disability, period and nature
	Loss of earning capacity
	Sport and leisure activity
SOCIAL HISTORY	Include marital status and dependants
THE CURRENT POSITION (use patient's own words)	Nature and degree of any disability, loss of function, scarring, pain
	Other symptoms
PREVIOUS MEDICAL HISTORY	General health; drug history; family history
	Dominance
	Contributory factors
	Intercurrent illnesses
EXAMINATION FOR REPORT	General condition
	Specific areas of injury:
	a. state of healing, scarring
	b. sensation, power
	c. active and passive joint movements
	d. functional assessment
	Investigations, e.g. current radiographs, etc.
OPINION	Causation
	Contribution of previous and current illness
	Assessment of disability — total and partial (a percentage assessment may help)
	Prognosis and outcome (including effect of any more medical or surgical treatment

Being a medical witness can be a daunting experience. It may be less formidable, however, if the doctor has prepared himself for the event and has refreshed his memory from the records of the details of the case. All relevant notes including the case record and the doctor's own hand-written notes made at the time of examination should be taken to the courtroom. 'Dress up: stand up: speak up: shut up' remains a useful adage to correct court behaviour. The scruffy, slouching doctor mumbling unintelligibly over his illegible notes or the brash, overconfident young man who is full of his own opinions are equally liable to experience the harsh lash of the advocate's tongue. Neither do credit to the doctor's reputation.

SPECIAL PROBLEMS FOR THE ACCIDENT AND EMERGENCY DEPARTMENT

Offences against the person

Victims of various crimes against the person such as woundings, battery, attempted strangulation, street muggings, poisoning and those with gunshot wounds, may attend A & E departments for treatment. Likewise, victims of rape and sexual assaults may present requesting treatment for injuries sustained, or because they feel that the hospital offers unbiased support, care and sympathy. A & E department staff often find themselves having to balance the overwhelming need to provide competent medical treatment for the victim against the personal, legal and social needs to investigate the crime, detect the perpetrator and prevent further offences. These are police duties which require meticulous attention to detail in the collection, retention, recording and presentation of evidence. However great these pressures, no process, legal or social, should be allowed to get in the way of the foremost consideration — the need for treatment. Nevertheless, staff should be particularly careful to ensure that their actions do not inadvertently or deliberately obstruct any criminal investigation.

When should the police be informed?

If the patient requests police involvement, then the local police duty room should be notified without delay. In the event of sexual assaults this action is likely to result in two immediate sequelae;

1. The mobilisation of a special police sexual offences unit. Most forces now employ especially skilled, non-uniformed women police officers who have received specific training in the care of victims of sexual offences. These policewomen are particularly experienced in all the problems of rape and can be of great benefit to the other people involved.

2. The involvement of the duty police surgeon. The police surgeon is a medical practitioner trained and skilled in the subject of clinical forensic medicine. The police surgeon is not employed by the police, but is retained as an independent medical adviser in matters of medical evidence. The surgeon is not 'on the police's side'. He or she will be the person who would normally carry out the forensic medical examination and obtain the necessary evidential samples. A & E specialists should develop a harmonious professional relationship with their local force surgeon for, after all, the patient's needs are their common interest. Joint consultations and examinations are sometimes needed, for example in cases of suspected sexual abuse in children. The police surgeon's involvement does not absolve the A & E department staff from their normal duties of patient care. For example one police surgeon recently reported two rape cases in which the victims had, unnoticed, lost substantial amounts of blood whilst awaiting her arrival.

When the victim states, categorically, that he or she does not wish the police to be involved, there is no dilemma. 'A doctor should preserve secrecy on all he has learnt about his patient in the course of his professional duties' (see the section on Confidentiality above).

There are, however, intermediate situations which are problematical and call for balanced judgement.

Sometimes the victim does not know what to do for the best and seeks advice. Any advice offered should be impartial and offered in the patient's interests. Genuine victims of sexual offences, for example, are usually relieved to be able to share their experiences and anxieties with people whom they can trust and who share empathy. A realisation that the police force is, in the main, courteous, sympathetic and discreet and an understanding of the role of the investigating officers and police surgeon will permit the involvement of the police force and a fair investigation of the offence.

Occasionally there are situations which call for preservation of information and evidential material until a. the victim has recovered sufficiently to decide if he or she wishes the assault to be investigated, or b. the victim dies, in which case all the evidential material becomes the property of the Coroner.

Evidence

Modern forensic science is based on the concept known as Locard's principle that every contact leaves a trace. In assaults this *contact trace material* may be in the form of:

1. Loose debris (textile fibres, hairs, fragments of paint, glass and metal)

2. Powder, e.g. gunshot residues

3. Stains of body materials (blood, semen, saliva, faeces, urine and vomit).

The contact trace material may be on the victim's clothing, hair or skin, be deposited in a body orifice or be left in a wound. It is important to retrieve this contact trace material as soon as possible as it may disappear or be removed and discarded in ignorance. Any debris which falls from the person's clothing or body is also important and should be retrieved.

The preservation of contact material; the description and interpretation of wounds, injuries and wounding instruments and the acquisition of body fluids (blood and/or urine samples for alcohol analysis, drugs assay and serological typing) will normally be the responsibility of the attending police surgeon. For sexual offences, many police forces employ a sealed 'sexual offences kit' for the use of the police surgeon, containing the appropriate specimen containers and examination materials. Spares of these, together with the accompanying forensic science laboratory check list form, could well be held in the A & E department.

Special considerations

1. When cutting off or removing clothing during a resuscitation procedure, hospital staff should avoid cutting through damaged areas such as stab holes and bullet holes.

2. Wet or damp clothing should be retained in brown paper packets, not in polyethylene bags. The latter encourage the growth of yeasts and moulds which destroy the evidence.

3. When the victim of a major crime is to be cross-matched for blood transfusion, a separate, pretransfusion blood sample should be retained for the police as a control sample for the forensic laboratory.

4. In most A & E departments the clothes and valuables of a patient who is to be admitted are listed in the department in the presence of a witness. Sometimes such property is required by the police, either as evidence or to aid in the identification of an unknown patient. It is good practice to request and retain a copy of an offical receipt. This is especially important when dealing with multiple unidentifiable victims from a major disaster.

5. Patients suffering from self-poisoning or self-injury, should have the weapon or poison removed from their possession on arrival. It is not common for such patients to demand the return of their property. If the A & E staff think that such a patient is likely to damage or poison himself again they may decline to return the weapons or tablets and, in certain circumstances, may hand them over to the police. If the property is to be retained, it should be properly labelled and placed in a secure place, in the presence of a witness, in case litigation should follow. Such patients may complain about losing their property, but usually do not persist with their complaints.

Legal continuity of evidence

It is important in criminal investigations to be able to establish who first took possession of items of evidential value and to trace their subsequent chain of possession and storage, until they are made court exhibits. All items have to be packed and sealed and a court exhibits label is affixed to show from whom or where the samples came, when and by whom they were taken and who has subsequently handled them. This is a responsibility of the police.

Drink–drive procedures

> A person who, when driving or attempting to drive, or when in charge of a motor vehicle on a road or other public place, is unfit to drive through drink or drugs shall be guilty of an offence (Road Traffic Act, 1972, Section 5).
>
> If a person drives or attempts to drive or is in charge of a motor vehicle on a road or other public place, having consumed alcohol in such a quantity . . . that this exceeds the prescribed limit . . . he shall be guilty of an offence. (Section 6).

The prescribed limit is
35 microgrammes per 100 ml of breath
80 milligrammes per 100 ml of blood
107 milligrammes per 100 ml of urine.

> If an accident occurs owing to the presence of a motor vehicle on a road or other public place, a constable in uniform may require any person whom he has reasonable cause to believe was driving or attempting to drive the vehicle at the time of the accident to provide a specimen of breath for a breath test (Section 8).
>
> A person while at hospital as a patient may be required by a constable to provide at the hospital a specimen for a laboratory test . . . if it appears as a consequence of a breath test . . . that the proportion of alcohol in this blood exceeds the prescribed limit (Section 9).
>
> . . . a person shall not be required to provide a specimen . . . if the medical practitioner in immediate charge of his case is not first notified of the proposal to make the requirements or objects to the provision of the specimen on the ground that its provision or the requirement to provide it would be prejudicial to the proper care or treatment of the patient.

Should the police wish to know whether a patient has taken an excess quantity of alcohol A & E department doctors are under no obligation to perform tests. Samples must be taken by a police officer or police surgeon. The drink–drive legislation is complex and the procedures for taking specimens clearly defined by statute. Nevertheless, hospital staff should assist the police in this part of their work, as long as this does not conflict with confidentiality or with the immediate treatment of the patient. The A & E doctor can indicate that a patient is fit to be breathalysed or to have a blood sample taken and he should record in the notes that the patient is fit to give consent. Rarely is a subject unfit for such procedures on medical grounds. If the patient is to be admitted great care should be taken with the patient's own sample. It should be secured for safe keeping as a valuable property item.

Samples of blood which may be taken by medical staff for the measurement of blood alcohol for clinical purposes probably would not, for technical reasons, be admissable in a court of law. Such estimations should, nevertheless, be carried out if they contribute to the patient's proper medical management (see Ch. 30).

Offences involving drugs

The laws controlling the supply and use of drugs of addiction are contained within the *Misuse of Drugs Act 1971* together with its associated regulations.

> A person is regarded as being addicted to a drug if, and only if, he has as a result of repeated administration become so dependent on a drug that he has an overpowering desire for the administration of it to be continued.

Within the above Act, the drugs of addiction are:
cocaine
dextromoramide

diamorphine
dipipanone
hydrocodone
hydromorphone
levorphanol
methadone
morphine
opium
oxycodone
pethidine
phenazocine
piritramide

The care of patients presenting to the A & E department as a result of addiction and its associated problems is discussed in Ch. 30. There are two main legal issues described in the Notification and Supply to Addicts Regulations 1973, relating to drugs misuse:

1. The requirement for the attending doctor to notify, in writing, the Chief Medical Officer of the DHSS of the details of the addict (see Disclosure, above).

2. The issue of drugs of addiction. No doctor may administer or authorise the supply of cocaine or diamorphine or their salts to addicted persons for the purpose of treating organic disease or injury unless he is licensed to do so by the Secretary of State.

The common practical problem remains the decision to inform the police of the presence of a suspected drug abuser in the A & E department seeking hard drugs. The balance lies between providing a confidential environment in which effective care can be given to the individual patient and the wider duty of care to the public in controlling the illegal activities of drug pushers.

Perhaps the only satisfactory solution to this dilemma is to build up a mutually trusting and professionally caring relationship with members of the local police drug squad such that professional confidences can be maintained yet the wider aspects of prevention go unhindered.

Mental health

The 1983 Mental Health Act contains those sections relating to the compulsory admission to hospital of patients suffering from mental disorder either in the interests of the patients' own health or safety, or with a view to the protection of others. The provisions and practical application of the Act are discussed in depth in Ch. 30 (Psychiatric Emergencies).

The violent or aggressive patient

Episodes of violence against members of staff of A & E departments are, regrettably, on the increase. When staff have satisfied themselves that the patient's aggressive behaviour cannot be explained on the basis of an underlying medical disorder (e.g. hypoglycaemia, psychotic illnesses, etc. — see Ch. 30) and that, in fact, the assault and damage to property has a criminal basis, then they should have no hestitation in asking the patient to leave the department, enlisting the assistance of the police where appropriate. Careful notes should be made on the patient's record

and in the departmental record of untoward incidents, the A & E consultant should be informed and a written report should be submitted to the hospital managers at the earliest opportunity.

Child abuse

The clinical features of this syndrome are detailed in Ch. 5. The A & E doctor's duty will be set out in the procedural guidelines laid down at local level by the Joint Child Protection Committee. If an A & E doctor suspects child abuse he should discuss the case with the senior doctor in the department and the paediatricians and admit the child to the paediatric ward. Sometimes when a child has been admitted to hospital with suspected non-accidental injuries, it appears unsafe to return the child home, either because the circumstances are the subject of an ongoing investigation, or because there is indisputable evidence of physical abuse.

Section 28(1) of the Children and Young Persons Act, 1969 gives the authority to a Justice:

' . . . to detain the child in a place of safety if there is reasonable cause to believe that his/her proper development is being avoidably prevented or neglected or his/her health is being avoidably impaired or neglected or he/she is being ill-treated.'

In the event of the parent refusing to allow the child's admission to hospital, the consultant should be informed and the police and social services involved so that an emergency order can be obtained. A Place of Safety Order may run for 28 days during which time investigations can be carried out and a case conference held to determine further action. The A & E doctor may be required to attend. His opinion concerning the circumstances at the time of admission may prove very valuable.

Sudden death

All deaths in the A & E department should be reported to HM Coroner. The report should be made by telephone to the Coroner's officer, who can be contacted via the local police station. When reporting a death, the following items of information should be given:

patient's name
address
date of birth
date and time of death
cause of death and relevant history
name, address and 'phone number of next of kin.
name, address and 'phone number of general practitioner.

Brain death

One of the hardest decisions to be faced by doctors striving to sustain life using advanced resuscitation techniques is when to accept the futility of continuing life-support measures, i.e. when to accept that the moment of death has occurred. The decision is all the more important when the possibility arises of using the deceased's organs as homografts in transplantation operations under the provisions of the Human Tissue Act 1961. Usually this decision is faced in the intensive care unit with the patient being supported on a mechanical ventilator. Rarely the question arises in the A & E department. Accordingly staff should be familiar with the rules and guidelines for diagnosing brain death and instituting organ salvage procedures.

By 'brain death' is meant brainstem death, the diagnosis of which can be made using simple clinical tests (Statement 1976).

All the following should coexist:

1. Patient deeply comatose
   a. exclude drugs, especially narcotics, hypnotics and tranquillisers
   b. exclude primary hypothermia
   c. exclude a metabolic or endocrine cause for the coma.
2. Patient is being maintained on a ventilator because spontaneous respiration had previously become inadequate or had ceased altogether.
3. There should be no doubt that there is irremediable, structural brain damage. The diagnosis of a disorder which can lead to brain death should have been fully established.

The tests for confirming brain death

1. Absence of all brain stem reflexes
   a. pupils fixed in diameter with no response to sharp changes in intensity of incident light
   b. absent corneal reflex
   c. absent vestibulocochlear reflex ie no eye movements during or after slow injection of ice-cold water into each external auditory meatus in turn, clear access to the tympanic membranes having being established
   d. absent motor response within the cranial nerve distribution
   e. absent gag reflex or reflex response to bronchial simulation.
2. Absent respiratory movements on disconnecting the patient from the ventilator.

The suggested procedure is to administer 5% CO_2 through the ventilator and disconnect when the $PaCO_2$ reaches 5.3–6.0 kPa (40–45 mmHg). The patient should remain disconnected for long enough to enable the $PaCO_2$ to reach 6.7 kPa (50 mmHg), i.e. greater than the threshold for stimulating respiration.

Other considerations

The decision to withdraw artificial support should be made after all the above criteria have been fulfilled and would normally be made by the consultant who is in charge of the case and one other senior doctor.

Possible organ donors are patients who have sustained brain damage to the extent of possible or imminent death and who are maintained on a mechanical ventilator. Suitable cases would include:
1. Cranial trauma
2. Intracranial haemorrhage or thrombosis
3. Primary intracranial tumour.
Unsuitable cases would include:
4. Patients with malignancy (excepting a primary nervous system tumour)
5. Patients with established infection
6. Patients with kidney disease.

Do not even consider organ donation from a patient whose death or impending death is likely to be the subject of criminal proceedings, in particular murder, manslaughter or death due to abdominal trauma.

The consultant in charge of the A & E department should know the local arrangements for contacting the organ transplant team when a suitable case arises. It should be stressed that the doctors in charge of the potential donor must remain totally independent of the transplant team. The two doctors who decide brain death must make their decisions separately and record them separately in the notes. The responsibility for obtaining consent for cadaveric organ transplantation is that of the transplant team. The relationship of involved parties to the Coroner and the Coroner's appointed pathologist must be clearly understood.

RELEVANT LEGISLATION

Note: The examples cited in this chapter refer to the application to the practice of Emergency Medicine in *English law.* Different legislation may be in force in other countries within the United Kingdom (for example, in Scotland the role of the Coroner is taken by the Procurator Fiscal) and, obviously, in the rest of the world. The following statutes of English Law form the basis for those general principles of medical practice discussed.

Abortion Act 1967
Children and Young Persons Act 1933, 1969
Criminal Justice Act 1986
Data Protection Act 1986
Family Law Reform Act 1969

Human Tissue Act 1961
Mental Health Act 1983
Misuse of Drugs Act 1971
National Health Service Act 1977
Notification and Supply to Addicts Regulations 1973
Offences against the Person Act 1861

Police and Criminal Evidence Act 1984
Reporting of Injuries, Diseases and Dangerous Occurrences
 Regulations 1985
Road Traffic Act 1972
Sexual Offences Act 1956, 1967
Sexual Offences Amendments Act 1976.

FURTHER READING

General reading
The new police surgeon: a practical guide. Burgess S H, Hilton J E (eds) 1978 Hutchinson Benham, London

Professional conduct and discipline; fitness to practise. General Medical Council 1983 GMC, London

Legal aspects of medical practice, 3rd edn. Knight B 1976 Churchill Livingstone, Edinburgh

Butterworths medico-legal encyclopaedia. Mason J K, McCall Smith R A 1986 Butterworths, London

The doctor and the law, 2nd edn. Taylor J L 1983 Pitman Medical, London

Symposium — doctors and the courts 1985 Medicine, Science and the Law 24(2): 81–126

Professional competence and the accident and emergency department
Missed diagnoses in an accident and emergency department. Guly H R 1984 Injury 15: 403–406

Mishap or malpractice. Hawkins C 1985 Blackwell Scientific, Oxford

Symposium — Problems in the accident and emergency department. Medical Protection Society, London

Pitfalls in the management of accidental injuries. Stevens J Medical Protection Society, London

Medical malpractice. Taylor J L (ed) 1980 John Wright, Bristol

Professional secrecy and consent
Handbook of medical ethics. British Medical Association 1980 BMA, London

Statement — Jehovah's Witnesses and the question of blood. Watchtower Bible and Tract Society of Pennsylvania, USA

Consent, confidentiality, disclosure of medical records. Palmer R N 1985 Medical Protection Society, London

The duty of confidence Parks R 1982 (leading article) British Medical Journal 285: 1442–1443

What the doctor must tell the patient. Samuels A 1982 Medicine, Science and the Law 22: 41–46

The medical report
Report of the Joint Committee of British Medical Association, Senate of the Inns of Court and the Bar and Law Society 1981 Medical evidence. BMA, London

The medical report and testimony. Pearce G H 1979 George Allen and Unwin, Beaconsfield

A doctor's guide to court. Simpson K 1967 Butterworths, London

Offences against the person
The criminal law — book 2. Offences against the person. Greaves A, Pickover D 1979 Police Review Publishing, London

Rape. McLay W D S (ed) 1983 Association Police Surgeons of Great Britain, Creaton House, Northampton

Mental health
The Mental Health Act 1983. The psychiatric emergency — notes for casualty officers. Responsibility for the suicidal patient. Bradley J J 1986 The Medical Protection Society, London

Mental illnesses and the law. Whitehead T 1982 Basil Blackwell, Oxford

Brain death
ABC of brainstem death. Pallis C 1983 BMJ Publications, London

Diagnosis of brain death. Statement 1976 British Medical Journal ii: 1187.

Anthony D. Redmond

Social aspects

A & E departments do not exist in isolation. They are part of a small hospital community but more importantly, a larger urban/rural community. The relationship between the staff of the A & E department and these other communities will determine the quality of care for the patient. Communication within the hospital is discussed further in Ch. 3. The A & E department is the bridge between the community and hospital services. The circumstances in which a person lives within that community will shape and often cause the condition with which the patient presents.

HOMELESSNESS

To have 'no fixed abode' or permanent address renders the individual impotent in society. You may not actually be living on the streets (though many are), but without an address you have no family doctor, no school provision and no state benefit. The logistics of living from a temporary address makes it difficult to establish any of the normal social supports. Such people are more prone to illness and paradoxically have more difficulty in securing any help.

A homeless person may present to the A & E department, either because of, or as a result of his homelessness. Merely asking for help in finding an address is an unusual reason for attendance, but it is helpful if the department has a list of local agencies who can help in these matters. The homelessness, however, may be the reason behind some trivial or imaginary complaint which the patient uses as an excuse to find shelter. Exclude a serious medical condition before referring the patient to the social worker. Occasionally the patient may be referred to the police. However, a thorough medical approach first will prevent any subsequent unnecessary suffering for the patient.

Many homeless people are single. The middle-aged may have been married once but are now without a partner. There has been a recent dramatic rise in homelessness amongst the very young. This is linked in part to unemployment — another potent factor in ill-health. It has long been established that pulmonary disease and, in particular, tuberculosis is increased in those of no fixed address. This is not just amongst those who live in common lodging houses, but amongst anyone who lives in poor surroundings. Overcrowding in temporary accommodation increases the risk of all infectious disease and respiratory disease in particular. The middle-aged and elderly, homeless, single person has a significant incidence of mental illness. This may have contributed to their homelessness in the first place but must be considered in his assessment. This 'chicken and egg' argument also extends to homelessness and drug abuse. It is well established that many homeless people misuse a variety of drugs, including alcohol. However, the cause and effect of one to the other is not as clear as it might at first seem. Regardless of the underlying reason the emergency doctor must be aware of this association and appreciate the risks of hepatitis B and HIV infection (see Ch. 25). Actually to 'live rough' has in the past been uncommon. However, the incidence is increasing. There are obvious risks such as hypothermia and frostbite, but perhaps the greatest risk is violent injury. The combination of drug/alcohol abuse and homelessness renders people easy victims.

Infestation with lice occurs but is easily treated. What is of greater importance is the fact that the person tolerated the infestation. Head lice can be remarkably well tolerated and, if the hair is never combed, will easily flourish. Pubic lice are extremely irritant when they burrow into the skin, but alcohol and other sedatives will reduce the discomfort. Widespread body lice imply a serious deterioration in personal hygiene. Alcohol has usually facilitated the tolerance of the vermin by the patient but more serious organic pathology may be present. A radiograph of the chest is mandatory and a head injury should be considered.

The infestation is easily treated with γ-benzene hexachloride or lindane BP 1%. It should be repeated in 10 days to destroy the product of any eggs. However, the physical condition of the patient is likely to be poor.

Unlike pubic or head lice, scabies is highly infectious and can easily be passed from patient to doctor. It causes intense itching. The mite burrows under the skin often between the fingers. Thread-like burrows may be seen in these areas. The treatment is as for other infestations.

The risks of homelessness have been outlined and chest infections and injury will be treated accordingly. More difficult is the patient who presents to the emergency department because he has no family doctor. There can be no counsel of perfection but certain guidelines can be proferred:

1. Any patient who insists on seeing a doctor should see a doctor. This need not be immediately.

2. Listen to and examine the patient *before* you decide on the appropriateness of their attendance.

3. Any treatment must be accompanied by attempts at establishing a family doctor for the patient. In the UK general practitioners will be paid for taking on any patient as a 'temporary resident' and this can be explained to the patient. Arrange an appointment with a social worker if any difficulties are envisaged.

There has to be somewhere within a health service where patients can secure medical advice at any time. The emergency department is it. It is not possible to stem the flow of 'inappropriate attendances' with any degree of safety or compassion, but rapid redirection will go some way to preventing such attendances detracting from the primary function of the department in treating the seriously ill and injured.

THE ELDERLY AND INFIRM

A visit to the emergency department is never an isolated event. It is only one of many which shape and form the health of an individual. The increasing age of a patient and, much more importantly, his mobility and general health will determine his response to any subsequent illness or injury. In fact one study has shown that, for cardiac arrest, it was underlying disease alone and not age that determined outcome. But even for far less dramatic conditions it is important to establish what effect the illness or injury will have on the patient's overall health, mobility and *dependence*. Establish how the patient sleeps, dresses, uses the toilet and who helps with any of this. If the patient used a walking stick can they still do so after the accident? The level of dependence must encompass the effects of any treatment options. Indeed, great care must be taken if the effects of treatment are not be worse than the final effects of the condition. Furthermore, the mere presence of a condition is not in itself an indication for treatment. For example, immobilising a wrist in plaster will significantly increase the dependence of a patient on others, particularly if they have injured their dominant hand. Ultimate anatomical alignment may be of secondary importance to independence.

If the patient lives alone it may be necessary to admit them for a short while in order to allow them to adjust to the effects of your treatment. This will also allow a home assessment and the mobilisation of the primary care team. If the patient can go home or insists on going home, then inform the general practitioner and arrange for the health visitor to call. When repeated dressings are

necessary it may seriously disrupt a patient's life if he repeatedly returns to the department. The district nurse will arrange dressings either at a local health centre or the patient's home and supervise the wound. It is of great benefit if a relationship is established which allows the district nursing service to decide when a wound is healed, rather than insisting that the patient returns merely to be told that things are doing well.

The assessment of an elderly patient must include mobility. Ask the patient to sit on the side of the trolley with his feet on low steps and if this is well tolerated, to stand on the floor and then take a few steps. A patient who lives alone and is incapable of walking across an examination cubicle unsupported is not fit to go home. This test will often reveal a previously unsuspected fracture of the neck of the femur. When there is pain on walking and a radiograph shows no such fracture, the pubic rami should be carefully scrutinised for the presence of a fracture. Unexplained pain may also be due to pathological fractures.

After a full medical assessment the doctor should turn to the assessment of the social situation, discussing it fully with the nurses, medical colleagues and relatives.

Medical social workers are of special help in assessing the nature of the patient's housing needs and in arranging help from relatives and neighbours, home helps, district nurses, community social workers and volunteers. Often the social and medical problems have been present for a long time and precarious independence maintained with outside help. This independence may be threatened by a minor illness or accident to the patient or to another elderly person who has, until that time, provided the support at home.

SOCIAL STRESS

It is not merely the presence of a problem that is stressful. Many people find this stimulating. It is the inability to deal with it effectively that is stressful. This coping ability depends on many factors, but socioeconomic status is perhaps the most important. The more socially stable, the more financially secure, and the higher up the social scale you are the more easily you can deal with life's problems. Stress is not exclusive to the poor and disadvantaged, but it does accumulate there. Stress will precipitate acute medical and social problems and predispose to many more. Furthermore, the effects of stress are cumulative. Each individual problem may not in itself be insurmountable, but layer upon layer will combine to form a serious problem complex. Important measures of stability are:

1. Age — the very young and the very old are more at risk.

2. Isolation — living alone or losing a partner are potent factors.

3. Finance — ability to cope with the majority of social problems is largely determined by the money available to you.

4. Sexual relationships — difficulties in interpersonal relationships and lack of a stable relationship predispose to many social problems.

5. Employment — difficulties at work are potent stress factors.

More important is the lack of a job. This increases the risk of suicide and illness significantly.

Each of the above may seem unimportant individually, but in combination with each other and associated with intermittent psychiatric, or physical illness will precipitate a serious mental, social or physical crisis.

VIOLENCE WITHIN THE FAMILY

The cumulative effect of social, psychological and physical pressures can precipitate violence in many forms but in particular towards 'helpless' dependents. 'Granny bashing' is perhaps uncommon but must be considered in any old person where injuries cannot be fully explained. The violence of neglect is probably more common. When this is physical it is more easily remedied than when it is emotional. What is of most importance to the emergency doctor is to recognise those at risk, rescue the victims and appreciate that any relative who has brought the patient has made the first move in asking for help.

Child abuse

Non-accidental injury to children and child neglect are relatively common problems for the A & E department. In Britain alone as many as a hundred children each year may die in this way.

'An abused child is a boy or girl under the age of 17 years who has suffered from *physical injury, physical neglect, failure to thrive, emotional or sexual abuse* which the person who had custody, charge or care of the child either caused or knowingly failed to prevent.'

It is essential to be able to identify the families 'at risk' and recognise the types of injury most commonly incurred. Each department must have a published 'plan of action' for these children and senior doctors should be involved ab initio.

Families at risk

Any adult can deliberately injure a child. However, certain factors will increase the likelihood of this occurring. As outlined above the event is usually the expression of an underlying series of stresses and no one event may be solely to blame. There are some warning signs however:

The parents.   1. Young, immature parents, particularly those who have children before the age of 20. Such parents may not appreciate the needs of children and even expect them to meet some of their own emotional shortcomings.

2. Failure to attend antenatal classes or prepare for the birth. Such information may be gained from the health visitor or family doctor.

3. A partner is not a parent.

4. Poor educational background of parents and/or low intelligence. The demands of parenthood are less likely to be met by those less equipped to deal with life in general.

5. Parents who abuse alcohol or other drugs.

6. Mental illness in a parent.

7. If parents are violent to each other they are more likely to be violent to their children.

8. Social isolation. Single parenthood and lack of an extended family will mean all of the above problems are unrelenting and obvious mistakes will go uncorrected.

9. Inappropriate expectations.

10. Poverty and low socioeconomic status. The rich are not without stress, but the poor have more stress. Unemployment in particular is a potent factor in all social problems. Overcrowding and poor housing make child rearing particularly difficult. Insufficient privacy may add the burden of complaints from neighbours to the anguish of a crying child.

The factors above may combine and contribute to a parents unrealistic demands on a child's development. Feeding and 'potty training' are the two commonest functions which produce undue stress in vulnerable parents (Fig. 5.1). If you do not know when children should achieve continence or appreciate the natural difficulties of weaning, then you place 'adult' values on a child's behaviour. Incontinence is interpreted as deliberate and punished 'appropriately'. Difficulties with feeding are similarly misinterpreted. This lack of appreciation of the child as different from an adult is a fundamental theme in abuse and is a function of all the above factors. In a similar way, such parents cannot cope with the 'crying child' in a reasonable way. They may give 'never stops crying' as a reason for attending an A & E department.

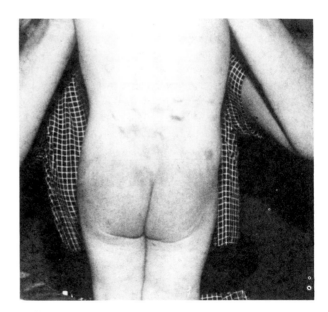

Fig. 5.1 Child who was severely chastised for bed wetting.

The children.   1. The children of those who themselves were abused are at a greater risk.

2. Premature babies and those who were separated from their parents at birth because of ill-health.

3. Clearly, a child that was unwanted or is different in some way must be considered to be at risk.

The story

Particular injuries are in themselves always suspicious of abuse. Any injury in a child but particularly in a child under the age of 5 years, must be considered 'suspicious' and steps taken to refute this. The essential points to establish are:

1. Was the accident witnessed? It is not, of course, only parents who abuse children. Other siblings, relatives and neighbours may be responsible. If the event was unwitnessed this cannot be excluded.

2. Does the story fit the injury? Are several differing explanations offered? If parents are trying to mask a non-accidental injury, errors and inconsistencies in the history may become apparent.

3. Is the injury recent? Delay in presentation can, in itself, indicate neglect even if the injury was accidental. However, many deliberate injuries are characterised by the parents' attempts to delay treatment, presumably in the hope that recovery will precede discovery.

4. Have all the injuries present (new and old) been volunteered in the history?

5. Is the family history free from any incident of non-accidental or suspicious injury?

6. Is the child an infrequent attender or non-attender at the A & E department?

If the answer to all the above questions is 'yes' then the injury is likely to be accidental.

The examination

Children are naturally apprehensive in hospital and usually seek refuge with their parent. A happy, healthy child who is active and at ease with its parent is usually not at risk. Children will naturally cry and struggle when strangers examine them. Abused children often have a passivity when examined. They do not resist but exhibit an almost 'waxey flexibility'. The fact that the child is easy to examine and a 'model patient' is not necessarily a good thing.

The child must be examined completely, including the perineum. However, this can be done 'piecemeal' rather than in toto. Inspect the clothing and nappies and form an opinon on the general level of care. Several non-accidental injuries may be discovered, characteristically in different sites, of different ages and different types.

A detailed record of the examination must be made and retained. Any injuries must be clearly described and measured. Photographic records should ideally be taken at the time of presentation. A Polaroid camera is extremely useful in this respect.

Abused children are often the victims of violent outbursts, but some are subjected to premeditated acts. Twisting injuries to the limbs will result in epiphyseal and joint injuries. Shaking the child will cause bilateral injuries to limbs that are gripped. It will also cause damage to brain and eyes. Dislocation of the lens and retinal detachment and haemorrhage must be excluded. Subdural haematoma can occur and CT scanning may be required.

Children bite each other; but adults bite children as well. If a bite mark is observed, measure it (Fig. 5.2).

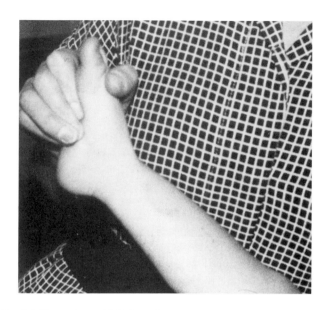

Fig. 5.2 Bite mark on child's leg. Measurement shows that the bite was made by an adult.

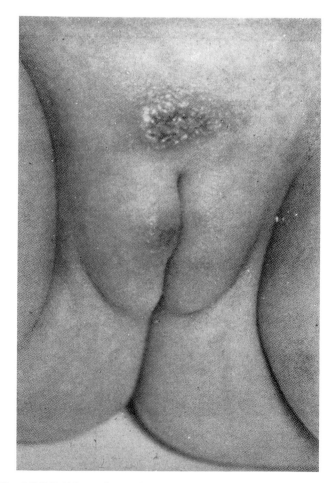

Fig. 5.3 Full-thickness cigarette burn close to genitalia.

Cigarettes may be used deliberately to burn a child, often in the genital area (Fig. 5.3). Children may be forced to stand in hot baths or even on cookers. Anyone who is burned will attempt to withdraw from the source of heat. A full thickness burn implies that the skin remained in contact with the heat for some time. For instance, it is reasonable, though regrettable, to assume that a cigarette might cause a superficial burn, but contact will be withdrawn as soon as heat is felt. However, if a full or deep partial thickness cigarette burn occurs the withdrawal from the heat must have been prevented (Fig. 5.4).

Children must first walk before they can fall. Skull fracture and long bone injury in children who cannot walk are highly suspicious. Furthermore, any bony injury is suspicious and non-accidental injury (NAI) must always be excluded before discharge home.

Slaps around the face will create bruising in the pattern of a hand or finger (Fig. 5.5). When the pinna of the ear is involved the rise in pressure in the external auditory meatus may lead to perforation of the tympanic membrane. The frenulum of the upper lip can occasionally be torn by a fall onto the face. This is unusual and will be accompanied by obvious blunt injury to the nose and face consistent with the history. This can occur accidentally in active older children who, for instance, fall from a bicycle. In young

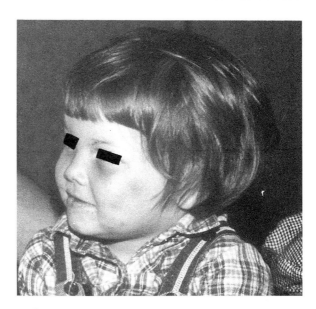

Fig. 5.5 Child slapped on face — bruises from finger imprint.

children and as an isolated finding it represents NAI until proven otherwise.

Poisoning in children may not be accidental. Deliberate harm may have been intended or 'Munchausen by proxy' have been attempted.

Many instances of abuse may, in fact, be more correctly termed 'neglect'. This of course may still be deliberate. Emotional neglect of children is a serious concern but it is difficult for the emergency doctor to evaluate.

There are conditions that will mimic child abuse. Only some of these can be identified in the A & E department. Commonsense is required.

Pathological fractures do occur in children but they are unusual. Osteogenesis imperfecta is usually associated with diaphyseal rather than metaphyseal injuries. If the diagnosis is known, the parents will tell you. Osteopetrosis will be revealed by the radiograph. Spina bifida will lead to disuse osteoporosis of the lower limbs which may fracture with relatively trivial injury.

Thrombocytopenia will lead to bruising and eventually to spontaneous haemorrhage. This may be as part of an already diagnosed blood dyscrasia, or as a presenting feature of a new condition. Idiopathic thrombocytopenic purpura is perhaps the commonest. It may have been preceded by a viral illness and the spleen is sometimes palpable. Leukaemia may also present in this way and it is important that bruised children are screened both sociologically and haematologically. Inherited haemoglobinopathies, such as haemophilia and Christmas disease, produce haemarthroses but the diagnosis is usually already known.

Pigmented naevi in the cheek can cause diagnostic difficulty but a phone call to the family doctor should resolve it. 'Mongolian blue spot' (Fig. 5.6) is too often mistaken for the effects of chastisement. It is a common birthmark in the lumbar region of Asian children.

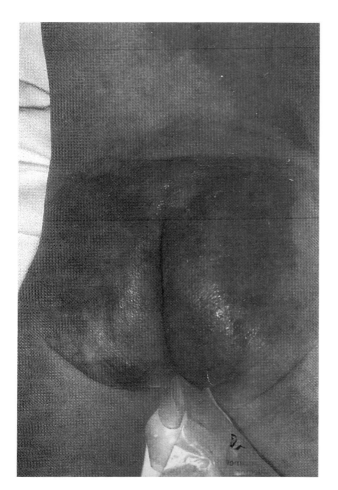

Fig. 5.4 Scalds to buttocks. Child held in over-hot bath.

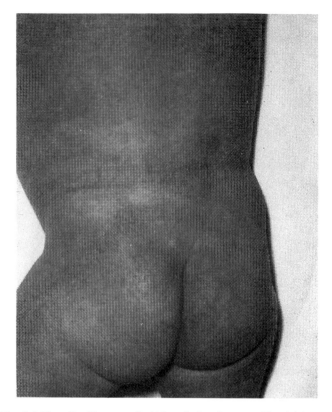

Fig. 5.6 Mongolian blue spot. Could be mistaken for non-accidental injury.

Radiological examination

A skeletal survey is often used to investigate children who are thought to have been abused. It involves a fairly high dose of radiation for a small child, but it might reveal older, unaccounted for, healing fractures. In fact the presence of multiple fractures at different stages of healing is almost pathognomonic of child abuse. Osteogenesis imperfecta may produce a similar picture and must be *excluded*. A skeletal survey is part of a planned investigation programme. It will not exclude child abuse. It is therefore usually inappropriate to conduct such an investigation in the A & E department. (Some departments have an arrangement whereby the investigation is done in A & E, but for/by the inpatient team.) Any child thought to be sufficiently at risk to warrant this investigation clearly requires admission to a paediatric unit. If the family doctor feels the investigation is appropriate, he should discuss the case directly with the departments of paediatrics and radiology.

Fractures in children usually leave one or both cortices intact — the 'greenstick' fracture. Disruption of both cortices requires considerable force and the history must support this.

A chronic rise in intracranial pressure will separate the sutures and be visible on a skull radiograph. Subdural haematomata may present in this way.

Pulling and twisting injuries to the limb result in injuries around and to the metaphyses of long bones. Calcified haematomata may be seen, but metaphyseal avulsion fractures are more common.

Plan of action

Admit all children with injuries which are suspicious or highly suspicious of non-accidental injury (see Table 5.1).

Table 5.1 Indications to non-accidental injury

Suspicious injuries
Story doesn't fit the injury
Delay in presentation
Presentation only at request of social worker
Repeated attendances of patient or siblings
Family background of abuse or deprivation
Burns and scalds
Bruises that might be in the pattern of fingers
Bite marks

Highly suspicious injuries
Skull fracture
Long bone fracture in a child who cannot walk
Metaphyseal injury
Cigarette burn
Scalds from bath water
Torn frenulum
Ruptured tympanic membrane
Facial bruising
Retinal haemorrhage
Lens dislocation
Genital injuries

Inform the paediatric department if the patient has been referred elsewhere and arrange for a social worker to be involved. It may be that, after investigation, it becomes clear that the child was a victim of a genuine accident. However, this must be established with the child in a safe environment. Execute great skill and compassion in explaining the reason for admission. Although ultimately a place of safety order may be involved it is always better for the long-term management of the child if this can be avoided.

If the child appears to be 'at risk' or neglected, but a non-accidental, serious or highly suspicious injury is not found, then the child may be allowed home if the following criteria can be fulfilled:

1. There is no evidence of serious, highly suspicious or deliberate injury.

2. The parents are with the child.

3. The child does not appear on the 'at risk' register or child-abuse register of either the A & E department or the social services.

4. There is no history of child abuse involving siblings.

5. Social services, health visitor and family doctor have all been contacted and agree that discharge is appropriate.

6. Adequate follow-up arrangements can be made.

If any *one* of these criteria cannot be met then the patient must be admitted.

Frequent attendances by children, often with trivial complaints, may mean that the parents cannot cope and may be a thinly concealed cry for help. Furthermore, whenever the reason for attendance is unclear ask the parents if they would like the child to be admitted. Most parents resist separation from their children, but some will readily give them up. Whatever the reason, if a parent is willingly forfeiting a child there is a serious underlying problem which must be faced. Admission of the child to a paediatric unit is the first step.

Spotting the child at risk from his previous attendances and those of his siblings requires adequate records. A computer will greatly help in this and can be programmed to scan automatically for previous attendances by the patient, siblings or anyone of that address. If a computer is not available then the records of the under-fives should be filed in such a way that it is relatively easy to search for previous attendances. All attendances by the under-fives should ideally be followed up by a health visitor, if only to advise on prevention of future accidents. The local community soon learns to expect such a visit and any stigma or suspicion is quickly removed.

Each local social services department maintains a register of children who are thought to be 'at risk' of non-accidental injury. A child's name can be placed on the register only after an official and duly constituted case conference. Similarly the maintenance of the child's name on the register is subject to review and it can be formally removed.

Sexual abuse

It is becoming increasingly more apparent that, in addition to the above, many children are subjected to sexual abuse.

This is defined as:

'the involvement of children *under 17* in sexual activities with any person having custody, charge or care of them, which they do not fully comprehend or to which they are unable to give informed consent, or that violate the social taboos of family rules'.

The investigation of this is usually carried out by paediatricians, family doctors, gynaecologists and police surgeons. However, particularly when injury is involved, a child may present to the emergency department. The examination must be done with tact, care and caution. Expose only those areas you are actually examining although you must ensure that you examine everywhere. Pelvic examination will clearly be interpreted by the child as yet another act of abuse. It should be carried out by someone with experience. The child will invariably require admission and such detailed examination can usually be carried out in the relative calm and privacy of the ward. Suspicion may be roused by overt sexual precociousness in the child or sometimes by direct allegation by the child. This cannot be passed off as a 'childish' remark and the problem must be addressed. Injuries to the perineum are clearly suspicious but persistent urinary tract and mouth infections or vaginal discharge must also be considered suspicious (see Ch. 22).

Further action

If there is a strong element of doubt or question at the time of admission, a *case discussion* should be organised by social services as soon as possible. Otherwise, a *case conference* will be organised as soon as practically possible. The A & E consultant will be asked to attend when the child is presented to the A & E department. The minutes of the meetings are *strictly confidential*. The purposes of the meetings are to determine risk, plan future strategies for the family, consider placing the child's name on the 'child protection' register and determine who (including those involved) should be informed of any conclusions and whether the police should be involved.

BEREAVEMENT

The very nature of the work of an A & E department dictates that staff have to deal on a daily basis with death and bereavement. The technical nature of the resuscitation room should not prevent staff from showing due respect to the body once attempts at resuscitation have failed. The patient should be quickly laid out and relatives allowed to see the body as soon as possible.

The grieving process can often only begin once the dead body has been seen. Relatives require time and privacy for this basic human act. As far as is possible, any religious needs of the patient and family should be met. The department should have a list of chaplains who can be contacted on these occasions. When the relatives have had time with the body then it can be moved to the mortuary. Distress and upset is normal after bereavement. Weeping and sorrow are part of the grieving process and eventual recovery. The sooner grief starts the sooner the sorrow will lift. Sedatives and tranquillisers will only postpone what is a natural and healing emotion. They may be required but, it is better if they are prescribed by the physician who will have long-term care of the relative throughout their bereavement.

The death of a child is a particularly tragic event and one that parents in western countries are unaccustomed to. When the death is sudden and unexpected it brings with it a particular group of problems.

The sudden infant death syndrome (cot-death) is used to describe the sudden and unexpected death of a small child, usually within the first few months of life. No family is immune, but bottle fed boys of mothers of low socioeconomic status are particularly at risk. Siblings of victims are also at risk and the incidence for all groups is increased during the winter months.

When a child is found dead in its cot an ambulance is often summoned and the baby is rushed to hospital. If the ambulance personnel were performing CPR throughout the journey then the baby should be admitted to the resuscitation room. Intubation, ventilation, venous access and cardiac monitoring can be quickly instituted. Any remedial condition will then be apparent. Unfortunately it is usually clear that the child is dead. All attempts at resuscitation should then be stopped. In this way the ambulance personnel are encouraged to attempt resuscitation, the baby is given (and seen to be given) every chance, but unnecessary procedures and consequent distress are avoided. This sequence need only take a few minutes and can usually have been completed by the time the parents arrive. On most occasions the parents can simply be informed that their baby has died.

Parents will blame themselves. They will have put the baby down and perhaps left it to sleep longer. They will naturally feel that if had they gone to the baby at any time events might have been different. Tell them nothing could have been done. The baby appears to have had a 'cot-death'. Let them see and hold their baby as soon as possible. Privacy and time are essential. Summon a chaplain if requested. Men must not be excluded from opportunities to express their grief and should be encouraged to hold the baby if they so wish.

Contact the family doctor and arrange for a visit. Ensure that any other children are safe. Siblings of similar age should be admitted to a paediatric unit as coincidental cot-deaths can occur. Make arrangements with the family doctor to cancel future appointments for the dead child. Parents have often recovered from their grief only to receive a reminder about vaccination for the dead child. When the child has been removed to the mortuary direct the parents to the 'distressed relatives room'. Explain to them the need for a postmortem (it is legal requirement) and that the police are obliged to interview them. This is routine and implies no guilt. They will not be aware of hospital procedure in these matters and someone should explain funeral arrangments and death certificates.

They require unparallelled support, particularly in the months to come. Many paediatricians take a special interest in counselling parents and they should be contacted.

Finally, whenever you inform someone of the death of a friend or relative there are a few important points:

1. Establish the identity of the person with whom you are speaking and their exact relationship with the deceased. Identify the deceased by their full name.

2. Make sure that your words can be clearly understood and that there can be no doubt that the person is dead.

3. There is no painless way of imparting bad news. Endless perambulation increases anxiety, so come quickly to the point. For example, having completed 1. above, say: 'I have some very bad news for you . . ., I am afraid that . . . has died'. Once this has clearly, fully registered, and you may have to repeat it, do not feel afraid of offering words of condolence and physical touch. Encourage them to weep.

4. Ensure that you have a senior nurse with you. They will know exactly what you said and be able to add any more information or advice as required.

Prehospital care

Doctors who work in A & E departments, by the very nature of their work, have close contact with the emergency services and are in a strong position to influence and control the provision of services for prehospital care. Occasionally they will be required to exercise their skills in the prehospital arena – an environment which, without training, can appear alien and hostile. For these reasons prehospital care is considered an important part of the A & E department specialist's 'stock-in-trade'. This section will examine, from the viewpoint of A & E department, those areas in which prehospital care can be practised and some of the ways in which it can be organised.

THE SCOPE OF PREHOSPITAL CARE

Prehospital coronary care

Within the past 20 years, since the pioneering work of Pantridge and his colleagues in Belfast, the importance of prehospital care in the emergency management of coronary artery disease has been realised. Coronary artery disease is the most common cause of sudden cardiac death outside hospital in western civilisations. Many people who die suddenly from heart disease have no previous symptoms. The percentage mortality from heart attacks is related to the time from onset of the symptoms; 50% of deaths occur within 15 minutes and 75% within the first hour. Many patients die before reaching hospital and so having excellent resuscitation facilities in the A & E department or on the wards can only affect the outcome in a minority of cases. The ideal coronary care unit is one which can provide care as soon as the heart attack has taken place.

The commonest mode of sudden death from heart disease is ventricular fibrillation and the most important treatment is defibrillation. With the availability of lightweight, fully portable defibrillators, prehospital coronary care and the prevention of sudden death have become realities. Of course survival is dependent upon the speed at which that care can be provided. Eisenberg and colleagues have established that, for optimum

salvage, basic life-support by a relative or bystander should be started immediately and a fibrillating heart defibrillated by the advanced life support team within, at most, 12 minutes. Recently, relatively low-cost automatic or *semiautomatic ('advisory') defibrillators* have been developed which can be used by ambulancemen after only a few hours training (Fig. 6.1). They appear to be accurate and reliable.

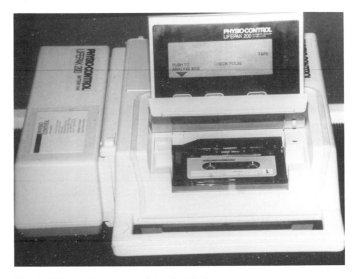

Fig. 6.1 The semiautomatic (advisory) defibrillator.

Prehospital coronary care encompasses more than a service to provide cardiac resuscitation and should include the stabilisation of the patient for transport, the relief of pain, the administration of prophylactic antidysrhythmic drugs where appropriate, and careful electrocardiographic monitoring before and during transfer to hospital.

Prehospital trauma care

In contrast, the role of prehospital care for the trauma victim is less clearly defined. For the critically injured casualty a sophisticated advanced trauma life-support service would strive to convey the patient to the local trauma centre as smoothly and rapidly as possible with the minimum of delay. Time spent at the scene in putting up intravenous lines and infusing fluids may, at the least, be wasteful; at the most it may cost the patient his life, for nothing can be achieved when the patient is bleeding internally at a greater rate than fluids can be infused. The only essential manoeuvres are the establishment of a clear airway, respiratory support including, if necessary, the relief of a tension pneumothorax, and the control of gross external bleeding.

However, there are circumstances where greater on-site intervention may be required:

1. The entrapment of a victim in, for example, motor vehicle wreckage, industrial machinery or a fallen building.

2. Where long distances are involved in reaching hospital care. In such cases the techniques of prehospital care for the trauma victim might include:

1. Emergency anaesthesia
2. Antishock trousers
3. Nerve blocks
4. Cervical splintage
5. Intravenous fluid and blood administration
6. Traction splintage
7. (rarely) Emergency amputation.

At all times during the rescue the attendant must weigh the merits and necessity of intervention at the scene against any advantages of intensive resuscitation at hospital and the potential risks of delay.

The crush syndrome

This is a name, coined by Bywaters in 1941, to describe the condition, frequently seen in World War II, of acute renal failure following the release from prolonged entrapment. It is usually the lower limbs which are crushed. The ensuing stagnant hypoxia and acidosis lead to compartment syndromes and tissue necrosis. Muscle breakdown products including myoglobin are released into the circulation following rescue; renal failure develops as a result of the myoglobinaemia and dehydration and sepsis is frequently a complicating factor. Members of rescue teams should be alert to the possibility of the development of this syndrome; dehydration should be avoided by adequate intravenous fluid therapy and, prior to release, pretreatment with 50 mmol sodium bicarbonate should be considered. The mainstay of prophylaxis in hospital is early fasciotomy and the extensive excision of dead tissue, including limb amputation, where necessary. ECG monitoring should alert clinicians to the development of hyperkalaemia.

Rescue from remote places

There are particular problems where the geographical setting makes access difficult, requires long journeys or causes unusual delays. The problems of snow, storms, flood and cold often hamper rescue operations. Added to these factors may be the additional problems of exposure and hypothermia (see Ch. 27). For mountain, cave, mine and sea rescue there are specialised services which have gained experience in these areas. Equipment and techniques have been specially developed for specific jobs (Fig. 6.2):

1. Mountain and ski rescue stretchers
2. Lifting devices, e.g. Paraguard and Neil Robertson stretchers
3. Insulating body bags of neoprene or fibre-pile material

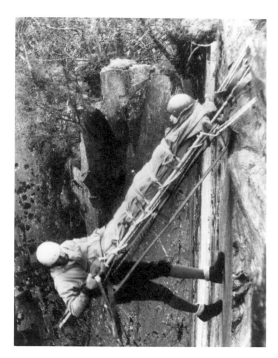

Fig. 6.2 A mountain rescue stretcher in use as rescuer abseils down rock face.

4. The 'Reviva' apparatus for inhaled air rewarming.

Those A & E departments situated close to a remote or inclement environment should know the special problems, services and resources relevant to their area.

Multiple casualties

The major incident, with its inherent problems of mass casualty sorting, rescue organisation and public, security and forensic interests, is the subject of the next chapter.

Long-distance transportation and interhospital transfer

Transportation of the patient long distances to hospital or between hospitals may be by land or air using surface transport (ambulances or specialised mobile intensive-care units), helicopters, or fixed wing aircraft.

Air transport will be required only under special circumstances such as accidents in mountain areas, on oil rigs and for island communities. In the UK, regulations for the use of aircraft are laid down in the DHSS circular no. HSC (IS) 196, 1975. There is a clear distinction between interhospital transfers and emergency flights. (The former are charged to the Health Service, the latter are not.)

Emergency flights have two functions. The first is to carry the emergency team to the patient, who will then be resuscitated on the ground until his condition is stabilised. A decision will then be made by the emergency team as to whether the patient should go to a local hospital or be transported to the major accident centre by conventional ambulance. The second function is to airlift the patient to the major accident hospital. This requires a larger aircraft with more complex facilities and entails dangers inherent in emergency landings, especially at night or in bad weather. In helicopters there are particular problems of noise and vibration which make the monitoring of patients in flight very difficult — everything possible should be organised and decided in advance of the helicopter's arrival. Every major accident centre should have landing facilities for helicopters. Communications and landing exercises should be held regularly (Table 6.1).

Table 6.1 Dos and don'ts in and around helicopters

ALWAYS
1. Obey the winchman's instructions
2. Switch off radios
3. Carry long equipment horizontally
4. Secure loose items especially headgear
5. Remain strapped in until told otherwise
6. Lower your head in the rotor disc area

NEVER
1. Smoke within 50 m of a helicopter
2. Enter or leave the rotor disc area without permission
3. Go near the tail rotor
4. Throw equipment, especially sharp or heavy items, on board
5. Carry on board fuels, acid, weapons, mercury thermometers
6. Wear crampons inside the cabin
7. Inflate life-jackets inside the helicopter
8. Touch yellow and black handles except for emergency egress
9. Anchor the winch cable

BOARDING
Kneel in a line with equipment secured at the 2 o'clock position 30 m from the aircraft. Do not approach the helicopter or rotor disc area without permission, which is the thumbs up signal from the pilot

STATIC ELECTRICITY
The Sea King generates considerable static electricity. Never touch the winch cable until the earthing lead has contacted the ground and the electric charge dissipated

---

The decision to hover or land is that of the Captain. Certain basic criteria must be fulfilled before a landing is attempted. Emergency teams can help by:
1. Selecting an area which:
   a. is clear of tall structures for 100 m diameter
   b. has an approach clear of trees
   c. has a central 15 m diameter of firm ground
   d. does not slope more than 12%.
2. Removing loose articles such as equipment or broken branches.
3. Controlling crowds and animals.
4. Indicating the landing point when the helicopter is in sight.
5. Flares or a small fire will indicate the wind direction.

(From Nicholson PJ 1986 BASICS monograph — search and rescue, reproduced by courtesy of the author and publishers.)

Interhospital transfer of patients to specialised units (such as neurosurgery, burns, spinal injuries and cardiothoracic units) will usually be made by surface transport. Air transport should be considered only if land or sea transport would be prolonged or uncomfortable, since air travel may not only be bumpy but usually involves additional patient transfers at both ends of the journey. Transfer of seriously ill or injured patients to specialised units requires careful advance planning so that the necessary facilities for ventilation, monitoring and transfusion en route can be made available at short notice. This may be by using special vehicles or by introducing modification to all standard front-line ambulances, e.g.
1. Points for central mounting of the stretcher
2. Medical rail attachment for monitors, etc.
3. Additional holders for intravenous infusions
4. Equipment for ventilation and suction
5. Housing for additional medical gas cylinders with reducing valves and plug-in fittings interchangeable with those carried on hospital trolleys.

Special vehicles are generally wider than front-line vehicles and, in addition to the above changes, may incorporate modifications to the suspension and/or 'floating' stretcher bases to reduce the harmful vibrations suffered by the patient.

A & E consultants should be involved in discussion of these problems so that adequate arrangements for these difficult and potentially dangerous journeys can always be made at short notice.

THE PROVISION OF PREHOSPITAL CARE

Several levels of skill are available for the provision of care outside the hospital. There will often be overlap and interplay between the tiers of care. Teamwork is essential at all times and, to facilitate good co-operation, the providers of care should be aware of their own and others roles and limitations.

First aid

First aid training in the UK is usually provided by one of the three voluntary aid societies:
1. The St John Ambulance
2. The British Red Cross Society
3. St Andrew's Ambulance Association.

In addition, training in resuscitation, especially where it involves water rescue, is part of the remit of The Royal Life Saving Society.

The standard *adult certificate* of the voluntary aid societies is based on their *first aid manual* and follows a minimum of six one-hour lectures integrated with practical training. Under the requirements of the 1983 First Aid At Work Act the number and disposal of trained and accredited first-aiders operating at all places of work is controlled by statute.

Shortened first aid courses, e.g. *Essentials of First Aid* are available for children and young people. The Emergency Aid Course has been pruned down to the bare necessities, with practical cardiopulmonary resuscitation training on manikins provided in one single, short session. Such classes form the basis of the United Kingdom *Save a Life* campaign, which links media advice with the encouragement of all citizens to receive practical training about what should be done in an emergency.

The uniformed first-aid organisations, e.g. St John Ambulance Brigade, are well organised to offer first-aid support to public events ranging from attendance at football matches to the establishment of forward aid centres and the provision of medically staffed resuscitation ambulances at large gatherings, e.g. motor-racing events and royal occasions.

In factories and other work-places there may be special first-aid teams to provide rescue or to deal with any specific hazards to which employees might be exposed. The mining industry is a good example of this. Arrangements made to deal with special hazards should be known to the local A & E department and lines of communication with the occupational health services established so that they can be used in an emergency.

Emergency services

The level of knowledge of prehospital emergency care possessed by police and fire officers ranges considerably from force to force. In some areas very specialised resuscitation skills and equipment may be available whereas in others only rudimentary arrangements exist.

In the UK it is the ambulance service with which the A & E department will have the greatest contact. All front-line emergency ambulances are provided with resuscitation facilities, suction, oxygen, Entonox, emergency childbirth equipment, splints, cervical collars, carrying chairs, etc. The training of ambulancemen to the appropriate standard is vested in the National Health Service Training Authority (NHSTA) (for the Ambulance Service National Staff Committee). To be able to practise 'on the road' as an independent ambulanceman in a front-line vehicle the officer must be the holder of the *Millar proficiency certificate.* This requires attendance at a 6-week residential course in an approved ambulance training school, a 2-week advanced driving course, a 1-week period of in-hospital experience and 12 month's experience, under continuous assessment, of emergency work. Some ambulance authorities have schemes whereby young people are appointed from school as cadets before undertaking Millar training.

The requirements for the *extended training of ambulance personnel* are also defined by the NHSTA. Candidates are accepted from practising ambulancemen and women following an examination and an aptitude test. A 4-week intensive residential course at an approved centre covers instruction in the basic sciences and the theoretical aspects of cardiac care, respiratory care, fluid and drug administration, etc. After the successful completion of two examinations the trainees attend hospital for a minimum of 4-weeks for clinical training in, for example, defibrillation and e.c.g. monitoring in the departments of cardiac care, anaesthesia and A & E medicine. It is difficult to arrange the placement of extended trained ambulancemen and women to provide the most effective use of their skills within the operational needs of the service and to obtain sufficient exposure to maintain their skills. Where this can be achieved, however, the Service should witness the realisation of a recent Health Economics Research Unit's prediction of the saving of 5 lives per year from a vehicle fully staffed and maintained 24 hours a day.

The term 'paramedic' is not restricted to the extended trained ambulanceman. Registered members of the Association of Emergency Medical Technicians include rig and diving medics, Royal Navy sick berth attendants, paramedics from the other armed forces, aeromedical transport attendants and members of other specialised rescue squads.

Immediate care schemes — general practitioners and hospital flying squads

Hospital based doctors

In some areas cardiologists are members of cardiac ambulance teams. In others a casualty officer, an anaesthetist and a nurse may go from the A & E department to accident sites. The first such *Accident Flying Squad* was started at Derby in 1955 and now over a dozen units operate with their own specialised vehicles and equipment. Some hospitals treat both cardiac and traumatic emergencies using the same team.

General practitioners

In many parts of the country groups of specially trained and equipped family doctors can be summoned to accidents at the same time as other rescue services. GPs have the advantage that they know the area well and are often on the spot before other emergency personnel. A wide net of such GP services now exists, many being modelled on Easton's original Road Accident After Care Scheme in North Yorkshire. Such *Immediate Care doctors* appreciate the interest and support of the A & E department staff in their area.

The British Association for Immediate Care Schemes (BASICS) acts as a co-ordinating body between all prehospital care schemes. It has accumulated a wealth of knowledge and understanding of the difficulties in the provision of emergency care. It seeks to define and promote standards of organisation, equipment and training. Membership is open to individuals and to groups and therefore includes associate members of the rescue services as well as doctors. Since its foundation in 1977 it has increased its membership to 300 individuals and over 70 immediate care schemes incorporating 1500 doctors. A regional organisation ensures effective representation nationwide. BASICS supports a library and a publications department and includes several committees each offering expertise in specialised areas:
1. Research and data collection
2. Interservice and disaster planning
3. Radiocommunications and emergency equipment
4. Aeromedical evacuation.

THE REQUIREMENTS FOR PREHOSPITAL CARE

Organisation

Any scheme involving emergency treatment outside the hospital requires careful organisation — and in this we have much to learn from our colleagues in the armed forces. It was Baron Larrey (Napoleon's chief of surgery) (Fig 6.3) who proved in successive campaigns what good organisation of facilities for the evacuation and medical treatment of the injured could do for the morale of an army. He showed that mortality and morbidity could be reduced, not only by early definitive amputation (where his results compare favourably with those of today), but also by the use of what he called *ambulances volantes* (flying ambulances), horse-

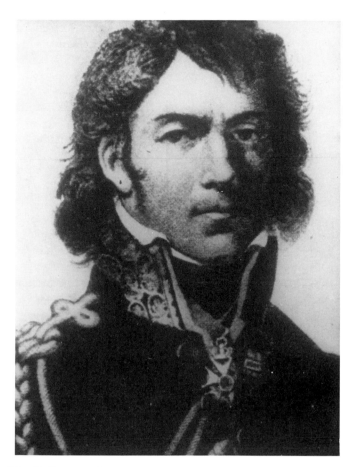

Fig. 6.3 Baron von Larrey.

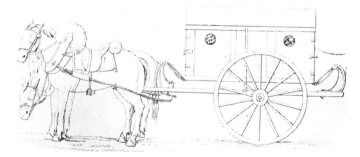

Fig. 6.4 Larrey's 'flying ambulance'.

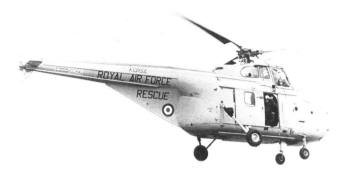

Fig. 6.5 Casevac using a helicopter.

neighbouring services are compatible and equipment is interchangeable. The three rescue services (police, fire and ambulance) should be represented on a 'joint rescue service planning committee', which should decide on such matters as how many teams are required in the area, what their function should be, what transport should be used, where they should be based, who should staff them and what equipment and communications should be carried.

It was in the United Kingdom that the first comprehensive civilian accident service was established. In 1888 Sir Robert Jones was appointed Consultant Surgeon to the Manchester Ship Canal, a major project linking the port of Liverpool with the city of Manchester. The canal employed 20 000 workers on its 35-mile stretch. It took many years to build and there were many serious accidents; 3000 recorded in one 5-year period. Sir Robert Jones divided the canal into three operational sectors for the provision of emergency care (Fig. 6.6). Each section had a chain of first-aid

drawn vehicles which followed close behind the front-line to remove the injured (Fig 6.4).

Successive wars have refined the development of forward primary care (e.g. the field surgical teams of World War II) and a modern airborne unit is now self-contained as far as urgent resuscitation is concerned. The addition of massive air support has, under certain circumstances (e.g. the Vietnam war) allowed the primary care to be carried out further back in a field hospital to which helicopters are able to take patients with the most severe injuries within minutes of wounding (Fig 6.5).

In civilian life the organisation for emergency care outside the hospital should be area based so that radio frequencies between

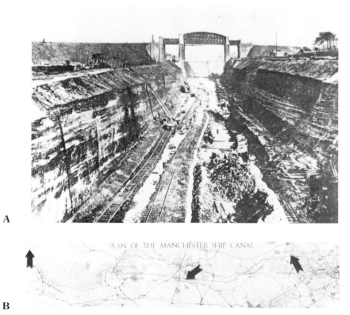

Fig. 6.6 A Photograph of the Manchester Ship Canal under construction. **B** Map of the Manchester Ship Canal. The sites of the three hospitals serving injured workers are arrowed.

stations and its own hospital. The hospitals were linked by a railway which ran the length of the canal and was used to convey the injured to the hospitals. They were also linked by wireless telegraphy to Sir Robert's hospital in Liverpool in order that he could be summoned whenever needed.

Equipment (Table 6.2)

Equipment for prehospital care should be simple, reliable, resilient, self-contained and portable. It should be waterproof. It needs to be clearly labelled, easily identifiable and accessible. In many circumstances as much thought should be given to the container for the equipment as its contents.

Table 6.2 Equipment for prehospital emergency care

Module 1: AIRWAY AND VENTILATION MANAGEMENT
Resuscitation bag and mask (adult and child)
Laryngoscope and batteries (and spares)
Endotracheal tubes and connectors
Tube introducer and Magill forceps
Syringes and artery forceps
WOW bandage — 1.25 cm and tapes
Oropharyngeal airways
Oxygen cylinder, reducing valve and flowmeter
Oxygen tubing and masks
Suction apparatus and catheters
Chest drains, one way flutter valve, scalpel and sutures
Cricothyrotomy device or large-bore cannulae
Stethoscope

Module 2: FLUID REPLACEMENT
Intravenous infusion-giving sets
Assorted intravenous cannulae
Syringes, needles, mediswabs, cross match bottles
Bandages, tapes, film dressings
Venous tourniquet, elbow immobiliser splint
Intravenous fluids: 0.9% saline
     5% dextrose
     Hartmann's solution
     Plasma protein fraction
     Polygelatine plasma expanders
     Dextran 70 in saline plasma expander
Emergency drugs pack (prefilled syringes preferred)
Sphygmomanometer

Module 3: DRESSING AND SPLINTS
Bandages and assorted dressings
Assorted burns dressings
Scissors
Surgical instruments
Cervical splint
Traction splint
Inflatable/vacuum/box splints
Fracture straps

E.C.G. MONITOR/DEFIBRILLATOR AND ACCESSORIES

MISCELLANEOUS ITEMS
Warm packs
Foil blankets
Heavy duty scissors
Rescue tools
Protective clothing
Fire extinguisher
Green beacon
Lighting equipment

Patient report forms

Personal protection will include comfortable, easy-to-wear working clothing (e.g. pull-on overalls), a set of waterproofs (e.g. storm jacket or cagoule with overtrousers), head protection, kneepads for scrambling work, good footwear, and cold-weather gear (e.g. gloves and mufflers). A good light source e.g. headlamp or heavy duty handlamp is essential. The clothing should identify the wearer — for example, by a tabard or label utilising 'Scotchlite' or other reflective material. Emergency clothing is not cheap and should be selected with care. The same can be said for *vehicle protection* and identification. Home Office regulations allow the use of a rotating flashing green beacon by doctors providing emergency care; in some areas this device has been distinctly successful.

Resuscitation equipment is available in preassembled emergency cases, produced by the major manufacturers. Though these are excellent in concept, they should be tailored to individual needs — often the most needed item is overlooked. Spare plastic bags are useful for collecting unused equipment at the incident scene. Standardisation of airways and transfusion fittings is obligatory. Oxygen fittings, masks and suction attachments should be interchangeable with the fittings in the ambulances and A & E department.

Little attention has been paid in the past to the design and manufacture of *stretchers* for everyday use. The carrying sheet with poles is the easiest means of transporting multiple casualties (Fig 6.7). The material should be washable, non-shrinkable and antistatic. It should have slots for poles and handholds at suitable intervals along each side so that it can be used when the patient has to be moved in confined spaces, such as down a narrow staircase. Tensionable spreaders which do not slip on the poles should be available to convert a carrying sheet into a semirigid structure on which a patient can be carried comfortably and with ease and safety. The patient should be moved on this stretcher during the various transfers within the hospital.

Communications

No emergency aid scheme can function without effective communications. Usually a radiotelephone will be needed. For this there will be a base station (comparable to a telephone exchange) and a number of mobiles (Fig. 6.8). The mobiles may be fitted in vehicles or be carried personally by the user as a portable handset. The base station will always have a transmitter and a receiver. The mobiles may be receiver only (signal or voice 'pagers') or receive/transmit units. The 'duplex' radio system allows communication between base and mobiles but not, normally, between mobiles; mobile users have to be 'controlled' from base and await their turn for radio airspace. Often they can be called up by selective signalling. Under certain circumstances (laid down in DHSS circular no HSC (15) 186, 1975) communication is permitted between base, mobiles and other radio systems. It is an advantage when the ambulance and emergency team networks can switch on to the common *Emergency Reserve Channel*. This should be used only on receipt of specific instructions from the ambulance control. It is a national frequency which can link neighbouring ambulance services.

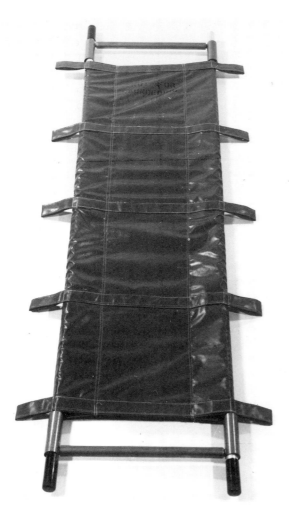

Fig. 6.7 Carrying sheet and poles.

It is vital that staff using radios be familiar with their controls and the radiocommunications procedure and phonetic alphabets which have to be used (Table 6.3). The basic difference between an ordinary telephone and a radiotelephone is that, in the latter, simultaneous listening and speaking facilities are not normally employed and more than two parties are using the same line. The requisites for clear communication are, therefore:

1. Identification of speaker by call-sign
2. Brevity of message
3. Occasional use of coded message for privacy
4. Identification of end of message expecting reply by 'OVER'
5. Identification of end of message not expecting reply by 'OUT'.

The same communications system will, of course, be employed in the event of a major disaster, in which case all personnel likely to be involved (including administrators and nurses) should be familiar with its operation.

Table 6.3 Radiotelephone procedure

Standard phrases

Go ahead	pass your message
Stand by	wait until called
Wait	you are interrupting another call
Roger	message received and understood
Wilco	will comply with instructions
Repeat (from)	repeat (from specified part of) message
ETA	estimated time of arrival
Priority	urgent message

Specimen message

Alpha base	base station call sign
Medic	mobile call sign

Alpha base from Medic, do you receive, over
Medic from Alpha base, receiving, over

Signal strength

1 Barely audible	4 Good but not full strength
2 Faint	5 Loud and clear
3 Weak but discernible	

Phonetic alphabet

A	Alpha	F	Foxtrot	K	Kilo	P	Papa	U	Uniform
B	Bravo	G	Golf	L	Lima	Q	Quebec	V	Victor
C	Charlie	H	Hotel	M	Mike	R	Romeo	W	Whisky
D	Delta	I	India	N	November	S	Sierra	X	X-ray
E	Echo	J	Juliet	O	Oscar	T	Tango	Y	Yankee
								Z	Zulu

Numbers

Numbers causing difficultly should be pronounced clearly as follows:

5 fife	7 sev-en	9 niner	0 zero

Say 'fife-niner' rather than 'fiftynine'

(From Snook R 1974 Medical aid at accidents Update, London. Reproduced by courtesy of the author and publishers)

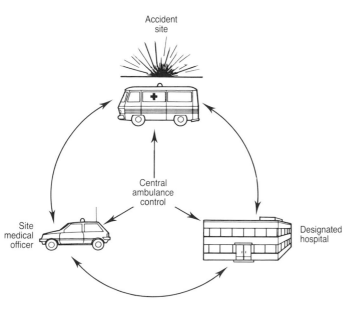

Fig. 6.8 Radiotelephone communications network between ambulance control (base station), accident site, hospital and 'site medical officer' (mobiles).

FURTHER READING

Rescue emergency care Easton K (ed) 1977 Heinemann Medical, London

Sudden cardiac death in the community Eisenberg M S, Bergner L, Hallstrom A P 1984 Praeger, New York

Extended training in ambulance aid 1987 National Health Service Training Authority, Bristol

Monographs on immediate care The British Association for Immediate Care. BASICS, 31C Lower Brook Street, Ipswich, Suffolk IP33 IAQ

Medical aid at accidents Snook R 1974 Update Publications, London

Disaster management

DEFINITION AND CLASSIFICATION

Disaster is a word with several meanings in ordinary parlance. In relation to the organisational aspect of A & E medicine it means an event which creates large numbers of casualties simultaneously. This sudden unexpected load requires special mobilisation procedures to obtain sufficient staff to deal with the extraordinary load of patients. There was a time when it was common to specify a number of casualties, and to say that any event with more casualties than a specified number was a disaster. The difficulty in practice with this approach is that often action must be taken without knowing exactly what the numbers are. From an academic point of view it may be helpful to classify disasters by number. One simple system is to count disasters with 10–99 casualties as small, 100–999 moderate and 1000 and above as large. In comparing a number of different disasters, this may be useful. However, it does not help in the early stages of responding to disasters.

Disasters may be classified in several other ways as well as size. For example, they may be classified by cause. A distinction is usually made between natural and artificial disasters. Examples of natural disaster are earthquakes, typhoons and floods. Examples of artificial disasters are air or road crashes, industrial accidents, fires and rioting or explosions during civil disorder.

Disaster management is very different where the disaster, though creating many casualties, still leaves the emergency services and facilities intact. Under these circumstances, very many patients can be dealt with comparatively quickly. If, however, roads, communications, hospitals and ambulance stations are involved in the destruction (as in an earthquake) then the ability to respond and the method of proceeding has to be quite different. The former type of disaster is sometimes called a simple disaster and the latter a compound disaster.

A somewhat similar yet different distinction may be drawn on the basis of the balance between the casualty load and the medical facilities. In the early stage the important facility is the ability to transport casualties. At a later stage it is the facility to treat patients in hospital, and here the most usual critical factor is the number of casualties upon whom a hospital could reasonably be expected to operate on each day for which the disaster lasts. This is a very fundamental distinction for it affects the way in which casualties should be sorted (triage) and methods of treatment. It has even been suggested that where the load is smaller than the capacity, the term 'disaster' should not be used at all. However, these smaller and simpler events still require good management arrangements, and most hospitals within 5 or 10 years will face at least one or more such events. It would seem that books and conferences deal with both large and small events and this, indeed, has been the practice of the World Association for Emergency and Disaster Medicine. The two types of disaster do, however, need to be clearly distinguished and this is probably best done by calling the smaller (when the load is less than the capacity) a compensated disaster and the larger (when load exceeds capacity) an uncompensated disaster (Figs 7.1 and 7.2).

Four distinctions have been made, depending on the number of casualties, the cause, the condition of the environment and the balance between load and capacity. There is considerable overlap between these different categories. Artificially caused disasters tend to have small to moderate numbers, to be simple and to be compensated. Natural disasters tend to be large, compound and uncompensated.

It is sometimes also useful to distinguish between rural and urban disasters. Urban incidents are more common and often occur very close to hospitals. Ease of evacuation is another useful distinguishing feature. A disaster in an underground railway may be urban, yet evacuation may be very difficult.

ORGANISATION AT HOSPITAL LEVEL

The basic organisational problem in a hospital is to mobilise the

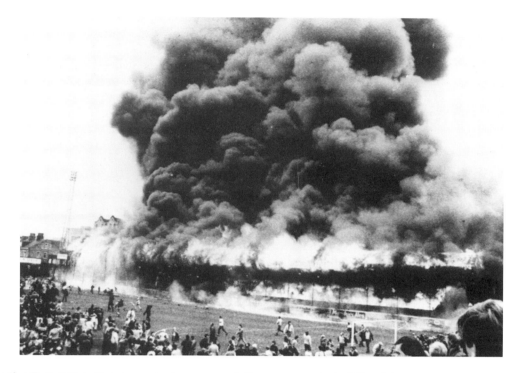

Fig. 7.1 Fire at Bradford Football Club. Typical example of a compensated disaster, common in the UK and throughout Europe.

right number and the right kinds of staff for the particular disaster which has occurred. It is important to be able to call in sufficient workers, but also important not to call in far too many. Some disasters will produce many patients with burns, another many with fractures and another a large number of people in emotional shock. Not only is there endless variety of numbers, but the

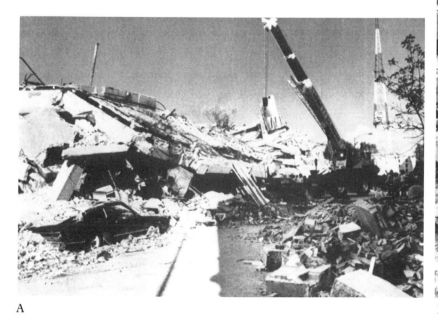

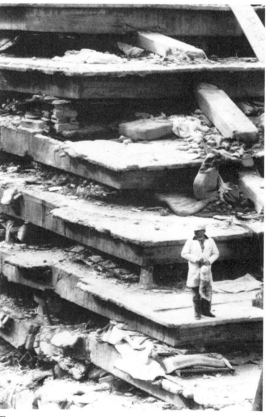

A   B

Fig. 7.2 A Earthquake in New Mexico City. Compound uncompensated natural disaster. **B** All that remained of the General Hospital in Mexico City after the earthquake.

proportion requiring hospital admission differs. Therefore, it is not possible to detail in advance the number of doctors or surgeons of any particular speciality, nor the number of beds, required. The nature of the staffing and bed requirements will gradually become evident as the size and the nature of the disaster become known. What is necessary is a command structure of people with sufficient experience, who will be able to call up staff and resources as required.

Command structure

This is made up of a senior doctor and nurse for the A & E department, and a senior doctor, nurse and administrator working with a senior surgeon for control of events in the hospital as a whole.

Accident and emergency department

In the evolution of a disaster there is usually some time lag between the event and the arrival of ambulances at hospital. The speed with which patients arrive will depend on how near the disaster is, how easily evacuation of casualties can be performed and how much transport is available. On occasion the first patients may arrive in taxis or private cars before any warning has been received. Similarly, it takes time to resuscitate, diagnose and document patients in the A & E department, and there is, therefore, some time before operating theatres and ward beds are needed. There is usually a short but valuable period between the receipt of news that a disaster has occurred and the arrival of the first patients. The first priority at this time is to make arrangements in the A & E department. A doctor and a nurse of suitable experience and authority must be summoned to take charge. The larger the disaster, the more valuable it will be to have the senior consultant and sister of the department in charge. Their function is not to treat individual patients but to organise the whole work of the department.

Often in a disaster there is a spontaneous response and doctors, nurses and lay volunteers turn up wanting to help. The doctor and nurse in charge have to form a picture of what is happening, what numbers of patients are arriving with what types of injury. They should direct patients to the most suitable areas of the department and delegate doctors and nurses to manage specific patients. They have tactfully to turn away unneeded helpers and, where help is inadequate, summon more staff. There is considerable overlap between the functions of the doctor and the nurses in charge. Initially, at least, the nurse is more likely to concentrate on sorting out patients so that they can be examined in the most suitable area of the department. This may seem to be a job for a doctor but A & E sisters do this every day with patients entering the department and are very skilled at it. The severely injured will go to the resuscitation room and the next worst in cubicles adjacent to this. Those with minor injuries should be furthest from this region. There may be patients obviously shocked and weeping and apparently uninjured. They can be directed to a single large room which may be outside the department. Medical notes should be recorded for all patients, including the apparently uninjured, both to assist immediate enquiries and to give a factual basis for later legal claims.

In a disaster the desire for privacy disappears. People are reassured by being able to talk to others in a similar condition. So four to six patients with minor complains can be dealt with in cubicles reserved for one patient in more normal times, and even two seriously ill patients can be seen in a cubicle which would be reserved for one in normal working.

The hospital as a whole

There are four functions to be fulfilled:

1. The mobilisation and co-ordination of doctors and supervision of medical policy. If there is a doctor-administrator in the hospital, he will best manage this aspect. Otherwise, it should be undertaken by the chairman or the secretary of the medical staff. He will gather information from the A & E department, the police and the medical administrators of the area. This will give him an idea of the number of patients likely to need admission. He must take steps to make the necessary beds available. The doctor in charge of the A & E department will be concerned mainly about the medical staff required in the A & E department. The medical administrator will consider the medical needs for the theatres and wards. He will direct and co-ordinate the whole hospital response, and keep in touch with medical authorities outside the hospital.

2. The oversight of nursing staff. The chief responsibilities of the principal nursing officer (PNO) are in mobilising as many nurses as possible and directing them to where they will be of most use. As far as possible, senior nurses should work in areas where they are used to the routines and more junior nurses can be transferred to make up numbers. A senior nurse in an area she does not know is inhibited by the small details with which she is unfamiliar and junior nurses of that department are embarrassed in having to direct her.

The responsibility for collecting information about the bed state of each ward and the details of who can and who cannot be discharged or transferred may be given to the PNO (Figs 7.3 and 7.4). The medical administrator will then make specific decisions about discharges and transfers.

3. Providing technical support. This will be carried out by the hospital administrator or his deputy. His responsibility is to direct all the other resources of the hospital. He will see that there are sufficient porters, clerical staff, maintenance and security staff and, if necessary, staff for the pharmacy. He may have to get the central sterile supply department to produce a special issue. In a disaster the demands on the hospital can never be fully foreseen. An administrator of sufficient seniority with intimate knowledge of the day-to-day running of the hospital is the person who can best help to solve the unusual problems which arise.

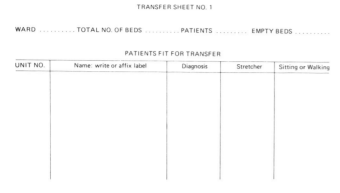

Fig. 7.3 Form for collecting information about patients fit for discharge or transfer. Each ward completes a form and returns it to the principal nursing officer.

TRANSFER SHEET NO. 2

WARD . . . .

PATIENTS FIT FOR TRANSFER ONLY IN EXTREME CIRCUMSTANCES

UNIT NO.	Name: write or affix label	Diagnosis	Stretcher	Sitting or Walking

Fig. 7.4 Form for collecting information about patients who may be transferred if situation becomes very critical.

4. The clinical supervision of patient care.   This function will be carried out by a senior surgeon. His main responsibilities are in deciding operative priorities, for allocating operating teams to theatres and patients to these teams.

The mechanism of the call-up (Figs 7.5, 7.6 and 7.7)

Some system must be devised for contacting the five or six officers in the command structure very rapidly after news of a disaster. This may be by paging machines, in which case they must have a radius which will encompass the homes of those involved. A special telephone line with an ex-directory number may be kept for these officers to report that they have received their call. The known details of the disaster can then be given to them. This part of the disaster drill should be rehearsed frequently.

The next most urgent call-up is for staff to work in the A & E department. It is useful to have a pro forma listing the people likely to be wanted. The sister or doctor in charge can then tick off those required and leave a clerk or volunteer to call them. The clerical and radiological staff may be asked to telephone for any extra staff they need. If hospital phones are blocked, the patients' coin box phones can be used.

Finally, doctors, nurses and paramedical staff may be needed for the wards, theatres and the general running of the whole hospital.

It will be the responsibility of the command team officers to supervise the call-up of these grades of staff.

TRIAGE OR SORTING

There is a widespread understanding that as patients arrive at hospital they should be seen near the entrance by a doctor called the triage officer. He will perform triage. This is understood as a categorisation according to the likely prognosis. Different authorities give somewhat different categories, but the following is a fairly widely accepted list.

Category 1. Patients in an extremely critical condition.
Category 2. Patients with major injuries, not too serious and with good prognosis.
Category 3. Patients with minor injuries, not needing inpatient treatment in hospital.
Category 4. Dead.

The triage officer will allocate one of these categories to each patient on arrival and indicate the category with a label. On the basis of this label, the patient will be taken to an appropriate area in the department. This will also indicate the priority for examination and later for operating. The correct order is said to be 2,1,3. This method is probably correct in large compound uncompensated disasters. In the UK and the rest of Europe such disasters are extremely uncommon.

In the simple compensated disaster, which is commonly encountered in the UK, there are objections to this method of proceeding. Examinations have to be in a corridor, rapidly and without complete removal of clothing. The patient is then going to be taken to a cubicle or examination area where another doctor will do a more complete examination. It is likely that radiological examination will be required. If separation of the patients into strict categories is felt to be helpful, this is better done at the end of this process rather than before.

The difficulty in having a doctor called triage officer is that it is then thought that it is he who is responsible for triage, and other doctors are not concerned with this aspect. It should be remembered that triage is just the French word for sorting. A disaster is a very confused situation and it is of prime importance to sort and re-sort patients so that eventually order is brought out of chaos.

It is necessary to do a triage or sorting as patients enter the A & E department. The object of this sorting is to place the patient at the most suitable position within the department. Patients with life threatening injuries go to the resuscitation room. Those with major, but not life-threatening, injuries go into nearby cubicles. Three or four patients with more minor injuries can go to a cubicle usually used for one patient. A weeping room is a suitable area for emotionally shocked but uninjured patients. Sorting of this type is done every day by the nursing staff, and they will do it very efficiently in a disaster.

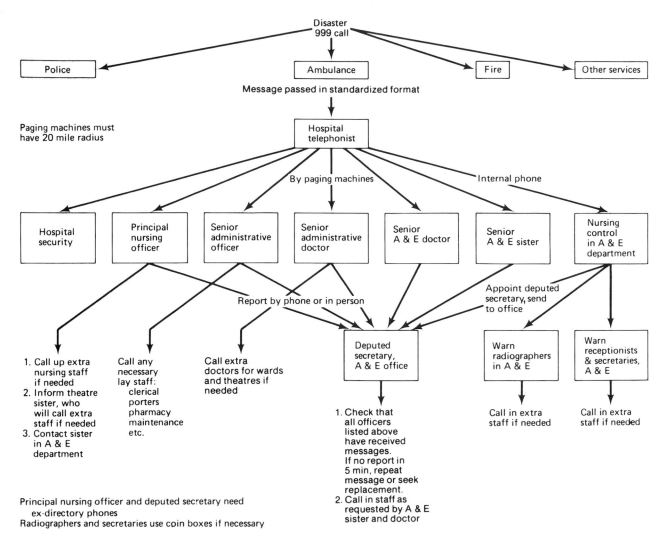

Fig. 7.5 Diagrammatic representation of mobilisation of staff. This scheme is suitable for a large hospital with a major A & E department.

Sister, Accident & Emergency Department

Rehearsal . . . .

For real disaster . . . .

Disaster information received at . . . . hours by . . . .

Source   Ambulance Control . . . .

                Other . . . .

Site of disaster . . . .

Type of disaster . . . .

No. of ambulance sent out . . . .

Possible no. of casualties . . . .

Deputed secretary, Accident & Emergency Department

Notice received at . . . .

By . . . .

Contacted
A & E sister . . . . hours

A & E senior doctor . . . . hours

Medical administrative
officer . . . . hours

Senior administrative
officer . . . . hours

Principal nursing
officer . . . . hours

Fig. 7.6 Forms for A & E sister receiving information from a disaster, and for deputed secretary recording acknowledgement of call-up messages by members of the control team.

CALL-UP INSTRUCTIONS FROM SISTER
TO THE DEPUTED SECRETARY

Please call such staff as are indicated

☐ A & E sisters
☐ A & E registrar
☐ A & E senior house officer
☐ A & E housemen
☐ Fracture clinic sister
☐ Fracture clinic consultant
☐ Fracture clinic registrar
☐ Fracture clinic senior house officer
☐ Fracture clinic housemen
☐ Other available doctors on site
☐ Laboratory – inform technician of disaster
and possible demand for blood

Fig. 7.7 Form for A & E sister or doctor to indicate to deputed secretary the staff members to be called in for A & E department.

Once patients are in cubicles, the examining doctors sort them into those needing admission and those who may go home. It is helpful if they classify admission cases into 'critical' 'serious' and 'not serious'. This is a great help in answering telephone enquiries.

There is often a problem when a queue forms near the radiology department. A senior doctor should go and scrutinise the requests. He may send some patients to theatre without radiology. For some of the less serious cases, he may postpone taking radiographs until the following morning. The remainder he will place on a list with the most urgent first and least urgent last.

Once there is a group of patients ready for admission the senior surgeon should arrange the operating lists and decide which patient is to go to which theatre and surgeon and in which order. If he finds it helpful to categorise patients into strict grades he should do so. Often patients are ranked in descending priority without saying exactly which patient is in which grade.

Orthodox teaching states that those cases with good prognosis should be taken first. In the common type of simple, compensated disaster this is unnecessary. Unless bad cases are taken early they will die unnecessarily. However, in compound uncompensated disasters, it becomes essential to reverse normal working procedures and to do short simple operations with good prognosis first.

INFORMATION

The police should set up a central office and the public should be informed by radio and television to contact this centre. The more quickly the hospital can transmit its patient lists showing who is being admitted and who treated and discharged the more quickly will the police centre begin to function (Fig. 7.8).

In spite of this, many phone calls will be made to the hospitals, so three or four people should be issued with photocopies of the list of patients who have been brought to the hospital and placed at phones to answer these enquiries. The public may also come direct to the hospital with their enquiries. Arrangements must be made for answering their questions. The condition of all inpatients should be gathered every six hours over the first day or two, and this will provide sufficient information for most enquiries.

The press and broadcasting reporters may want to report details from hospital. The care of patients must always have priority over news and much of the reporting can be organised through either the police information centre or the offices of the district health authority. However, public interest is often intense and if it is possible to co-operate with reporters rather than fighting them, the results may be beneficial to the hospital and to society at large.

Doctors have a special responsibility in protecting any patients

PATIENTS RECEIVED FROM DISASTER

Date _____

A & E No.	Unit No.	Name	Address	Nature of injury	Condition Critical: C Fair: F Satisfactory: S	Disposal Home: H Admitted: write ward number	Age	6 am	6 pm	6 am	6 pm

Fig. 7.8 Form for collecting information about all patients arriving from a disaster, their injuries, their disposal and the seriousness of those patients who are admitted.

or relatives who do not wish to be interviewed. However, if they can help to find a few people who do not object to being interviewed, this will be much appreciated. Often a period of very intense work at the start of a disaster is followed by a lull. A press conference may be held at this time.

Documentation

While it may be necessary during a disaster to simplify some documentation routines in the A & E department, it is essential that the central features of the ordinary documentation procedures are maintained. It is of supreme importance the laboratory specimens, reports on radiographs and patient identification in ward and theatre are free from doubt or confusion. People's lives depend on avoiding errors in this field.

THE DISASTER SITE

Inside a hospital the medical response to the disaster may be erroneously considered the whole response. At the disaster site it is obvious that several different emergency services are involved.

Police

In a disaster of any size the police will have a large control vehicle at the site. The senior police officer at the site is accepted by all members of all emergency services as being the man whose authority is final. The police will control the site to prevent members of the public getting injured or hampering rescue attempts and to direct the evacuation of injured persons.

Fire service

A fire may break out at a disaster site. The fire services are experts in helping in the evacuation of the injured by cutting away obstacles in which they are entrapped, in rescue from heights and can also be helpful by providing lighting.

Ambulance service

Ambulancemen will arrive at the same time as the police and firemen. In the beginning they will be the only people with any medical training at the site. A special ambulance control vehicle may bring stretchers and first aid supplies and act as a communication centre for ambulances, hospitals and the district health authority.

The public

It may be wrong to count the public as a service. To some extent the public are the enemy of the services, rushing in with ghoulish interest and blocking the roads and, at the site, giving way to frenzied panic. It is the task of the uniformed services to bring order into the chaotic situation which may arise. On the other hand among the public will be found quick-witted, courageous and indefatigable helpers who may already have saved lives before the services arrived. It is part of the duty of the services to decide how much the public is to be repelled and excluded, how much to be welcomed and utilised.

Triage at the site

If sorting large numbers of patients at hospital seems a daunting task, this is even more true at the disaster site. Orthodox theory states that doctors, ambulancemen or paramedics should search the site for casualties, should categorise them and should tie an appropriate label indicating their category. It should be remembered that the object of the exercise is to save the maximum number of lives. Patients injured in a disaster deteriorate like those injured in ordinary accidents. Dr Adams Cowley of the Maryland Institute for Emergency Medical Services Systems has stressed the great importance of transporting severely injured patients to a hospital capable of treating them within an hour of injury — 'the golden hour'. There is no physiological difference between patients injured in single accidents and those injured in disasters. Although in a disaster there may be difficulties, which at times are insuperable, the correct aim should still be to transport all except the trapped or unreachable to hospital within an hour. Triage procedures on the site, if carried through to any elaborate extent, will increase the injury–treatment interval and with it the mortality.

Some sorting, of course, must be done. However, there is much to be said for collecting areas for different groups of patient, rather than tying labels. One drawback of labelling is that it tends to be done early on in conditions of very great difficulty where thorough examination is impossible. Once patients are labelled, inordinate importance is attached to the label and recategorising is difficult. If floor space is used instead of labelling, patients can be arranged in a sliding scale of urgency without attributing any prearranged categories. It is then easier on re-examination to move a casualty up or down the line a few places. This also allows for categories which cannot be anticipated. For example, taxis or buses may be available to transport some casualties. It is easy to designate separate floor spaces for patients suitable for such transport. It may be helpful also to sort out patients by the hospital of destination.

As with triage in hospital, orthodox teaching suggests that cases with good prognosis must be transported first, the life threatening cases second and the minor cases last. In real life this is often impossible to carry through. Those with minor injuries are usually available for transport first. They do not require ambulances. The sooner they are cleared from the site the easier the remaining task becomes. In urban disasters which are simple and compensated it is probably best to look on the hospitals as the correct site for definitive triage and to attempt to transport casualties immediately they become available. Some people will be trapped and extrication will take time. Ambulances will have made one or two quick runs to hospital and back before these patients are available for transport. In rural areas the ambulance turn around time may be measured in hours rather than minutes. In this case, it may be necessary to set up a holding area, and to start resuscitative proceedings for waiting patients. It is in such situations that careful triage is most important. However, even then there are distinct advantages in clearing the site of minor casualties at the earliest possible moment. Sometimes they may be sent to hospitals not involved with the care of major casualties.

The role of doctors at the site

Site medical officer

In small to moderate urban disasters which are simple and compensated, the main aim at the site is to transport casualties as they become available. This can often be done expertly by a senior ambulance officer and it may not be necessary to have a doctor at the site. In large uncompensated disasters, especially if sited at some distances from hospitals, it becomes essential to have a doctor in overall charge of medical services at the site. Ambulance personnel will work under his guidance, as will all doctors who arrive at the disaster offering their services. He will decide what kind of triage will be employed, whether a holding area is necessary or not. He should aim to guide and direct, building up a picture of the overall situation. He will be the channel of communication with medical authorities, with hospitals and with the senior officers of other services at the site. He should try to avoid getting drawn into resuscitating patients as it is essential that he exercise control and this is virtually incompatible with individual patient care.

One of the problems of disaster management is making provision for appointing such a man and getting him mobilised quickly and efficiently. Only in places where doctors are involved on a day to day basis with the work of the ambulance service is there likely to be a simple and obvious choice. In rural disasters, helicopters may be of great help in evacuation, and a doctor from the Royal Air Force is an ideal choice for site medical officer. He is specifically trained for such work.

Site medical team

There are occasions when it is very valuable to have the help of a small team for the treatment of patients on or close to the site. This is less likely in urban disasters, especially if there is no obstruction to rapid evacuation of patients. In disasters which occur is isolated areas far from large hospitals, patients may be kept waiting for considerable periods before transport can be arranged. The best teams for going to such a site are those who do the same work on a daily basis (see Ch. 5). They may be either hospital based or based in general practice. The clothing and equipment necessary is the same as that used on everyday rescue work. If the hospital which sends out such a team daily happens to be the main receiving unit, it should look for assistance from another unit in a neighbouring city.

Helicopters

These can be of great value for disasters in outlying areas, especially where there is no easy road access. The time taken to transport a patient to hospital and return to the site is likely to be dramatically shorter than by ambulance. The armed services are very co-operative in such situations and may be able to supply a doctor and some paramedics. Hospitals likely to receive disaster patients should know how to summon such help. Helicopter pads need to be designated and marked out in advance.

DISASTER MANAGEMENT AT DISTRICT, AREA, REGIONAL AND NATIONAL LEVELS

While doctors who work in hospitals or at the site are likely to be directly involved with patient care, the bodies responsible for medical services as a whole in cities, districts, regions and in any country at national level will have organisational responsibility towards disaster preparedness and management. This will include both ensuring that contingency plans exist for different types of disaster and also executive action during such an event. It is obvious that the organisation for both these aspects will be dependent on the nature of medical services organisation in the country. These are bound to be different in countries which use largely private medicine from those in countries with state medical services. Even inside state medical systems there may be considerably different structures. Thus, in the United Kingdom, in England and Wales services are organised at regional and then district level, whereas in Scotland and Northern Ireland there are area boards between region and district. In the smallest disasters, some organisation at district level is all that will be necessary. As the size increases one may expect involvement at area, regional, inter-regional and national level. The very worst disasters will also require international help. At every level arrangements are necessary so that a number of officers with responsibilities in different fields can be contacted. It is important that at each level these officers are well acquainted with the procedures for communicating upwards to an authority at a higher level. Such action will rarely be necessary, but when it is necessary it will need to be carried through with great speed. It is also important that, at each level, there are good channels of communication between the medical services and the other emergency services.

In Great Britain it is very rare for disasters to affect more than a single region. Disaster management is looked on as an important responsibility of local government at the regional level and in each region there is an emergency planning officer whose responsibility it is to see that all regional services have disaster plans and that these plans are exercised and revised at the regional level.

At a national level in the United Kingdom, there is a Civil Defence Advisor at the Home Office who has a responsibility to monitor and co-ordinate the work of emergency planning officers. The Cabinet also has an Emergency Committee which can be called to respond to various types of emergency situations (for example, the seige of a foreign embassy). Disasters are one type of emergency to which the Cabinet's Emergency Committee might respond. It has the authority to take all necessary measures once a disaster is happening. It does not, however, anticipate disasters, nor is it involved in monitoring preparedness in the country as a whole, or ensuring that co-operative machinery exists to co-ordinate the work of such emergency services as the medical, ambulance, police, fire and armed services, all of which are responsible to different ministries. Routine co-ordinating responsibilities of this nature are left in the hands of the Civil Defence Advisor to the Home Office.

EXERCISES

Committees responsible for disaster management draw up plans. It is likely that those who write the plans will be involved in discharging them should occasion arise. However, there will be many other people involved in responding to a disaster who are not on the disaster committee yet who will have duties to perform. It is important that they are aware of the plan and of their role in it. In hospital this will partly be achieved by having copies of the disaster plan distributed to all the offices where those involved work. It is helpful if the plan has a distinctive eye catching cover and its position should be near the phone in a special small shelf or transparent container. It is essential that, from time to time when work is slack, the plan will be taken from the container and read. New medical and nursing staff should read through the plan in their first day or two in the department.

This alone is unlikely to be a reliable method of dissemination. The other method which is frequently used is to have exercises. The best known and most common type of test is to simulate a disaster with, for example, a crashed plane, dummy corpses and live casualties acted by volunteers. The most usual place for such exercises is at airports, where the airport licence may depend, among other things, on carrying through such exercises annually. There is no doubt that such exercises may demonstrate weaknesses in a plan. Especially the communication network may fail, and good disaster management is highly dependant on good communications systems.

There are, however, considerable drawbacks to this form of exercise, it is a very expensive activity requiring weeks and months of preparation by a small staff and repeated attendance at committee meetings by officers whose time is very valuable. The emergency services must so arrange the exercise that they can still cope with current responsibilities. Organising this between a number of

different services usually results in the expected date and time being very widely known. In this respect it is very different from a real life disaster. During the exercise participants often enter into the proceedings like teams competing for a first aid prize. The conditions are very different from real life, and it is far from certain that participants would behave in the same way in the heat and emotional pressure of real life.

As long as international airports insist on this type of exercise, it is likely that many hospitals with disaster responsibilities will be able to get involved in some way and there is little doubt that they will derive some benefit from so doing.

A second form of exercise is what is called a table top exercise. Here a hypothetical disaster is presented to a group of people with disaster responsibilities, and they are asked to explain exactly what response they should make. This may be done at many different levels and may involve either players with in a single emergency service, or more usually a number of officers from different services. This is an exercise for those holding responsible positions rather than workers from the rank and file and in real disasters the major mistakes are usually made by bosses rather than workers. As long as those in authority make wise decisions, it is unlikely that others will seriously undermine their efforts.

A simpler level of exercise can be made by breaking up a disaster management plan into component parts and exercising each part separately. The most obvious exercise of this type is the initial call up of the disaster management team in the hospital. This should probably be exercised on a monthly basis. Other parts of the plan — like gathering classified bed states and planning the clear-out of beds to accommodate disaster patients, or the setting up of a disaster ward — can be carried out once or twice a year.

Finally, it has been found possible to have the provisions of a disaster plan programmed into a computer. Members of staff can then be faced with questions relating to various situations and key in the action which they would take. The computer responds, informing whether this was or was not appropriate. Reaction with the computer has proved a more stimulating way of involving staff than asking them to read a printed plan.

None of these forms of exercise is without disadvantages, and it is probably best to use all of them. It takes time to develop skills in preparing and organising good exercises and, at the end of exercises, assessment sessions should be organised so that on the next occasion for a test the same mistakes need not be made.

FURTHER READING

The Journal of the World Association for Emergency and Disaster Medicine

Disasters. Medical organisation De Boer, Baillie T W 1980 Pergamon Press, Oxford

Types and events of disasters. Organisation in various disaster situations Frey R, Safar P 1980 Springer-Verlag, Berlin

Disaster medicine MacMahon A G, Iooste M 1980 A A Balkema, Cape Town

A handbook for the caring professions Raphael B 1986 Hutchinson, London

Disaster planning Richardson J W 1975 John Wright, Bristol

Disasters, hospital planning Savage P E A 1979 Pergamon Press, Oxford

Disaster management Spirgi E A 1979 Hans Huber Publishers, Bern

Trauma management Wiener S L, Barrett J 1986 W B Saunders, Philadelphia

Accident and emergency burns: lessons from the Bradford disaster Wood C 1986 Royal Society of Medicine Services, London

Radiology and imaging

THE DEPARTMENT

Radiographic examination is requested in approximately 50% of all patients attending accident and emergency departments. The radiological facilities should therefore be as close as possible to the patient treatment areas.

Although the size of X-ray department required will depend on the number of patients, there should be one room large enough to accommodate the monitoring and life support equipment and extra personnel required for severely ill patients. All rooms should have oxygen and suction. A 'panic button' is essential to summon medical help from the A & E department, particularly when the radiographer is single handed. A regularly updated emergency drug box must be available. Accident trollies should be available to minimise patient handling. Movable table tops in the department are also of great assistance in this respect. Radiographic examination of the severely ill patient should be of the highest quality, and fixed apparatus with short exposure times and adequate power permit this. Portable examinations are of limited value and should be avoided where possible. Fixed apparatus in the resuscitation room will overcome the problem. Strict adherence to radiation protection measures and personnel monitoring are, however, required. This can give rise to difficulties, especially when the room is busy.

THE STAFF

Close liaison between the radiology and A & E departments is essential. Regular consultation at an individual level is necessary and joint meetings are most beneficial. Sadly, scant attention is often paid to radiological interpretation and diagnosis at undergraduate medical courses. These skills can be improved by giving basic instruction to junior A & E staff, who are usually the first and often the only doctors to see the patient. Radiologists should be available for consultation at all times and should provide reports on all examinations within 24 hours, if not sooner. The referring doctors should be promptly informed of any significant discrepancy between their and the radiologists' opinion. One method is to insert a code or word on such reports, so that they can be readily identified by the clerical or medical staff for separate filing and drawn to the attention of the doctor concerned. Radiologists also make mistakes, and this method of 'double checking' will minimise diagnostic errors.

As the time spent in the A & E department is closely related to the time taken in obtaining radiological examination, the elimination of unnecessary radiography will improve the turn-round times for all patients.

REQUESTING A RADIOLOGICAL EXAMINATION

A full history must be taken and physical examination carried out before any request is made. The pertinent facts should be available to the radiologist when reporting. Clinically unstable patients should not be sent for a radiological investigation unless adequately supervised. Examination should not be requested simply to placate the patients or relatives, or for purely medicolegal reasons. The decision to carry out an X-ray examination is made on clinical grounds alone. It is well worth asking: 'will the results of radiological investigation alter management?'. If not, then no request should be made. The referring doctor should also consider whether there is any risk to the patient by delaying the examination until the following day. This particularly applies to the drunk or uncooperative patient who is being admitted to hospital for overnight observation and whose behaviour may have improved sufficiently to allow more diagnostic studies the next day. Often symptoms and signs have ameliorated so that radiological examination is no longer necessary.

Having decided to proceed with radiological examination, indicate clearly which anatomical area is to be examined. This greatly reduces the radiographer's time and minimises repeats. Avoid unnecessary irradiation at all times. For example, do not request a study of the foot and ankle, when symptoms and signs are related to a toe. Similarly, supplementing an adequately penetrated chest film with rib views for possible rib fractures is unnecessary. When there is doubt concerning the particular view required, consult a radiologist or radiographer.

Women of child bearing age should be asked if they are, or may be, pregnant. If the answer is 'yes' and radiological examination is clinically indicated, the information should be clearly conveyed so that the appropriate protective measures may be undertaken.

HOW TO LOOK AT A RADIOGRAPH

First check that the name on the film corresponds with the patient. Then ensure that the area in question is clearly demonstrated. If not, consult with a radiographer: there may or may not be good reasons for an inadequate study. Look at the radiographs on a proper viewing box. Holding the film up to ceiling lights or windows is to be deprecated. Develop a system of looking at all features initially, including the soft tissues. 'Bright light' any dark areas, as unsuspected dangers often lurk in such places. Beware of obvious abnormalities, which tend to distract the observer from noticing less obvious lesions, which can be important in arriving at a more accurate diagnosis. When possible, obtain previous films. This can be extremely useful in determining whether the abnormality is recent, or whether it is improving, or otherwise.

DISASTERS

The simultaneous arrival of large numbers of injured patients, many of whom have severe trauma, can pose serious problems to the X-ray department. Disasters can cause dangerous delays and bottle-necks in the early vital stages. It is imperative that the radiology department is an integral part of every disaster plan. Senior radiographers and radiologists should be informed as soon as possible, in order that life threatening delays and confusion may be avoided. It may be necessary to restrict radiographic examination to the chest, spine and pelvis initially, and examine limb injuries later.

SPECIAL PROCEDURES

In the vast majority of cases plain film studies are all that are necessary for initial diagnosis and treatment. In certain circumstances immediate recourse to further radiological investigations is necessary to obtain an early diagnosis. This will help reduce mortality and morbidity. A delay in diagnosis of even a few hours may prolong the patient's illness by weeks or even months. It is important that the A & E doctor maintains a high index of suspicion for those conditions which require urgent investigation. After consultation with an X-ray department, special procedures may be undertaken without delay. The investigation employed will vary between hospitals, depending on the level of sophistication of available equipment, and radiological expertise.

Tomography

Conventional tomography is most useful in delineating injury to the vertebral column, when plain film studies are equivocal or unhelpful. It will usually demonstrate the area in question more clearly. This particularly applies to the craniocervical, cervical–dorsal junctions and upper thoracic vertebrae. The technique will also give excellent demonstration of facial fractures and should be employed when blow-out injuries are suspected (Fig. 8.1), even when no fracture is identifiable on conventional films. A similar rule applies to the elderly osteoporotic patient with suspected fractures of the femoral neck region.

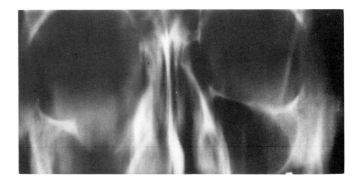

Fig. 8.1 AP tomograms of the facial bones following a blow to the right eye. There is depression of the medial two-thirds of the infraorbital margin and protrusion of the orbital contents into the antrum.

Intravenous urography

High-dose urography is most helpful in evaluating patients with suspected renal trauma (Fig. 8.2). Nephrotomography will delineate the renal outlines, and may demonstrate parenchymal tears. The examination may reveal coincidental contralateral disease, which could have a significant bearing on subsequent surgery (Fig. 8.3). The possibility of tears of the renal pedicle may be raised by non-function on the affected side. The examination is also useful in demonstrating extravasation due to rupture at any point in the renal outflow tracts and it may show blood clots or haematomata (Fig. 8.4).

Small ureteric calculi may pass unnoticed in the early stages of renal colic, leaving no residual abnormality on i.v.u. It is therefore important that the i.v.u. is performed urgently so that the correct diagnosis is documented. When renal colic is present the i.v.u. will usually indicate the degree, level and nature of the obstructing lesion. It may be necessary to obtain delayed films up to 24 hours to demonstrate the exact level of obstruction. A postmicturition film should be routine as the distal ureter can be masked by the filled bladder.

If i.v.u. injections are administered by A & E staff they should be fully cognisant of treatment of allergic reactions. If a patient

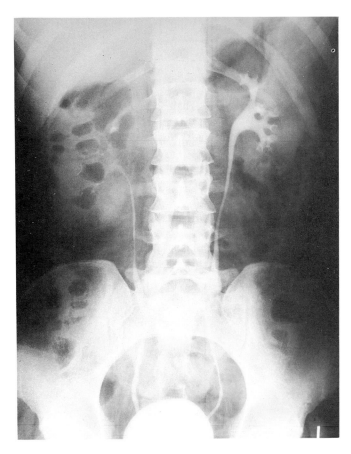

Fig. 8.2 A young man kicked in the back playing rugby. High dose i.v.u. demonstrates a normally functioning left renal tract. On the right side there is diminished concentration and poor filling of the collecting system. Laceration of the kidney and intrarenal haematoma.

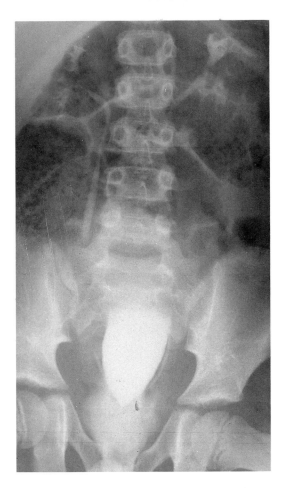

Fig. 8.4 Blunt trauma in a young boy; i.v.u. shows normally functioning kidneys. A rupture of the bladder base has occurred, with extravasation of contrast. The bladder is elevated and compressed on both sides by pelvic haematoma.

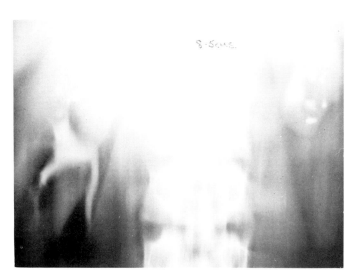

Fig. 8.3 Nephrotomography in a patient who had sustained significant right renal trauma, with haematuria. This study reveals a small shrunken, poorly functioning, chronic pyelonephritic kidney on the opposite side.

claims to be allergic to contrast media the possibility of pethidine addiction should be considered.

Gastrointestinal studies

Upper gastrointestinal perforation

Perforation of the stomach or duodenum is usually manifested by the presence of free gas in the abdomen, most readily identified on the erect chest film or decubitus abdominal studies. In doubtful cases, this may be confirmed by administering water soluble contrast orally, placing the patient right side down for 15–20 minutes and then taking an abdominal film or screening the abdomen. Confirmation of a leak, and often the site of perforation, will thus be made in the majority of cases.

Spontaneous perforation of the oesophagus is rare, but this may also be shown by screening the oesophagus after the administration of water-soluble contrast (Fig. 8.5). If this is negative and a tear is still suspected, it is then safe to give barium. The administration of barium is also useful in demonstrating gut herniation due to rupture of the left hemi-diaphragm.

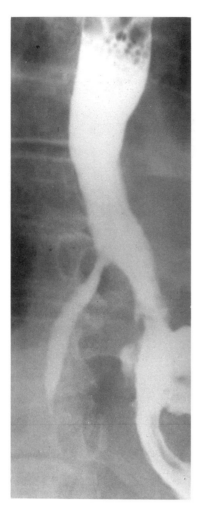

Fig. 8.5 A middle-aged male patient who felt something 'pop' and complained of severe chest pain after several episodes of vomiting. Water-soluble contrast administered orally shows rupture of the distal oesophagus.

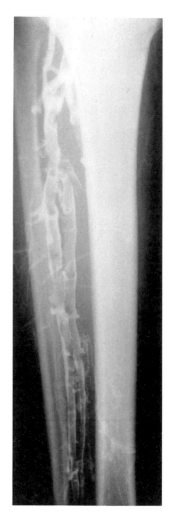

Fig. 8.6 Lower leg ascending venogram. There is non-filling due to complete occlusion of the posterior tibial vein. The perineal and anterior tibial veins are poorly filled with contrast, due to extensive recent thrombosis.

Colonic obstruction

Where acute large bowel obstruction is present, a single contrast 'instant enema', without preparation, will demonstrate the level and nature of the obstruction prior to surgery. It is perfectly safe and will help eliminate unnecessary surgery in other conditions such as pseudo-obstruction, which may mimic the condition both clinically and radiologically.

Ascending venography

Lower limb venography is a reliable method of demonstrating deep venous thrombosis, enabling the appropriate therapy to be instigated immediately (Fig. 8.6).

Ultrasound

Abdominal sonography has the advantage of being more widely available than computerised tomography (CT), and can be rapidly performed by the bedside or in the A & E department. The quality

of examination may however be impaired by the presence of large amounts of gas, which are frequently present in A & E patients. Acute inflammatory conditions such as cholecystitis and pancreatitis, may be demonstrated (Fig. 8.7). In trauma, small amounts of free intraperitoneal blood may be seen along with lacerations and haematomata of solid viscera (Figs 8.8, 8.9). Ultrasound is also extremely useful in the diagnosis of leaking abdominal aneurysm and ectopic pregnancy.

'Mid-liner' ultrasound is also helpful in demonstrating a shift in head injuries, and can be performed in theatre if necessary.

CT scanning

The accuracy of CT is well established in the demonstration of a wide variety of acute intracerebral conditions, whether due to disease or trauma (Figs 8.10, 8.11, 8.12). It is probably also the most reliable and accurate investigation in abdominal trauma. In experienced hands, specific organ injuries, both intra- and retroperitoneal, can be detected with a high degree of accuracy

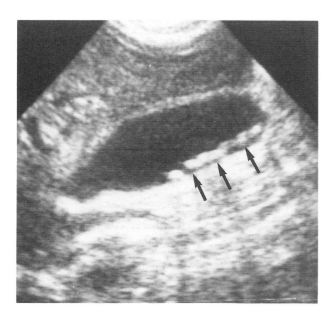

Fig. 8.7 Middle-aged female with pain in the right hypochondrium. Ultrasound examination shows multiple gall stones lying within the gall bladder (arrowed), with typical acoustic shadowing posteriorly. (Courtesy of Dr P. Hanley.)

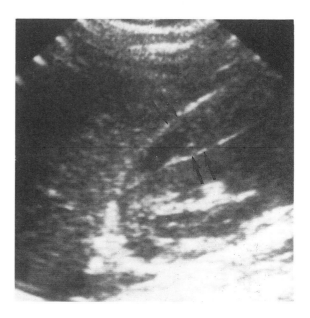

Fig. 8.9 Ultrasound right kidney following blunt trauma. There is separation of Gerota's fascia due to perirenal haematoma (arrowed). (Courtesy of Dr G. Crothers.)

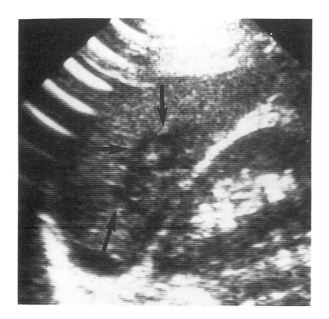

Fig. 8.8 Ultrasound scan of the spleen and left kidney. A fairly well-defined echo-poor area (arrowed) at the splenic hilum, in keeping with a haematoma. (Courtesy of Dr G. Crothers.)

(Figs 8.13, 8.14, 8.15). Where there is clinical doubt, it is a valuable asset in acute non-traumatic conditions, such as pancreatitis and leaking abdominal aneurysm. It is probably as accurate, and certainly less invasive, than aortography in the diagnosis of non-traumatic rupture of the thoracic aorta (Fig. 8.16). CT gives excellent demonstration of spinal fractures and dislocations. Computer reconstruction to the coronal or sagittal planes gives useful additional information, without further patient manipulation or radiation. The integrity of the spinal canal can accurately be

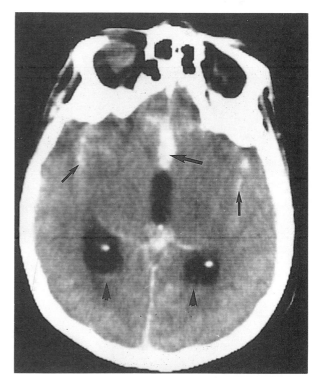

Fig. 8.10 Head CT showing acute subarachnoid haemorrhage. This was due to rupture of an anterior communicating aneurysm. Note blood (arrowed) in the interhemispheric fissure (large arrow). Blood in the sylvian fissures (small arrows) and blood layering in the ventricles (arrow heads). (Courtesy of Dr K. Bell.)

assessed. Fractures of the posterior elements are well seen and encroachment by bony fragments on the canal or foramina can be clearly shown. These abnormalities are not usually appreciated on plain film studies.

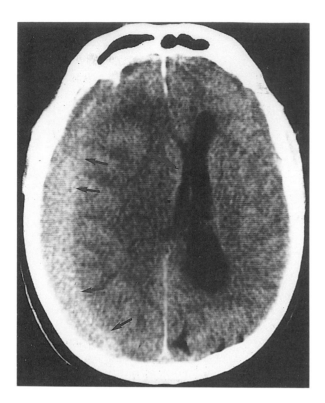

Fig. 8.11 Head CT scan showing a large left subdural haematoma (arrowed). Note the high attenuation indicating that this is recent. There is a concave inner margin in contradistinction to an extradural haematoma. There is also compression of the left hemisphere and lateral ventricle, with midline shift to the right. (Courtesy of Dr K. Bell.)

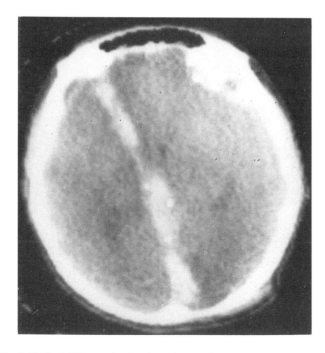

Fig. 8.12 Head CT scan showing the trajectory of a low velocity bullet.

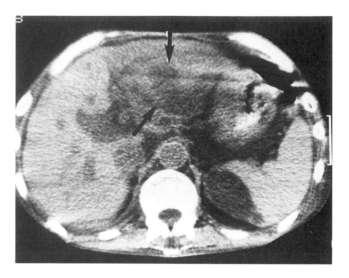

Fig. 8.13 Subcapsular haematoma on the posterior aspect of the spleen, with rupture of the left lobe of the liver (arrows). (Reproduced with permission from H K Lewis & Co.)

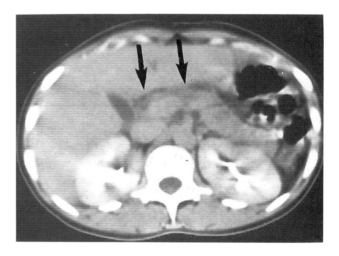

Fig. 8.14 A small amount of fluid outlines the anterior surface of the head and neck of the pancreas following blunt trauma (arrows). (Reproduced with permission from H K Lewis & Co.)

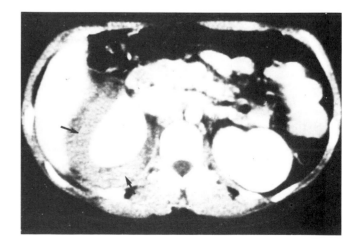

Fig. 8.15 Abdominal CT scan following blunt trauma. A large perinephric haematoma is clearly seen on the right side (arrows).

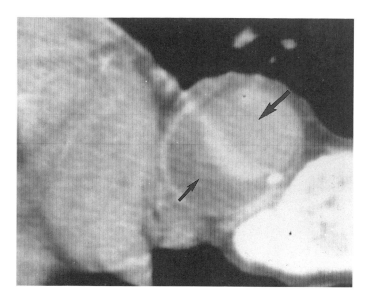

Fig. 8.16 CT scan thoracic aorta showing dissection. Following administration of contrast the true lumen (large arrow) is more dense than the false lumen (small arrow).

The availability of CT scanning will obviously determine referral for immediate investigation. Irrespective of this, the decision to use it should be based on sound clinical indications and after close consultation with the radiologists and surgeons.

Angiography

Rupture of the aorta, whether due to trauma or atherosclerosis, carries a high mortality if untreated. Early recourse to angiography will usually provide a definitive diagnosis.

A flush aortogram should be carried out as a matter of urgency when acute occlusion of a major vessel is suspected as a result of trauma, embolism or thrombosis.

Selective angiography may be required to study more distal or smaller vessels. In expert hands this can be performed rapidly with little risk to the patient.

Immediate operative intervention is usually indicated when rupture of a major vessel is firmly diagnosed. If, however, the location is uncertain, and the patient is clinically stable, selective angiography will usually demonstrate the site accurately (Fig. 8.17). When surgery or anaesthesia are contra-indicated, control of bleeding may be possible by the introduction of Gelfoam, wire coils or balloons inserted via the arterial route.

CT will usually demonstrate the presence and site of subarachnoid haemorrhage due to ruptured aneurysm (Fig. 8.10). If it does not, then complete cerebral angiography within the first 24–48 hours is indicated.

RADIOLOGICAL TIPS AND TRAPS

Head and neck

A fractured skull usually demonstrates well defined non-branching translucent linear shadows, sometimes sharply angular in places

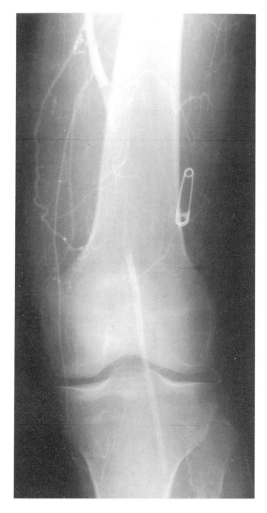

Fig. 8.17 A young male patient with a gun shot wound to the thigh and diminished peripheral pulses. Femoral arteriogram demonstrates complete transection of the lower superficial femoral artery. The popliteal artery is reconstituted by collaterals.

(Fig. 8.18). Stellate fractures may be seen and are due to local impact (Fig. 8.19). Where a depressed fracture is present, it may cause a dense curvilinear shadow due to overlapping of bone fragments (Fig. 8.20). Tangential views are then helpful. Dried blood in matted hair can also produce similar appearances. When there is doubt about whether a line is indeed a skull fracture, it often helps to examine the relevant area of the scalp for evidence of trauma.

On the lateral 'brow-up' film, a frontal aerocele may be seen indicating sinus fracture. A fluid level in the sphenoid sinus may be the only evidence of basal skull fracture (Fig. 8.21).

Old fracture lines can persist in adults for years. It is important to compare the films with previous studies.

Cervical spine

All patients who have sustained head injuries and are still unconscious in the A & E department should have cervical spine films taken.

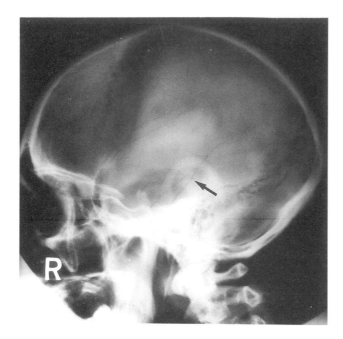

Fig. 8.18 Fracture through the right temperoparietal region (arrowed). Compare with the normal vascular markings elsewhere.

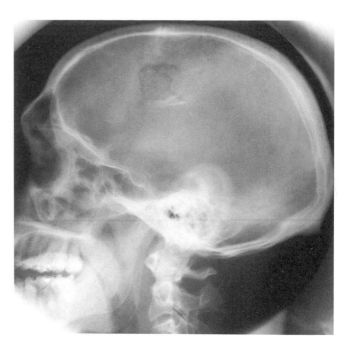

Fig. 8.20 Struck on the head with a hammer following a domestic argument! There is a circular and stellate fracture in the parietal region. Note the dense inferior margin, indicating a depressed fracture.

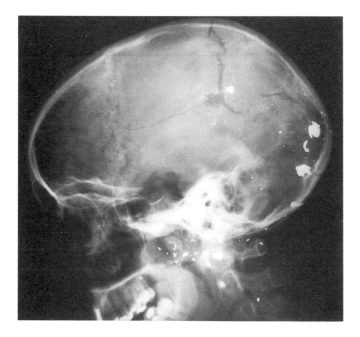

Fig. 8.19 A large stellate fracture in the left parietal region due to a low velocity gun shot wound. A frontal aerocele is noted and there is air around the base of the skull. Metallic bullet fragments are also clearly seen.

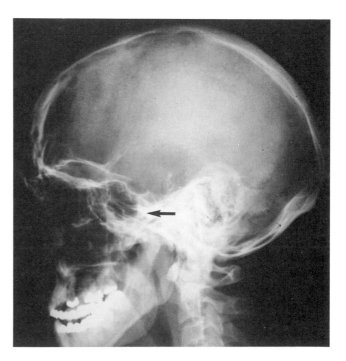

Fig. 8.21 Lateral brow-up skull film following a fall from 15 feet. There is a comminuted fracture of the frontal region extending through the sinus. A frontal aerocele is present. A fluid level is seen in the sphenoid sinus (arrowed). This usually indicates a fracture through the base of the skull. However, in this case it is probably due to the frontal sinus fracture.

The presence of prevertebral soft tissue swelling (>7 mm) in the cervical spine (Fig. 8.22), and paravertebral swelling in the thoracic spine, raises the index of suspicion for bony injury.

C1/C2 and the cervicodorsal junction should be clearly demonstrated on all examinations (Figs 8.23, 8.24). This may require tomography. Oblique views may be necessary to evaluate the neural arches and articular facets. When instability is suspected and the standard views are normal, consideration may then be given to obtaining flexion and extension views, performed in the presence of an experienced doctor (Fig. 8.25).

Anterior dislocation in the cervical spine of 50% or more indicates bilateral facet dislocation and is unstable. Displacement

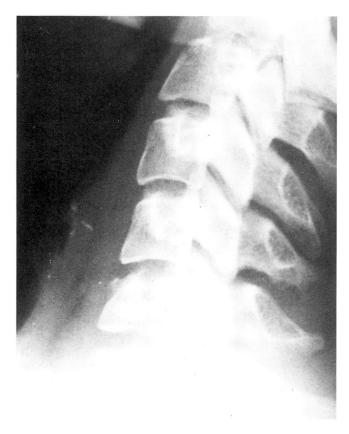

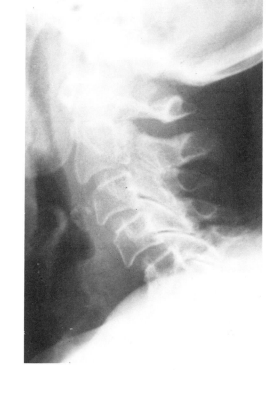

A

Fig. 8.22 Lateral view of the cervical spine showing anterior wedge compression of C6 due to forward flexion injury. The prevertebral soft tissues are increased, measuring 12 mm.

of less than 50% indicates unilateral facet dislocation and is usually stable.

Hyperflexion injuries of the thoracic spine usually cause anterior compression. Tomography may be necessary, particularly of the upper thoracic spine. Look also for internal injuries and fractures of the sternum.

Fish bones or other foreign bodies impacted in the upper oesophagus may be difficult to see. Soft tissue studies are required. Swelling and/or an air-fluid level will suggest abscess formation. Barium swallow or endoscopy should be employed where the diagnosis is in doubt.

Lumbosacral spine

As in the thoracic region, forward flexion injuries usually cause anterior compression fractures (Fig. 8.26). Minor forms of this injury can be easily missed. Look carefully for fractures of the spinous and transverse processes. When the latter is present suspect renal damage.

Spondylolysis is best seen on oblique projection (Fig. 8.27).

Fractures of the sacrum are easily missed. They are best seen on lateral tomography and are often associated with other pelvic fractures especially of the pubic rami.

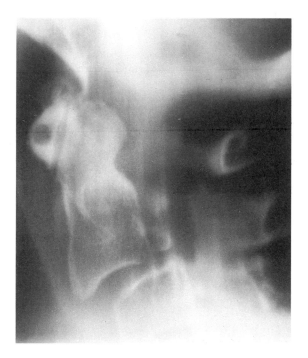

B

Fig. 8.23 An elderly female patient who fell down stairs, complaining of severe neck pain and restricted movement. **A** Lateral view shows a suspicious area in the lamina of C2. **B** Lateral tomography confirms a complete fracture through the laminae, with marked separation and slight forward subluxation.

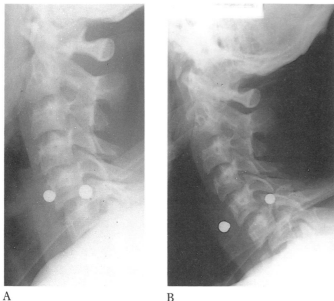

A   B

Fig. 8.24 A A lateral view of the cervical spine following a road traffic
accident. The spine is visualised as far as C6. No other abnormality is
evident. **B** With the shoulders pulled down, an unstable fracture/dislocation of
C6/7 is revealed.

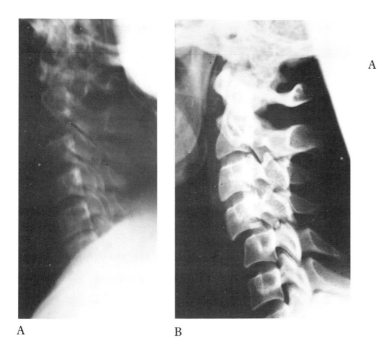

A   B

Fig. 8.25 A An apparently normal cervical spine carried out in the A & E
department, following neck trauma. **B** Forward flexion study shows anterior
dislocation of C4 on C5.

Chest

In the severely injured patient, frequently only an AP supine film
is possible. This causes magnification of the heart and aortic
shadows, giving rise to diagnostic difficulties, particularly when
aortic injuries are suspected (Fig. 8.28). Further widening of the
mediastinum on sequential studies in the same projection should

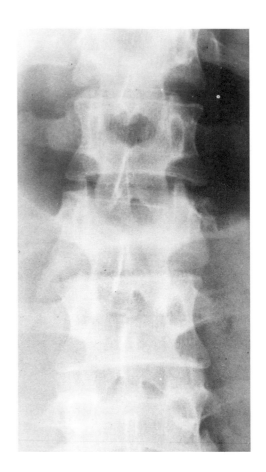

A

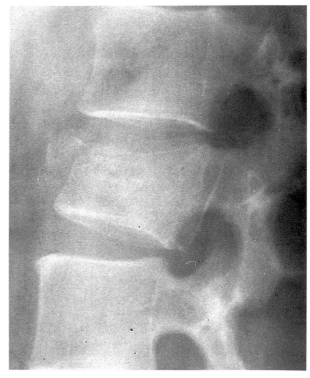

B

Fig. 8.26 Road traffic accident. Forward flexion injury. **A** AP view showing
loss in the vertical height of L2. **B** Lateral view confirms the presence of a
stable fracture with anterosuperior compression of the body and avulsion of a
small fragment anteriorly.

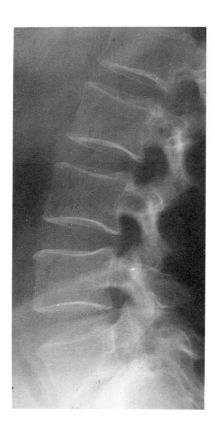

A

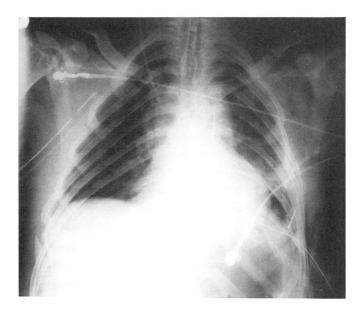

Fig. 8.28 An AP chest film following a road traffic accident shows widening of the mediastinum, fractures of the left upper ribs and a small left basal pneumothorax. Subcutaneous emphysema is present. Right lower rib fractures are also identified. Suspected aortic rupture.

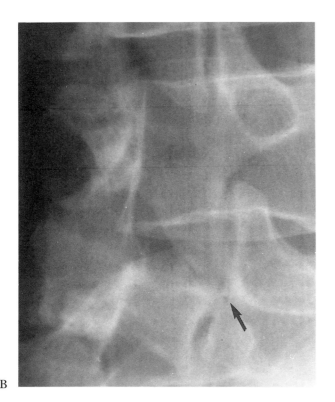

B

Fig. 8.27 A A young male complaining of persistent low back pain. The only abnormality is slight forward slipping of L5 on S1. B Same patient. The oblique view shows a break in the pars at L5 (arrowed). Compare with the intact pars above.

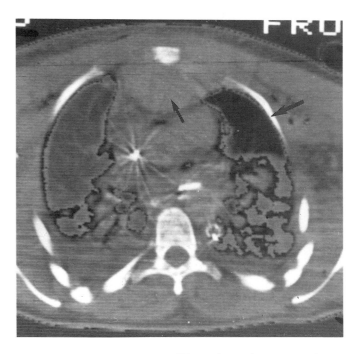

Fig. 8.29 Same patient as Fig. 8.28. CT scan shows a large retrosternal haematoma (small arrow) responsible for the mediastinal widening. The left-sided pneumothorax is also clearly identified (large arrow). The aorta was intact.

be treated with grave suspicion. Additional clues to aortic trauma are fractures of the sternum, upper ribs and clavicle, particularly when left sided, and fluid in the left pleural space. Sternal fractures per se can produce apparent mediastinal widening due to retrosternal haematoma formation (Fig. 8.29). Sternal injuries are best seen on the lateral view (Fig. 8.30), supplemented by

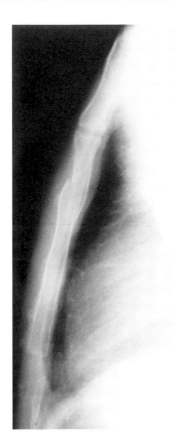

Fig. 8.30 Fracture through the upper sternum clearly seen on the lateral view. There is a small retrosternal haematoma.

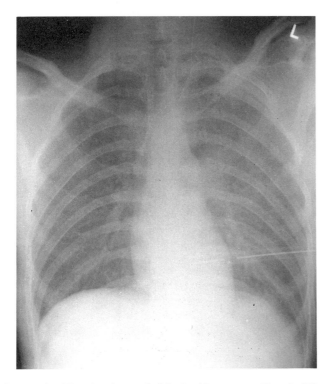

Fig. 8.31 An AP supine chest study following blunt trauma. There is diffuse haziness of the left lung field, compared with the right side. A chest drain·has been inserted. There is a small pleural 'cap'. Two litres of blood were aspirated from the left pleural cavity.

tomography. Blood in the pleural cavity does not show as a fluid interface on the supine radiograph. The blood tracks posteriorly producing a diffuse increase in density on the affected side, which can be easily overlooked (Fig. 8.31). Pneumothorax/haemopneumothorax may also be difficult to detect on supine films. Horizontal beam studies will readily demonstrate gas and gas/fluid levels, when the patient is supine, or in the lateral decubitus position with the affected side upwards. Small pneumothoraces are best seen on expiration films.

Diaphragmatic rupture

The chest film may be normal. Valuable clues are lower left rib fractures, apparent elevation of the diaphragm and haemothorax (Fig. 8.32). Splenic trauma is often present. Loops of gut are occasionally visible in the left lower hemithorax.

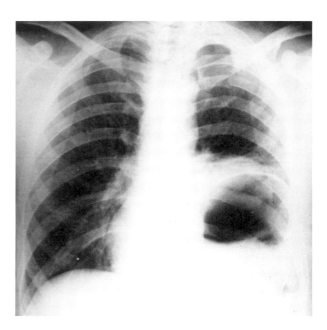

Fig. 8.32 Road traffic accident victim complaining of dyspnoea. The gastric air bubble is in an abnormally high position. There is compression of lung tissue above it. At operation the stomach had in fact herniated through a major tear in the left hemidiaphragm.

Abdomen

Perforation

Free gas is best demonstrated on the upright chest film. Horizontal beam studies of the abdomen with the right side raised for 15–20 minutes will usually show even small amounts of free gas lying in the right flank or under the liver.

Supine film findings:

1. Small collections of gas in the right hypochondrium.

2. The falciform ligament may be outlined as a dense linear oblique shadow several centimetres long, lying in the right hypochondrium (Fig. 8.33).

3. Both sides of gut wall may be visualised (the double wall sign) (Fig. 8.33).

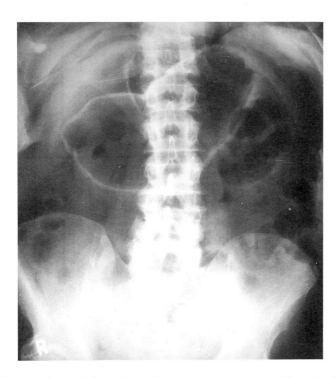

Fig. 8.33 Supine abdominal film of a patient on steroid therapy. The walls of the stomach and the falciform ligament are clearly identified. There are also collections of free gas in the subdiaphragmatic areas. Perforated gastric ulcer. (Reproduced with permission from H K Lewis & Co.).

Intestinal obstruction

The supine film is usually the most helpful. This may show distended loops of bowel proximal to the site of obstruction, with collapsed bowel distally (Fig. 8.34). The presence of fluid levels is not a good discriminator between mechanical obstruction and paralytic ileus. Distinction between distended small and large gut is usually possible. The valvulae conniventes completely traverse the lumen, whereas the haustral markings do not. Gas in the rectum does not preclude large gut mechanical obstruction. Look out for distension of the caecum in large gut obstruction. There is a greatly increased risk of perforation of the caecum when its diameter exceeds 12 cm. High small gut obstruction may present as a 'gasless' abdomen on the plain films.

Toxic megacolon

The transverse colon is most frequently distended in this condition and may be mistaken for stomach. Look for a diameter in excess of 5.5 cm and thickened oedematous mucosa (Fig. 8.35). 'Thumb printing' is due to mucosal oedema and may occur in severe inflammatory bowel disease or gut ischaemia. Identical appearances may be seen as a result of submucosal bleeding due to trauma or disease. The characteristic 'thumb printing' in *ischaemic colitis* is frequently identified around the splenic flexure.

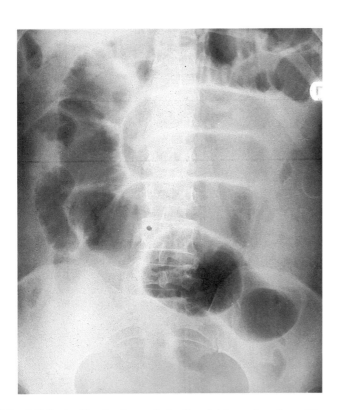

Fig. 8.34 Supine film showing markedly distended loops of small gut. There is little gas or faecal residue in the colon. Obstruction of the distal ileum due to adhesions. (Reproduced with permission from H K Lewis & Co.).

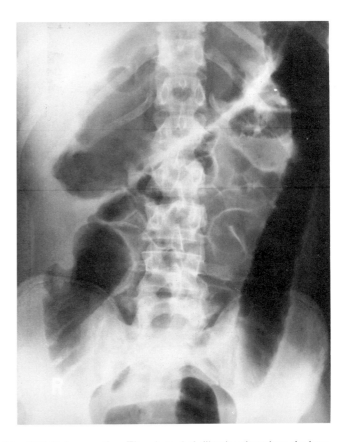

Fig. 8.35 Toxic megacolon. There is marked dilatation throughout the large gut. Thickening of the walls can be identified, and islands of inflamed mucosa are seen in the transverse colon, which measures 12 cm in diameter.

Leaking abdominal aneurysm

A fine curvilinear rim of calcification is identifiable in the lower lumbar spine region in 50% of cases. There may be loss of the psoas shadow, particularly on the left side, and displacement of the left kidney. When there is doubt a lateral view may confirm the diagnosis.

Abdominal trauma

Radiographic examination is of limited value, especially in penetrating trauma. CT scanning, ultrasound or angiography may be necessary to enable a definitive diagnosis. In severe abdominal trauma the patient usually goes straight to theatre, without recourse to further radiology.

On the abdominal film look for blurring of the flank stripe, enlargement or displacement of viscera and/or separation of loops of bowel, all caused by bleeding. Intraperitoneal bleeding may displace the colon medially due to its accumulation in the paracolic gutters. There may be generalised haziness of the abdomen, indicating an increase in intraperitoneal fluid. The renal and psoas shadows may be enlarged, displaced or indistinct due to retroperitoneal bleeding (Fig. 8.36).

Fractures of the lower ribs should raise the suspicion of injury to the liver, duodenum and kidney on the right side, and of the spleen and kidney when the fractures are on the left side.

The high incidence of accompanying damage to the thorax makes chest X-ray examination mandatory (Fig. 8.37, 8.38).

Peripheries

Upper limb

Acromioclavicular dislocation can be completely missed if weight bearing views are not taken.

Posterior dislocation of the shoulder

This is rare, but frequently missed. It often follows severe muscle spasm (e.g. epilepsy, ECT) or a direct blow to the front of the shoulder. Look for loss of parallelism between the humeral head and glenoid rim. There may be overlap of the medial aspect of the humeral head on the glenoid. An axial view will confirm the diagnosis. The humeral head assumes a characteristically round appearance due to fixed internal rotation (Fig. 8.39).

Elbow and forearm injuries

The numerous ossific centres around the elbow up to the age of 18 can cause confusion. When in doubt, take contralateral views for comparison. If a fracture of the shaft of the radius or ulna is present look for another fracture or a dislocation at the elbow or wrist.

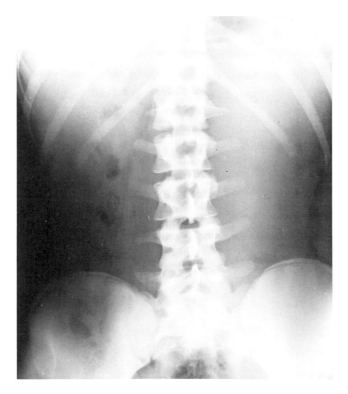

Fig. 8.36 Abdominal film of a young male patient following a sports injury. He presented with left-sided abdominal pain, tenderness and haematuria. There is loss of the normal soft tissue interfaces and obliteration of the psoas shadow. At operation a severely lacerated kidney and extensive retroperitoneal haematoma was found. A splenic laceration was also present.

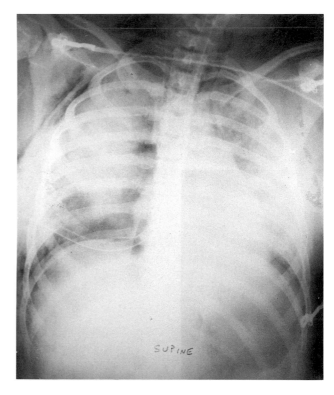

Fig. 8.37 Supine chest film of a patient with multiple intra-abdominal injuries. There is gross bilateral pulmonary contusion, with very little normally aerated lung. Subcutaneous emphysema is seen on the right side.

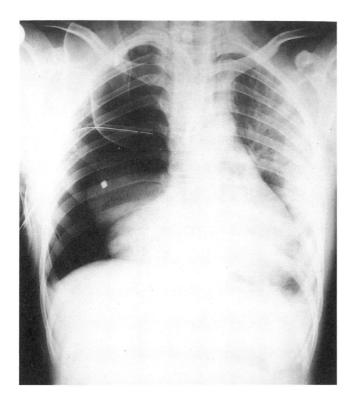

Fig. 8.38 A 14-year-old boy who had fallen off a tractor. He was admitted to A & E with marked abdominal tenderness and guarding. A tension pneumothorax was also suspected and a chest drain inserted. Despite this a chest film one hour later shows a large right-sided pneumothorax, with collapsed lung adjacent to the right heart border. There is also evidence of left-sided pulmonary contusion and mediastinal emphysema. At operation a complete transection of the right main bronchus was successfully repaired.

Avulsion of the medial epicondyle

This ranges from minor dislocation to entrapment within the joint. Such injuries are easily overlooked (Fig. 8.40).

Fractures of the radial head

Small fractures are often difficult to see. Displacement of the anterior fat pad will be seen in this and other elbow injuries, especially supracondylar fractures, and should prompt a review of the apparently normal film. The position of the posterior fat pad should also be carefully sought in all injuries around the elbow joint.

Dislocation of the distal radioulnar joint

This is not always appreciated. A fracture of the radial shaft should be sought (Galeazzi fracture).

Carpal injuries

The commonest is the scaphoid fracture. Scaphoid views should be requested when suspected. If negative, the patient should be re-examined out of plaster in 2–3 weeks and again later if tenderness persists. Tomography may be necessary to identify hairline fracture.

Dislocation of the lunate

On the AP views, the lunate assumes a triangular outline (Fig. 8.41). Dislocation of the lunate anteriorly is best seen on the lateral

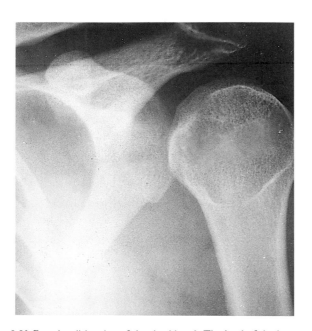

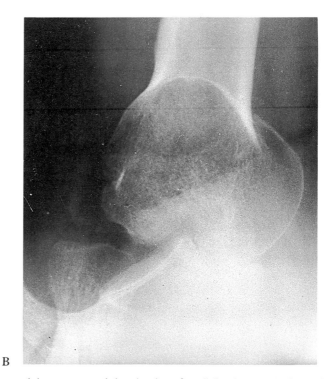

Fig. 8.39 Posterior dislocation of the shoulder. **A** The head of the humerus has a rounded appearance and there is a loss of parallelism between the humeral articular surface and the glenoid. **B** The axial view shows the degree of posterior displacement from the glenoid.

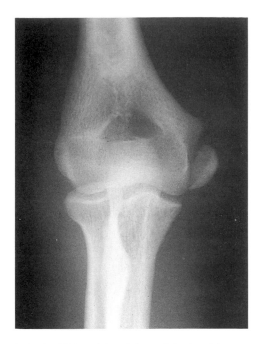

Fig. 8.40 A clearly visible avulsion of the medial epicondyle.

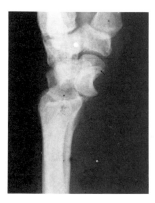 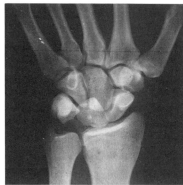

Fig. 8.41 AP and lateral views of the wrist. On the AP view the lunate has a triangular configuration, with incongruity of the adjoining joint surfaces. On the lateral view the characteristic 'C' shape of the dislocated lunate is clearly seen.

view. Look particularly for this, or perilunar dislocation, if there are signs of post-traumatic median nerve compression.

Perilunar dislocation

This is frequently missed. The lunate maintains its normal position, the rest of the carpus being displaced backwards. Best seen on the lateral view. Accompanying fracture through the waist of the scaphoid can occur (Fig. 8.42). Although fractures of the remaining carpal bones are rare, careful scrutiny of the region is mandatory. If the wrist is painful and tender and no fracture is seen, look for a dislocation.

Bennett's fracture/dislocation

This is easily missed if the X-rays are centred on the hand or distal thumb.

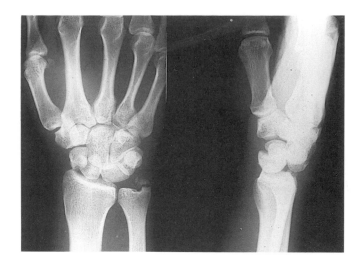

Fig. 8.42 AP and lateral views of the left wrist. Trans-scaphoid perilunar dislocation. Note that the lunate lies in a normal position on the lateral view, with backward displacement of the carpus. There is a fracture through the waist of the scaphoid and the ulnar styloid.

Fingers

Collateral ligament injuries of the first MCP joint. Instability is demonstrated by stressing the ulnar collateral ligament.

Phalangeal fractures producing unstable subluxations of the IP joints. It is essential to obtain coned true lateral views of the affected joint. Open reduction may be required.

Foreign bodies

X-ray examination in two planes, with a marker and using soft tissue technique, is required. Radiography should always be employed when glass foreign bodies are suspected.

Lower limb and pelvis

Pelvis. Always look for more than one fracture or dislocation of the pelvic ring. Diastasis of the sacroiliac joints or symphysis may be overlooked (Fig. 8.43).

Posterior fracture of the acetabulum. This should be suspected when there is a history of force applied along the flexed femur, followed by pain on hip rotation. Small fragments are difficult to see. Look for associated posterior dislocation of the femoral head and sciatic nerve injury on clinical examination.

Fractures of the acetabular roof or floor. These usually arise as a result of central dislocation of the femoral head (Fig. 8.44). Tomography may be necessary.

Os acetabuli. These may persist into adult life unfused to the superior margin of the acetabulum. They are frequently mistaken for a chip fracture and are characteristically rounded.

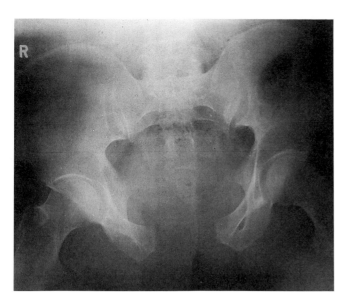

Fig. 8.43 This middle-aged man fell astride his horse. There is wide separation of the symphysis. Note in addition diastasis of the sacroiliac joints. There was also a ruptured bladder.

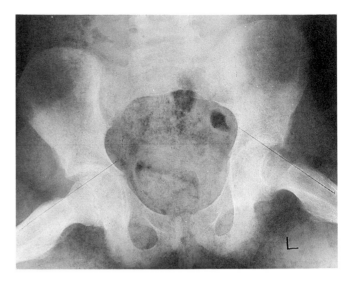

Fig. 8.45 Thirteen-year-old boy complaining of left hip pain. Note the femoral epiphysis lying medially to a line drawn through the superior margin of the femoral neck. Part of the medial aspect of the epiphysis lies outside the acetabulum. Normal appearances are seen on the right.

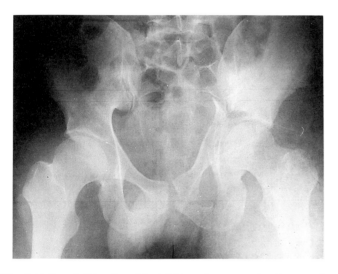

Fig. 8.44 Central dislocation of the left hip and accompanying fractures of the acetabulum are seen. There are also fractures of the left inferior pubic ramus.

Slipped upper femoral epiphysis. This usually presents in young males aged 10–15 who complain of thigh or knee pain. Abduction views show the abnormality more clearly. Downward dislocation of the epiphysis, with extrusion of its medial portion from the acetabulum, is present. There is usually widening and sometimes sclerosis of the epiphyseal plate. A line drawn along the superior margin of the femoral neck normally transects the epiphysis. When slipping occurs, the epiphysis lies medial to this line (Fig. 8.45).

The knee

Osteochondritis dissecans. Occurs in young people without any clear history of injury. There is often pain and locking. Tunnel

views may be required to show the fragment of bone detached from the inner aspect of the medial femoral condyle.

Fracture of the upper tibia or its epiphysis. Even if there is no visible displacement of the epiphysis, it may have occurred at the time of injury, and damage thus sustained to the popliteal/posterior tibial vessels.

Bipartite patella. This is often mistaken for a fracture. Affects the upper outer quadrant, frequently bilateral. Fractures of the patella are usually best seen on skyline views.

Fabella. This may be mistaken for a loose body lying posterior to the joint, usually round and smooth.

Intra-articular fractures of the knee, e.g. tibial plateau injuries. Subtle fractures may be difficult to see. A horizontal beam lateral view will often show a fluid level in the suprapatellar pouch, due to lipohaemarthrosis. Such a finding should prompt a careful search for an intra-articular fracture.

Tears of the cruciate ligament. Sometimes avulsion of the intercondylar eminence may be seen with accompanying joint effusion.

Stress fractures of the tibia. These may be invisible initially. Delayed studies may reveal callus around the fracture site (Fig. 8.46). A bone scan is diagnostic.

Ankle and foot

Fracture of the talus. Fractures of the neck are sometimes difficult to see on standard views. Oblique views are often helpful.

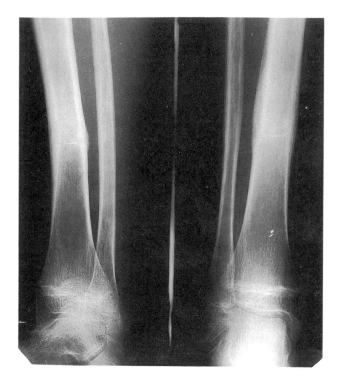

Fig. 8.46 AP and lateral views of the tibia. There is a typical stress fracture, with prominent fusiform new bone formation around a faint transverse fracture.

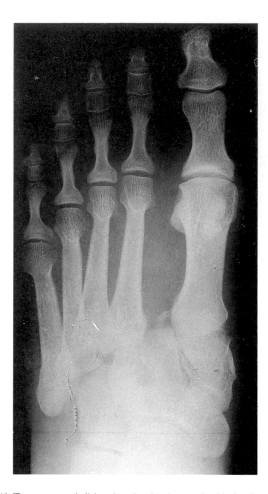

Fig. 8.48 Tarso-metatarsal dislocation showing increased widening between the first and second metatarsals.

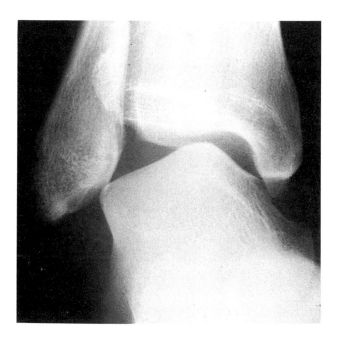

Fig. 8.47 Forced inversion study showing complete tear of the lateral ligaments producing a talar tilt of 30°.

Fractured calcaneum. This usually follows a fall on the heels. Lateral views supplemented by axial studies will usually show fractures of the posterior portion. Subtaloid views may be required for further evaluation of the anterior portion and the subtaloid joint. If a fracture of a calcaneum is found look for a similar contralateral injury and also injury to the spine.

Lateral ligament injuries: forced inversion views will show an abnormal talar tilt (Fig. 8.47). Comparative views of the uninjured side are necessary.

Tarso-metatarsal dislocation. Minor degrees of dislocation are easily missed. Look for widening of the gap between the bases of the first and second metatarsals (Fig. 8.48).

Stress fractures of the metatarsals. Delayed radiography in 2–3 weeks time usually shows new bone formation around the previously invisible fracture site (Fig. 8.49).

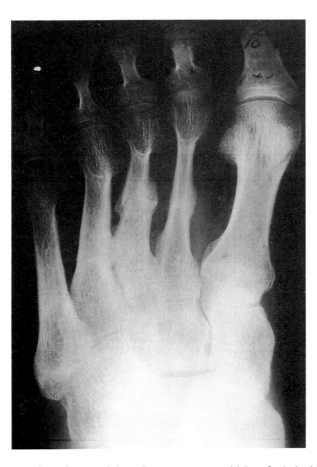

Fig. 8.49 Stress fractures. A long distance runner complaining of pain in the feet. Faint fracture lines are seen through the mid-shafts of the second and third metatarsals with prominent callus formation.

FURTHER READING

Plain X-ray diagnosis of the acute abdomen 2nd edn. Gough M H, Gear M W L, Doar A S 1986 Blackwell Scientific, Oxford

Casualty radiology Grech P 1981 Chapman and Hall, London

An atlas of normal roentgen variants that may simulate disease, 3rd edn. Keats T E 1985 Year Book Medical Publishers Inc, Chicago

Use of X-rays in trauma Mills J O M 1981 In: Odling-Smee W, Crockard A (eds) Trauma Care 9: 127-152

Emergency radiology self-assessment Mueller C F, Rund A D 1982 Williams and Wilkins, Baltimore

Radiology of skeletal trauma, vols I & II Rogers L F 1982 Churchill Livingstone, Edinburgh

Symposium on emergency department radiology Emergency Medicine Clinics of North America 3(3) Aug 3. Dalinka M J (ed) 1985 W B Saunders, Philadelphia

Anaesthesia and pain control

GENERAL ANAESTHESIA

General anaesthesia may be needed in an A & E department for the manipulation of fractures and dislocations, the incision of abscesses, the management of head injuries, cardioversion and acute respiratory problems such as asthma and epiglottitis.

Basic techniques of general anaesthesia

Anaesthesia is usually induced by an intravenous anaesthetic agent such as thiopentone, methohexitone or etomidate, but inhalational agents, such as halothane may be used instead. Anaesthesia is maintained using nitrous oxide and oxygen supplemented by an inhalational agent (e.g. halothane, enflurane) or by intravenous agents (e.g. fentanyl plus droperidol). Spontaneous breathing on a mask may be used when the airway is not at risk and the operation will be relatively short. Endotracheal intubation is usually required if the airway is at risk. Muscle relaxants, such as suxamethonium, are commonly used to aid intubation in emergencies, but other more specialised techniques may be needed. Once intubated, muscle relaxation is often maintained using a long acting muscle relaxant, such as atracurium or pancuronium, and controlled ventilation is required.

Many factors influence the choice of anaesthetic technique and some are relevant to A & E practice. The use of preoperative analgesia may reduce the amount of anaesthetic agent required. Intubation may be required for operations on the face or if the patient must lie prone. Intubation is essential for the unfasted patient. There is a risk of causing cardiac dysrhythmias if adrenaline is used on a patient receiving certain inhalational agents, e.g. halothane or enflurane, and so the surgeon must consult the anaesthetist if he needs to use adrenaline. Repeated anaesthetics can affect the type and amount of anaesthetic used and every effort should be made to keep these to a minimum.

General anaesthesia in the A & E department

Any room where a general anaesthetic is given must have standard resuscitation equipment immediately available. Responsibility for checking and maintaining anaesthetic equipment must be clearly defined. Routine and emergency drugs are likely to be spread throughout the department in cupboards, both locked and unlocked, and some require storing in a refrigerator. Some drugs will rarely be needed so expiry dates must be checked regularly. Nursing staff assisting at operations should have some anaesthetic training and know where all the necessary drugs and extra equipment are kept. Treatment regimes for uncommon emergencies, such as malignant hyperpyrexia (p. 86), should be readily available. Precalculated doses of emergency drugs, particularly for children, should also be clearly displayed.

The A & E doctor can help reduce the incidence of anaesthetic problems. A concise history, including past illnesses, medication and time of last eating, will help in case the patient later changes his story. Drug administration should be clearly recorded as this may affect the choice of anaesthetic technique. Where there are multiple injuries these should be recorded and brought to the attention of the anaesthetist. For example, a general anaesthetic may be required to reduce a Colles' fracture. However, if the anaesthetist was unaware of an associated head injury the usual anaesthetic technique could cause the patient serious harm. Early communication with the anaesthetist is important. It allows maximal time for preoperative assessment, lists can be rearranged and extra help brought in as required. Above all, the A & E doctor must be capable of helping the anaesthetist should an emergency arise.

Mortality

The commonest causes of anaesthetic deaths are:
1. Major disturbance of the respiratory system
   a. Intubation problems
   b. Inhalation of gastric contents
   c. Hypoventilation and airways obstruction
2. Major disturbances of the cardiovascular system
   a. Unrecognised hypotension, e.g. hypovolaemia, drug overdose

3. Mechanical failure
   a. Failure of oxygen supply
   b. Disconnection
   c. Leaks
   d. Obstruction
4. Inadequate monitoring
5. Human failure
   a. Inadequate training
   b. Error: particularly when tired, distracted or in a hurry
6. Organisational failure
   a. Inadequate supervision or assistance
   b. Inadequate recovery facilities.

Many of these problems are pertinent to anaesthesia within an A & E department. Aspiration of gastric contents is more likely during emergency surgery than elective surgery. Unrecognised hypovolaemia may also be a problem. General anaesthetics are often delegated to junior doctors in an A & E theatre, which may be separate from the main operating theatres and thus away from ready supervision or help. There may be no recovery room in the A & E department or it may be shared by non-surgical patients, thus restricting the care which the recovery nurse can give.

Particular problems of anaesthesia in an A & E department

Patient.   Patients of any age may require emergency surgery and some will also have conditions unrelated to their present problem. Children may have undiagnosed congenital abnormalities. As age increases so does the number of associated medical problems both treated and untreated. The elderly provide their own particular anaesthetic problems. A & E patients may have single or multiple injuries.

It is sometimes difficult to obtain a full history of the present complaint, past illnesses, medication or timing of the last meal. Difficulty in obtaining previous hospital notes or contacting the general practitioner may add to the problem. Some patients have grown wise to the rules regarding preoperative fasting and unfortunately may deliberately mislead the doctor so they can have an anaesthetic at a time convenient to themselves. Likewise some patients may withhold information about a present medical condition fearing that this will prevent them having an anaesthetic. The patient's condition and absence of accompanying relatives may present problems in obtaining consent for operation. (For further discussion of consent see Ch. 4.) Poor social conditions may necessitate admission of the patient postoperatively.

Environment.   Many A & E departments have their own fully staffed emergency operating theatres. Others have only small theatres or rooms for minor surgical procedures which may be some distance from the main theatres and backup teams. The A & E department can be a very lonely and isolated place for a junior anaesthetist.

Staffing.   Multiple emergencies may occur at night when medical, nursing and ancillary staffing is limited. The associated stress and fatigue may predispose to anaesthetic accidents.

Emergency operations.   Problems described previously may limit the extent of the preoperative assessment. Time may prevent the stabilisation of medical conditions or improving preoperative status.

Induction of anaesthesia is a particularly hazardous time. The patient is often unpremedicated and anxious. However there may have been recent alcohol ingestion or a narcotic analgesic may have been given. All these factors complicate judging the dose of induction agent. A stormy induction increases the risk of laryngospasm and aspiration.

Vomiting and aspiration are major problems in emergency anaesthesia. Anxiety, trauma, pain and narcotic analgesics delay gastric emptying and some conditions, such as intestinal obstruction, are associated with stasis or vomiting. If an operation can be delayed, waiting for 4–6 hours will give time for the stomach to empty. However, the stomach respects neither time nor textbook and complete emptying cannot be guaranteed after this time even in normal circumstances.

The anaesthetist has various techniques to reduce the risk of vomiting and aspiration. The A & E doctor must be competent at assisting at induction, particularly in providing cricoid pressure if requested and acting quickly if vomiting and aspiration occur.

The risk of vomiting continues through emergence from the anaesthetic and diligent management is required postoperatively.

Cricoid pressure (Sellick's manoeuvre) (Figure 9.1)

This manoeuvre aims to prevent regurgitation by occlusion of the oesophagus between the cricoid cartilage and the vertebral column. The tips of the thumb and first two fingers of one hand are placed either side of the cricoid cartilage and backward pressure is applied, when directed by the anaesthetist. The pressure may be applied

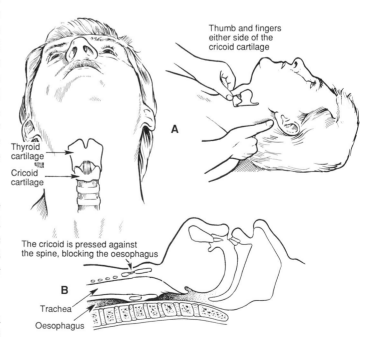

Fig. 9.1 Cricoid pressure.

just before or just as the patient goes to sleep. In either case it is wise to warn the patient beforehand that he may feel some pressure on his neck as he goes off to sleep. The pressure should not be released until the airway is safely secured.

This method should not be used during active vomiting as it may lead to oesophageal rupture.

Fitness for anaesthesia

The anaesthetist is the person who must decide whether a patient is fit for an anaesthetic, since it is he who will have to choose the correct technique and take responsibility for the outcome. If an operation needs to be done urgently an anaesthetist should be contacted immediately. If there is any doubt, a senior opinion should be sought.

Recovery from anaesthesia

Transfer of the patient from the operating theatre to the recovery room is a critical time since observation may be difficult and equipment less easily accessible. The patient should be assumed to have a full stomach and be allowed to recover from anaesthesia in the lateral position with head-down tilt. Suction should be immediately available. The patient should be cared for by an experienced nurse capable, in particular, of identifying and starting initial management of airway problems. The blood pressure and pulse should be monitored every 15 minutes for the first half hour and then every 30 minutes until the patient has fully recovered.

Fitness for discharge after general anaesthesia

The patient may be considered for discharge if there have been no anaesthetic complications and none is expected. There should also be no surgical indication for admission. The patient must remain under observation for at least 2 hours postoperatively and must have regained full consciousness and normal co-ordinated movements. Patients who have been intubated must be free from laryngeal stridor. If suxamethonium (a short-acting muscle relaxant) was used, activity during the following 24 hours should be limited to minimise muscle pains and so overnight admission to hospital may be preferable. The dangers of taking alcohol, driving, or operating dangerous machinery during the subsequent 24 hours should be stressed both preoperatively and on discharge. Ideally, written instructions should be given. The patient should be accompanied by a responsible relative or friend and should rest for the next 24 hours. Mild analgesics only should be needed and an adequate supply should be provided. The patient should contact his own doctor or the hospital if he is at all worried. A brief discharge summary would be helpful to the general practitioner in this situation.

Emergencies complicating general anaesthesia

The inference that a 'short' anaesthetic is a 'safe' anaesthetic is untrue since the emergencies described below may occur, albeit rarely, during the briefest and simplest of anaesthetics. It is thus essential that the A & E doctor is competent at assisting in anaesthetic emergencies. It is essential to know how to raise the foot of the trolley and how to operate all the resuscitation equipment. The exact location of emergency drugs and extra anaesthetic drugs (some of which may be kept in the refrigerator) must also be known. When staffing at emergency operations is limited the surgeon should remain in the operating theatre until the anaesthetist is happy with the patient's condition.

Intra-arterial injection of irritant solutions

Pain is felt distal to the injection site and there is associated blanching or discolouration of the skin. The distal pulse may be absent and hypotension sometimes occurs.

Treatment

1. Leave the needle in situ.
2. Postpone the operation unless the surgery is lifesaving, in which case treatment should proceed during the operation and a second anaesthetist will be required. Inform the consultant anaesthetist on call.
3. Inject into the artery 10–20 ml 0.5% plain procaine or 10–40 mg papaverine in 5 ml normal saline.
4. Provide sympathetic blockade with a brachial plexus or stellate ganglion block.
5. After performing the block give 10 000 units heparin intra-arterially.
6. Elevate the limb and keep it warm.
7. Use additional analgesia as required.
8. Consider using a systemic vasodilator (e.g. tolazoline) if the nerve block is incomplete.

Adverse drug reactions

An anaphylactic reaction may occur with anaesthetic agents, e.g. barbiturate induction agents. Most adverse drug reactions to intravenous anaesthetic agents are anaphylactoid in type and can occur without previous exposure.

Predisposing factors

Age. Adverse reactions are comparatively rare in young children, but the incidence gradually increases as repeated exposure occurs.

Atopy. Hypersensitivity is more common in this group.

Pregnancy. Pregnancy appears to produce an increased incidence of adverse reactions.

Previous exposure. This is likely to predispose to an adverse reaction on subsequent administration of either the same drug or one with similar constituents.

Stress. An increase in catecholamine release due to stress may increase the risk of an adverse reaction.

Preservatives and solubilising agents. The widespread use of these agents makes repeated exposure and thus adverse reactions more likely. (Management of anaphylactic reaction: see Ch. 13.)

Laryngospasm

This is a reflex response commonly brought about by an irritating stimulus to the airway when the patient is only lightly anaesthetised. Such stimuli may include secretions, vomit or blood in the airway, oropharyngeal or nasopharyngeal airway placement, laryngoscopy and endotracheal intubation. Painful peripheral stimuli can also trigger this reflex and it is thus essential that the surgeon leaves the patient undisturbed until the anaesthetist says that the patient is ready.

Untreated laryngospasm leads to hypercapnia, hypoxia and acidosis and eventually to cardiac arrest. Small children are particularly at risk.

Treatment requires immediate removal of the stimulus (e.g. by suction, removing an airway, stopping peripheral stimulation) and administration of 100% oxygen. If after 1–2 minutes the laryngospasm persists, steady positive pressure on the airway using 100% oxygen with a well fitting mask may succeed. Failing this, a small dose of suxamethonium may be required to relax the striated laryngeal muscles. The patient should be ventilated with 100% oxygen and then anaesthesia must be deepened before any surgery can proceed.

Bronchospasm

This is a reflex response to stimuli similar to those causing laryngospasm. It is also associated with asthma or anaphylactic reactions and is more common in smokers and chronic bronchitics.

Bronchospasm is best prevented by ensuring a smooth induction and obtaining a deep level of anaesthesia before surgery commences. Halothane produces bronchodilatation and may be useful for the maintenance of anaesthesia. If bronchospasm occurs, noxious stimuli should be removed. Bronchospasm can usually be controlled by deepening the plane of anaesthesia, but occasionally a bronchodilator may be required.

Inhalation of gastric contents

Any patient having an emergency operation is at risk of inhaling gastric contents. Fasting the patient may reduce the risk, but it offers no guarantee of safety.

Immediate management of aspiration involves placing the patient head down in the lateral position. The pharynx should be sucked out and then the patient should be intubated and the cuff of the endotracheal tube inflated as soon as possible. The patient should be ventilated with 100% oxygen and the pulse checked, since reflex cardiac arrest may occur. The trachea should be alternately sucked out and ventilated with 100% oxygen until it is clear. The pH of the aspirate will give some indication of the prognosis. Subsequent management will usually include elective ventilation and hypovolaemia or acidosis may require correction. Bronchoscopy and the use of methyl prednisolone may be considered. Unless the operation is life-saving it should be postponed or curtailed.

Cardiac arrest

Anaesthetic agents should be discontinued and any mechanical cause for the arrest be treated (e.g. draining a pneumothorax). (For further management see Ch. 10.)

Pneumothorax

This may be related to chest trauma or an undiagnosed bulla. The surgeon must be ready to put in a chest drain, while the anaesthetist makes appropriate changes to the anaesthetic.

Malignant hyperpyrexia

This is a rare autosomal dominant disease characterised by a rise in temperature of up to 1°C every 15 minutes. In the UK it occurs approximately once every 190 000 anaesthetics. It is commonest in young adult males and is seen most frequently during anaesthesia for trauma and appendicitis as well as squints and spinal deformity. It is often triggered by suxamethonium or halothane, but other anaesthetic agents have been implicated. Always be suspicious if there is a history of an unexplained anaesthetic death in the family.

Clinical features. 1. Extreme pyrexia which may immediately follow the trigger or may be delayed by 30–45 minutes.
2. Cyanosis
3. Tachycardia
4. Metabolic and respiratory acidosis
5. Hyperkalaemia
6. Muscle rigidity.

Treatment. 1. Discontinue inhalational agents, call for extra help and notify the consultant anaesthetist on call.
2. Change to a vapour-free anaesthetic machine and circuits if possible.
3. Complete surgery as soon as possible.
4. Hyperventilate with oxygen (two or three times the predicted minute volume).
5. Start surface cooling with tap water and fans. Use cold intravenous fluids, such as 0.9% saline, which should be kept permanently in the theatre refrigerator.
6. Commence intravenous dantrolene giving 1 mg/kg every 5 minutes up to a total of 10 mg/kg. (Dantrolene is an expensive drug and will probably be kept centrally in the pharmacy or main operating theatre. It is important to know exactly where it is kept and how it may be obtained, particularly at night.)
7. Check plasma urea and electrolytes. Correct hyperkalaemia with 50 ml of 50% dextrose plus 20 units of soluble insulin i.v.

8. Check blood gases. Correct any metabolic acidosis with 8.4% sodium bicarbonate. 100 ml or more may be required.

9. Arrange transfer to the intensive care unit.

Particular hazards

Anaesthesia for cardioversion

Emergency cardioversion is sometimes required for conscious patients who have a life-threatening supraventricular or ventricular tachycardia. Any anaesthetic procedure on this group carries added risks. Increased sensitivity to induction agents will be caused by associated myocardial ischaemia or other medical problems. The reduced cardiac output will also produce the same effect. The patient may be unable to lie flat thus complicating induction and airway management. Vomiting and aspiration of gastric contents are real hazards since the patient will not have been fasted and may have had an opiate which would delay gastric emptying.

Anaesthesia for cardioversion should always be performed in a room with full resuscitation equipment and by a doctor capable of performing tracheal intubation and managing routine anaesthetic problems. It is preferable to anaesthetise the patient with a short-acting intravenous induction agent which causes minimal cardiac depression, such as methohexitone or etomidate, using a reduced dose as appropriate. Although diazepam causes relatively little cardiac depression and provides some amnesia, it is not an ideal induction agent. In normal circumstances the induction time may be up to 2 minutes but this may increase to 4–5 minutes when cardiac output is reduced. In this situation a reduced dose will be needed but it is very easy to get impatient and give an overdose in an effort to speed up induction. Diazepam has the disadvantage of having a long recovery time.

Intubation and severe head injuries

Except in cases of cardiorespiratory arrest, head injured patients should be anaesthetised using an appropriate induction agent and muscle relaxant before endotracheal intubation is performed. The temptation to see if an endotracheal tube will go down without any anaesthetic should be avoided whenever possible.

Intubation of a head-injured patient may be required if the patient is unconscious. It is mandatory for gunshot wounds of the head and it may also be required in the management of respiratory failure or convulsions, or to provide safe transfer to a neurosurgical unit. Such patients will have raised intracranial pressure and coning may be precipitated by hypoxia, hypercapnia, uncontrolled pain and overstimulation of the patient by rough pharyngeal suction or incompetent endotracheal intubation. The only way to reduce this risk during elective intubation is to use a neuroanaesthetic technique.

The patient is presumed to have a full stomach and thus suction, already switched on, must be at hand, and preoxygenation is performed. Although the patient is unconscious, it is assumed that the pharyngeal and laryngeal reflexes are still active and so an induction agent is required to depress these reflexes. Thiopentone

may be used for induction, with a reduced dose being given if the cardiac output is reduced, for example due to hypovolaemia. Cricoid pressure may raise the intracranial pressure, but is probably worthwhile because of the risk of aspiration. A short-acting muscle relaxant such as suxamethonium is given and intubation should not be attempted until the patient is totally relaxed. Once the airway is safely secured, a full dose of a long-acting muscle relaxant such as pancuronium is given. There is no place for waiting to confirm that the suxamethonium has worn off, since the associated straining could raise the intracranial pressure. Anaesthesia may be maintained with nitrous oxide, oxygen and increments of an intravenous analgesic such as morphine. (For further discussion of head injuries see Ch. 14.)

Sedation and anaesthesia for the patient in transit

Portable resuscitation equipment should be available throughout the journey. Analgesia must be given if the patient is conscious and in pain. Entonox (p. 103) could be used, but it creates difficulties of bulk and supply on a long journey. Prolonged use may also make the patient restless or confused. Incremental, low dose, intravenous morphine is probably the safest and most effective analgesic. An antiemetic should also be given. Naloxone should be available in case respiratory depression occurs. The effect of the chosen agent should always be assessed before the journey commences.

Patients who are intubated and receiving controlled ventilation should have a completely painfree and amnesic journey. An intravenous analgesic in an adequate dose may be given. Muscle relaxants will often be required and should only be given when the patient is neither in pain nor emotionally distressed. Ketamine may be of value in this situation since its dose/response relationship is predictable and its cardiovascular side-effects are minimal. Diazepam should not be used if the patient is in pain since it has no analgesic properties. It produces unpredictable sedation and cardiorespiratory effects.

Sedation using pethidine and diazepam

The use of intravenous diazepam and pethidine, either intravenously or intramuscularly, for procedures such as reducing dislocated shoulders is very popular. The combination aims to provide analgesia, sedation and perhaps some reduction in muscle spasm. However, it must be realised that if given in excess these are potent anaesthetic drugs. The dose of diazepam in particular may be difficult to judge. After intravenous injection the maximum effect of diazepam usually occurs after two minutes, but this time may be increased in the elderly or those with heart disease and it is tempting to give too much at this stage. The elderly show an increased sensitivity to diazepam and the dose should be reduced to half or a quarter of the normal adult dose. On the other hand, it is sometimes difficult to obtain the required effect with obese or very muscular patients. When using diazepam intravenously it is preferable to use the formulation in a lipid-water emulsion ('Diazemuls') as this reduces the incidence of pain and thrombophlebitis after injection. Supplementation with Entonox may help, but it is probably better to change to a more controlled anaesthetic sooner rather than later.

The patient having an emergency procedure is likely to have a full stomach and be at risk of vomiting and aspiration. Pethidine itself may cause vomiting and both diazepam and pethidine may cause depression of consciousness and respiration. The procedure must always be performed in a room with full resuscitation facilities and the patient must be on a trolley allowing head-down tilt. Appropriate postoperative observations should always be recorded and the advice about fitness for discharge home (p. 000) should be observed.

Children and general anaesthesia

General anaesthesia should only be administered to children by those who have had training in paediatric anaesthesia or are under the supervision of a trained person. Specially designed paediatric anaesthetic circuits are usually used. The child should be weighed and drug doses calculated carefully. Endotracheal intubation and venous access require extra expertise, particularly in the very young. Specialised nursing care is required, particularly during the immediate postoperative period where incorrect airway management could prove disastrous. In general hospitals which have isolated emergency theatres with very limited paediatric equipment, it is usually best to admit the child and operate in the theatre where routine paediatric lists are carried out.

Anaesthetic expertise

An experienced anaesthetist can offer assistance in the A & E department in a wide variety of ways including:
1. Administration of emergency anaesthetics.
2. Management of airway obstruction, e.g. facial trauma, epiglottitis, inhaled foreign bodies, burns.
3. Airway management during gastric lavage on an unconscious patient.
4. Management of chest injuries.
5. Management of head injuries.
6. Management of the unconscious patient.
7. Management of respiratory failure.
8. Problems with obtaining venous access.
9. Transfer of patient to a specialised unit, e.g. neurosurgery.
10. Admission to the intensive care unit.

LOCAL ANAESTHESIA

Local anaesthesia is the most common form of anaesthesia used in the A & E department. It is simple, cheap, relatively safe and it can usually be used in an unfasted patient. It is often the technique of choice for patients in poor general health. Many local anaesthetic techniques can be performed by adequately trained A & E doctors without needing an anaesthetist. However, local anaesthesia is not as reliable as general anaesthesia, particularly in obese patients. Operations may be restricted by the limited dose of local anaesthetic which may be used and some patients will not tolerate being awake for an operation.

Unfortunately, many doctors are unaware of the value of using local anaesthesia primarily as an analgesic. The use in prehospital care is discussed in Ch. 6.

Anyone giving local anaesthetics should know about the possible complications, how to minimise the risks and how to manage any problems that might occur.

Indications

1. Any situation where local anaesthesia will provide adequate operating conditions or satisfactory analgesia.
2. Previous reactions to general anaesthetic agents.
3. Patients with poor medical history, e.g. pulmonary disease.
4. Anticipated problems with maintaining the airway.

Contraindications

1. Refusal by patient.
2. Allergy to local anaesthetic.
3. Infection. Local anaesthetic should not be injected directly through infected tissue. However, it is possible to anaesthetise small abscesses by circumferential local infiltration without any adverse reaction or clinical sign of spread of infection.
4. Bleeding diathesis.
5. Anticoagulant therapy.

Special caution

1. Impaired cardiac conduction.
2. Low cardiac output states.
3. Hepatic impairment.
4. Epilepsy.
5. Extremes of age.
6. Debilitated patients.
7. Myasthenia gravis.
8. Neurological disease where an exacerbation may be blamed on the local anaesthetic.

Patients who are at greater risk of developing local anaesthetic toxicity require particular care in the choice of local anaesthetic and the type of block used. The dose of local anaesthetic should generally be reduced.

Factors affecting anaesthetic activity

Physicochemical properties

The potency, duration of anaesthesia and speed of onset of a local anaesthetic agent are related to the lipid solubility, degree of protein binding and pKa respectively. A comparison of the resulting pharmacological properties is shown in Table 9.1.

Table 9.1 Local anaesthetic agents

Local anaesthetic (amides)	Onset	Relative potency	Duration	Metabolism	Comments	Maximum dose mg/kg	
						Plain	With adrenaline
Lignocaine	Fast	2	Moderate	In liver	Most versatile agent	3.0	7.0
Prilocaine	Fast	2	Moderate	By plasma cholinesterase	Methaemoglobinaemia occurs at high doses (e.g. 600 mg in adult) Drug of choice for IVRA	3.0	7.0
Bupivacaine	Moderate	8	Long	In liver	Useful where prolonged anaesthesia required	2.0	2.0

Dose of local anaesthetic

The dose of drug given affects the onset, depth and duration of anaesthesia. Increasing the dose will generally shorten the time of onset, increase the depth of anaesthesia and prolong the action.

Addition of vasoconstrictor

A vasoconstrictor will reduce the rate of vascular absorption and thus prolong the duration and improve the depth of anaesthesia. Adrenaline is the commonly used vasoconstrictor with local anaesthetics and for infiltration and peripheral nerve blocks is best used in a concentration of 1:200 000. Its effects are sometimes modified by the local anaesthetic or type of block. Vasoconstrictors should never be used around end arteries.

Site of injection

The latent period (time before onset of anaesthesia) varies with different sites of injection. Local infiltration has the shortest latent period followed by minor nerve blocks, topical anaesthesia and then major nerve blocks, which have the longest latent period. Obviously, a poorly sited injection will increase the latent period. Injection into a vascular area will reduce the depth and duration of block, unless a vasoconstrictor is used, due to rapid absorption of the local anaesthetic.

Mixtures of local anaesthetics

These have no significant advantage over single drugs.

Differential blockade

Most peripheral nerves contain a mixture of autonomic, sensory and motor fibres. The sensory fibres carry the modalities of pain, temperature, touch and pressure. The extent and order in which these fibres are blocked depends on many factors. These include the type and dose of local anaesthetic, the type of nerve block and the time since injection. It is important for the patient to realise that sensations of pressure may still be felt even when a local anaesthetic block is providing adequate analgesia.

Local anaesthetics and vasoconstrictors

Vasoconstrictors are used to retard the absorption and reduce the toxicity of a local anaesthetic, so allowing a larger dose to be used safely. They also prolong anaesthesia and produce local ischaemia which is helpful in vascular areas such as the scalp.

Adrenaline

This is the most commonly used vasoconstrictor. For infiltration the optimal concentration is 1:200 000 (500 micrograms/100 ml) with a maximum dose of 500 micrograms of adrenaline.

Serious complications due to the use of adrenaline in surgical and local anaesthetic procedures are rare. They are more likely to occur when high concentrations are used. Intraosseous injections of small volumes of adrenaline 1:80 000 during dental procedures have been associated with a high incidence of tachycardia, palpitations and feelings of tightness in the chest. Inadvertent intravascular injection may also cause serious complications, especially tachycardia, dysrhythmias and hypertension.

It is wise to avoid the use of adrenaline in patients with cardiac disease. It should not be used in patients taking tricyclic and related antidepressants because of an increased risk of hypertension and dysrhythmias. Adrenaline should be used with caution in patients receiving certain inhalational anaesthetic agents such as halothane, enflurane, trichloroethylene and cyclopropane, as cardiac dysrhythmias may occur.

Management of adrenaline toxicity

This will depend upon the patient's haemodynamic state. Monitor the pulse, blood pressure and electrocardiogram. Oxygen and sublingual glyceryl trinitrate should be given to patients who develop angina. Beta-adrenergic blocking drugs may be useful for persistent tachycardia. Infusion of a short-acting vasodilator such as nitroprusside may control arterial pressure and allow rapid withdrawal of this therapy once the blood pressure falls. This treatment would require monitoring in an intensive care unit.

Adrenaline and local ischaemia

Adrenaline should never be injected around end arteries such as in fingers, toes, nose or penis, since this could cause irreversible ischaemia. This should be prevented by careful checking of ampoules and storing local anaesthetic solutions containing adrenaline in locked cupboards. If adrenaline is given around an end artery the patient should be admitted for observation and the consultant should be informed. Analgesia may be needed. Treatment such as anticoagulation with heparin, vasodilators and sympathetic blockade should be considered.

Complications

Local anaesthetic toxicity

Overt toxicity is seen most commonly following the accidental intravenous injection of local anaesthetic. Toxicity due to overdose is less common but does occur. This is more likely in situations where maximum safe doses are reduced such as the elderly, in liver and renal diseases. A bolus effect occurs when a large dose of drug is given over a short period of time. The factors affecting the initial high concentration may be described by the following relationship (Scott 1986):

$$\text{Peak plasma concentration} \propto \frac{\text{dose}}{\text{cardiac output} \times \text{speed of injection}}$$

This means that a severe reaction might be anticipated when a large dose is given very quickly to a person with a low cardiac output (e.g. elderly, hypovolaemic).

The main toxic effects are seen on the brain and heart.

Signs and symptoms of central nervous system toxicity

1. Numbness of the tongue and mouth (a local effect due to local anaesthetic leaving the vascular space and affecting sensory nerve endings)
2. Lightheadedness
3. Tinnitus
4. Visual disturbance
5. Slurring of speech
6. Muscle twitching
7. Confusion
8. Grand mal convulsion
9. Coma
10. Apnoea.

It should not be assumed that the patient will demonstrate all these stages. The first sign of toxicity may be immediate convulsions, or they may not occur until 1–2 minutes after completion of the injection.

Provided local anaesthetics are injected slowly and the doctor maintains a continuous dialogue with the patient, early signs of toxicity should not be missed. Irrational behaviour may have to be distinguished from neurotic or hysterical reactions. Muscle twitching may be caused by shivering due to nervousness or cold. Fainting is also quite common during local anaesthetic procedures. The presence of cardiovascular signs may help to make the correct diagnosis.

Signs of cardiovascular toxicity

1. Bradycardia
2. Hypotension
3. ECG changes: prolonged PR interval and widened QRS, AV block, cardiac dysrhythmias of re-entrant type
4. Cardiac arrest.

Treatment

Toxic reactions are potentiated by hypoxia and acidosis. It is essential to maintain adequate ventilation and thus prevent hypoxia and respiratory acidosis.

Central nervous system toxicity. Place the unconscious patient in the coma position. Give oxygen by face mask or ventilate the patient if apnoea occurs. If convulsions do not stop within 15–30 seconds an anticonvulsant drug should be given.

The drugs of choice are:
Diazepam 5–10 mg i.v. slowly (0.1–0.2 mg/kg)
Paraldehyde 10 ml i.m.
Thiopentone 150–200 mg i.v. slowly (1–2 mg/kg)

Diazepam is the drug of choice for those not trained in the use of thiopentone. However, thiopentone is probably the best drug in this situation because of its rapid effect and short duration of action. In the absence of a massive overdose the convulsions do not last longer than a few minutes and seldom recur when the anticonvulsant has stopped them. After thiopentone the patient will be awake and rational within a few minutes.

Cardiovascular toxicity. 1. Hypotension: Give oxygen by face mask. Elevate the legs. Monitor the blood pressure. If the systolic blood pressure is less than 90 mm Hg in an adult give 500 ml of plasma expander (e.g. polygeline). This may be repeated if the hypotension persists. In a child treat if the systolic blood pressure falls below 70 mm Hg giving an initial bolus of 20 ml/kg of plasma expander.

2. Cardiac dysrhythmias: Give oxygen by face mask. Monitor the pulse and blood pressure. The dysrhythmia may resolve spontaneously and treatment should be reserved for cases where cardiac output is severely reduced. Atropine may be of value for bradycardia with severe hypotension. Cardiac pacing may be required for complete heart block. Bretylium may be of value in treating ventricular fibrillation unresponsive to DC shock.

Correct any concomitant hyperkalaemia which potentiates the cardiotoxic effects.

3. Cardiac arrest: see Ch. 10.

Serious toxicity from local anaesthetics is usually preventable. The maximum safe dose should always be known (Tables 9.2, 9.3) and the emphasis should be on scrupulous local anaesthetic techniques.

Allergic reactions

Allergic reactions to local anaesthetic agents are rare, but both local and systemic reactions may occur. They need to be distinguished

Table 9.2 Maximum dose of lignocaine for 70 kg man

Concentration	ml
Without adrenaline: 200 mg lignocaine i.e.	
0.5%	40
1.0%	20
2.0%	10
4.0%	5
With adrenaline: 500 mg lignocaine i.e.	
0.5%	100
1.0%	50
2.0%	25

Table 9.3 Maximum dose of lignocaine in children

Age	Average weight kg	1% lignocaine without adrenaline ml	1% lignocaine with adrenaline ml
6 months	7.5	2.0	5.0
1 year	10.0	3.0	7.0
3 years	14.5	4.0	10.0
5 years	18.0	5.0	12.0
7 years	23.0	7.0	16.0
10 years	30.0	9.0	21.0
12 years	40.0	12.0	28.0

from anxiety, simple fainting, systemic toxicity or reactions to adrenaline.

The ester group of local anaesthetics (e.g. procaine, amethocaine) are much more likely to produce allergic reactions than the amide group (e.g. lignocaine, bupivacaine, prilocaine). Patients who are allergic to one ester are likely to show cross-sensitivity with the whole group, but not to the amides. Patients who are allergic to an amide may not react to other amides or to esters. Testing for hypersensitivity with small doses has not proved reliable.

Multidose vials of both types usually contain the preservative methylparabens. This may be responsible for allergic reactions to local anaesthetics and other drug preparations. (For further discussion of anaphylaxis see Ch. 13.)

Nerve and muscle damage

The risk of nerve damage may be increased in the presence of pre-existing neurological disorders or systemic disease (e.g. diabetes mellitus).

1. Faulty positioning of the patient. Nerves may be damaged when they are stretched or compressed by equipment, e.g. tourniquets, arm rests, retractors or simply the position itself.

2. Surgical trauma. This may cause division, compression, stretching or ischaemic damage to nerves. Traumatic damage can be reduced by using needles with a short bevel. Deliberately eliciting paraesthesia will increase the risk of traumatic neuropathy and should be performed gently. If paraesthesia occurs the needle should always be withdrawn slightly before injection, which should be done slowly and stopped immediately if pain is felt.

Needle breakage

This is most likely to occur where the needle joins the hub. A needle of sufficient length should always be used and it should never be inserted up to the hub. Redirecting the needle may also cause the needle to break. Always withdraw the needle sufficiently so that minimal leverage is applied to the shaft.

Infection, haematoma and necrosis

A variety of local complications may occur. Possible sources of infection include contaminated equipment or local spread from the patient. Necrosis and gangrene may occur after the incorrect use of a vasoconstrictor, especially around an end artery. Haematoma formation is probably quite common but usually causes little additional discomfort. Bleeding can usually be controlled by direct pressure.

Local and systemic reactions to adrenaline

See the section on vasoconstrictors (p. 89).

Psychogenic reactions

Pain and fear can give rise to reflex vasomotor disturbances. Pallor, nausea, sweating and hypotension causing syncope may occur. These reactions are more common if the patient is sitting up. Cerebral hypoxia with loss of consciousness and tremors or convulsions may occur before the patient can be laid horizontal. Oxygen should be given by face mask and the patient's legs elevated.

Failed nerve block

Always believe the patient who says he can feel pain despite the presence of an apparently satisfactory nerve block.

There is usually a fault in technique due to:
1. Failing to wait long enough for the block to work
2. Waiting until the block has started to wear off
3. Using the wrong dose or volume of local anaesthetic
4. Injecting the local anaesthetic inaccurately.

Procedure for failed nerve block

Check the time of injection: it may be that the block has not had time to work or has worn off. Next check the amount of drug given and whether this is less than the maximum dose and volume (Tables 9.2, 9.3). If the injection was made at the correct site it is acceptable to repeat it giving half the initial dose, as long as the maximum dose or volume is not exceeded. Sometimes it is difficult to locate the nerve, particularly in an obese patient. In this case consider starting the procedure again or use a more proximal block, but only if the maximum dose is not exceeded. Once this amount has been reached 8 hours must elapse before any more drug may be given. It is often possible to obtain good analgesia by supplementing an incomplete nerve block with Entonox (p. 103). Occasionally it will be necessary to resort to a general anaesthetic, in which case the operation may need postponing until the patient is fasted.

If the block is beginning to wear off before the operation is completed a 'top up dose' of half the original amount may be given, provided the maximum dose or volume is not exceeded.

Local anaesthesia and children

Some doctors avoid using local anaesthesia in young children due to problems in obtaining the child's co-operation. It is certainly true that local anaesthesia should not be used without the correct indications and environment, but there are certain situations where the technique may be of value even in small children. The most compelling situation is the use of a femoral nerve block to provide analgesia for a fractured shaft of femur (p. 97). This commonly occurs after a road traffic accident and there may be an associated head injury. The management of the head injury is facilitated by the safe and effective analgesia given by the femoral nerve block.

Local anaesthetic techniques should only be performed in children by experienced doctors, ideally with an experienced nurse assisting. The confidence and co-operation of the patient and accompanying adult are vital. The procedure should be explained simply and honestly. There is no point saying something will not hurt if it will. Preconditioning with tales from friends or parents may make explanation and acceptance more difficult. If satisfactory conditions cannot be obtained and an anaesthetic is required, then a general anaesthetic would be the method of choice.

There is little information regarding the pharmacology and pharmacokinetics of local anaesthetic agents in children. Most information has been extrapolated from work done in adults. Toxicity of local anaesthetics is limited by their metabolism. The amide type are metabolised by hepatic microsomal enzymes. In early childhood, once these enzymes are fully developed, this metabolism is proportionally greater due to the relative size of the liver and thus much larger doses are tolerated. Higher maximum safe doses of local anaesthetic agents for children compared with adults have been quoted (Arthur & Nicol 1986). However, for standard local anaesthetic techniques used in an A & E department it is probably safer having one dose range for the whole of the population (Tables 9.2, 9.3). It is important to calculate accurately the dose and volume of drug to be used and check these do not exceed the maximum dose. Any necessary emergency drugs should also be immediately available and the doses known (Ch. 10). All the drugs and equipment must be prepared before the child is brought into the room and kept out of view.

Local anaesthesia is rarely used in some paediatric A & E departments. This is partly due to the ease of obtaining a general anaesthetic but also because of expertise in treating conditions without the need for any anaesthetic. The most obvious example is the widespread use of adhesive skin closure (e.g. Steristrips) to close wounds which in some departments would be sutured under local anaesthesia. However, in some cases local anaesthesia will still be required to enable adequate wound toilet.

General principles of local anaesthetic techniques

Always obtain a brief medical history and record medication and drug allergies. Explain the procedures simply to the patient. Tell the patient that the initial injection may be uncomfortable, but that once the local anaesthetic is working there should be no pain, although sensations such as pressure may be experienced. Outline the anticipated distribution of sensory block. Patients often expect a very large area to be anaesthetised and get worried if they have normal sensation near the site of operation.

Choose the appropriate drug and decide whether adrenaline is necessary. If adrenaline is contraindicated double check the drug label before drawing up the solution. (Some multidose vials are remarkably badly labelled.) Carefully calculate the maximum dose of local anaesthetic which may be given (Tables 9.2, 9.3 and Fig. 9.2) and then the amount actually to be used. Check that this does not exceed the maximum safe volume.

Before starting the procedure check all the necessary apparatus. Know what to do if a vessel is punctured, the block fails, or if there is a toxic or anaphylactic reaction (p. 90).

Clean the skin and note the time of injection. Inject slowly and aspirate frequently to prevent intravascular injection. Resistance to injection may be due to periosteum, tendon sheath or nerve and the needle should be repositioned. Estimate when the block should be working and only then test sensation. Testing before the block has had a chance to work will only damage the patient's confidence. It is often useful, where possible, to let the patient check for himself that the block is working. A needle is commonly used to confirm analgesia, but always distract the patient whilst this is being done. Many people, in particular children, will complain of pain while watching a needle being stuck into the skin despite there being a good block. Again, never ask the patient if he feels pain when the operation commences, he invariably will, and it will be perfectly apparent anyway if the block is not working.

Decide whether the patient will need analgesia after the operation and, if so, give the first dose before the block has worn off.

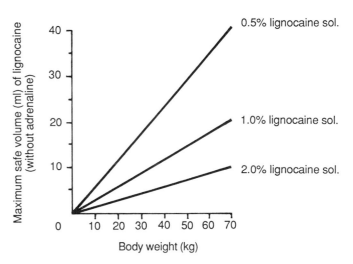

Fig. 9.2 Local anaesthetic dosage chart.

Always write complete, legible and concise notes on the anaesthetic procedure, no matter how simple it may be.

LOCAL ANAESTHETIC TECHNIQUES

This section contains a selection of local anaesthetic techniques which would be used routinely by A & E doctors after appropriate training. Other techniques, such as nerve plexus blocks, may also be useful but are usually done by anaesthetists. The doses quoted are for adults.

Local infiltration of the skin (Fig. 9.3)

Indications

1. Suturing lacerations
2. Minor surgical procedures, e.g. excision of cyst
3. Supplementing a nerve block
4. Cleaning and debriding wounds.

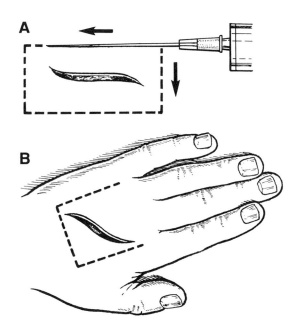

Fig. 9.3 Local infiltration of the skin.

Anatomy

Distal nerve endings and filaments are blocked at the operative site.

Dose

Up to 20 ml of 1% lignocaine or 40 ml of 0.5% lignocaine, with or without adrenaline.

Technique

Using a 23G (0.6 mm) or 25G (0.5 mm) needle, inject the local anaesthetic subcutaneously around the area to be treated. If a second puncture is required, always reintroduce the needle through anaesthetised skin. The patient should feel only one injection.

Onset and duration

Commences after 2 minutes and lasts up to 45 minutes depending on whether a vasoconstrictor is used.

Important aspects

1. NEVER use a vasoconstrictor near end arteries, e.g. finger, toe, penis, nose.
2. When the nerve supply to an area comes from one side, this alone need be blocked, e.g. dorsum of hand.
3. When using large volumes of local anaesthetic ensure that the maximum doses of anaesthetic and adrenaline are not exceeded.
4. Injection of local anaesthetic through a wound edge is less painful and thus may be indicated in children. It may introduce infection directly into the wound and should not be used if the wound is contaminated.

Digital nerve block (at base of digit) (Fig. 9.4)

Indications

Simple operations on fingers or toes.

Anatomy

A dorsal and palmar (plantar) nerve run along each side of the digit.

Dose

2–5 ml of 1% plain lignocaine.

Technique

Using a 23G (0.6 mm) needle, approach the nerves from the dorsal aspect of the base of the digit. Inject 1–1.5 ml of 1% plain lignocaine around each palmar digital nerve and then 1–1.5 ml across the dorsum of the digit to block the dorsal branches. Do not attempt to identify the nerve by eliciting paraesthesia since the small nerve may be damaged.

Onset and duration

Commences after 2–5 minutes and lasts 45 minutes to 1 hour.

Important aspects

1. NEVER use a vasoconstrictor.
2. Some people call this technique a 'ring block', implying that the local anaesthetic is put all around the digit and not specifically by the digital nerve. Such a method should be avoided since the

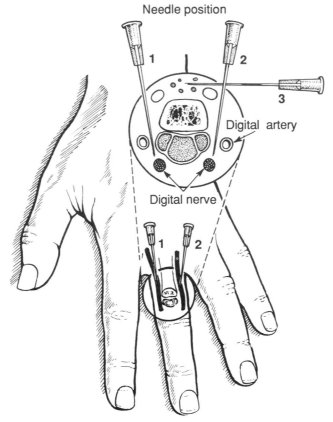

Fig. 9.4 Digital nerve block (at base of digit).

use of large volumes of local anaesthetic in a confined space may produce vascular insufficiency.

3. The maximum volume of local anaesthetic which should be used at the base of a digit is 5 ml. This should be reduced in small digits, e.g. toes, children.

Digital nerve block (at metacarpal level) (Fig. 9.5)

Indications

1. Analgesia for injured fingers.
2. Simple operations on fingers.

Anatomy

The digital nerves are formed from the median and ulnar nerves

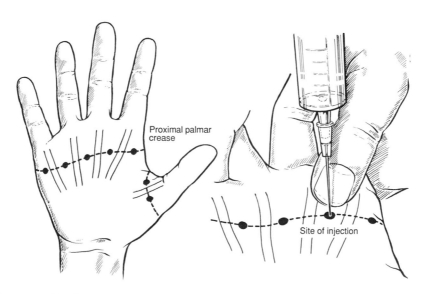

Fig. 9.5 Digital nerve block (at metacarpal level).

in the proximal palm and pass distally between the flexor tendons lying on the lumbrical muscles.

Dose

5–7 ml of 1% plain lignocaine.

Technique

Use a 23G (0.6 mm) needle. The digital nerves lie about 0.5 cm deep to the distal palmar crease and can be blocked at this level with 1.5–2 ml of 1% plain lignocaine. Do not attempt to elicit paraesthesia. The digital nerve on either side of the appropriate metacarpal should be blocked. 1–2 ml of 1% plain lignocaine may be infiltrated over the dorsum of the metacarpal spaces to block small dorsal nerves.

Onset and duration

Commences after 2–5 minutes and lasts 45 minutes to 1 hour.

Important aspects

1. NEVER use a vasoconstrictor.
2. A block at this level usually catches the digital nerve to the adjacent finger. This may be of value if more than one finger requires treatment.
3. A dorsal approach for this technique may be used instead, but there is an increased risk of venepuncture. The digital nerves lie deep and may be difficult to block. The dorsal approach is said to be less painful than the palmar one but if the needle is introduced through the palmar crease discomfort appears to be minimal.
4. A digital nerve block may be achieved by injecting 2–3 ml local anaesthetic into the appropriate web space.

Median nerve block (Figs. 9.6, 9.7)

Indications

Minor surgery to the areas of the hand innervated by the median nerve.

Anatomy

At the level of the proximal skin crease of the wrist the median nerve lies superficially either just below or radial to the tendon of palmaris longus. If this is missing the nerve is found just medial to flexor carpi radialis.

Dose

4–7 ml of 1% lignocaine with or without adrenaline.

Technique

Insert a 23G (0.6 mm) or 25G (0.5 mm) needle at right angles to the skin at the proximal skin crease of the wrist between the tendons of palmaris longus and flexor carpi radialis. Landmarks are more easily identified by flexing the wrist. Move the needle fanwise up and down in a plane at right angles to the long axis of the forearm until paraesthesia is elicited. Withdraw the needle slightly and slowly inject 2–4 ml of 1% lignocaine, with or without adrenaline, and a further 2 ml subcutaneously. If paraesthesia is not elicited, 5–10 ml of 1% lignocaine with or without adrenaline, may be injected slowly in the area where the median nerve is thought to lie.

Onset and duration

Commences after 5–10 minutes and lasts up to 1.5 hours.

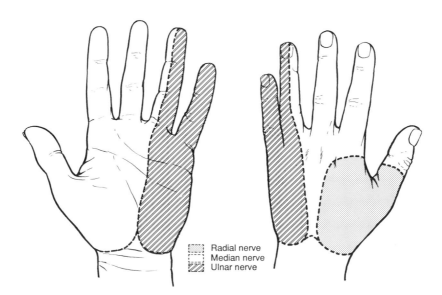

Radial nerve
Median nerve
Ulnar nerve

Fig. 9.6 Cutaneous distribution of peripheral nerves to the hand.

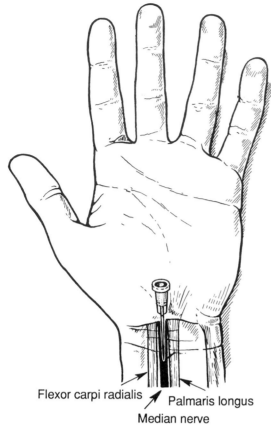

Fig. 9.7 Median nerve block.

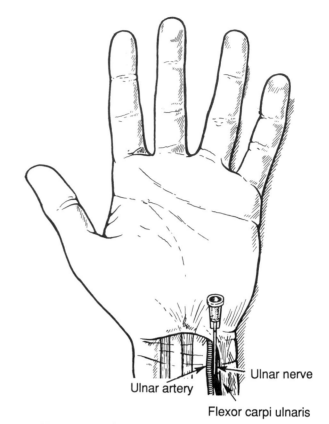

Fig. 9.8 Ulnar nerve block.

Important aspects

Do not use this block if there is a history of carpal tunnel syndrome.

Ulnar nerve block (at the wrist) (Figs. 9.6, 9.8, 9.9)

Indications

1. Minor surgery to areas of the hand innervated by the ulnar nerve.
2. Closed manipulation of fracture, e.g. displaced fracture of neck of 5th metacarpal.

Anatomy

In the distal forearm the ulnar artery is immediately lateral to the nerve. About 5 cm proximal to the wrist the ulnar nerve divides into a dorsal and a palmar branch whilst lateral to the flexor carpi ulnaris. The dorsal branch is purely sensory and proceeds dorsally under flexor carpi ulnaris. The palmar branch is mixed and continues distally alongside the tendon of flexor carpi ulnaris.

Dose

1. Palmar branch: 2–4 ml of 1% lignocaine, with or without adrenaline.
2. Dorsal branch: 5 ml lignocaine, preferably with adrenaline.

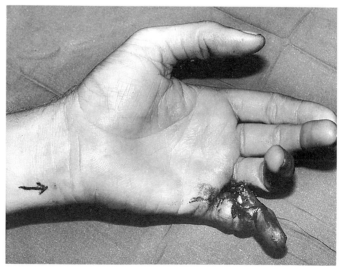

Fig. 9.9 Compound fracture of little finger treated under ulnar nerve block (Site of injection of local anaesthetic is marked.)

Technique

The palmar branch is blocked on a level with the ulnar styloid process. Insert a 23G (0.6 mm) or 25G (0.5 mm) needle at right angles to the skin between the lateral aspect of flexor carpi ulnaris and the medial side of the ulnar artery. Flexion of the wrist helps to identify landmarks. If paraesthesia is elicited withdraw the needle slightly and inject 2–4 ml of 1% lignocaine, with or without adrenaline. If no paraesthesia is elicited insert the needle to the deep fascia and then inject 5–10 ml of 1% lignocaine, with or without adrenaline, whilst withdrawing the needle to the skin.

The dorsal branch may be blocked by a subcutaneous infiltration of 5 ml of 1% lignocaine with adrenaline extending from the tendon of flexor carpi ulnaris around the ulnar aspect of the wrist.

Onset and duration

1. Palmar branch: commences after 5–10 minutes and lasts up to 1.5 hours.
2. Dorsal branch: commences after 2 minutes and lasts up to 45 minutes.

Important aspects

1. The presence of a radial pulse at the wrist should be confirmed before using a vasoconstrictor next to the ulnar artery on the same side.
2. When performing the palmar branch block, a vasoconstrictor should not be used if there is a history of peripheral vascular disease.
3. Since the dorsal branch block has a much shorter time of onset and duration of action it should only be performed once the palmar block is working.

Radial nerve block (Figs. 9.6, 9.10)

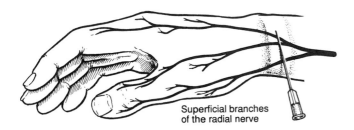

Fig. 9.10 Radial nerve block.

Indications

Minor surgery to areas of the hand innervated by the radial nerve.

Anatomy

The superficial branches of the radial nerve pass under bracheoradialis in the distal half of the forearm and come to lie subcutaneously on the extensor aspect of the forearm at the level of the wrist. Here they divide to supply the dorsal aspect of the hand.

Dose

5 ml of 0.5% or 1% lignocaine, preferably with adrenaline.

Technique

Using 5 ml of 0.5% or 1% lignocaine with adrenaline, raise a subcutaneous ring starting at the level of the tendon of flexor carpi radialis and extending around the radial border of the wrist to the dorsal aspect of the ulnar styloid.

Onset and duration

Commences after 2 minutes and lasts up to 1 hour.

Important aspects

1. The area to be infiltrated has a prominent venous network and care must be taken to avoid venepuncture or intravenous injection.
2. The area of infiltration should never extend around the whole of the wrist as mechanical occlusion could cause marked venous stasis.

Combined nerve blocks at the wrist

These are very useful for minor operations to the hand, such as suturing lacerations of the palm, or closed reductions, such as a dislocation of the 1st metacarpophalangeal joint (Fig. 9.11). The radial block has a much shorter onset and duration of action than the ulnar and median nerve blocks, and when used in combination, should only be performed after these are working.

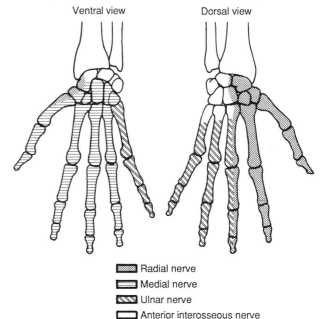

Fig. 9.11 Peripheral nerves supplying bones of the hand.

Femoral nerve block (Fig. 9.12)

Indications

1. Analgesia for a fractured shaft of femur.
2. Analgesia for a fractured patella.
3. Reducing quadriceps spasm.
4. Applying skin traction.
5. Anaesthetising donor area for skin graft (often in combination with a block of the lateral cutaneous nerve of the thigh, see below).

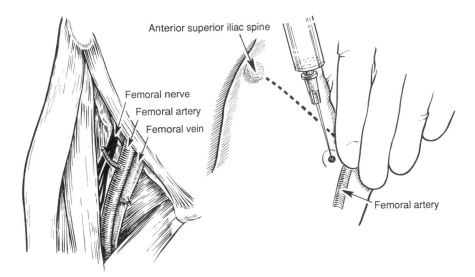

Fig. 9.12 Femoral nerve block.

Anatomy

The femoral nerve passes under the inguinal ligament to enter the thigh where it lies lateral to the femoral artery.

Dose

10–15 ml of 1% lignocaine with or without adrenaline.

Technique

The femoral artery is palpated and a 21G (0.8 mm) or 23G (0.6 mm) needle, at least 4 cm long, is inserted perpendicular to the skin and just lateral to the artery as it emerges under the inguinal ligament. If paraesthesia is elicited, 10 ml of 1% lignocaine with adrenaline is injected after withdrawing the needle slightly. Otherwise 10–15 ml of 1% lignocaine with adrenaline is injected whilst the needle is moved from a depth of 4 cm up and down gradually moving laterally to about 3 cm from the artery.

Onset and duration

Commences after 5–15 minutes and lasts up to 1.5 hours, or longer if adrenaline is used.

Important aspects

1. This technique uses a large dose of lignocaine and thus care must be taken to ensure the maximum dose is not exceeded (Tables 9.2, 9.3).

2. Bupivacaine is a useful alternative to plain lignocaine since it has a longer duration of action.

3. If the femoral artery is punctured compress it for 5–10 minutes then continue with the procedure if necessary.

4. This techniques is ideal for providing analgesia in children and adults for a fractured shaft of femur. It is most effective for middle third fractures. Analgesia may be less good for distal third fractures and the block is least effective for fractures of the upper third.

5. This block is usually easy to perform except in situations where the femoral artery is difficult to palpate, such as in the obese or those with peripheral vascular disease.

6. A paravascular approach for the femoral nerve is described which blocks the femoral, obturator and lateral cutaneous nerve of the thigh. The femoral nerve is located under the inguinal ligament and then 20 ml of local anaesthetic is injected whilst applying pressure immediately distal to the needle to force the solution proximally to the lumbar plexus. The needle must lie within the fascial compartment containing the plexus and this can only be guaranteed by eliciting paraesthesia. The needle should be of adequate length, at least 7 cm long, and use of an extension set will help immobilise the needle (Winnie 1973).

Tibial nerve block (Figs. 9.13, 9.14, 9.15)

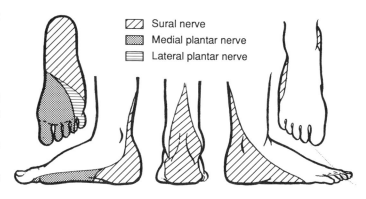

Fig. 9.13 Cutaneous distribution of peripheral nerves to the foot.

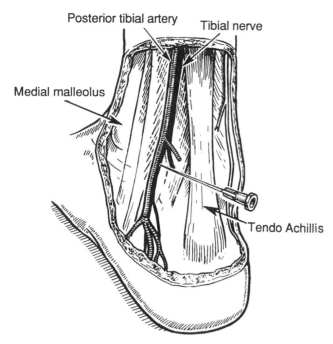

Fig. 9.14 Tibial nerve block.

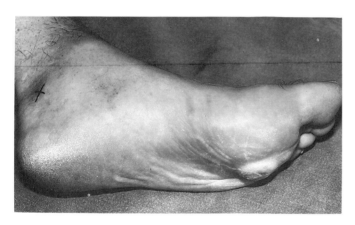

Fig. 9.15 Plantar abscess drained under tibial nerve block (Site of injection of local anaesthetic is marked.)

Indications

Minor operations to the part of the sole of the foot innervated by the tibial nerve.

Anatomy

The tibial nerve approaches the ankle at the medial border of the tendo Achillis. Here it lies behind the posterior tibial artery and between the tendons of flexor digitorum longus and flexor hallucis longus, covered by the flexor retinaculum. It divides at the back of the medial malleolus into the medial and lateral plantar nerves which supply the sole of the foot. A small branch supplies the medial aspect of the heel.

Dose

5–12 ml of 0.5% or 1% lignocaine with or without adrenaline.

Technique

The patient should lie prone with the ankles supported by a pillow. A small weal is raised at a level with the upper border of the medial malleolus either just lateral to the posterior tibial artery or, if this is impalpable, immediately lateral to the tendo Achillis. A fine gauge 6 cm long needle is inserted just lateral to the posterior tibial artery and at right angles to the back of the tibia. Movement of the needle in a mediolateral direction may elicit paraesthesia in which case the needle is withdrawn slightly and 5–8 ml of 0.5% or 1% lignocaine, with or without adrenaline is injected slowly. If paraesthesia is not elicited, 10–12 ml solution may be injected at the posterior aspect of the tibia whilst withdrawing the needle 1 cm.

Onset and duration

Commences 5–10 minutes (up to 30 minutes if paraesthesia is not elicited) and lasts up to 1.5 hours.

Important aspects

1. Lignocaine without a vasoconstrictor should be used if the patient has peripheral vascular disease.
2. Some patients cannot tolerate lying prone. In such cases it is possible, with careful positioning and identification of landmarks, to perform the block with the patient on his side.
3. This block is useful since it avoids the need for painful injections into the sole.

Sural nerve block (Figs. 9.13, 9.16)

Indications

Minor operations to the part of the sole of the foot innervated by the sural nerve.

Anatomy

The sural nerve proceeds with the saphenous vein behind and below the lateral malleolus to supply the outer margin of the foot.

Dose

5–8 ml of 0.5% or 1% lignocaine with adrenaline.

Technique

Using 5–8 ml of 0.5% or 1% lignocaine with adrenaline, infiltrate the subcutaneous tissue between the lateral malleolus and the tendo Achillis.

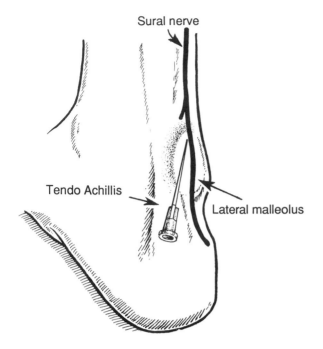

Fig. 9.16 Sural nerve block.

Onset and duration

Commences after 2 minutes and lasts up to 1 hour.

Important aspects

Care should be taken to avoid venepuncture of the prominent venous system in this area.

Combined nerve blocks at ankle

Tibial and sural nerve blocks are often required for operations on the sole of the foot. The sural nerve block has a shorter onset and duration of action than the tibial nerve block and should be performed once the tibial nerve block is working.

Superficial peroneal, deep peroneal and saphenous nerve blocks are occasionally of value (Eriksson 1979).

Supraorbital and supratrochlear nerve block (Fig. 9.17)

Indications

Minor surgical procedures on the forehead.

Anatomy

The supraorbital nerve forms two branches which leave the orbit through two holes or notches on the upper border of the orbit about 2.5 cm from the midline.

The supratrochlear nerve leaves the orbit medial to the supraorbital nerve.

Dose

3–6 ml of 1% lignocaine, with or without adrenaline.

Technique

Raise a weal over the root of the nose and then advance a 23G (0.6 mm) or 25G (0.5 mm) needle along the upper border of the eyebrow and inject 3–6 ml of 1% lignocaine, with or without adrenaline.

Onset and duration

Commences within 2 minutes and lasts up to 1 hour depending on whether a vasoconstrictor is used.

Important aspects

The lateral extremes of the forehead may be outside the field of this block, in which case supplementary local infiltration may be used.

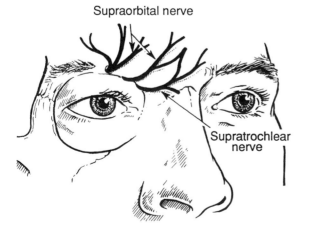
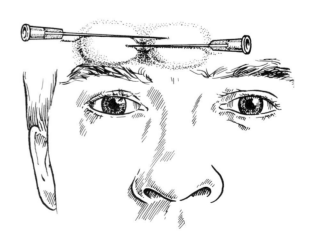

Fig. 9.17 Supraorbital and supratrochlear field block.

Intravenous regional anaesthesia (IVRA), Bier's block

Indications

1. Operations on the hand or forearm.
2. Reducing fractures below the elbow.

Contraindications

1. Known sensitivity to local anaesthetic agents
2. Peripheral vascular disease, including Raynaud's disease and scleroderma
3. Sickle cell disease or trait
4. Poor co-operation of patient
5. Children under 7 years old
6. Procedures exceeding 1 hour
7. Cellulitis
8. Operations on blood vessels
9. Inadequate equipment.

Special caution

1. Children
2. Elderly
3. Very thin patients
4. Obese or very muscular patients
5. Hypertension
6. Patients with a history of allergy, epilepsy or heart disease
7. Neuropathy (where anaesthetic may be blamed for a deterioration in the condition).

Anatomy

The local anaesthetic diffuses from the veins and acts on the peripheral nerve endings and nerve trunks.

Dose

0.5% plain prilocaine, 3 mg/kg.
Precalculated volumes based on above dose (Wallace 1982):

	(0.5% plain prilocaine)
Adult	40 ml
Very thin or elderly	30 ml
Adolescents (14–17 years)	30 ml
Children (11–13 years)	20 ml
Children (7–10 years)	15 ml

Equipment

1. Full monitoring and resuscitation equipment should be immediately available.
2. A specially designed tourniquet with a 15 cm wide cuff (for adults) and locking device to prevent accidental release of the cuff should be used, together with an efficient means of inflating the cuff, e.g. a bicycle pump (not a sphygmomanometer bulb). The manometer must be accurate.
3. All equipment must have frequent maintenance checks.

Technique

1. The patient should have a full preoperative assessment. Ideally, the patient should be fasted for 4 hours prior to the procedure.
2. Fully expose the arm to be operated on and apply the tourniquet to the upper arm over some padding. Identify the radial pulse.
3. Insert a 'butterfly' cannula into a vein on the dorsum of the hand on the affected side.
4. Insert a venous cannula in the other arm.
5. Elevate the affected arm for 3 minutes to drain the veins. (An Esmarch bandage or inflatable splint could be used instead if they did not cause any discomfort.)
6. With the arm still elevated inflate the tourniquet to 300 mmHg, or in hypertensive patients 100 mm Hg above the systolic pressure. Record the inflation time.
7. Check that the radial pulse is no longer palpable.
8. Lower the arm. With the arm resting comfortably slowly inject the calculated volume of 0.5% plain prilocaine (taking about 90 seconds). Record the time of injection.
9. Test for anaesthesia after 5 minutes. Remove the 'butterfly' needle when anaesthesia is established.
10. The cuff pressure must be continuously monitored. The cuff must not be deflated until at least 20 minutes after the injection to ensure the prilocaine is fully tissue bound and it must not be inflated for more than 1 hour. Record the deflation time.

Onset and duration

Commences after 2 minutes and lasts up to 2 hours.

Important aspects

1. IVRA has been associated with at least 7 deaths, 2 cardiopulmonary arrests, 10 generalised convulsions and many milder toxic symptoms. Unintentional leakage under the tourniquet appears to be an important factor in many of these cases. This can be reduced by using a wide cuff, exsanguinating the arm as efficiently as possible, using the correct cuff pressure and injecting the local anaesthetic slowly into a distal vein.

Other avoidable factors contributing to complications include the lack of immediately available monitoring and resuscitation equipment. Failure to notice, or satisfactorily manage, unexpected complications may also occur if the operator is inexperienced or operating alone.

2. Prilocaine has remained free from reported major side effects during its use in IVRA and is thus the drug of choice. The use of bupivacaine appears in many articles, but it has been associated with a small number of severe reactions, including 4 deaths. Although there was no direct evidence to indicate that its use affected the outome, the indication for use in IVRA was voluntarily withdrawn.

3. Some believe it is always advisable to use the minimum effective dose, e.g. 20 ml of 0.5% prilocaine for most adults. In this case, it may be necessary to give a further 10 ml of local

anaesthetic if anaesthesia has not occurred 5 minutes after the initial injection.

4. Double cuffs were designed so that a cuff could be inflated over anaesthetised skin. However, they cannot be relied upon to prevent leakage and should not be used.

5. If the cuff is accidently deflated within the first 20 minutes immediately reflate it. If this is not possible apply an ordinary cuff proximal to it and inflate this to the required pressure. Monitor and be prepared to treat any toxic reactions. It may be possible to complete simple procedures, e.g. reduction of Colles' fracture, with the analgesia already established, but this should not be done at the expense of more urgent resuscitation procedures.

6. Some recommend that on deflating the cuff it should be immediately reflated and then deflated again after 2 minutes in order to bind unbound drug and reduce the plasma concentrations which result.

7. Peak plasma concentrations of local anaesthetic after tourniquet release are lower when the tourniquet inflation time is prolonged, low concentrations of drugs are used and muscle activity in the limb is avoided after cuff deflation.

8. There is commonly some reactionary swelling after IVRA and thus it is advisable, when immobilising fractures, to apply only plaster back-slabs which can be completed when the swelling has subsided.

9. Inadequate analgesia may occur in 7% to 15% of cases. These are commonly due to poor technique such as injecting the local anaesthetic into a proximal forearm vein.

10. The Casualty Surgeons' Association has published a code of practice on the use of IVRA.

TOPICAL ANAESTHESIA

This is used most commonly in the A & E department for procedures on the eye (see Ch. 43). It is also used during urethral catheterisation (see Ch. 23), ENT procedures (see Ch. 44) and occasionally endotracheal intubation. Topical anaesthesia is sometimes used while cleaning dirty abrasions, such as gravel burns, but the analgesia is often inadequate and thorough cleaning is impossible. In such circumstances other means of anaesthesia should be used, with a general anaesthetic if necessary.

Topical anaesthesia requires high concentrations of local anaesthetic (e.g. 4% lignocaine) and it is essential to ensure that the maximum dose is not exceeded (Table 9.2). Adequate time must also be given for the anaesthetic to work, since absorption is often quite slow.

Infiltration of fracture haematoma

Indications

1. NOT for routine use.
2. Reduction of wrist fractures in a mass casualty situation.

Anatomy

Nerves supplying the surrounding soft tissue, periosteum and bone are blocked by local infiltration.

Dose

15 ml of 1% plain prilocaine or lignocaine.

Technique

A 23G (0.6 mm) needle is introduced into the fracture haematoma and its position confirmed by the aspiration of blood. The local anaesthetic solution is injected very slowly, since rapid injection is painful.

Onset and duration

Commences after 5 minutes and lasts up to 1 hour.

Important aspects

1. The technique converts a closed fracture into an open fracture and is thus contraindicated when the skin is dirty or other circumstances prevent complete asepsis.
2. NEVER use a vasoconstrictor.
3. Analgesia by this method is often barely adequate.
4. It is difficult to tell whether aspirated blood is, in fact, coming from a punctured vein, thus always be alert for the signs of toxicity (see p. 90).
5. Rapid absorption of local anaesthetic from the haematoma may cause toxicity.
6. Haematoma reorganisation will prevent the spread of local anaesthetic, thus the technique should not be used in fractures over 24 hours old.

Ethyl chloride

This is stored under pressure as a liquid in glass containers. It is highly inflammable. Local analgesia is obtained by spraying the liquid onto the skin where it vapourises causing a localised area of skin to be rapidly cooled. In the past it was used to provide analgesia for minor surgical procedures such as incision of a small abscess. However, it does not provide adequate analgesia for definitive treatment and should not be used for this purpose.

PAIN CONTROL

Most patients who attend A & E departments are suffering from pain. This pain may be very distressing, not only for the patient but also for the relatives and staff.

Pain may present acutely as in a myocardial infarction or may be chronic as in many lower back problems. Occasionally pain may form part of an intricate web of family, social, personal or other problems and a specific organic cause is sometimes difficult to find. It may be considered to be of 'psychogenic' origin. People's responses to pain differ widely and may be affected by factors such as personality, ethnic origin or environment.

It is important to avoid predicting the severity of the pain by the visual appearance of the injury. Some patients remain conscious and remarkably pain free despite extremely severe facial injuries, whereas the innocuous looking subungual haematoma may be excruciatingly painful.

Pain is valuable in warning the patient that something is wrong and helping the doctor in his diagnosis. However, this pain should be relieved as soon as possible. In some circumstances it may have a direct deleterious effect. For example, in a patient with a head injury pain may increase the risk of coning by causing a rise in intracranial pressure. Pain may restrict coughing and respiratory movement after a chest injury, resulting in atelectasis and possibly respiratory failure. Pain also increases oxygen consumption.

Pain prevention

It is worthwhile remembering than pain prevention forms part of an A & E department's practice. This may vary from health education, such as accident prevention, to ensuring that all procedures are as pain-free as possible, or just checking that the patient is comfortable on the trolley.

Methods of pain relief

Many factors require consideration when choosing the method of pain relief and the type and dose of analgesic agent which might be used. These include the patient's age, size, personality and pre-existing medical conditions or medication. The cause, severity and nature of the pain are important and plans to admit or operate on the patient will also affect the choice.

Explanation

Some people believe that a single visit to the A & E department will cure their pain. They often return worried because they are not completely better, although their progress is just as might be expected for their particular problem. A simple explanation of the diagnosis, expected time until recovery and appropriate use of analgesics or other measures should help prevent unnecessary worry.

Splintage

The immobilisation of fractures or dislocations often provides adequate analgesia, although pain may persist until reduction has been performed. Analgesia such as Entonox may be required for the application of a splint. The persistence of severe pain despite correct splinting should raise the question of some associated problem such as a vascular injury or the plaster being too tight.

Dressings

Pain due to minor burns or finger tip injuries often settles once an appropriate dressing is applied.

Definitive treatment

Some procedures, such as trephining a nail for a subungual haematoma or manipulating a pulled elbow will provide immediate relief of pain without any analgesic being required.

Entonox

Entonox is a 50:50 mixture of nitrous oxide and oxygen. When correctly administered it can provide analgesia comparable to 10–15 mg morphine.

The specially designed Entonox apparatus comprises a cylinder containing the premixed gases and a two stage demand valve. The cylinder is colour coded with a white neck and French blue body. The first stage of the valve is pressure reducing and this is followed by a tilt valve which opens under negative pressure (during inspiration) and closes under positive pressure (during expiration). At temperatures below $-7°C$ the nitrous oxide will liquify: if the cyclinder is used in this state initially almost 100% oxygen will be given followed by gradually increasing amounts of nitrous oxide until this appears in almost pure form. Separation should be prevented by storing the cyliners away from severe cold. If separation is suspected ideally a 'safe' cylinder should be obtained, or the original cylinder should be allowed to rewarm for at least two hours at a temperature not less than $10°C$ and then the cylinder should be inverted a few times.

Entonox may be given by the patient or attendant. The patient should be warned that he may feel dizzy or become drowsy. The face mask should form a comfortable and complete seal around the nose and mouth. The patient is encouraged to take relaxed, deep breaths until adequate analgesia is obtained. Facial injuries may prevent the use of this apparatus. An assistant will be required to hold the mask for those with upper limb injuries. Some patients find a mouth-piece easier to use than a face mask. If the pain returns more Entonox may be given.

Entonox has the advantage of providing 50% oxygen as well as good analgesia. It has a rapid onset of action and the analgesia quickly subsides once the drug is withdrawn. With correct use there is neither a reduction in blood pressure nor loss of consciousness. However, prolonged use may sometimes cause confusion and restlessness. The high oxygen content may cause respiratory depression in those who depend on a hypoxic drive for respiration (e.g. chronic obstructive airways disease), but in practice this problem is rare. The efficacy of Entonox depends on good patient compliance and for those unable to tolerate the face mask or work the demand valve some other form of analgesia will be required.

Nitrous oxide rapidly diffuses into air-containing spaces, causing expansion of air in pleural cavity, bowel, middle ear, cranial cavity and air emboli. Entonox should not be given to a patient with a confirmed pneumothorax until it has been drained. It is also best avoided in patients with intestinal obstruction and must not be used in patients with decompression sickness (Ch. 28). Entonox is a valuable analgesic in prehospital care in cases of trauma or in myocardial infarction, where it may have some coronary artery vasodilatory effect (Chs. 14 and 18).

In the A & E department Entonox continues to be a valuable analgesic whilst the patient is being moved and initial assessment is being made. It may also provide adequate analgesia for simple manipulations (e.g. reduction of a dislocated shoulder or patella). However, if it does not provide adequate analgesia for the manipulation the procedure must be stopped and a different analgesic or anaesthetic used. In these situations Entonox often fails because it cannot overcome the associated muscle spasm or the patient is unable to use the apparatus effectively. Entonox can prove a useful supplement to local anaesthesia.

A 50:50 mixture of nitrous oxide and oxygen can be given from an anaesthetic machine. In this case there will be no demand valve and the person administering the gases should be fully conversant with the use of the machine.

Local anaesthesia

Local anaesthesia is often used to provide anaesthesia for surgical procedures, but its value as an analgesic deserves more widespread recognition. Its major advantage is that, when used correctly, it does not affect the level of consciousness nor cause cardiovascular or respiratory depression. The main disadvantages are that the duration of analgesia is often shorter than that seen with a parenteral analgesic and expertise in performing the nerve blocks is required. Techniques such as femoral (p. 97) or digital nerve block at the metacarpal level (p. 94) are particularly useful.

Nerve blocks may be used immediately after initial assessment and emergency treatment has been given. Recording neurological status is particularly important because the local anaesthetic will mask these signs for a time. Once analgesia is obtained it is then possible to make a more thorough examination. Wounds can be explored and a patient will be much more willing to co-operate, for example, with testing movement in a crushed finger. Splints such as a Thomas splint can be applied at this stage. Analgesia should last long enough to give the patient a pain-free passage through the radiology department and definitive treatment may even be possible before the local anaesthetic action wears off.

Oral analgesics

Oral analgesics are very commonly prescribed in the A & E department, yet there are very few studies on their use in this situation. One recent study of four drugs used for the relief of mild to moderate pain showed no significant variation in therapeutic effect, side effects or patient compliance. It was suggested that drug choice should be based on side-effects and cost (Yates et al 1984).

Before prescribing an oral analgesic it is important to check the patient's present medication. The elderly often have a supply of one or more analgesics already. A history of allergy or peptic ulceration should also be sought. Instructions regarding dose and frequency of use should be given. Physiotherapy and splintage may reduce the need for analgesia.

There are many oral analgesic drugs from which to choose. It is best to use a few and get to know their side-effects and drug interactions well, such as paracetamol for mild pain and co-dydramol (paracetamol and dihydrocodeine) for moderate pain. A non steroidal anti-inflammatory drug such as naproxen will also be useful. The type, dose and amount of drug prescribed should always be clearly recorded on the patient's record card.

Parenteral analgesics

A patient requiring immediate analgesia for severe pain should be given the appropriate analgesic by the intravenous route. This has the advantage over the intramuscular route of providing a predictable and rapid onset of drug action which produces prompt analgesia. Peak plasma levels are rapidly attained, enabling easy assessment of need and appropriate titration of the drug. A decline in the initial peak level limits the time during which a toxic reaction may occur. Patients with a low cardiac output, such as in hypovolaemic shock, should never be given analgesia intramuscularly because the associated vasoconstriction will cause poor absorption and there will be no pain relief. Erratic absorption when vasodilatation occurs later may produce toxic effects. Although the intravenous route should be used for these patients it must be remembered that they are very sensitive to the drug's actions and toxicity can easily occur. The drug should always be given very slowly in small increments, e.g. 1 mg morphine, or 10 mg pethidine.

Morphine is one of the commonly used narcotic analgesics and is suitable for relieving severe pain. It also provides some sedation. Some cardiorespiratory depression may occur and in the shocked patient oxygen should be administered and an intravenous infusion started before the drug is given. Nausea and vomiting may occur and can be controlled with an antiemetic such as prochlorperazine or metoclopramide.

Intravenous morphine provides analgesia for up to two hours. If at any time it causes problems with diagnosis, or respiratory depression, its effect can be reversed with intravenous naloxone (Ch. 16).

Morphine should be given in a dose which will relieve pain. This may be 3 mg in a frail elderly patient or 20 mg or more in a fit adult.

When morphine is given in small incremental intravenous doses it should be prepared by diluting 10 mg morphine up to 10 ml with 0.9% saline, i.e. 1 mg morphine per ml. The syringe should be clearly labelled. Initially half the normal adult dose should be given and then 1 mg supplements added until analgesia is obtained.

In the elderly, shocked, or head-injured patient it is better to give 1 mg increments every minute until analgesia is obtained.

The use of a narcotic analgesic in the presence of abdominal or head injuries has been the cause of some concern because it was feared that this would mask valuable clinical signs. This problem is discussed in the relevant sections.

Morphine is just one of a number of parenteral analgesics which may be used. Choice may be swayed by personal preference or hospital policy. Pethidine may be of value in treating biliary or renal colic although parenteral diclofenac has recently been shown to be of benefit in these cases. Diamorphine is often preferred in the management of pain due to myocardial infarction. It produces euphoria and relieves anxiety. Analgesia is greater than with morphine and side effects are less.

Analgesia and special situations

Children

Some visually severe injuries, such as finger-tip injuries, require little or no analgesia. In many situations fear rather than pain is the main cause of the child's distress. This may be potentiated by the attitude of the accompanying parent who may feel anxious, guilty, helpless, or angered by what has happened. Most children will settle with patient, sensitive handling and appropriate analgesia if required. It is important to calculate the drug dosage carefully. Antiemetics are not routinely required with narcotic analgesics in children. If a child does not settle he should be reassessed to exclude any other injury and also to ensure that the analgesic is working. Sedation, for example using trimeprazine tartrate, should only rarely be required. Simple, clear instructions should be given to parents regarding the use of analgesics on discharge. Many parents are reluctant or afraid of giving analgesics to their child, particularly if he has had a head injury. Some parents believe that paracetamol is a 'sleeping tablet', probably because, since the child feels better with analgesia, he is at last able to sleep. The parents are thus reluctant to give paracetamol when it is needed. Such fears should be allayed and appropriate advice given. Salicylate should not be given to children because of the reported association with Reye's syndrome.

Acute abdominal pain

For many years it has been common practice to withhold analgesia from patients with acute abdominal pain due to the fear that analgesia will mask important diagnostic signs (Anon 1979). Some doctors still believe that it is preferable to leave the patient in pain, although patients and relatives may think otherwise (Salter 1985). Analgesia is likely to do more good than harm. A comfortable patient is able to give a clearer history and examination is often facilitated with tenderness and rigidity becoming more localised and masses more readily palpable (Angell 1978). In the very restless patient with renal colic or a perforated ulcer it may be impossible to obtain satisfactory radiographs until analgesia has been given. Incremental intravenous doses of a narcotic analgesic such as

morphine or pethidine should be given until the patient is pain-free at rest. Further analgesia should be given if the pain recurs.

Naloxone may be given if signs of overdose occur or the surgeon is unhappy assessing the patient while pain-free.

Diclofenac is valuable in relieving pain due to biliary colic (Broggini 1984) and renal colic (Hetherington 1986). It is more effective than pethidine and has fewer side effects.

Head injuries

Headache due to a minor head injury may be treated with oral analgesics such as paracetamol or co-dydramol. Stronger analgesia may be needed in the conscious patient with a more severe head injury. There is a fear that narcotics will mask the signs of an expanding intracranial lesion by depressing the conscious level and constricting the pupils. Some would withhold its use altogether and others would wait an hour to take a series of head injury observations and assess the general trend of the patient. However it is well recognised that pain will cause an increase in intracranial pressure which will aggravate secondary brain damage. Pain may produce signs which mimic cerebral oedema by making the patient restless and unco-operative. This must be distinguished from other causes such as hypoxia and gastric dilatation. Pain may also have detrimental effects on other injuries such as in chest injuries. It should be possible, by the judicious use of analgesia, to make the patient comfortable and still monitor conscious level, making allowances for some change due to the analgesic (Bewes 1983). This can be done by giving small incremental intravenous doses of a narcotic analgesic such as morphine and is described further in the section on parenteral analgesia. If there is any concern, the analgesic can be reversed using naloxone.

Chest injuries

It is essential to prevent hypoxia. Entonox may be used whilst initial assessment and emergency treatment is being given, but 100% oxygen should be used as soon as possible. It is essential to identify and drain a pneumothorax quickly, since diffusion of nitrous oxide may cause it to enlarge. Severe pain should be treated with a narcotic analgesic such as morphine, given intravenously in small incremental doses and repeated as required. This is essential since pain not only increases tissue oxygen consumption but also restricts respiratory movements and may prevent coughing, thus predisposing to atelectasis. Signs of respiratory depression, hypercapnia and hypoxia should be looked for and a blood gas estimation should be obtained. Pain from fractured ribs may be relieved by infiltration with local anaesthetic at the fracture sites. Longer term analgesia can be provided by a continuous local anaesthetic technique, e.g. thoracic epidural or paravertebral block. This would usually be performed and supervised in the intensive care unit. Adequate analgesia and oxygen therapy may be sufficient to manage a severe chest injury but occasionally satisfactory control is not obtained and ventilation will be required (see Ch. 14).

'Minor' chest injuries may be very painful and the appropriate oral or parenteral analgesic should be given. Strapping tends to restrict respiratory movement and should not be used.

Multiple injuries

Entonox is the analgesic of choice for initial transport, assessment and emergency treatment. However the patient should be given 100% oxygen as soon as possible. Local anaesthesia should be used where possible, such as a femoral nerve block for a fractured shaft of femur (p. 97), since this does not cause cardiorespiratory depression or affect conscious level. Incremental doses of a narcotic analgesic such as morphine may be given slowly intravenously, but it should be remembered that shocked patients are very sensitive to such drugs and overdose can easily occur without due care.

The problems regarding an associated head injury are described in the relevant section.

Chronic pain

Patients commonly come to the A & E department seeking advice on some chronic problem. The A & E department is not the appropriate place to deal with this, but it is worthwhile checking that no new problem requiring immediate treatment has developed before referring the patient back to his general practitioner.

Munchausen syndrome

Some patients with Munchausen syndrome will present with acute conditions seemingly requiring analgesia and it is often easy to be misled. Suspicion and experience are the key to anticipating the problem. It is always worthwhile listening to the nursing staff, because they often develop a particular expertise at recognising this syndrome. (For further discussion of this topic see Ch. 31.)

Drug addiction

Some drug addicts are becoming wise to analgesic practice within A & E departments. As in Munchausen syndrome fictitious histories are given, such as renal colic, in this case to obtain a 'fix'. Physical signs of the underlying problem may be present. The use of diclofenac for renal colic is valuable in this situation. (For further discussion of drug addiction see Ch. 30.)

REFERENCES

Angell J C 1978 The acute abdomen for the man on the spot, 3rd edn. Pitman Medical, Tunbridge Wells

Anonymous 1979 Analgesia and the acute abdomen. British Medical Journal ii: 1093

Arthur D S, McNicol L R 1986 Local anaesthetic techniques in paediatric surgery. British Journal of Anaesthesia 58: 760–778

Bewes P 1983 Letter. British Journal of Hospital Medicine 30: 138

Broggini M, Corbetta E, Grossi E, Borghi C 1984 Diclofenac sodium in biliary colic: a double blind trial. British Medical Journal i: 1042

Eriksson E 1979 Illustrated handbook in local anaesthesia, 2nd edn. Lloyd-Luke, London

Hetherington J W, Philip N H 1986 Diclofenac sodium versus pethidine in acute renal colic. British Medical Journal 292: 237–238

Salter R H 1985 Diagnosis before treatment? Lancet i: 863–864

Scott D B 1986 Toxic effects of local anaesthetic agents on the central nervous system. British Journal of Anaesthesia 58: 732–735

Wallace W A, Guardini R, Ellis S J 1982 Standard intravenous regional anaesthesia. British Medical Journal ii: 554–556

Winnie A P, Ramamurthy S, Durrani Z 1973 The inguinal paravascular technique of lumbar plexus anesthesia: the 3 in 1 block. Anesthesia and Analgesia 56: 852

Yates D W, Laing G S, Peters K, Kumar K 1984 Mild analgesics and the accident and emergency department — cost and safety more important than potency? Archives of Emergency Medicine 1: 4 197–203

FURTHER READING

A synopsis of anaesthesia, 10th edn. Atkinson R S, Rushman G B, Lee J 1987 John Wright, Bristol

Illustrated handbook in local anaesthesia 2nd edn. Eriksson E 1979 Lloyd-Luke, London

Peripheral nerve block Jenkner F L 1977 Springer-Verlag, Vienna

Life-threatening Conditions

INTRODUCTION

One of the prime functions of A & E specialists is the resuscitation of the severely ill or badly injured patient. An area specifically designed and equipped for this purpose is best situated near the main entrance to the ambulance area. There should be a direct radio link between the department and individual ambulances, if necessary via the ambulance control centre. This enables interchange of information concerning the nature of the patient's illness or the seriousness of injuries and the number injured.

The importance of a well organised, multidisciplinary approach to the severely injured patient cannot be overstressed. Once a warning of the imminent arrival of such a patient is received, the appropriate specialists should be alerted, equipment made ready, drugs drawn up and blood and plasma removed from the refrigerator.

In the following pages the reception and management of patients with common life-threatening conditions are detailed. Often obtaining the history, carrying out the examination and starting treatment will proceed simultaneously. The conditions present as clinical problems, and are described under the following headings:

Cardiorespiratory arrest (Ch. 10)
Acute respiratory distress (Ch. 11)
The unconscious patient (Ch. 12)
The shocked patient (Ch. 13)
The severely injured patient (Ch. 14)
Other life-threatening conditions (Ch. 15)

This approach renders a certain amount of repetition and cross-referencing inevitable (e.g. the severely injured or poisoned patient may also be shocked and unconscious). However, each clinical presentation carries a different emphasis regarding diagnosis and management. A few basic resuscitative techniques are generally applicable, and are described in detail where first appropriate.

This is a book about the practice of medicine in the A & E department. No attempt, therefore, is made to describe the further management of dangerously ill patients in an intensive care unit.

Cardiorespiratory arrest

INTRODUCTION

Cardiorespiratory arrest is a sudden, potentially reversible, failure of cardiac action to supply adequate blood to the brain. It is the gravest emergency which a patient may experience. It may often be prevented by immediate expert resuscitation.

It has been shown that optimum survival from cardiac arrest is likely when:
1. The event was witnessed.
2. A bystander commenced resuscitation (ideally within 3 minutes).
3. The rhythm was ventricular fibrillation (VF – see below).
4. Defibrillation was carried out at an early stage (ideally within 8 minutes).

Staff working in A & E department must be trained, equipped and prepared to face this condition efficiently, competently and caringly as it arises. Patients requiring resuscitation in the A & E department for cardiorespiratory arrest may fall into one of two categories:
1. The patient may have arrested before arrival at the department. The arrest may have been witnessed or unwitnessed. Resuscitation measures will have been commenced by the ambulancemen, although the circumstances of the arrest, including the immediate cause and the period of cerebral ischaemia, will, in the case of an unwitnessed arrest, be unknown.
2. The patient arrests in the A & E department. Fortunately this is likely to occur after the patient has been received, details ascertained and, hopefully, base-line monitoring and intravenous access established. The results of resuscitation are usually very good

— over 70% immediate survival if the patient arrests in VF in the A & E department (Robertson 1984) and 30% overall survival to leave hospital (Wardrope 1986). Unwitnessed arrests in the A & E department indicate a poor level of care. Most arrests following myocardial infarction occur within the first hour after the onset of symptoms (63% of deaths relating to ischaemic heart disease amongst middle-aged and younger male patients occur within one hour). Any patient with chest pain suspected of being of cardiac origin should be seen in an emergency bay with resuscitation facilities to hand and should *never* be left unattended.

The common causes of cardiac arrest relevant to the A & E department are:
1. Ischaemic heart disease
2. Hypoxia.
Other causes include:
1. Pulmonary embolism
2. Electrolyte and acid-base disorders
3. Hypothermia
4. Drug overdose
5. Electrocution
6. Conduction system disorders.

WHEN TO START RESUSCITATION

A circulatory arrest, for example due to ventricular fibrillation, will be marked by the immediate loss of major arterial pulses. Consciousness is lost within 10–20 seconds, the patient will 'collapse', and, as the cerebral circulation diminishes, the breathing will cease. The pupils will often dilate but this sign is of little diagnostic or predictive value. The patient may appear pale or blue.

In the circumstances of an unwitnessed cardiac arrest it is difficult to ascertain exactly when the heart and/or breathing stopped. It may sometimes be clear either from the appearance of the patient, or as a result of information from the accompanying persons that continued resuscitation is inappropriate. For example, it would be inappropriate where there is a very long known delay without any attempt at revival (e.g. for more than 20 minutes, except in hypothermia); in patients with incurable or terminal diseases, advanced cerebrovascular insufficiency and very elderly individuals. However, it is extremely difficult to lay down 'conditions' in the A & E department and, if there is any doubt at all, full resuscitation procedure should be instigated.

The time of commencement of resuscitation should be recorded, when known, and, as soon as possible, information should be obtained from the ambulance attendants of the time when the arrest occurred and the nature of any resuscitation carried out before arrival at hospital.

THE PROCESS OF RESUSCITATION

There are two phases of cardiac resuscitation — basic life support, in which no special equipment, drugs nor special techniques are used, and advanced life support, which involves special apparatus and skills. In practical terms, for A & E departments, the division is academic for resuscitation equipment is readily available and used from the commencement of the resuscitation attempt. The single most important technique of advanced life support is that of defibrillation of a heart arrested in ventricular fibrillation. Where this is the electrocardiographic diagnosis, defibrillation is an absolute priority and must take precedence over all other advanced cardiac life support procedures (Fig. 10.1). For descriptive purposes the two phases of resuscitation will be described separately.

BASIC LIFE SUPPORT

The sequence of basic life support follows the A–Airway, B–Breathing, C–Circulation scheme. This system is logical, educationally attractive and applicable to most circumstances appertaining to accident and emergency work.

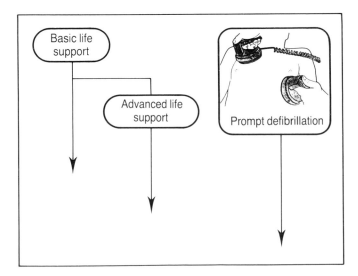

Fig. 10.1 The sequence of CPR.

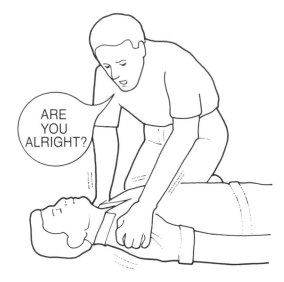

Fig. 10.2 Establishing unresponsiveness.

Preliminary considerations

A rapid assessment should precede any hands-on manoeuvres:

Assess — are the surroundings safe? This question is important in the prehospital phase. Is there any danger from electricity, gas, falling masonry, traffic, etc.?

Assess — is the victim conscious? Shake gently and shout to the patient (Fig. 10.2).

Assess — is the airway clear?

Assess — is the patient breathing? Look, listen and feel for breathing.

Assess — is there a pulse?

Help should be sought straight away. In well staffed emergency departments with senior doctors immediately available, the resuscitation should be managed in house. Otherwise the hospital cardiac arrest team should be summoned by using the designated emergency telephone number. There should be no delay in starting resuscitation whilst waiting for the arrest team. If the airway is blocked it should be opened; if the patient is not breathing he should be ventilated and if there is no pulse chest compressions should be performed.

Airway

Airway obstruction in an unconscious patient may occur because the flaccid tongue falls back against the posterior pharangyeal wall and the jaw sags (Fig. 10.3). The *triple airway manoeuvre* is the most effective postural technique for 'opening the airway' in unconsciousness (Fig. 10.4). It comprises:

1. **Head tilt.** With the palm of one hand on the subject's forehead and the other supporting the neck the head is tilted into full extension.

2. **Chin lift.** The fingers are placed under the bony part of the chin and the chin lifted upwards and forwards.

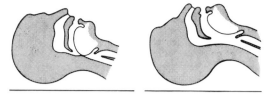

Fig. 10.3 The airway in unconsciousness. Tilting the head back opens the airway.

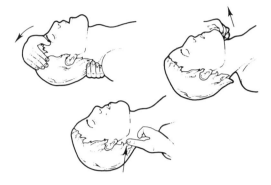

Fig. 10.4 The triple airway manoeuvre.

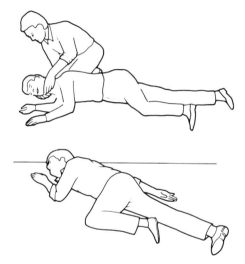

Fig. 10.5 The recovery position.

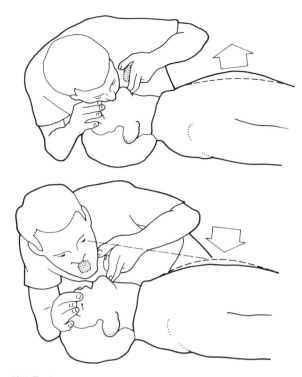

Fig. 10.6 Expired air resuscitation.

usually, the mouth-to-mouth method (Safar et al 1950) (Fig. 10.6). In hospitals unpleasant intimate patient contact is avoided by using interpositioned devices or bag-valve-mask techniques (see 'advanced life support' below).

Circulation

In the absence of major arterial pulsation (the carotid or femoral pulses felt for over at least five seconds) the circulation must be supported by the technique of *closed chest cardiac compression* (Kouwenhoven et al 1960). If performed efficiently a cardiac output of over 30% normal could be achieved. Chest compressions are

3. **Jaw thrust.** The index fingers are placed under the angle of the mandible on each side and the entire jaw is thrust upwards and forwards. This manoeuvre is useful in suspected spinal injury cases when hyperextension of the neck, as in head tilt, is unwise.

Management of the obstructed airway is described below.

If the patient is unconscious but breathing he should be placed in the recovery position (Fig. 10.5) in which the tongue will fall away from the back of the throat and any vomit or respiratory secretions will drain out of the mouth rather than be aspirated into the lungs (see Ch. 12).

Breathing

Ventilation in basic life support is by *expired air resuscitation* using,

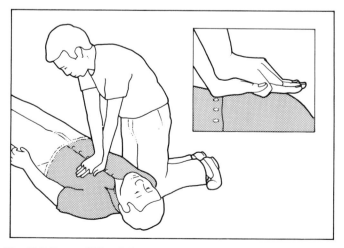

Fig. 10.7 Correct CPR technique.

performed with the victim lying on a hard surface; the compressions should be over the lower third of the sternum and the pressure coming from the rescuer's shoulders with the elbows straight, the fingers locked together and the fingers clear of the chest (Fig. 10.7). The compressions should be regular and smooth with an excursion of 4–5 cm; the downstroke should take slightly longer than the release.

In a cardiac arrest both chest compressions *and* ventilation are required. The combination of ventilation and chest compression is known as *CardioPulmonary Resuscitation* (CPR). When working alone, 15 compressions are given for two breaths. When working in pairs five compressions are given for each breath. Synchronous compression–ventilation resuscitation ('New CPR') is only possible when a cuffed endotracheal tube is in situ.

ADVANCED LIFE SUPPORT

The organisation of advanced life support

The delivery of advanced life support in the A & E department is best provided through teamwork with each member of the team responsible for his or her own role. Kaye (1981) has described a team approach which can be readily adapted for accident and emergency care (Fig. 10.8). A disinterested observer should be able to identify which person is the leader of the team. The leader will assess priorities, direct resuscitation, prescribe therapy according to the electrocardiographic diagnosis and arrange disposal and aftercare. At no stage should CPR be discontinued for longer than 10 seconds except for the passage of an endotracheal tube. The effect of each therapeutic manoeuvre should be assessed *on the patient* rather than on the ECG monitor. It is of the utmost importance to diagnose and treat VF rapidly and so the attachment of a cardiac monitor becomes a priority. Most modern defibrillators have the facility of monitoring the ECG through the paddles or chest pads. Rarely, when there is access to a defibrillator but not to a monitor, it is necessary to administer a 'blind' shock. With the patient connected to a monitor the diagnosis of the mode of the arrest should become apparent.

> There are four forms of cardiac rhythm associated with cardiac arrest:
>   1. Rapid dysrhythmias, including ventricular fibrillation, typical and atypical ventricular tachycardia.
>   2. Slow or absent rhythms, including complete heart block and sinus arrest and ventricular asystole.
>   3. Normal or near normal cardiac rhythms with little or no cardiac output ('electromechanical dissociation').
>   4. Bizarre, broad, slow and usually irregular complexes known as 'agonal rhythms'.

A flat trace on the monitor screen is not necessarily due to asystole: remember to check the lead connections, the selector position and the gain before excluding a fine VF. There should be no delay for endotracheal intubation though, as time passes, secural of the

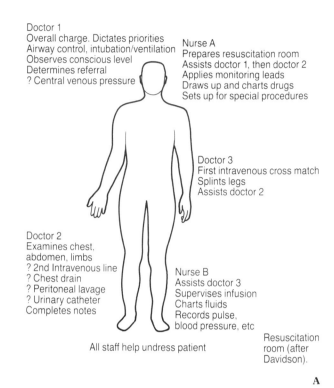

Doctor 1
Overall charge. Dictates priorities
Airway control, intubation/ventilation
Observes conscious level
Determines referral
? Central venous pressure

Nurse A
Prepares resuscitation room
Assists doctor 1, then doctor 2
Applies monitoring leads
Draws up and charts drugs
Sets up for special procedures

Doctor 3
First intravenous cross match
Splints legs
Assists doctor 2

Doctor 2
Examines chest,
abdomen, limbs
? 2nd Intravenous line
? Chest drain
? Peritoneal lavage
? Urinary catheter
Completes notes

Nurse B
Assists doctor 3
Supervises infusion
Charts fluids
Records pulse,
blood pressure, etc

All staff help undress patient

Resuscitation room (after Davidson).

A

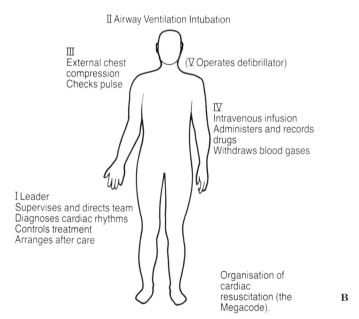

II Airway Ventilation Intubation

III
External chest
compression
Checks pulse

(V Operates defibrillator)

IV
Intravenous infusion
Administers and records
drugs
Withdraws blood gases

I Leader
Supervises and directs team
Diagnoses cardiac rhythms
Controls treatment
Arranges after care

Organisation of
cardiac
resuscitation (the
Megacode).

B

Fig. 10.8 A Organisation of the resuscitation room. (from Davison H A 1983 Resuscitation room routine. British Journal of Accident & Emergency Medicine 1:15-16.) **B** Co-ordination of cardiac resuscitation.

airway with a cuffed endotracheal tube becomes increasingly urgent. Through this route some of the cardiac resuscitation drugs can be administered (see below).

The techniques of advanced life support

Advanced airway care

The efficiency of expired air resuscitation may be improved by

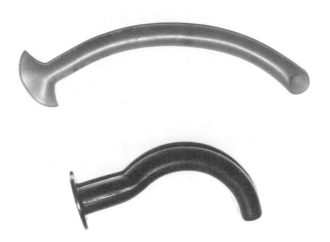

Fig. 10.9. Oropharyngeal and nasopharyngeal airways.

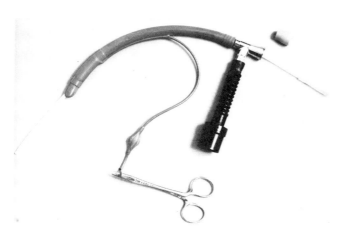

Fig. 10.10 The passage of a cuffed endotracheal tube establishes a watertight seal between the patient's airway and the ventilator device and allows endotracheal suction of secretions.

the use of artifical oropharyngeal or nasopharyngeal airways or valved airways designed to protect the rescuer from contamination. (Fig. 10.9). *No evidence exists that the HIV virus has been transmitted by saliva* and, in an emergency, direct mouth-to-mouth respiration should not be withheld. Nevertheless airway adjuncts are preferable for use by trained personnel. No simple airway can in any way substitute for endotracheal intubation and this important technique should be mastered by every A & E doctor. The equipment required for endotracheal intubation should always be laid out in readiness in the resuscitation room (Fig. 10.10).

Ventilation

There are two forms of bag-valve-mask device available in the A & E department for advanced life support: the self-expanding 'resuscitator' bag, e.g. the Ambu or Laerdal bag and the Water's oxygen circuit utilising a Heidbrink expiratory valve (Fig. 10.11). The latter facilitates the delivery of 100% oxygen provided it is washed through with a high flow rate (at least 10 L/min) of oxygen.

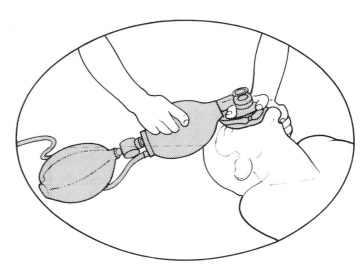

Fig. 10.11 Bag-valve-mask with oxygen reservoir.

The former will not permit high oxygen concentrations unless the optional oxygen reservoir bag is attached. Automatic ventilators (preferably of the manually triggered variety for cardiopulmonary resuscitation) should only be used in the intubated patient otherwise leaks occur, gastric distension may develop and the patient will be underventilated.

The use of circulatory adjuncts

An automatic chest thumper is available, which is extremely effective in the A & E department for maintaining an adequate cardiac output whilst freeing one operator from performing chest compressions (Fig. 10.12).

Defibrillation

The only effective treatment for established venticular fibrillation is electrical defibrillation utilising a direct current shock.

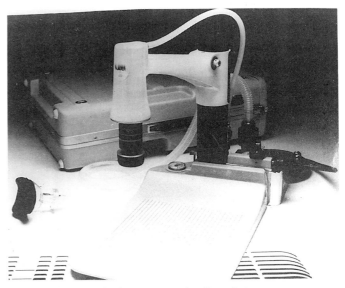

Fig. 10.12 An automatic chest compressor/ventilator device.

Mechanical 'thump-version' using a *precordial thump* has been shown to reverse VF on occasions. It should be attempted when no defibrillator is to hand.

> The factors contributing to successful defibrillation include the following:
>
> *Speed.* The shorter the period of VF the greater the chance of long term success.
>
> *Correct paddle position.* This is depicted in Figure 10.13.
>
> *Good electrical contact.* The paddles should be applied firmly to the chest wall. Electrical conductivity can be increased by the use of a conducting gel or, preferably, defibrillator pads.
>
> *An appropriate charge.* The initial charge in an adult should be 200 joules. This figure refers to stored energy and is equivalent to 160 J calculated delivered energy marked on the selector switch of some defibrillators. In refractory VF it is sometimes useful to deliver a second shock immediately after the first.
>
> *The state of the patient.* Successful defibrillation is inherently more difficult if the patient is hypoxic and/or acidotic. Chest compressions should continue whilst the defibrillator is being charged for the second and subsequent shocks so that interruption of basic life support is minimised.

Drug therapy in advanced life support

With an arrested circulation the selection of route for drug administration can be critical. As the circulation time from a peripheral site may be five minutes or even longer, then clearly a central route is preferable. The internal jugular vein is the vessel frequently chosen (Fig. 10.14). Intracardiac injections are of little value and are potentially hazardous. Some of the drugs used in resuscitation: lignocaine, adrenaline and atropine (but NOT bicarbonate or calcium) are known to be well absorbed through the respiratory endothelium; the endotracheal route should be considered when an endotracheal tube is in place before vascular access has been secured. Endotracheal injections may be given

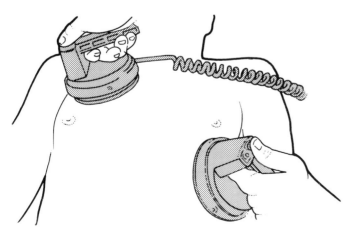

Fig. 10.13 Defibrillator paddle position.

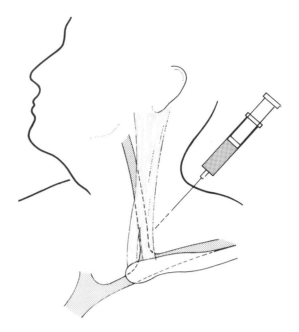

Fig. 10.14 Internal jugular cannulation.

through a cardiac needle provided that it is swaged onto the syringe and cannot become detached.

The following groups of drugs have particular roles in cardiopulmonary resuscitation:

Catecholamines. The vasopressor effect of adrenaline 10 ml of 1:10 000 is beneficial in all modes of cardiac arrest for maintaining adequate coronary perfusion. α Adrenergic stimulation produces intense peripheral vasoconstriction preventing coronary and cerebral arterial collapse during chest compression. Adrenaline and isoprenaline may be administered for their β effect (enhanced chronotropic and inotropic activity) in asystole and electromechanical dissociation.

Atropine. The anticholinergic agents should theoretically lift the vagal brake in the sinus and atrioventricular nodes and there is now fairly convincing evidence that atropine given in a minimum dose of 1 mg should be the first-line drug used in the management of asystole.

Antidysrhythmic agents. Lignocaine is the agent of choice for tachydysrhythmias. Given in a loading dose of 100 mg, this drug is used for the management of VF after three initial electrical shocks. In refractory VF a more effective agent might be bretylium tosylate given as a 500 mg injection. Following successful defibrillation an infusion of lignocaine at 3 mg/min is erected.

Sodium bicarbonate. Alkalis should not be used as a routine in cardiac arrest, but reserved for refractory cases or prolonged arrests in which there is a high likelihood of significant metabolic acidosis. Respiratory acidosis can almost always be corrected by

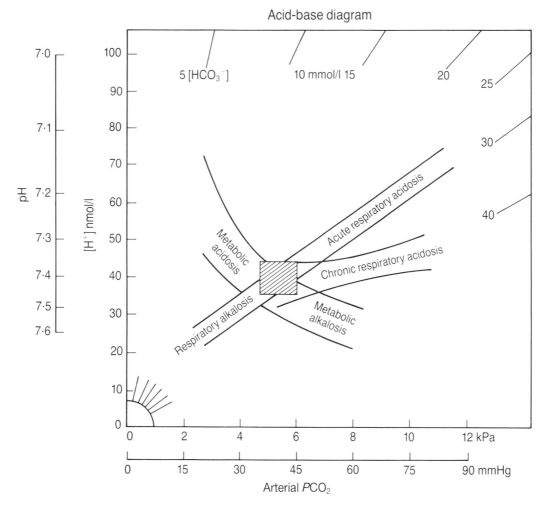

Acid-base diagram

Fig. 10.15 An acid-base nomogram for establishing the metabolic deficit from arterial blood gas measurements (from Flenley D C 1971 Lancet 921).

adequate ventilation; the risk of overdosing with alkali in the poorly ventilated patient is of producing a secondary metabolic alkalosis with a (paradoxical) intracellular acidotic state. Bicarbonate is hyperosmolar and an overdose gives rise to a large sodium load with hypokalaemia. Whenever possible the use of sodium bicarbonate should be guided by arterial blood gas analysis. An appropriate nomogram (Fig. 10.15) would give an indication as to the nature of the metabolic disturbance and the Astrop formula may be used to calculate how much bicarbonate would be needed to correct the base deficit. Usually half this requirement is given — hence the working formula:

$$\text{ml of 8.4\% bicarbonate} = \frac{\text{wgt (kg)} \times \text{base deficit}}{5}$$

Calcium salts. Calcium chloride or calcium gluconate (10 ml of 10% solution) have a limited role in cardiac resuscitation. They are indicated in cardiac arrest associated with hypocalcaemia, hyperkalaemia and calcium antagonist toxicity. They are occasionally useful in primary (cardiac) electromechanical dissociation.

Inotropic agents. In centres having haemodynamic monitoring, dopamine might be used to provide inotropic support after successful cardiopulmonary resuscitation. An infusion can be prepared by mixing 800 mg with 500 ml of 5% dextrose. It is infused slowly by burette, the rate being adjusted according to the response.

The management of ventricular fibrillation. The term ventricular fibrillation refers to wild, random uncoordinated electrical activity of the heart (Fig. 10.16). Each cardiac fibre continues to contract but independently and without the control of the sino-atrial node. The exposed heart would be seen to quiver, an action greatly consumptive of energy, yet pumping no blood. Rarely, VF can recover spontaneously or as a result of a precordial thump. The only sure treatment is electrical defibrillation using a d.c. countershock. Defibrillation stops this activity in all the fibres together. When spontaneous activity returns it will hopefully be synchronous and co-ordinated.

The algorithm recommended for the management of ventricular fibrillation is shown in Figure. 10.17. After each shock, chest

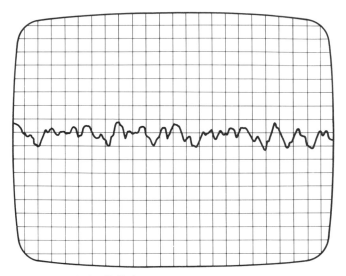

Fig. 10.16 Ventricular fibrillation.

compressions are resumed while the defibrillator is recharged for the next shock.

> The management of refractory VF can be summarised.
>   1. The hopeful phase: three shocks at 200 J, 200 J, 400 J.
>   2. The struggling phase: three shocks at 400 J after, respectively, lignocaine, adrenaline and bicarbonate. Patient intubated.
>   3. The desperate phase: three shocks at 400 J with different electrode positions or different defibrillator.

If VF remains refractory to nine shocks, then the chances of a successful outcome are extremely poor. Where VF is terminated by countershock then lignocaine should be administered, initially as a bolus, or 100 mg or 50 mg depending upon whether lignocaine has been given previously, followed by an infusion of 3 mg per minute reducing according to the reponse. Staff should be alert to the signs of lignocaine toxicity — hypotension and an increasing PR interval on the ECG leading to complete heart block.

The management of asystole

Asystole or ventricular standstill will usually produce a flat trace on the monitor. It is a condition with a gloomy prognosis for frequently in the A & E department it represents the end stage of VF. It may be the terminal mode of death in hypoxia, whether from respiratory obstruction, respiratory arrest or drowning, etc. Rarely it may arise from a conducting system defect, or when strong cholinergic activity suppresses the heart's pacemaker functions. Under these circumstances atropine may be beneficial and this is the first drug listed in the flowchart (Fig. 10.18). Pacing, whether externally or by the transvenous route, is only likely to

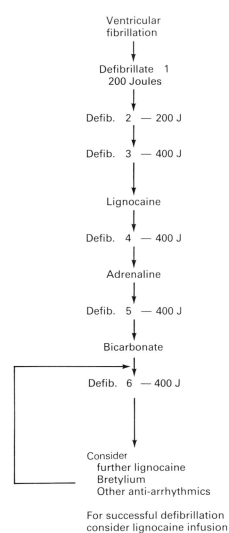

Fig. 10.17 Flow chart for the management of ventricular fibrillation (The Resuscitation Council, UK).

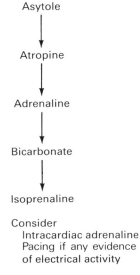

Fig. 10.18 Flow chart for asystole.

be of value when there are P waves in evidence or when there is electrocardiographic evidence of ventricular activity.

The management of electromechanical dissociation

Electromechanical dissociation (EMD) represents, as its name implies, a state of electrical cardiac rhythmic activity in the absence of a mechanical cardiac output. There are some important, remediable causes which require exclusion in the A & E department. These include mechanical embarrassment, acute hypovolaemia and drug overdose.

Mechanical embarrassment may be from a tension pneumothorax (p. 137), a cardiac tamponade (p. 179), massive pulmonary embolism or intracardiac thrombus. The first two are treatable within the arena of a cardiac arrest, the last two never are.

When hypovolaemia is considered as the cause of the arrest, cardiopulmonary resuscitation should be maintained whilst an attempt is made at rapid infusion. Sometimes the infusion of even half a litre of colloid is effective.

The commonest drug overdose to produce arrest in EMD is poisoning from β-blocking drugs. An attempt may be made at treatment using intravenous glucagon (see p. 214) whilst CPR is continued.

When such causes have been excluded, the diagnosis is of primary electromechanical dissociation and pressor agents are administered (Fig. 10.19), hopefully whilst the condition recovers. Primary (cardiac) EMD is almost always fatal.

Open chest cardiac compression

The proven success of external chest compression techniques has rendered the once popular practice of emergency thoracotomy and internal cardiac massage largely obsolete. However, there remain a few circumstances where the performance of an emergency thoracotomy in the A & E department is necessary and may be life-saving. The absolute indication is a cardiac arrest in the presence of penetrating cardiac trauma.

Other conditions in which, in expert hands, open-chest resuscitation *might* be used include the following:
1. Cardiac tamponade
2. Cardiac arrest secondary to severe hypothermia
3. Gross deformity of the chest
   a. anatomic deformity
   b. massive flail chest injury
4. Severe hypovolaemia (e.g. from ruptured aortic aneurysm) to allow compression of the thoracic aorta and control of the bleeding. Facilities for cardiopulmonary bypass should be close by.

The technique of emergency thoracotomy (Fig. 10.20)

An incision is made through the left fourth or fifth intercostal space extending 2–3 cm from the sternal border to the midaxillary line. In the female the incision should be just below the breast. The first pass of the scalpel incises the skin, the second pass divides the intercostal and pectoral muscles. The ribs are spread to their widest extent using Finochietto rib retractors. The pericardium is opened by a vertical incision, carefully made to avoid damage to the underlying epicardium and coronary vessels. Any blood or clots in the pericardial cavity should be removed by a sweep of the fingers. If there is a wound to the heart and the heart is not contracting then the wound should be repaired before attempting to restart the heart — otherwise torrential haemorrhage may occur before wound closure can be effected. Internal cardiac compression is performed by cradling the heart in the palm of the hand with the fingers posteriorly at the base and massaging the ventricles, either with the thumb of the same hand placed over the apex or with the palm of the other hand. The rate of cardiac massage should be approximately 100 times per minute.

When the initial decision to open the chest is made, the help of a surgeon skilled in intrathoracic procedures should be sought. With goodwill and organisation there should be, even in the least sophisticated centres, a few patients with penetrating cardiac trauma salvaged who would undoubtedly have died without intervention.

Electromechanical
dissociation
(No heart beat but ECG shows QRS complexes)

Consider
Drugs
Cardiac tamponade
Tension pneumothorax
or other physical causes

Adrenaline

Isoprenaline

Consider Calcium

Fig. 10.19 Flow chart for electromechanical dissociation.

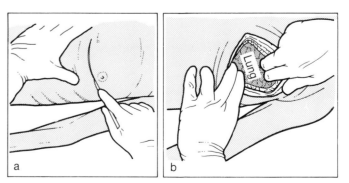

Fig. 10.20 Emergency thoracotomy and internal cardiac massage.

WHEN TO STOP RESUSCITATION

The decision as to when resuscitation should be discontinued can only be made on the merits of an individual case. As a general rule, it would be futile to attempt to prolong the life of a person suffering from an unwitnessed, asytolic cardiac arrest by CPR in the A & E department much beyond 20 minutes. Similarly, officious strife at survival in inappropriate cases (see When to start resuscitation, above) would be unethical. With children and young persons the capacity for survival is greater — provided that resuscitation has been started promptly and vigorously continued, then life support beyond one hour would not be unreasonable. The same holds true for resuscitation from near drowning (see below). With good training and modern technology there is no limit to the time during which the brain can be artifically perfused. The real skill in resuscitation is in deciding when this technology is uncalled for. Such a decision should be made by a senior, experienced doctor.

POST-RESUSCITATION CARE

A successful immediate outcome from cardiac arrest does not guarantee ultimate survival. A number of principles should be followed as part of the duty of the A & E department in postresuscitation care:

1. **Identify the need for elective ventilation.** Although spontaneous respiratory effort may return quite soon after a heart beat, it is rarely adequate. The absence of a gag reflex requires the retention of the endotracheal tube. Its placement should be rechecked. 100% oxygen should be administered. Controlled *elective* ventilation allows hyperventilation to be used to reduce cerebral oedema.

2. **Correct any electrolyte and acid-base abnormalities —** in particular, abnormalities of the serum potassium Note the comments about sodium bicarbonate on p. 114.

3. **Check for any complications of the resuscitation.** A chest radiograph is required to exclude an iatrogenic pneumothorax and to confirm the correct siting of any venous lines, pacing wires or tracheal tube.

4. **Treat any heart failure.** A Swan-Ganz catheter will be required for haemodynamic monitoring.

5. **Correct dysrhythmias** if the underlying cause.

6. **Commence treatment for the underlying cause.** A twelve-lead diagnostic ECG is required.

7. **Institute measures for cerebral protection.** This is a contentious area with a number of claims for agents offering cerebral protection. Corticosteroids may have a place, but short-

term hyperventilation is currently, the only feasible manoeuvre worthy of consideration.

8. **Make adequate arrangements for after-care.** This should be to a critical care area; the intensive therapy or coronary care unit. The doctor should escort the patient to the clinican who has agreed to continue care, taking with him drugs and equipment lest the patient should rearrest en route.

SPECIAL CONSIDERATIONS

Airway obstruction

Obstruction to the upper airway carries with it a grave risk of respiratory and ultimately cardiac arrest. Every doctor working in an A & E department should be able to recognise and treat airway obstruction including, if necessary, an emergency laryngotomy or tracheotomy to bypass the obstruction.

The causes of airway obstruction include:
1. Inhalation of foreign bodies
2. Corrosive injuries to the mouth and throat
3. Burns to the mouth and throat
4. Injuries to the face and neck
5. Acute upper respiratory infections
6. Allergic oedema
7. Tumours, especially following radiotherapy.

Facial injuries are discussed in Chapters 14 and 42 and burns in Chapters 14 and 37.

Clinically, the obstructed patient is recognised by continuing respiratory efforts which fail to produce chest expansion. Unchecked, this leads to deep central cyanosis. Complete obstruction will be silent, incomplete obstruction produces noisy breathing, the nature depending on the level of the obstruction. When the glottis is partially blocked there will be intermittent inspiratory stridor.

Foreign body airway obstruction

Foreign body airway obstruction usually occurs during eating. Meat is the most common agent in adults, the presentation often being mistaken for a heart attack and giving substance to the term 'café coronary'. In children a whole variety of objects — sweets, grapes, toys, bottlecaps, etc. — can be introduced into the mouth only to be inhaled into the respiratory tract. Most inhaled foreign bodies will pass through the vocal cords and become impacted lower in the tracheobronchial tree (see Ch. 39). They do not usually cause airway obstruction and can be dealt with electively by the ENT department.

Foreign bodies may cause either partial or complete obstruction of the airway. When partial obstruction allows adequate air exchange the patient is able to cough. The patient should be bent forwards to allow the assistance of gravity and encouraged to cough.

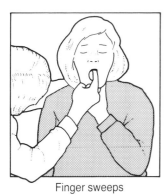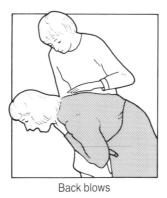

Finger sweeps   Back blows

Fig. 10.21 Backblows for the adult choking emergency.

In this position backslaps may help to free the obstructing object which can be coughed out (Fig. 10.21).

Foreign bodies which produce complete obstruction do so not because of their size, but because the irritation caused by their presence produces acute glottic spasm. In small children the best first aid treatment is to lay the child head-down along the outstretched arm and attempt to dislodge the foreign body by sharp blows with the flat of the hand to the child's back (Fig. 10.27).

Subdiaphragmatic abdominal thrusts described by Heimlich (1976), by elevating the diaphragm, can force air from the lungs in sufficient quantity to create an artificial cough intended to move and expel an obstructing foreign body from the airway. The doctor stands behind the patient and places his clasped hands on the patient's epigastrium. A rapid compression of the epigastrium should then expel the foreign body from the larynx (Fig. 10.22).

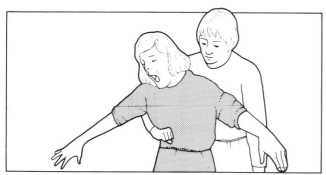

The abdominal thrust - form a fist with one hand

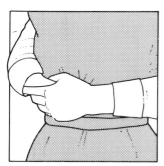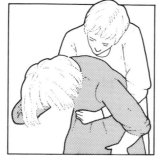

Grasp the fist and pull sharply upwards and inwards

Fig. 10.22 Abdominal thrust (Heimlich) manoeuvre.

If these methods fail, it is sometimes possible to dislodge the offending object from the larynx with a finger. If this fails and if the foreign body cannot be removed with Magill's forceps using direct laryngoscopy, then resort should be made to emergency laryngotomy as described below.

Acute epiglottitis

This serious condition can occur at all ages, but is commonest in young children. It is described in the next section.

Allergic glottic oedema

Allergic glottic oedema may occur either as part of a generalised anaphylactic reaction (see Ch. 15), or as a reaction to a local allergen, such as may occur when a bee or wasp is accidentally ingested.

> The treatment is:
> 1. Adrenaline 1:1000 0.5 ml subcutaneously then 0.1 ml/min i.v. over 5 minutes
> 2. Chlorpheniramine maleate 10 mg i.v.
> 3. Hydrocortisone 200 mg i.v.
> 4. 100% oxygen
> 5. Monitor ECG

When the cause is hereditary angioedema (see Ch. 45) an infusion of fresh frozen plasma should be administered.

Surgical relief of airway obstruction

The lives of many patients with acute upper airway obstruction have been saved by the performance of a timely tracheotomy. In the past, tracheotomy has been regarded as an heroic measure to be avoided at almost any cost. This is a perilous philosophy; the patient may die while the doctor deliberates. The operation is not difficult; the only requirements are a sharp knife and the courage to use it.

In adults the easiest emergency procedure is that of *laryngotomy* — the creation of an opening through the cricothyroid membrane. The patient is laid flat with a pillow or similar support under the shoulders to flex the neck and extend the head, thus bringing the larynx and trachea as far anteriorly as possible (Fig. 10.23). The thyroid and cricoid cartilages are identified by palpation and a vertical stab incision is made between these two cartilages (Fig. 10.24). When the airway is entered there is usually a bubbling of blood in the wound. The knife blade should then be twisted, a suitable tube, e.g. a 5 mm endotracheal tube, is inserted alongside the blade and the blade withdrawn. Kits for the performance of laryngotomy are available commercially (Fig. 10.25). Alternatively, one or more (four may be required) large-bore needles can be pushed through the cricothyroid membrane. A 12 gauge intravenous cannula is suitable; with the needle withdrawn the cannula hub can be connected by way of a 3.5 mm endotracheal tube connector to an oxygen-enriched bag-mask device. Both these

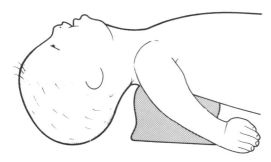

Fig. 10.23 Position for emergency laryngotomy.

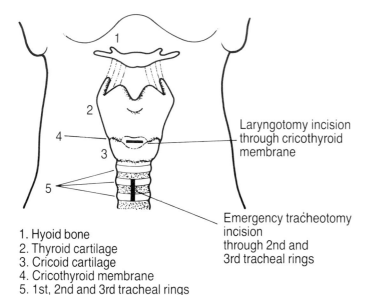

Laryngotomy incision through cricothyroid membrane

Emergency tracheotomy incision through 2nd and 3rd tracheal rings

1. Hyoid bone
2. Thyroid cartilage
3. Cricoid cartilage
4. Cricothyroid membrane
5. 1st, 2nd and 3rd tracheal rings

Fig. 10.24 Emergency laryngotomy.

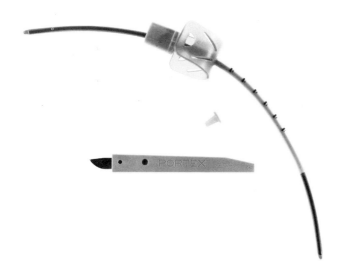

Fig. 10.25 A device for emergency cricothyrotomy.

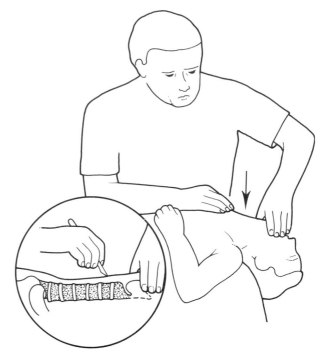

Fig. 10.26 Emergency tracheotomy in a small child.

procedures are temporising and a formal tracheotomy should be arranged without delay.

In children the cricothyroid membrane is small and often difficult to identify. It is usually easier to perform a tracheotomy. With older children the positioning is the same as for adults, but in the infant and small child it is easier for the surgeon to be seated with the child laid across his lap in such a way as to leave the head hanging (Fig. 10.26). The larynx is steadied with the left hand while a vertical stab incision is made in the midline approximately midway between the cricoid cartilage and the suprasternal notch. Intubation is effected in the same way as in the adult. In an extreme emergency it is a secondary consideration if the larynx is damaged or if the oesophagus is accidently incised during the procedure. The important thing is to establish the airway as rapidly as possible.

Children

Resuscitation techniques must be modified for the variations in size, shape, function and pathological processes which occur in childhood and infancy. Table 10.1 sets out the essential differences

Table 10.1 The differences in resuscitation parameters between infants, children and adults

	Baby	Child	Adult
Heart rate (beats/min)	120	100	60
External chest compressions (per min)	120	100	60
Depth (cm)	1–1	2–3	4–5
Respiratory rate	30	20	12
Expired air resuscitation (per min)	24	20	12

in resuscitation parameters between infants, children and adults. Primary cardiac arrest in childhood is a rare event and survival seldom occurs. By contrast, airway obstruction and respiratory arrest are frequent in children and deserve special mention.

Young children cool very rapidly and are readily prone to hypothermia; they should be adequately insulated during the resuscitation process.

The airway in children

Head tilt is performed as for the adult, with care being taken not to overextend the neck as this may cause kinking of the soft trachea, nor to press on the soft tissues in the floor of the mouth.

Airway obstruction may occur from a toy or a sweet and might be cleared by inverting the child along the outstretched arm and applying back blows (Fig. 10.27). Heimlich abdominal thrusts can be applied in the older child. Blind probing or finger sweeps might cause further impaction of the foreign body or result in damage, oedema or haemorrhage to the pharynx or larynx.

Infectious diseases affecting the upper airway in children, e.g. diphtheria or croup, may have serious or even fatal consequence if not carefully handled. An inspiratory stridor may be present in the conditions of acute *epiglottitis* and *laryngotracheo-bronchitis*. Table 10.2 sets out the main differential features of these two conditions. Acute epiglottitis is a fulminating bacterial infection of the supraglottic structures, particularly affecting children between the ages of 3 and 6 years. The causative organism is usually *Haemophilus influenzae*. The child will present with a history of sore throat progressing rapidly (over 2–6 hours) to respiratory distress and dysphagia. He will usually adopt a tripod position (Fig. 10.28) and will resist attempts to lay him down. Saliva will be seen to dribble from the mouth in severe cases and the child will have an anxious drawn look. Unlike most other cases of respiratory obstruction, respiratory efforts are often not very marked because the child quickly learns that, in attempting to

Table 10.2 Differential diagnosis of acute stridor

	Epiglottitis	Laryngotracheobronchitis
Incidence	Uncommon 3–6 years	Common 3/12–3 years
Onset	Rapid progression	12–36 hrs after URTI
Aetiology	*H. influenzae*	Virus
Severity	Child ill, toxic, temp 39.5	Not usually ill
Sore throat	Present	Absent
Voice	Muffled	Hoarse
Dysphagia	Present	Absent
Air hunger	Present 'Tripod sign'	Absent
Lateral neck X-ray	Epiglottic swelling	Subglottic narrowing

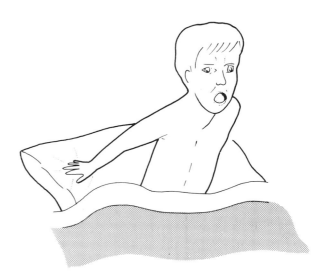

Fig. 10.28 The tripod position in acute epiglottitis — the following features should be noted: (1) the child is sitting up; (2) the chin is pushed forwards, the mouth open and the tongue protruded; (3) saliva tends to pool in the pharynx; and (4) breathing is slow and difficult.

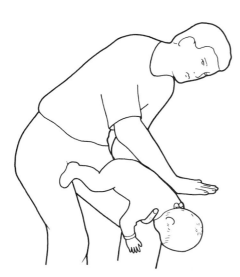

Fig. 10.27 Backblows in infants and children.

breathe, he simply decreases his laryngeal airway by drawing in the inflamed and grossly swollen supraglottic tissues. Although the diagnosis may sometimes be confirmed by asking the child to protrude his tongue, whereon the typical cherry-red swollen epiglottis will be seen to rise up from the base of the tongue, *on no account should an attempt be made to depress the tongue forcibly*. To do so is likely to precipitate total laryngeal obstruction by forcing the swollen epiglottis down over the glottic inlet. Lateral radiographs of the neck may show the grossly swollen epiglottis, but are both unnecessary and dangerous; unnecessary because the diagnosis is almost always clinically obvious and dangerous because the child may succumb while in the X-ray department. The patient with epiglottitis must be admitted to an intensive care unit or at least kept under the strictest possible observation. The most senior doctors available in the departments of paediatrics, anaesthesia and otolaryngology should be summoned. The patient will require airway protection either with endotracheal intubation or tracheotomy. Intubation is, however, sometimes impossible and should only be attempted in the operating theatre where there is someone standing by ready to perform a tracheotomy. *In no circumstances should a wait-and-see policy be adopted,* especially if drooling from the mouth is apparent.

> The technique for airway management of acute epiglottitis is summarised below:
> 1. Oxygen
> 2. Avoid erecting a drip or giving injections, etc. since anxiety may precipitate spasm and complete obstruction
> 3. Call anaesthetist and ENT surgeon
> 4. Gas induction with halothane until deep ... then oral intubation (range of thin tubes and stilettes needed) ... then change to nasopharyngeal tube if possible.

A loading dose of ampicillin (100 mg/kg i.v.) may be administered once the airway has been secured. Although the benefit of corticosteroids in this condition is not proven, it would seem wise to prescribe a short course at high dosage (e.g. dexamethasone 1 mg/kg 4-hourly).

Advanced airway support in children, as with all advanced paediatric resuscitation techniques, highlights the difficulties of using the equipment. It is essential that, before the emergency, all items are inspected. A wide range of tube sizes should be made available and the standardisation of connectors checked. Operators should have familiarised themselves with the special techniques and items of equipment required (Fig. 10.29, Tables 10.3 and 10.4).

Table 10.3 Endotracheal tube sizes for infants and children

Age	Endotracheal tube internal diameter (mm)	Length (cm) Oral	Length (cm) Nasal	Suction catheter (F)
Premature	2.5–3.0	11	13.5	6
Newborn	3.5	12	14	8
1 year	4.0	13	15	8
2 years	4.5	14	16	8
4 years	5.0	15	17	10
6 Years	5.5	17	19	10
8 years	6.0	19	21	10
10 years	6.5	20	22	10
12 years	7.0	21	22	10
14 years	7.5	22	23	10
16 years	8.0	23	24	12

$$\text{Tube size mm} = \frac{\text{Age of child} + 4.5}{4}$$

Table 10.4 Self-inflating bag volumes for infants and children

Age and weight	Bag volume (ml)	Tidal volume (ml)
< 2 years (< 7 kg)	240	205
2–10 years (7–30 kg)	500	350
> 10 years (> 30 kg)	1600	1000

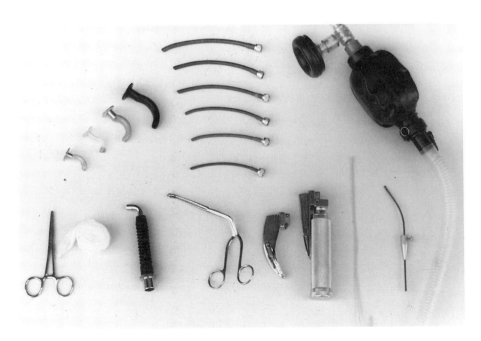

Fig. 10.29 Equipment for airway care in children.

Ventilation in children

If the child is not breathing expired air resuscitation will be necessary, usually by the mouth-to-mouth and nose method. The correct volume is adjusted by watching the chest movements. Ventilation is adjusted by altering the rate of breathing, not the tidal volume.

Paediatric resuscitation bags come in different sizes. They should incorporate a pressure limiting valve which prevents overpressurisation of the child's lungs. Oxygen supplementation through a reservoir is always required.

The circulation in children

The brachial pulse is the easiest to feel in children. A slow pulse may indicate hypoxia, which should be corrected by adequate ventilation. If the pulse be absent, chest compressions are applied to the junction of the lower and middle third of the sternum. The rate and depth of compressions varies with the child's age and size — a recommended range is given in Table 10.1. A ratio of 5 compressions per ventilation with a compression rate of at least 100 per minute is advised for young children. In small babies, two fingers only are used for the compressions — in larger children the heel of one hand.

Intravenous access in children is difficult and the choice of technique will vary with the skill of the operator. Generally, most resuscitations can be carried out through a 20 or 22 gauge cannula. Children do not tolerate even small degrees of hypovolaemia and it may be necessary to administer appropriate volumes of intravenous fluids though keeping a watchful eye out for the earliest signs of fluid overload.

Rarely, ventricular fibrillation might occur in children. The recommended defibrillation energy level is 2 joules/kilogram delivered through special paediatric paddles.

A list of drugs for cardiopulmonary resuscitation in infants and children, their dosages and routes is shown in Table 10.5. Paediatric

dosages relate to the weight of the child in kilograms — if, in an emergency, the child's body weight is unknown, then the age should be estimated and the dose of resuscitation drug read off from a standard paediatric nomogram (see Table 13.1).

The collapsed child

When faced with a child in a state of cardiovascular or respiratory collapse, time should not be wasted in the A & E department on the esoterics of diagnosis but, instead, a checklist should be followed which would be applicable to the majority of life-endangering conditions:

1. Clear the airway. Aspirate secretions. Ventilate on oxygen bag and mask then intubate if necessary.
2. Call the paediatrician.
3. I.v. infusion:
   a. No peripheral pulses
      PLASMA or SALINE
      10–20 ml/kg i.v. stat. then
      7–10 ml/kg/h depending on response
   b. Peripheral pulses present
      Dextrose 4% / saline 1/5N
      5–10 ml/kg stat or over 10 minutes, then
      7–10 ml/kg/h
4. Urgent investigations:
   Full blood count
   Electrolytes, blood glucose, dextrose-stick
   Blood cultures
   Rectal temperature
   Chest radiograph
   Monitor ECG
5. HYDROCORTISONE 100 mg i.v.
6. AMPICILLIN 250 mg plus CLOXACILLIN 250 mg i.v.
7. DEXTROSE 25%; 1–2 ml/kg i.v. if necessary.

Near drowning

The management of cases of near drowning and hypothermia are described in Ch. 28.

There is a fundamental difference in the mechanism of cardiorespiratory arrest in drowning from that which occurs in ischaemic heart disease. In the latter, circulatory arrest occurs as a result of ventricular fibrillation and breathing stops soon afterwards. In drowning this sequence of events is reversed with respiratory arrest occurring immediately after submersion, but the heartbeat continuing from some time. Human survival after 40 minutes total immersion have been recorded. Clearly protective mechanisms, as yet ill-understood, are at work. The inference in cases of drowning is that, especially in young people who appear to have an increased propensity for survival, rescue and resuscitation should persist even when the outcome initially appears gloomy. CPR should be tried for 1 hour at least.

Because of difficulties encountered in detecting the pulse, the

Table 10.5 Resuscitation drug dosages for infants and children

Drug	Dose	Route
Adrenaline	10 μg/kg (0.1 m/kg of 1 in 10 000)	Intravenous or endotracheal
Atropine	0.02 mg/kg (maximum 0.6 mg)	Intravenous or endotracheal
Sodium bicarbonate	1 mmol/kg (1 ml/kg of 8.4%)	Intravenous
Calcium chloride	5–10 mg/kg (0.3 ml/kg of 10%)	Intravenous
Lignocaine	1 mg/kg (0.1 ml/kg of 1%)	Intravenous or endotracheal
Dextrose	1 g/kg (2 ml/kg of 50%)	
Frusemide	1 mg/kg	

Infusions (usually in 5% dextrose solution)
Adrenaline — 0.02–0.05 μg/kg/min
Isoprenaline — 0.05–0.1 μg/kg/min
Dopamine — 1.10 μg/kg/min (calculate by adding 3 × bodyweight in mg of dopamine to 50 ml of 5% dextrose → infusion in ml/h equivalent to μg/kg/min)

carotid pulse should be felt for over at least 10 seconds, after first having successfully inflated the chest. If absent, combined heart-lung resuscitation should ensue for at least 1 hour without interruption. Two-rescuer CPR is much more effective because of the problems of exhaustion. In those uncommon cases where water has been taken into the lungs, chest inflation may be difficult. Bag-mask ventilation employing a PEEP (positive end expiratory pressure) valve may be beneficial for PEEP helps to prevent atelectasis due to loss of surfactant.

All patients who have been nearly drowned should be admitted for at least 24 hours, even if they appear perfectly well in the A & E department. The severe cases should be placed on the intensive care ward for elective ventilation, because of the problems of pulmonary and cerebral oedema which may develop at a later stage.

Hypothermia

The cerebral protection afforded by hypothermia to an arrested circulation is well known. Hypothermic patients should not be pronounced dead until a determined attempt has been made at rewarming. The method of rewarming will depend on the circumstances and resources available (see Ch. 27), but in an extreme case might include open chest cardiac massage, irrigation of the heart with warmed fluids and the use of cardiopulmonary bypass.

Throughout the resuscitation attempt, patient-handling should be kept to a minimum because ventricular fibrillation is easily provoked. It is unwise to intubate hypothermic patients unless they are already fibrillating or apnoeic. Electrical defibrillation is unlikely to be successful unless the core temperature exceeds 30°C.

REFERENCES

Heimlich H J 1976 A life-saving manoeuver to prevent food-choking. Journal of the American Medical Association 234: 398–401

Kaye W, Linhares K C, Breault R V, Norris P A, Stamoulis C C, Khan A H 1981 The Mega-Code for training the advanced cardiac life support team. Heart and Lung 10: 860–865

Kouwenhoven W B, Jude J R, Knickerbocker G G 1960 Closed chest cardiac massage. Journal of the American Medical Association 176: 574–580

Robertson C E, Little K 1984 Cardiopulmonary resuscitation in the accident and emergency department. Archives of Emergency Medicine 1: 17–22

Safar P 1959 The failure of manual artificial respiration. Journal of Applied Physiology 14: 84–88

Wardrope J, Crosby A C, Ferguson D G, Edbrooke D L 1986 A computerised prospective audit of cardiopulmonary resuscitation in the accident and emergency department. Archives of Emergency Medicine 3: 183–191

FURTHER READING

ABC of resuscitation Evan T R (ed) 1986 British Medical Journal, London

Save a life — an instructor's guide Fisher J, Marsden A K, Rogers J 1986 BBC Publications, London

Advanced techniques in resuscitation Greenberg M I, Gernerd M D, Roberts J R 1985 Williams and Wilkins, Baltimore

Clinics in emergency medicine Jacobson S (ed) 1983 Resuscitation Churchill Livingstone, New York

The Resuscitation Council UK (Reg. Charity No. 286360) Resuscitation Council, Dept of Anaesthetics, Royal Postgraduate Medical School, Hammersmith Hospital, Ducane Road, London W12 OHS Tel: 01-749-9974

Maintains a library of source material on all aspects of cardiopulmonary resuscitation. Its publications include Resuscitation Guide, Resuscitation for the Citizen, posters and wallcharts on Cardiopulmonary Resuscitation and a reference pack on advanced cardiac life support. For information send S.A.E. to the above address

Resuscitation from cardiopulmonary arrest: training and organisation Royal College of Physicians Journal of the Royal College of Physicians, London, 21, No. 4

Standards and guidelines for cardiopulmonary resuscitation and emergency cardiac care American Heart Association 1986 Journal of the American Medical Association 255: 2905-2996

Acute respiratory distress

The management of the patient with severe chest and cervical cord injuries, and of the conditions causing acute upper respiratory tract obstruction, are considered in Chapters 14, 10 and 44. This chapter is confined to the other common medical conditions in which breathlessness is life-threatening. Septicaemia (see Ch.13) and severe metabolic acidosis are excluded because the overbreathing associated with these states is not, in itself, the threat to life. Whilst hysterical hyperventilation can be quite alarming, it is rarely dangerous and is described in Chapter 31.

Respiratory failure is said to be present when the gas exchange function of the lungs is significantly impaired. The causes range from interference with the neuromuscular control of breathing (e.g. central nervous system depression or polyneuropathy), and flail chest (see Ch. 14), to diseases associated with severe airflow obstruction. The final common product in the patient is hypoxaemia with or without hypercapnia. A PaO_2 of less than 60 mmHg (8 kPa) when the patient is breathing room air at sea level is arbitrarily accepted as indicative of respiratory failure.

Before dealing with specific conditions some general points are made about the clinical examination and medical management.

HYPOXAEMIA

Lack of oxygen produces central cyanosis, sweating, tachycardia, hyperventilation, initially a rise in blood pressure, restlessness and confusion. The patient becomes acidotic and heart failure may get worse. Central cyanosis occurs when the PaO_2 drops below 50 mmHg (6.7 kPa) and the presence of at least 2.6 g/dl of reduced haemoglobin in the arterial blood is necessary for it to be clinically detectable. It is best seen in the mucous membranes of the mouth, is accentuated by polycythaemia and lessened by anaemia. Ultimately with severe hypoxia the patient becomes comatose, the vasomotor reflexes are depressed, cardiac dysrhythmias occur and ventilation ceases.

HYPERCAPNIA

Early symptoms of hypercapnia include headache due to raised intracranial pressure, and daytime drowsiness. Coarse tremors, muscle twitching and peripheral vasodilatation are common. The retinae may exhibit venous engorgement, sometimes progressing to frank papilloedema. As the $PaCO_2$ rises, depression of the central nervous system occurs. At a $PaCO_2$ of 80 mmHg (10.6 kPa) the patient is frequently drowsy and confused; if it rises above 100 mmHg (13.3 kPa), coma is likely. This situation rarely occurs when the patient is breathing room air as hypoxia is usually fatal first. However, it may arise in patients with chronic respiratory failure who are treated with too high a concentration of oxygen (see below).

OXYGEN TREATMENT

In the A & E department decisions regarding the need for administration of oxygen are initially made on the basis of the patient's clinical state. In general, breathless patients and those in heart failure should be given oxygen. These patients should also be encouraged to cough to help clear their bronchial secretions. Cyanosis alone is not necessarily an indication for oxygen because many such patients are in a perfectly stable condition. As a rough objective guide, if the PaO_2 falls below 60 mmHg (8 kPa) oxygen is necessary. Correction of hypoxaemia helps to dampen excessive respiratory drive and consequently makes the patient more comfortable.

In most instances the administration of high concentration oxygen for short periods of time is unlikely to do harm. High concentrations are especially urgent in patients in whom hypoxaemia has already impaired cardiac output, i.e. the patient is pale and sweating with cold peripheries and a feeble pulse. Care must be exercised in the patient with chronic pulmonary disease who has become dependent on a hypoxic respiratory drive (i.e. his $PaCO_2$ is persistently elevated). If uncontrolled concentrations of oxygen are administered to such a patient, hypoventilation and eventual apnoea may follow rapidly. Therefore, if there is any suspicion that the patient may have chronic obstructive airways disease, controlled low concentrations of oxygen must be given. In practice this means 24–28% oxygen delivered via a face mask fitted with a Venturi device (e.g. 'Ventimask'). The oxygen flow rate for each particular model is stamped on the mask and normally varies between 2–4 litres/minute. Even 24% oxygen should not be regarded as absolutely safe and the patient's respiratory response should be carefully observed. In the critically ill patient frequent measurements of the *arterial blood gases and pH* will be necessary to monitor the effects of oxygen treatment. Blood samples are usually obtained from the radial artery. Electrodes for transcutaneous PO_2 monitoring are popular in children as they are non-invasive and give a continuous read-out of the state of oxygenation of the blood. However, they are not entirely reliable. A more recent advance is the pulse oximeter which can be attached to a finger tip and will continuously record the pulse rate and the oxygen saturation of the blood. This device is relatively unaffected by a poor cardiac output. A saturation level below 85% indicates an urgent need for active intervention. The aim of administering oxygen should be to raise the PaO_2 above 60 mmHg (8 kPa) without causing the arterial pH to fall below 7.25 or the hydrogen ion concentration to rise above 55 mmol/l.

High concentration oxygen can be given to all other patients via light, disposable, low volume masks. The inspired oxygen concentration will vary between 25–80% depending on the oxygen flow rate (2–10 litres/minute), variations in respiration and malpositioning of the mask. Using non-rebreathing systems in which the oxygen is first passed into a bag and then, via a one-way inhalation valve, to the mask (Fig. 11.1), high concentrations of oxygen (80–90%) can be achieved at relatively low flow rates. By omitting the one-way valve and allowing some of the patient's exhaled gases to enter the bag, the ratio of oxygen to air drops to 60–80%.

Some patients will not tolerate face masks. The alternative is to give oxygen via nasal cannulae (prongs), which have the advantage of permitting eating, drinking and coughing without hindrance. At a normal respiratory rate, 2 litres/minute of oxygen by nasal cannulae gives an inspired oxygen of 25–30%. The maximum tolerable flow rate is about 4 litres/minute.

All oxygen should be humidified before delivery to the patient, otherwise secretions rapidly become dry and viscid. This is of particular importance when nasal cannulae are being used, or in the delivery of oxygen to the intubated patient. The danger of pulmonary oxygen toxicity only occurs when high concentrations of oxygen are delivered for prolonged periods and do not therefore

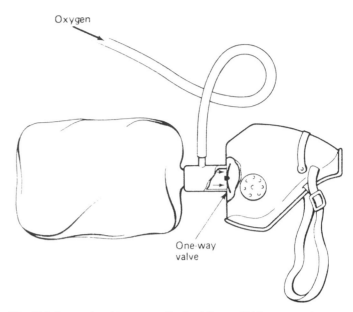

Fig. 11.1 A non-rebreathing system for the delivery of high concentration oxygen to the patient.

concern the A & E doctor. It is, however, sometimes forgotten that oxygen/air mixtures are explosive in the presence of inflammable materials and naked flames and any apparatus likely to cause sparks should be kept well away from the treatment area.

Mechanical ventilation is required for patients who have become too breathless, stuporous or exhausted to cough up secretions. The decision to ventilate should be made early rather than later. A patient who is suffering from a potentially reversible condition such as pneumonia, acute bronchial asthma, massive atelectasis or an overdose of a CNS depressant drug may come into this category. An inability to maintain the PaO_2 by administering high concentrations of oxygen by mask, plus a rising $PaCO_2$, are particularly ominous signs. Ventilation should also be instituted early in severe pulmonary oedema due to aspiration, inhalation, sepsis or acute heart failure. The patient's life may be saved by endotracheal intubation, vigorous tracheobronchial suction and a short period of assisted or mechanical ventilation. The key word in this decision making process is 'reversibility' and it is both inappropriate and inhumane to apply these extreme measures to a severe chronic respiratory 'cripple'. Relatives and the family doctor may be able to supply information regarding the patient's exercise tolerance prior to the acute episode. In a department where doctors of varying expertise may have to use the apparatus, ventilators should be simple to operate. In these circumstances, a volume-cycled machine is preferable to a pressure-cycled one because obstruction in the patient's air passages is more readily recognisable. The machine should be capable of providing a positive end expiratory pressure, be easy to sterilise and have means for accurate regulation of the inspired oxygen concentration.

The presentation and management of the common causes of life-threatening respiratory distress (Table 11.1) are described in the remainder of this chapter.

Table 11.1 Causes of life-threatening dyspnoea

Acute bronchial asthma
Cardiogenic pulmonary oedema
Massive pulmonary embolism
Spontaneous pneumothorax
Pneumonia
Acute exacerbations of chronic obstructive airways disease
Bronchiolitis
Non-cardiogenic pulmonary oedema (adult respiratory distress syndrome)
Miscellaneous — pleural effusions and neurological problems

ACUTE BRONCHIAL ASTHMA

The term 'status asthmaticus' has largely been dropped from the medical vocabulary and replaced by the more general term, acute bronchial asthma. Both expressions describe the clinical state of a patient dangerously ill as a consequence of severe bronchospasm. A rigid time scale is not an integral part of the definition. Some atopic patients become severely hypoxic within a matter of 20–30 minutes. Others, usually older patients, gradually deteriorate over days or weeks before arriving in the A & E department in a state of physical exhaustion. In practice, an attack of bronchial asthma which has not responded to one or two extra doses of the patient's usual bronchodilator within 1–2 hours is a medical emergency. In an acute exacerbation, asthmatic patients should be taught to seek help early rather than late. To this end, hospitals should operate an open door admission policy for these patients.

History

Immediate treatment with oxygen and nebulised salbutamol should be started before taking a history. Many patients will have had previous episodes of acute asthma. A knowledge of the pattern and severity of previous attacks is helpful, as it is often repeated. Did the patient require hospital admission previously and, more particularly, mechanical ventilation? Was there a previous pneumothorax?

A common story is that the patient has had to use his bronchodilator more often than usual, but with diminishing effect. Breathlessness has increased inexorably. Early in the attack inspiration tends to be more difficult than expiration, but later both become equally difficult. Breathlessness may have eventually become so severe that eating, drinking and talking were hindered. Due to the natural diurnal variation in airways narrowing many of these patients arrive in hospital in the early hours of the morning.

Other individuals will be seen during their first acute attack of wheezing. The diagnosis of bronchial asthma is not usually difficult. Many children and young adults will have a history of atopy (e.g. infantile eczema, hay fever or perennial rhinitis) and/or a family history of asthma. The possibility of an inhaled foreign body should be considered, especially in children. Problems can arise amongst older patients in deciding whether wheeze is due to late-onset (intrinsic) bronchial asthma or a reversible

bronchoconstrictive component in a person suffering from chronic bronchitis. A history of persistent sputum overproduction suggests the latter and should lead to care with oxygen administration (see under Management). Otherwise, the emergency medical management is the same in both cases. It may be possible to identify the precipitating cause of the acute attack from the patient's history, although this is not of great practical importance in the immediate management. Common precipitants include: respiratory tract infections (more often viral than bacterial), inhaled allergens such as pollens and animal danders, drugs such as aspirin, β-adrenergic blocking agents and non-steroidal anti-inflammatory preparations, food dyes such as tartrazine, mental stress, exercise and poor treatment compliance.

It is most important to find out if the patient has received any emergency treatment before being sent to hospital as any drugs already administered may have a substantial influence on the treatment plan in the A & E department. For instance, if the patient has been on oral treatment with aminophylline or has had an intravenous loading dose, it may be dangerous to inject more. A list of the patient's current medications and any drug allergies should always be recorded.

Occasionally wheezing may be the main presenting symptom of left heart failure and other rare conditions such as allergic bronchopulmonary aspergillosis, polyarteritis nodosa and the carcinoid syndrome.

Examination

The characteristic feature of bronchial asthma is wheeze which is heard in both phases of respiration but is more prolonged in the expiratory phase. There is no correlation between the loudness or pitch of the wheeze and the severity of the attack. In the typical patient all the accessory respiratory muscles will be in use and the chest hyperexpanded. Life may be endangered by hypoxia or physical exhaustion, most usually in combination, or rarely a tension pneumothorax.

The signs of severe asthma are:
1. The patient has become too breathless to speak.
2. The disappearance of wheeze — a silent chest indicates widespread bronchial obstruction (rarely a pneumothorax).
3. Evidence of hypoxaemia — tachycardia (over 110 beats per minute in an adult), mental confusion, vasoconstricted peripheries and central cyanosis.
4. Physical exhaustion — a diminishing amplitude of the paradoxical pulse is one objective sign.
5. Evidence of circulatory embarrassment such as hypotension.
6. A sudden increase in breathlessness which may signify a pneumothorax.
7. A falling PaO_2, rising $PaCO_2$ and persistent metabolic acidosis.

Management

The patient is most comfortable sitting up so that the accessory muscles of respiration can be used to best advantage. The ECG should be monitored continuously throughout the attack.

Oxygen

Patients with severe bronchial asthma are always hypoxaemic. In most there is no danger of causing hypoventilation and 100% oxygen can be safely administered. The exception is the older person who may have chronic bronchitis, to whom 24–28% oxygen should be given. The oxygen should always be humidified as the patient is often already dehydrated and further drying up of bronchial secretions can cause widespread inspissation of mucus and rapid death. Ideally a heated humidifier should be used to lessen the chance of cold-induced bronchoconstriction.

An arterial blood sample for gas and acid/base analysis should be obtained at the beginning of therapy to provide a baseline. The time and oxygen concentration being administered should be recorded. Typically the PaO_2 will be reduced and the $PaCO_2$ normal or low. Metabolic acidosis is also common and resolves spontaneously during recovery. Further blood gas measurements can be made according to the patient's progress. A rising $PaCO_2$ is a particularly ominous sign, indicating inadequate ventilation. Blood gas values should be correlated with the patient's clinical condition and decisions regarding therapy should take both into account.

N.B. High concentration oxygen must always be given before a bronchodilator otherwise underperfused areas in the lung may be opened up causing the PaO_2 to fall.

Bronchodilators

Selective β_2-adrenoceptor stimulants are now generally accepted as the first line bronchodilators. They can be given either by nebuliser or intravenously. Both methods are equally effective but nebulisation is preferable, especially in children. The nebuliser should be driven by oxygen at a flow rate of at least 4 l/min. The initial dose for adults is 5 mg salbutamol or its equivalent. Up to 10 mg may be used. If the patient has ischaemic heart disease the dose should be halved or angina may be precipitated. The drug should be diluted with normal saline to a total volume of 5 ml, as smaller volumes permit greater loss by deposition on the walls of the nebuliser chamber. The adult intravenous bolus dose is 0.5 mg and both salbutamol and terbutaline can also be given by continuous intravenous infusion. If there is no nebuliser available a high dose administered via a spacer device, such as a nebuhaler, is usually effective.

Children under 18 months can be relatively resistant to the bronchodilatory effects of β_2-stimulants and aminophylline or ipratropium (see below) are sometimes used instead as the initial therapy. Occasionally subcutaneous adrenaline (0.1–0.3 ml of 1 : 1000) is given to very young children.

Aminophylline is an effective bronchodilator but there are several problems associated with its use and it should only be given if β_2-agonists fail to produce an adequate response. It has a narrow therapeutic range and a high incidence of side effects, the commonest being agitation, nausea and vomiting. More serious side effects include ventricular tachydysrhythmias, convulsions, hypotension and occasional sudden death. The usual adult intravenous loading dose of aminophylline is 5.6 mg/kg injected over 20 minutes, which can be followed by an infusion of 0.5 mg/kg per hour. However, many patients are receiving long-acting oral theophylline derivatives as part of their maintenance therapy and will already have appreciable blood theophylline levels on arrival at hospital. If a patient has taken oral theophylline or been given aminophylline by injection within the previous 24 hours, the above doses should be halved. There should be a similar dosage reduction in the elderly or patients with cardiac, hepatic or renal disease and those taking erythromycin or cimetidine. Ipratropium bromide is an anticholinergic agent which acts synergistically with sympathomimetics and the combination will produce greater bronchodilatation than either used alone. In an adult 0.5 mg of the drug should be made up in saline and the solution given by nebuliser.

Steroids

All patients with severe asthma must be given intravenous hydrocortisone, the initial dose being 4 mg/kg body weight. The benefit of its action is not immediate but becomes apparent after several hours.

Other drugs

In the occasional patient in whom acute bronchospasm has been caused by the injudicious use of a β_2-blocker, intravenous glucagon can help to reverse the situation. Antibiotics are rarely necessary and do not need to be given in the A & E department.

Intravenous fluids

This aspect of treatment can easily be overlooked. Many patients become significantly dehydrated because they are too breathless to drink and because of increased fluid loss from the respiratory tract and through sweating. The dehydration not only produces hypovolaemia but also increases the viscosity of the bronchial secretions thereby increasing the likelihood of their plugging the airways. An intravenous crystalloid infusion should therefore be started. Some patients may also become markedly hypokalaemic from a combination of the effects of hyperventilation, sympathomimetic drugs and corticosteroids and potassium supplementation will then be necessary. An intravenous line also provides ready access to the circulation for the administration of drugs. The risk of overhydration, especially in children, should not be forgotten. Sodium bicarbonate should *never* be infused in the A & E department. As the patient's ventilation improves, acidosis will resolve spontaneously.

Investigations

A chest X-ray is mandatory as it may reveal a clinically undetectable pneumothorax, sometimes accompanied by mediastinal or subcutaneous emphysema. The chest film should be closely scrutinised. A shallow pneumothorax can be very difficult to see against the background of the hyperinflated lungs. An expiratory film may be required. Relief of even a small air leak by chest drainage may tip the balance towards survival. The typical radiographic findings are overexpanded lungs with peripheral air trapping (Fig 11.2) and occasionally signs of a superimposed infection. Patchy infiltrates and segmental, lobar, or occasionally whole lung collapse are found in allergic bronchopulmonary aspergillosis.

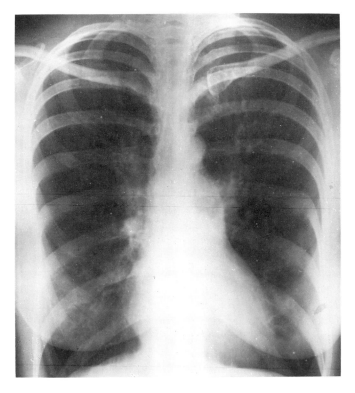

Fig. 11.2 Hyperexpanded lungs in acute bronchial asthma.

Monitoring the ECG is more important than obtaining a write-out. Sinus tachycardia is virtually invariable. Evidence of right heart strain and supraventricular rhythm disturbances are an occasional feature.

Serial blood gas measurements have already been mentioned.

Initially patients are often too breathless to provide peak expiratory flow readings. However, they may improve enough to enable a baseline reading to be obtained before going to a hospital ward. Finally, blood samples should be taken for measurement of serum electrolytes, the haemoglobin level and white cell count.

Controlled ventilation and bronchial lavage

If the asthma is very severe an anaesthetist should be summoned *early*. A small number of patients require mechanical ventilation because they suffer a sudden cardiorespiratory arrest or present in extremis with both circulatory and respiratory failure. Other patients may require ventilation because they fail to respond to treatment and become increasingly distressed with worsening hypoxaemia, exhaustion, a decreasing level of consciousness and a rising arterial carbon dioxide tension. 100% oxygen should be used. Induction of anaesthesia with halothane, ether or an intravenous infusion of ketamine produces bronchodilation and therefore has specific benefit in this dangerous situation.

The decision to ventilate should be based on clinical grounds, with analysis of arterial blood gas tensions being no more than supporting evidence. Suggested guidelines for the latter are an initially high $PaCO_2$ (greater than 50 mmHg or 6.7 kPa) despite oxygen therapy. Persistent metabolic acidosis is another ominous warning sign.

Some mechanically ventilated patients fail to improve because their lungs prove virtually impossible to inflate. Bronchial lavage should then be considered, the aim being to remove plugs of inspissated mucus. Aliquots of physiological saline are run into the lungs through the endotracheal tube, with the patient positioned to wash out each pulmonary segment. The mixture of fluid and bronchial plugs is then aspirated by mechanical suction. This procedure will normally be carried out in the intensive care unit by those experienced in the technique.

Beware of *tension pneumothorax* resulting from mechanical ventilation.

Acute bronchoconstriction may be part of a generalised *anaphylactic reaction* (see Ch. 13). These patients require an immediate subcutaneous injection of adrenaline (1 ml of 1 : 1000), repeated after 2–5 minutes if necessary, and followed by an antihistamine and hydro-cortisone given intravenously. Oxygen should be administered and the ECG monitored throughout.

There is NO place for the use of sedatives or tranquillisers in acute bronchial asthma.

CARDIOGENIC PULMONARY OEDEMA

The conditions which commonly underlie acute attacks of left heart failure include acute myocardial infarction, chronic ischaemic heart disease, hypertension, cardiac dysrhythmias, drug toxicity (e.g. β-blockers) and mitral or aortic valve disease. Among infants congenital heart disease, tachydysrhythmias and myocarditis associated with bronchiolitis are the usual causes. Occasionally a severe attack of rheumatic carditis will cause heart failure in an older child or young adult.

History

The attacks often occur at night when the patient is in bed but may be provoked at any time by exertion or emotion. Characteristically, the individual is awakened by a dry cough and a sensation of intense breathlessness to the point of suffocation. There is often a history of increasing orthopnoea, episodes of paroxysmal nocturnal dyspnoea, previous heart attacks, angina, hypertension or rheumatic heart disease. The presence or absence of cardiac-type pain is particularly important to establish, especially if the patient was previously well.

It is also important to find out what current medicines the patient may be taking, for several reasons: 1. they may be a useful pointer to the diagnosis, 2. the inappropriate prescription of β-blockers may have precipitated the attack and 3. it must be established if the patient is already taking digoxin, for if he is, it cannot be given as part of the emergency treatment regimen as a fatal dysrhythmia might be provoked.

Examination

The diagnosis is usually obvious on first sight of the patient. The bolt upright posture, rapid noisy respirations, profuse sweating, vasoconstricted cyanotic peripheries and foam-flecked lips are quite characteristic. Central cyanosis may also be present. On closer inspection most patients will have cold clammy skin, a tachycardia, pulsus alternans, a gallop rhythm and widespread pulmonary crepitations. The blood pressure is often increased but is sometimes low, especially after myocardial infarction. There may also be quite marked bronchospasm, hence the expression 'cardiac asthma'. In addition to the signs of left heart failure there may be evidence of systemic venous congestion, as right heart failure is often associated with left-sided failure

The cardinal signs of acute heart failure in small infants are tachycardia, tachypnoea and liver enlargement.

Management

The patient should be propped upright and 100% oxygen administered by face-mask unless chronic respiratory disease is suspected. The ECG should be monitored throughout treatment and an arterial blood sample obtained for blood gas analysis. Venous access should be established and the following drugs injected intravenously (except nitrates):

1. A quick acting diuretic such as frusemide (50–250 mg), bumetanide (1 mg) or ethacrynic acid (50–100 mg) — they act by producing rapid vasodilatation as well as by diuresis.

2. Morphine (5–15 mg) or diamorphine hydrochloride (2.5–5 mg). These drugs help to allay the acute anxiety caused by this condition and reduce cardiac work. They are particularly indicated for the relief of severe chest pain from myocardial infarction and immediately prior to the institution of mechanical ventilation. Naloxone must be immediately available in case of respiratory arrest.

3. Aminophylline (5.6 mg/kg given over 15–20 minutes) — this drug combines both positive inotropic and bronchodilatory properties and is especially suitable if there is any doubt about the relative bronchial and cardiac contributions to the breathlessness.

4. Sublingual glyceryl trinitrate (0.8–2.4 mg every 5–10 minutes) or isosorbide dinitrate (10 mg sublingually or orally) — nitrates cause venodilatation and reduce 'preload' on the heart.

5. Digoxin (up to 0.5 mg given over 2 minute) if the patient is in atrial flutter or fibrillation. The drug is contraindicated if

the patient is already receiving oral digoxin and after acute myocardial infarction when there is an increased risk of digoxin induced rhythm disturbances.

If these measures have not ameliorated the attack within 10–15 minutes and the patient remains acutely distressed, 500 ml of blood should be removed by venesection.

Cardiac output in severe heart failure can also be improved by combined vasodilator and inotropic therapy. If pulmonary congestion associated with a high venous filling pressure is the main problem, reduction of 'preload' with a nitrate may be of benefit. Nitrates can be administered intravenously and may be combined with an infusion of dopamine or dobutamine if the systolic blood pressure is below 100 mmHg. Dobutamine is preferred because the inotropic effects are more predictable. In low output heart failure the infusion of dobutamine, sometimes with the addition of an arteriolar vasodilator (e.g. hydralazine or sodium nitroprusside), may be life saving. Because the doses must be carefully titrated against the responses this type of combination therapy should only be given under conditions of full haemodynamic monitoring. In practice, this usually means in an intensive care unit with a Swan-Ganz catheter in situ.

Children in acute heart failure are usually treated with oxygen, intramuscular or intravenous digoxin (0.015 mg/kg) and frusemide (1 mg/kg) alone.

As a last resort mechanical ventilation may be necessary for unresponsive cardiogenic pulmonary oedema.

In severe hypertensive left heart failure, if the diastolic pressure has not fallen below 130 mmHg and the patient's general condition not shown any improvement after administration of intravenous frusemide and morphine, more morphine can be given. The best drug for lowering blood pressure is sodium nitroprusside, but it requires intensive care unit facilities for its administration. Less satisfactory alternatives, due to their unpredictability include hydralazine (10–20 mg intramuscularly or intravenously — even after intravenous administration the effect develops gradually over 15–20 minutes) and diazoxide (50–150 mg by slow intravenous injection). The aim of treatment is slowly to reduce the diastolic blood pressure to about 100 mmHg. The emphasis is on 'slowly' as unexpected extreme hypotension can precipitate a stroke, blindness or myocardial infarction.

When the patient's clinical state is sufficiently stable, an ECG write-out and chest X-ray can be obtained. A chest film is useful for later comparison.

The typical radiographic features of left heart failure are:
1. Overall cardiac enlargement.
2. Congestion of the upper lobe pulmonary veins.
3. Prominence of the pulmonary arteries.
4. Perihilar blurring.
5. Soft alveolar shadowing (oedema), typically bat's wing in distribution but occasionally unilateral (more often right sided than left).
6. Kerley's B lines.
7. Small basal pleural effusions.

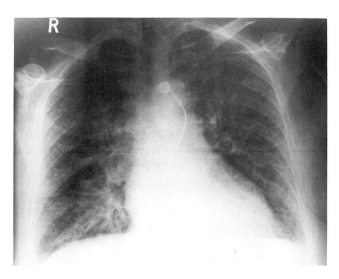

Fig. 11.3 A chest radiograph showing the typical features of acute left ventricular failure (see text).

Figure 11.3 illustrates many of these features.

Individuals who respond satisfactorily to the initial treatment, and who are not deemed to have had a recent myocardial infarction, can be admitted to a general medical ward.

MASSIVE PULMONARY EMBOLISM

Most large pulmonary emboli arise in the deep veins of the thighs and pelvis and as many as 50% of these venous thromboses are asymptomatic. Other occasional sources are the right side of the heart and arm veins of patients with indwelling central lines. Profound haemodynamic effects are produced when 50% or more of the pulmonary arterial tree is obstructed.

History

The following conditions predispose to venous thromboembolism: prolonged bed rest, cardiac failure, recent abdominal or orthopaedic surgery, leg trauma (including long journeys in a cramped position), varicose veins, previous thromboembolism, pregnancy and use of the contraceptive pill and disseminated malignancy. Obese patients over the age of 50 with these conditions are at special risk. One or more smaller 'herald' emboli quite often precede massive embolism and the symptoms they can produce should be recognised as possibly premonitory. For instance they may cause pleuritic pain and haemoptysis which are not essential features of the major event. The latter is characterised by sudden intense respiratory distress, cardiac-type chest pain, syncope and, in the worst cases, cardiorespiratory arrest.

Examination

The typical patient is severely dyspnoeic with evidence of acute right heart failure and a low output state. The blood pressure is low or unrecordable and the pulse rapid and of small volume.

Central cyanosis often has a peripheral component superadded due to marked vasoconstriction. The neck veins are distended. A right ventricular gallop rhythm, best heard at the left sternal edge, and absent pulmonary valve closure may be apparent on auscultation. The breath sounds are often unremarkable, but mild bronchospasm may occur. The patient is often confused and there may be evidence in the legs suggestive of deep venous thrombosis, such as swelling, tenderness and discoloration. Myocardial infarction with cardiogenic shock and left ventricular failure may produce a superficially similar clinical state except that those patients prefer to sit up. In contradistinction, after massive pulmonary embolism the patient prefers to lie flat and may lose consciousness if sat up.

Management

The patient should be placed supine, as the horizontal position helps to maintain right ventricular filling pressure and cerebral perfusion. 100% oxygen should be administered by face mask or endotracheal tube and the heart rhythm continuously monitored. A large intravenous dose of heparin (10 000–15 000 units) should be administered in an attempt to counteract serotonin-mediated vasoconstriction in the pulmonary vasculature. An intravenous infusion of 500 ml of Dextran 70 should be started with the aim of promoting venous return and supporting right ventricular output. In the severely collapsed patient external cardiac massage may help to disperse large emboli and should be maintained throughout the resuscitation attempt.

Arterial blood should be obtained for gas and acid/base analysis. Usually the PaO_2 and $PaCO_2$ are both low. If the pH is also low, the acidosis should be corrected by ventilating the patient.

Massive pulmonary embolism is primarily a clinical diagnosis. Electrocardiographic and chest X-ray findings may help but are often non-specific and both may be entirely normal. Suggestive ECG changes may be seen in about 85% of patients and may include one or more of the following:

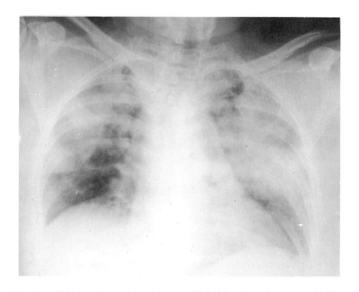

Fig. 11.4 Widespread opacities due to multiple bilateral pulmonary emboli.

1. Sinus tachycardia or atrial dysrhythmias.
2. Right axis shift.
3. Changes indistinguishable from those of inferior myocardial infarction.
4. T wave inversion in the right precordial leads.
5. Partial or complete right bundle branch block.

The combination of 2. and 3. is conveniently referred to as the S1, Q3, T3 pattern.

Suggestive radiographic findings (Figs 11.4, 11.5) are:
1. An area or areas of lung devoid of vascular markings due to patchy oligaemia.
2. A prominent right hilar shadow due to abrupt cut off of a slightly dilated pulmonary artery at the site of occlusion.
3. Visible thrombus in the descending branch of the right pulmonary artery (very rare).
4. An area of atelectasis, often at the right base, with elevation of the right haemidiaphragm and a small pleural effusion (or the last alone).
5. Evidence of previous peripheral thromboembolism such as a raised hemidiaphragm, a segmental opacity or plate atelectasis.

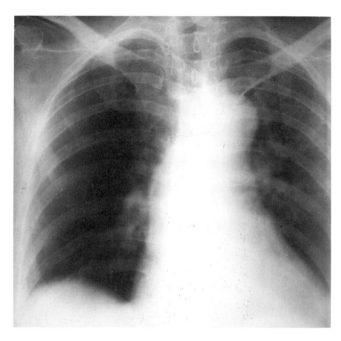

Fig. 11.5 Thrombus outlined in the descending branch of the right pulmonary artery, producing almost complete avascularity of the right lung field.

It must be re-emphasised that even after a large pulmonary embolus the chest X-ray may look entirely normal. If the diagnosis is in doubt, a ventilation/perfusion lung scan may be helpful.

In massive embolism with peristent shock and hypoxia, thrombolytic drugs or pulmonary embolectomy should be instigated. Unless there is a contraindication (see below), streptokinase can be given in a standard dosage of 250 000 units, administered intravenously over 30–60 minutes. The thrombin clotting time should be measured beforehand and 100 mg of intramuscular hydrocortisone given simultaneously to prevent allergic reactions. Contraindications to streptokinase therapy include active peptic ulceration, hypertension, acute cerebrovascular disease, recent surgery, severe renal or hepatic insufficiency and pregnancy and the immediate postpartum period (up to 10 days).

When thrombolytic therapy is contraindicated, or deterioration occurs despite the above measures, the patient should be considered for pulmonary embolectomy which necessitates cardiopulmonary bypass facilities. Prior to embolectomy the patient will require investigation either by selective pulmonary angiography or by simple venous angiocardiography. A new dimension in treatment is offered by interventional radiography in which the thrombus may be removed from the pulmonary artery by a suction catheter inserted via the femoral vein.

SPONTANEOUS PNEUMOTHORAX

Spontaneous pneumothoraces are categorised as primary (pneumothorax simplex) and secondary. The former is usually due to rupture of a small apical bulla or bleb, the rest of the lung being normal. More than three-quarters of these patients are tall, thin young males. Secondary pneumothoraces may be caused by a wide variety of either generalised or localised lung diseases, the most common being asthma, emphysema and subpleural neoplasia.

Life may be endangered if one of the following situations arises:
1. A tension pneumothorax develops.
2. A pneumothorax, however small, occurs in a patient with serious generalised lung disease (e.g. acute bronchial asthma or emphysema).
3. Simultaneous bilateral pneumothoraces occur (very rare).
4. If the pneumothorax is complicated by tearing of a blood vessel producing a haemopneumothorax (less than 5% of cases).

History

In uncomplicated pneumothorax there is a wide variation in the severity of symptoms. Chest pain may range from a slight localised twinge to oppressive substernal pain mimicking myocardial infarction. Breathlessness shows a similar variation. If tension develops, due to a flap-valve effect, breathlessness is rapidly progressive. A sudden increase of breathlessness in a person with pre-existing lung disease should also immediately suggest the diagnosis of pneumothorax. Specific questions should therefore be aimed at identifying patients with chronic pulmonary diseases. Some patients will have had one or more similar episodes in the past.

Examination

If a tension pneumothorax develops the patient becomes intensely dyspnoeic, tachypnoeic and cyanosed. The trachea is shifted to the opposite side and the affected hemithorax is hyper-resonant and silent. Due to the mediastinal displacement, venous return to the heart is rapidly obstructed resulting in engorgement of the neck veins and a rapid, small volume pulse. If the air is not released at this stage cardiovascular collapse will occur. This clinical situation is an ACUTE MEDICAL EMERGENCY. There is no time for radiographic confirmation.

Very rarely air escapes into the mediastinum producing an audible click and crunch in time with the beating of the heart (Hamman's sign). The air may also track upwards into the root of the neck and beyond, causing obvious surgical emphysema.

A combination of hypotension, basal dullness to percussion and a succussion splash should suggest a haemopneumothorax.

Management

Tension pneumothorax demands the immediate insertion through the second intercostal space anteriorly of whatever large-bore needle or cannula is to hand. Improvement in the patient's cardiorespiratory state should accompany the hiss of escaping air. Formal tube drainage can be instituted later.

Most other patients will be well enough to have a postero-anterior chest radiograph taken to confirm the diagnosis. The typical findings are shown in Figure 11.6. The collapsed lung appears as a dense clump close to the left hilum and left heart border. The periphery is devoid of bronchovascular markings and the line of the visceral pleura is easily seen. The upper lobe is usually the first to collapse. Subcutaneous or mediastinal emphysema appears as translucent linear streaks. The major differential diagnosis is a large emphysematous bulla.

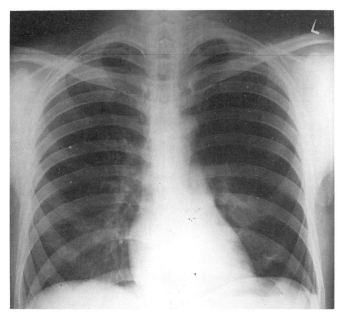

Fig. 11.6 A large primary pneumothorax producing almost total collapse of the left lung.

Occasional situations do arise when, because of acute breathlessness, it may be necessary to insert a chest drain before obtaining a chest X-ray. One simple method of confirming the diagnosis is to place a 21 G needle on a 10 ml syringe and aspirate while passing it through the second intercostal space in the midclavicular line. If there is a pneumothorax the air will aspirate easily. If, on the other hand, the needle enters the lung, aspiration will be difficult and some blood and air bubbles will appear in the syringe.

Chest drain insertion (see also Ch. 14)

The procedure should be briefly explained to the patient. In an emergency, the cannula is usually inserted in the second intercostal space in the mid-clavicular line. An alternative is the 4th or 5th intercostal space in the anterior or mid-axillary line just behind the lateral border of the pectoral muscles.

> The following equipment is required:
> 1. A chest drain, an introducer (24–32 French gauge) and clamps — the introducer or trocar should have a blunt tip.
> 2. Sterile towels, gloves and antiseptic solution.
> 3. 15–20 ml of 1% plain lignocaine.
> 4. A scalpel and silk suture material.
> 5. An underwater seal bottle containing 500 ml of sterile water — ensure that the top is on correctly and the correct tube below the water level.

The patient should be placed supine with his head turned away from the operative site. Full aseptic precautions must be applied. A point midway between the second and third ribs in the mid-clavicular line is located, using the sternal angle as a guide. A bleb of local anaesthetic is injected under the skin and the needle is advanced through into the chest while aspirating gently. When bubbles appear, the needle is withdrawn until the bubbling stops, which indicates that it has passed out through the parietal pleura. This is a very sensitive area and 4–5 ml of anaesthetic should be injected there. The remaining lignocaine is used to infiltrate the intercostal muscle. The operator should then scrub up and clean the operative field with chlorhexidine and iodine. The anaesthetised area is then surrounded with sterile towels. A 1 cm transverse incision is made in the intercostal muscle and the path can be enlarged by blunt dissection. The pleura is cut so that air escapes. The hole should be large enough that no force is required to push the drain into the chest. The drain and introducer are placed perpendicularly at the site of the incision. One hand placed at skin level should be used to control the length of tube entering the pleural cavity. There is usually a slight 'give' as it passes through the intercostal muscle. Both introducer and drain should be inserted approximately 5 cm and the introducer then removed. About 10 cm of the drain should be fed into the pleural space, then clamped and connected to the tube which goes under the water in the drainage bottle (Fig 11.7). When the clamp is released bubbles should appear in the bottle. The drain should be securely

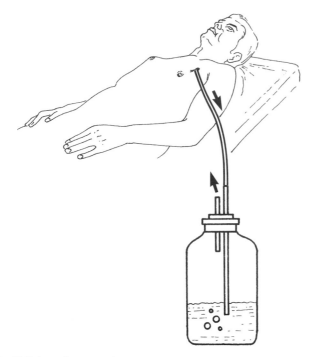

Fig. 11.7 An underwater seal.

tied to the sutures in the wound. The wound can then be cleaned and dressed and the drain firmly taped to the skin. The tube connections should all be checked and taped. Finally the position of the tube should be checked on a repeat chest X-ray.

PNEUMONIA

Pneumonia takes its most severe toll when it supervenes upon chronic illnesses such as long-standing pulmonary disorders, cerebrovascular disease, diabetes, alcoholism, immunoparesis (e.g. AIDS) and heart failure. The commonest pre-existing chronic respiratory disease is chronic bronchitis, but pneumoconiosis, bronchiectasis and carcinoma may all be complicated by secondary pneumonia. Previously fit young people sometimes develop such extensive pneumonia, which may be of either viral, bacterial or mycoplasmal origin, that ventilatory failure occurs. Pneumonia may also follow aspiration of either gastric contents or a foreign body.

History

An upper respiratory tract infection followed by the development of a productive cough, breathlessness and pleuritic pain is easily recognised as pneumonia. Old or debilitated patients may, however, exhibit few definitive respiratory symptoms. They may just become confused, lose their appetite and languish in bed.

A general medical history and a list of current medications should always be obtained. Opportunistic lung infections are one common and serious manifestation of the acquired immune deficiency syndrome (AIDS — see Ch. 25). The family doctor may have already started treatment with an antibiotic to which the patient has not responded and this information will be relevant to further therapy.

Examination

The typical patient is breathless, pyrexial and hypoxic, the last feature being mainly evidenced by mental confusion. An eruption of 'cold sores' around the mouth is a common accompaniment. Older patients do not always develop a pyrexia. Congestive heart failure with peripheral circulatory stasis and dehydration may complicate the clinical picture, especially in the elderly. Examination of the chest may reveal classic signs of consolidation, a pleural rub or evidence of a small effusion. More often the only abnormalities detected are reduced movement on the affected side and inspiratory crackles. Pre-existing lung disease may modify the clinical signs. Extreme prostration should suggest septicaemia.

Management

This is essentially supportive, namely correction of hypoxia, dehydration, acidosis and heart failure. Care must be taken with the concentration of oxygen administered if a background of chronic pulmonary disease is suspected. Arterial blood gas measurements help to guide the oxygen requirements. Intravenous fluids may be required, but again care should be exercised if there are signs of heart failure. A chest radiograph (Fig. 11.8), ECG recording and white cell count should be obtained routinely. The clinical and radiological differential diagnoses include pulmonary infarction, tuberculosis, acute alveolitis, pulmonary oedema, bronchiectasis, pulmonary eosinophilia complicating bronchial asthma, a pleural effusion or empyema and lung abscesses. If septicaemia is suspected, blood samples should be taken for culture. Apart from this last instance, antibiotics will rarely be started in the A & E department. Mechanical ventilation is sometimes required.

The indications for ventilation in an adult are:
1. Previously well, or at least no untreatable terminal condition.
2. A respiratory rate over 40 breaths minute.
3. Increasing drowsiness and exhaustion with inability to expel secretions.
4. A rising $PaCO_2$ above 50 mmHg (6.7 kPa).

ACUTE EXACERBATIONS OF CHRONIC OBSTRUCTIVE AIRWAYS DISEASE

These periodic infective exacerbations are the commonest cause of breathlessness during the late winter and early spring. Paradoxically, many of these patients may be in severe respiratory failure (PaO_2 below 60 mmHg or 8 kPa and $PaCO_2$ above 50 mmHg or 6.7 kPa), with concomitant cor pulmonale, yet remain relatively undistressed. One of the main dangers to the patient

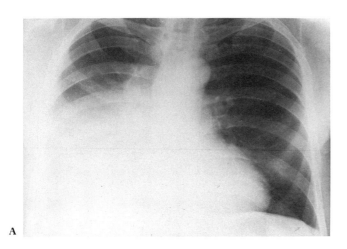

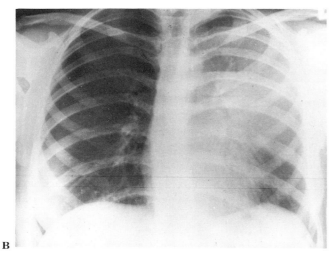

Fig. 11.8 Two examples of extensive pneumonic consolidation: **A** accompanied by an effusion and **B** showing an air bronchogram.

arises when the chronicity of the pulmonary disease goes unrecognised and uncontrolled oxygen is administered. Ventilatory failure may also follow inappropriate sedation and quite minor chest trauma. Although chronic obstructive airways disease is the commonest cause of recurrent respiratory failure it may also occur in the end-stages of any diffuse infiltrative lung disease.

History

The patient, usually a cigarette smoker and town-dweller, gives a history of chronic productive cough, often with previous winter exacerbations. The acute episodes are often initiated by upper respiratory tract infection, which are followed a few days later by expectoration of purulent sputum and increasing breathlessness. Shortness of breath is worse when the patient lies down due to the splinting effect of the abdominal contents on the diaphragm. This can lead to a mistaken diagnosis of acute pulmonary oedema.

Examination

There are two classic clinical types, one predominantly bronchitic ('the blue bloater') and the other predominantly emphysematous ('the pink puffer'). The former individual is cyanosed, oedematous and may exhibit signs of carbon dioxide retention (warm peripheries, a bounding pulse, bulging eyes, mental confusion and retinal venous distension which has sometimes progressed to frank papilloedema) — breathlessness may be minimal, in contradistinction to 'the pink puffer' who continues to hyperventilate, thus keeping his $PaCO_2$ at relatively normal or even low levels. Most patients lie somewhere between the two clinical extremes.

Chest signs may be limited to moist creptitations and sonorous rhonchi, mainly in the lower zones. A variable degree of generalised bronchospasm is common which has led to the term 'chronic reversible obstructive airways disease' replacing 'wheezy bronchitis' and 'late onset bronchial asthma'. Signs of right-sided cardiac failure (cor pulmonale) may be present, but it is not widely appreciated that severe hypoxia may precipitate left-sided heart failure in the patient with coexistent cardiac disease.

Management

Arterial blood gas measurements should be obtained at the start of therapy. If breathlessness is extreme, the ECG should be continuously monitored. The most important aspect of treatment is the administration of humidified low concentration oxygen (24–28%). Any tendency for the $PaCO_2$ to rise should be countered by a reduction in the oxygen concentration. If there is pronounced wheeze, bronchodilators and intravenous hydrocortisone should be given as for an acute asthmatic attack (see. p. 128). Right heart failure is initially treated with an intravenous diuretic. Digoxin is not indicated in cor pulmonale, unless atrial fibrillation is present, because of the increased danger of inducing cardiac dysrhythmias. Venesection may benefit both the heart failure and the polycythaemia which many of these patients develop.

A plain chest film must always be obtained or small pneumothoraces or unsuspected carcinomas will be missed. Drainage of even a small pneumothorax can be life-saving (cf. acute bronchial asthma). The chest radiograph can show a spectrum of abnormalities ranging from increased bronchovascular markings to frank pneumonic consolidation. The changes resultant from left heart failure may be superimposed. Typical radiographic features are shown in Figure 11.9.

1. Heart — the cardiac configuration is long and narrow.
2. Lung fields — the diaphragms are flattened. The lungs are over expanded and hypertranslucent.
3. Blood vessels — prominent pulmonary coni and peripheral pruning of the pulmonary vasculature is evidence of pulmonary hypertension. Blood is diverted to the upper lobes because the disease is predominantly basal. Prominence of the superior vena cava suggests right heart failure.

Surprisingly, many patients in severe respiratory failure have a remarkably normal chest film.

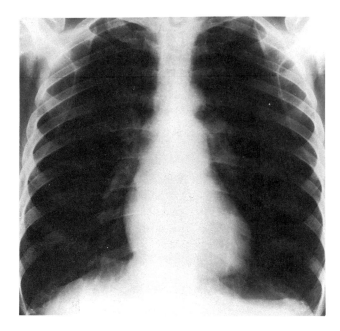

Fig. 11.9 Typical radiographic features of chronic obstructive airways disease.

If, in spite of the treatment outlined above, respiratory failure worsens — in other words, a deteriorating clinical state is paralleled by blood gas changes — endotracheal intubation and tracheobronchial suction should be tried. Controlled ventilation is a last resort and the decision to proceed to this form of therapy can be very difficult. It largely depends on the patient's previous degree of respiratory disability. Prospects for recovery are good if the patient has been able to venture out of the house unaided during the three months before the acute illness. They are extremely poor if he has been restricted to the bedside. The patient's relatives or family doctor may be able to provide valuable insight into whether the patient's recent life has been tolerable, which should also be taken into account before starting mechanical ventilation. The whole aim is to avoid ventilating a patient who later cannot be weaned off the ventilator.

BRONCHIOLITIS

Bronchiolitis is an epidemic viral illness occurring mainly in infants under 6 months. The illness starts with an upper respiratory tract infection. Wheeze is common and the child may become quite dehydrated, in which case an intravenous line should be set up. A careful watch should be kept for signs of heart failure.

The chest X-ray may show characteristic signs of thickened bronchi: perihilar ring shadows and a 'tramlining' effect extending out from the hila. Pneumatocoeles may also be seen. In most cases, however, the chest film is normal.

The upper air passages should be cleared using mechanical suction and high concentration humidified oxygen administered. The child's blood gases must always be monitored.

A small percentage (less than 5%) develop respiratory failure. As the sick infant becomes more distressed his cry becomes weaker.

Recurrent apnoeic attacks, often after pharyngeal suction or a feed, are another obvious danger signal.

> The criteria for respiratory support are:
> 1. Increasing respiratory effort with sternal recession, diminishing breath sounds and restlessness despite oxygen.
> 2. A rising pulse and respiratory rate.
> 3. Altered consciousness and lethargy.

Biochemical confirmation of respiratory failure is provided by a $PaCO_2$ above 50 mmHg (6.7 kPa) or a PaO_2 below 60 mmHg (8 kPa) or both.

Childhood asthma is virtually indistinguishable from bronchiolitis and wheezing is sometimes a symptom of congenital heart disease. More rarely it is caused by a foreign body (see Chs. 10 and 44). Laryngotracheobronchitis may also cause diagnostic confusion, although it tends to occur in an older age group (1–5 years) and inspiratory stridor (croup) rather than wheeze is the main clinical feature. The presentation and management of acute epiglottitis are described in Chapter 10.

NON-CARDIOGENIC PULMONARY OEDEMA (ADULT RESPIRATORY DISTRESS SYNDROME)

Adult respiratory distress syndrome (ARDS) occurs 12–48 hours after a number of severe insults which may or may not directly involve the lungs:

> *Causes of ARDS*
> *Direct lung injury*
> Inhalation of smoke or toxic fumes
> Aspiration of gastric contents (see Ch. 9)
> Near-drowning and secondary drowning (see Ch. 28)
> Atypical pneumonia
> Fat emboli — long bone fractures
> Blast lung and pulmonary contusions.
>
> *Other causes*
> Burns (see Ch. 37)
> Extrapulmonary sepsis
> Shock — multiple trauma
> Pancreatitis
> Overtransfusion
> Drug overdoses
> Disseminated intravascular coagulopathy
> Subarachnoid haemorrhage

By definition the patients have neither pre-existing pulmonary disease nor left ventricular failure. Transudation of protein rich fluid into the alveoli causes progressive hypoxaemia, vasoconstriction of the pulmonary vessels and reduced lung compliance. It is thought that conditions remote from the lung work via mediators and that ARDS represents a final common expression of multifactorial lung injury. Added to the pulmonary oedema there is mechanical obstruction of small vessels by leucocyte and platelet emboli. The pathophysiological changes in the lung are not uniform but tend to be self-perpetuating and continue long after the initial insult. The development of pulmonary hypertension and ventilation perfusion mismatch worsens hypoxia and causes further pulmonary damage.

A history suggestive of several causative factors is most uncommon.

> The characteristic clinical features of ARDS are:
> 1. Severe dyspnoea, tachypnoea and cyanosis.
> 2. Hypoxia resistant to supplemental oxygen.
> 3. Bilateral diffuse infiltrates on the chest film.
> 4. Increased lung stiffness which necessitates abnormally high inflation pressures during assisted ventilation.
> 5. A normal pulmonary capillary wedge pressure.

The mortality from ARDS is high, about 50%, death often being due to multiorgan failure. While the condition usually occurs in patients already being treated in hospital, the A & E doctor should be aware of this clinical syndrome as early recognition, or better still prevention, offers the best prospect for a reduction in mortality. The general principles of management are the maintenance of adequate circulation, acid-base balance and arterial oxygenation.

In the A & E department the patient should be given high concentration oxygen by mask, have an intravenous line erected and have blood taken for arterial gas analysis. Inotropic support with dobutamine may be required. High-dose intravenous steroids (30 mg methylprednisolone sodium succinate/kg body weight) may lessen the severity of some of the underlying processes if given early but the evidence in favour is arguable. Progressive respiratory distress with combined respiratory and metabolic acidosis is an indication for early ventilation. All these patients require management in an intensive care unit. The mainstay of treatment is intermittent positive pressure ventilation with positive end expiratory pressure. In order to assess the response to various vasoactive drugs it is essential to monitor the blood pressure, blood gases, cardiac output and pulmonary arterial wedge pressure.

MISCELLANEOUS

Occasionally a massive pleural effusion may produce a sense of suffocation and require aspiration in the A & E department. Various neurological diseases (e.g. motor neurone disease, acute postinfective polyneuropathy and poliomyelitis) can also cause severe breathlessness as their main presenting symtpom. Such patients frequently require mechanical ventilation.

FURTHER READING

Asthma, 2nd edn. Clark T J H, Godfrey S 1983 Chapman and Hall, London

Respiratory diseases, 3rd edn. Crofton J, Douglas A 1981 Blackwell Scientific, Oxford

Diagnosis and management of respiratory diseases, 2nd edn. Crompton G K 1987 Blackwell Scientific, Oxford

Pulmonary emergencies Sahn S A 1982 Churchill Livingstone, New York

The unconscious patient

THE UNCONSCIOUS PATIENT

An unconscious patient often needs treatment before any diagnosis is made. Whatever the cause of the coma, the patient may die or suffer brain damage due to airway obstruction, respiratory depression or circulatory failure. These matters, which require immediate attention, have been discussed in Chapter 10. An unconscious patient should be placed in the recovery position (Fig. 12.1) to reduce the risk of airway obstruction and aspiration of vomit. If there is any possibility of trauma, movement of the neck must be avoided, unless essential to clear the airway. Convulsions must be controlled (p. 141). Venous access should be obtained and the blood glucose concentration checked. Hypoglycaemia may cause permanent brain damage and so requires immediate treatment. Intravenous glucose may be given (p. 141) after blood has been taken for analysis and will reverse hypoglycaemia without seriously affecting other conditions. If no cause of coma is apparent, naloxone should be given as a therapeutic trial for opiate poisoning (p. 212).

The common causes of coma seen in an A & E department are listed below:

> Hypoglycaemia
> Drug overdosage
> Head injury
> Cerebrovascular accident
> Convulsions
> Alcohol intoxication.
>
> Other causes to consider include:
> Diabetic ketoacidosis
> Hepatic failure
> Respiratory failure
> Cardiac failure
> Hypothermia, heat stroke
> Meningitis, encephalitis
> Hypovolaemic shock
> Anaphylaxis
> Malaria
> Hysteria.

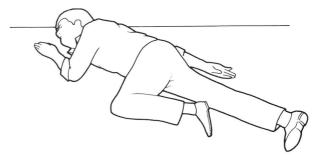

Fig. 12.1 The recovery position.

Many of these conditions are interrelated, for example hypoglycaemia may occur in alcohol intoxication (especially in children) and fits may result from hypoglycaemia, poisoning or hypoxia.

DIAGNOSIS OF THE CAUSE OF COMA

History

Any available information should be obtained from relatives, witnesses or ambulancemen. It is important to determine and record when the patient was last well, what he was like when he became ill or was found, and whether he is improving or deteriorating. Any history of injury, diabetes, fits, blackouts, poisoning or foreign travel may be relevant. Any drug therapy or allergy should be recorded. Useful information may be obtained from previous hospital notes and from the patient's general practitioner.

Examination

The patient should be undressed and examined all over for evidence of illness and injury. His clothes and belongings should be inspected for tablet bottles and for cards or bracelets warning about pre-existing disease.

Airway and ventilation

The adequacy of the airway and ventilation should be reassessed and the respiratory rate recorded. A raised respiratory rate may be caused by airways obstruction, pneumonia, salicylate poisoning, or by metabolic acidosis due to diabetic coma, hepatic or renal failure, methanol or ethylene glycol poisoning. Damage to the brain-stem by a stroke or compression may cause rapid or irregular respiration, sometimes with intermittent (Cheyne-Stokes) breathing. Respiratory depression is often caused by poisoning, especially by opiates, barbiturates and tricyclic antidepressants (Ch. 16).

Cardiovascular system

The pulse rate and rhythm and the blood pressure must be recorded. A bradycardia may be caused by hypoxia, complete heart block, raised intracranial pressure or by digoxin or beta-blocker poisoning (Chapter 16). Tachycardia may result from airway obstruction, hypoxia, hypovolaemia, ventricular or supraventricular tachycardia or anticholinergic poisoning. Atrial fibrillation may be associated with cerebral emboli.

Skin

The colour, temperature, degree of sweating, rashes and signs of trauma are noted. Pallor, cyanosis, jaundice or hyperpigmentation may be apparent. Injection marks may result from drug addiction or previous medical treatment. Erythema or blistering over pressure areas show that the patient has been unconscious for some hours, usually as the result of an overdose or hypothermia. Purpura may be due to septicaemia (especially meningococcal) or disseminated intravascular coagulation.

Temperature

The rectal temperature should be measured in an unconscious patient, using a low reading thermometer if the patient is cold. The temperature at which consciousness is lost varies between patients but coma is common at core temperatures below 30°C. Hypothermia and heat stroke are discussed in Ch. 28.

Neurological examination

The level of consciousness should be measured and recorded in a way that allows changes to be recognised: the Glasgow coma scale is intended for patients with head injuries (Ch. 14), but is also useful in other causes of coma. The responses to pain and commands should be noted. The strength of all limbs should be assessed and the muscle tone and reflexes recorded. The pupil sizes should be measured in millimetres, using a special ruler or the scale on the Glasgow coma chart, and the reactions of the pupils to light recorded. The scalp should be examined carefully for evidence of a head injury and the optic fundi and eardrums inspected. Neck stiffness should be assessed, except in patients who might have a neck injury, in whom meningeal irritation may

be elicited by Kernig's method (extension of the knee with the hip flexed). In young children the state of the anterior fontanelle and the head circumference should be recorded.

A lateralising sign, such as inequality of the pupils or unilateral facial or limb weakness, usually results from a stroke or from intracranial bleeding after a head injury. Such lateralising signs may, however, result from a pre-existing condition (e.g. eye drops or a previous Bell's palsy). Hypoglycaemia may cause localised weakness and coma, as in a stroke, but with rapid recovery following treatment with glucose. Coma without lateralising signs is usually due to drug overdosage, metabolic coma, a postictal state, a brain-stem stroke or a subarachnoid haemorrhage. Extensor plantar reflexes are common in these conditions. Poisoning with anticholinergic drugs, such as tricyclic antidepressants, often causes coma with increased muscle tone, clonus, extensor plantar reflexes and a divergent squint (Ch. 16). Poisoning with an opiate drug may cause coma with respiratory depression and small pupils: a therapeutic trial of naloxone should be performed in any patient with unexplained coma (Ch. 16).

Investigations

Glucose

The blood glucose must be checked in every unconscious patient. Reagent sticks, such as Dextrostix, are used initially. If there is any suspicion of hypoglycaemia, blood should be taken for laboratory measurement and intravenous dextrose should be given immediately (p. 141).

Arterial blood gases

Arterial blood should be taken for measurement of oxygen, carbon dioxide and hydrogen ion concentrations. When taking the sample, one should record how much oxygen was being given and whether the patient was breathing spontaneously or being ventilated. If a patient is pyrexial or hypothermic, the blood gas results may be misleading unless corrected for temperature: the laboratory should be able to do this if told the patient's temperature when the sample is sent.

Other laboratory tests

Measurement of urea and electrolytes, plasma osmolality, full blood count and prothrombin time are sometimes needed, depending on the clinical history and examination. Drug screening is discussed in Ch. 16. Screening for sedative and hypnotic drugs is never needed in an A & E department, but if the cause of coma is not clear blood should be kept for later analysis if necessary.

Radiographs

A radiograph of the chest may show evidence of aspiration, pneumonia, trauma or tumour. Radiographs of the skull and a lateral view of the cervical spine should be taken if there is any possibility of trauma. A Midliner ultrasound test may show midline shift due to an intracranial haematoma. A computerised tomogram scan is sometimes helpful, for example to exclude a treatable haematoma in a patient with localising signs and scalp trauma who has apparently fallen after suffering a stroke.

Electrocardiogram

The ECG may show cardiac arrhythmias or evidence of anticholinergic drug overdose (Ch. 16). ECG changes, such as T wave inversion, may occur in patients with subarachnoid haemorrhage, which may also cause severe pulmonary oedema.

MANAGEMENT OF SPECIFIC CONDITIONS

Convulsions

A patient who has a convulsion must be protected from injury and turned into the recovery position in order to reduce the risk of airway obstruction. Oxygen should be given via a face-mask. Nothing should be forced into the mouth but a nasopharyngeal airway may be helpful if obstruction occurs. Most convulsions stop spontaneously within a few minutes. If the convulsion continues this is *status epilepticus* and requires drug treatment. The drug of choice is diazepam, which is given intravenously or rectally (never intramuscularly). The lipid formulation of diazepam as Diazemuls causes less thrombophlebitis than Valium. The usual treatment for an adult is diazepam 10 mg intravenously over 2 minutes. Larger doses (up to 40 mg) are occasionally required but may cause respiratory depression requiring ventilation by a bag and mask. A child may be given intravenous diazepam (0.2–0.3 mg/kg or 1 mg per year of life), but in many cases venous access is difficult and rectal administration is preferable. Special rectal tubes (Stesolid) may be used, or alternatively the intravenous formulation in a syringe without a needle. The rectal dose of diazepam is 5 mg for children aged 1–3, or 10 mg for older children or adults. These doses may be repeated after 5 minutes if the fit has not stopped. In the rare cases of status epilepticus not responding to diazepam, one should give intramuscular paraldehyde (adult 10 ml, child 0.1 ml/kg or 1 ml per year up to 5 ml). Other drugs which may occasionally be useful are chlormethiazole (Heminevrin) and phenytoin. It is important, however, to maintain oxygenation and stop the fit as soon as possible and so, if diazepam and paraldehyde are ineffective, it may be best to ask an anaesthetist to give thiopentone and paralyse and ventilate the patient. The blood glucose must be checked and hypoglycaemia treated (see below). Febrile convulsions are discussed in Ch. 25.

Cerebrovascular accident (see also Ch. 26)

A cerebrovascular accident or stroke is a common cause of coma. Treatment in the A & E department consists of nursing care and excluding other treatable conditions, especially hypoglycaemia and head injury. The blood pressure may be high after a stroke, but rapid reduction is dangerous since it may cause further cerebral damage.

Hypoglycaemia

Hypoglycaemia most often occurs in diabetic patients who have missed a meal or taken too much insulin. It may also be caused by deliberate or accidental overdosage of sulphonylurea drugs, alcohol excess (especially in children), or due to strenuous exercise after taking alcohol but no food. Various rarer conditions, such as insulin-secreting tumours, may also cause hypoglycaemia. If the patient is unconscious dextrose should be given intravenously after a blood sample has been taken. The usual dose for an adult is 50 ml of 50% dextrose, which should be given into a large vein. In children 25% dextrose (2 ml/kg) is preferable since it is less irritant. It is important to minimise the damage to veins, especially in the non-dominant arm of a diabetic who may later need haemodialysis for renal failure. Intramuscular glucagon (1–2 mg in adults, 0.5–1 mg in children) may be used if venous access is difficult. Once consciousness is restored, oral glucose or food should be given and the cause of hypoglycaemia established. Many patients will need admission to hospital, especially those who have taken long-acting hypoglycaemic drugs.

Diabetic hyperglycaemia

Diabetic ketoacidosis is usually the result of an infection increasing the insulin requirement. It may be the presenting feature in a new diabetic. There is often a history of thirst, polyuria and vomiting. Abdominal pain and leg cramps may occur. Many patients are confused and a few are deeply unconscious. There is severe dehydration and hyperventilation (Kussmaul respiration) and often hypotension. The breath smells of acetone. Hypothermia is common, even with severe infection.

A large intravenous cannula must be inserted immediately and the patient rehydrated with 0.9% saline (in adults 1 litre in 30 minutes, then 1 litre in 1 hour, 1 litre in 2 hours; in children 20 ml/kg in 30 minutes, then reassess). Blood must be taken for measurement of glucose, urea and electrolytes, ketones, full blood count, arterial gases and hydrogen ion concentration. The ECG should be monitored for changes of hypo- or hyperkalaemia. The stomach should be emptied by a nasogastric tube. Blood cultures and a chest radiograph should be taken to look for infection.

The inpatient medical team must be informed immediately and should arrange further treatment. Insulin is usually given by continuous intravenous infusion in a dose of 6 units of soluble insulin per hour. If this is impractical, intramuscular injections may be used, 20 units of soluble insulin initially, followed by 6–10 units per hour until the blood glucose falls below 12 mmol/l. Rehydration and insulin therapy lower the plasma potassium and so potassium replacement should be started when insulin is given. Potassium chloride is mixed into the saline infusion in an initial adult dose of 20 mmol of potassium hourly, adjusted according to the plasma potassium concentration. Sodium bicarbonate is rarely helpful and may be dangerous in ketoacidosis, so it should not be given without specialist advice. It is occasionally used in patients who remain severely acidotic (pH less than 7) and have a poor cardiac output despite adequate fluid replacement.

Hyperosmolar non-ketotic coma is less common than ketoacidosis and usually occurs in elderly undiagnosed diabetics who have quenched their thirst with sugary drinks. Rehydration should be started with 0.9% saline but changed to 0.45% saline if the plasma sodium concentration is above 150 mmol/l. A central venous line may be needed to monitor fluid therapy. Insulin and potassium will be needed, as in ketoacidotic coma.

Lactic acidosis is a rare cause of severe metabolic acidosis in diabetics and is associated with the use of phenformin. Large amounts of bicarbonate are needed and sometimes haemodialysis.

FURTHER READING

Diabetic ketoacidosis Conalgen J V, Sonksen P H 1985 Medicine International 2: 546–548

The diagnosis of stupor and coma, 3rd edn. Plum F, Posner J B 1980 Davis, Philadelphia

Diabetic emergencies Wheatley T, Clark J D A 1987 Hospital Update 13: 31–41

The 'shocked' patient

INTRODUCTION

The word 'shock' is often accused of being an unsatisfactory term and many experts deprecate its use. However, it does have a use in the A & E department and, like the term 'collapse', has meaning for those of us who work there. It has medical and non-medical connotations. Its literal meaning is to 'startle', but it has additional clinical and physiological meanings. 'Treat the patient for shock' is a well used first-aid maxim, when what it usually meant is give comfort and allay fear.

Physiologists talk of shock as a failure of perfusion at a cellular level. Capillary flow is reduced and tissue hypoxia ensues.

Clinicians know shock to mean a patient who is hypotensive, sweating, agitated, pale and clammy and has a tachycardia.

This view of shock is really an observation of the general response to the cellular problem described by the physiologist. The general response to injury is triggered by several factors:

1. *Fluid loss* — either from haemorrhage or exudation into the damaged tissues.

2. *Afferent nociceptive stimuli* — from pain and deformity in limb fractures.

3. *Toxic factors* — the release of histamine, lactic acid and ions at the site of injury is not only proportional to the amount of tissue damage, but more importantly the amount of tissue hypoxia. Certain bacteria release toxins that produce vasodilatation and capillary leakage.

The 'local' response to injury has been recognised for nearly 2000 years: *redness, swelling, local heat* (Celsius, 1st century AD), *pain* and *loss of function* (Virchow, 19th century AD). The local injury may stimulate the 'general' response, either by the release of 'toxic' factors or, more dramatically, by loss of fluid. For example, a small penetrating injury to the heart will not involve a high degree of tissue damage but the general response will be profound.

When tissue is injured there is an increase in microvascular permeability. This increased permeability of small vessels occurs as a result of direct injury and the damaging effect of chemical mediators on venules. Histamine, 5-hydroxytryptamine and bradykinins are involved. Histamine is probably the most important of the toxic factors involved in triggering the general response. It is released from MAST cells, dilates arterioles (producing redness) and creates leaks in venules by contraction of small cells.

The final size of the injury incurred by the patient is determined by these triggering factors plus the degree of tissue hypoxia and the length of time the patient is exposed to them. The factors which determine the size of the injury are:

1. The degree of tissue hypoxia.
2. The extent of tissue damage.
3. The location of the tissue damage.
4. The amount of fluid lost from the circulation.
5. The duration and severity of pain.
6. The time from injury to definitive surgery.

Early oxygenation and security of the airway, rapid restoration of blood volume, reduction and splintage of fractures, and definitive surgery within the first 'golden hour' will significantly reduce both the degree of general response and the size of the final injury. In addition, multiple organ failure and 'shock lung', in particular, are late sequelae of major injury, largely untreatable but perhaps preventable if resuscitation is rapid and effective and the extent and duration of tissue hypoxia is reduced.

The clinical manifestations of shock described earlier are largely features of the response to haemorrhage. As blood is lost from the circulation the filling pressure of the heart falls. This stimulates compensatory actions via the sympathoadrenal axis, which largely accounts for the signs and symptoms of 'shock'. A fall in arterial pressure, plus peripheral vasoconstriction, leads to a fall in capillary pressure. This leads to tissue hypoxia which in turn stimulates further vasoconstriction. In *septic shock* tissue hypoxia is the starting point. This leads to leakage of fluid into the tissues and a fall in filling pressure in the heart. The responses to hypovolaemia are activated and the tissue hypoxia is made worse. If the septic heart cannot even cope with this reduced preload then the right atrial filling pressure may be high in the presence of a low systemic arterial pressure. In *cardiogenic* shock it is the reduction in contractility of the heart that is the fundamental problem. Cardiac output falls and tissue hypoxia ensues. Filling pressures are usually high.

THE RESPONSE TO HYPOVOLAEMIA

Normal circulatory homeostasis demands that blood pressure and pulse are inversely related to maintain a constant cardiac output. The sympathetic outflow of the startle reaction (fight/flight) ensures an increase in cardiac output by allowing blood pressure and heart rate to rise together. These changes can occur before the injury if the person can anticipate the accident. External stimuli are processed through the cortex to the hypothalmus and brain-stem. The final release of sympathetic output may be reduced if the patient is taking β-blocking drugs. The initial cortical response may be reduced or absent if the patient is sedated — most notably with alcohol.

The mechanisms whereby the body responds to hypovolaemia and becomes shocked involve both hormonal and neuronal pathways. When the circulating volume falls, high pressure stretch receptors in the aortic arch and carotid sinus are understimulated. Their inhibitory effect is reduced and sympathetic outflow is increased. This response is mediated through the nucleus tractus solitarius of the medulla oblongata.

The injury itself, inadequate airway control, hypotension and poor tissue perfusion all lead to *hypoxia*. This is detected by carotid body chemoreceptors and the information is again relayed to the nucleus tractus solitarius. This in turn relays to the autonomic preganglionic neurones and sympathetic outflow is increased. Pre- and postcapillary resistance is increased so hydrostatic pressure falls. Fluid then moves from the tissues into the circulation. However, only 400 ml in 30 minutes is available for transfer in this way. Clearly this response to trauma is meant for small injuries.

> The effects of increased sympathetic outflow are:
> 1. Adrenal catecholamines ↑
> 2. Cardiac contractility ↑
> 3. Heart rate ↑
> 4. Respiratory rate ↑
> 5. Renal blood flow ↓
> 6. Juxtaglomerular apparatus releases renin
>   This stimulates
>   a. Release of angiotensin I and II
>   b. Release of aldosterone

Vasoconstriction of venous capacitance vessels can provide an additional 'autotransfusion'. As 70% of blood volume is in these vessels then this mechanism can be a significant, if somewhat temporary factor in survival. Peripheral vasoconstriction conserves heat, but fortunately cerebral and coronary arteries are not sympathetically innervated. Sympathetic stimulation and outflow is of course limited and vasodilatory metabolites accumulate. The precapillary sphincters fail before the postcapillary sphincters and interstitial oedema develops. Fluid is now being lost into the tissues from the circulation as well as from the wound.

Low pressure volume receptors in the thorax and myocardium stimulate the release of antidiuretic hormone (ADH) via afferent vagal fibres to provide an additional fluid conserving mechanism to the renin/angiotensin system.

Finally, if the heart begins to empty then distortion receptors in the myocardium stimulate the Bezold-Jarish reflex and parasympathetic slowing of the heart occurs.

There are hormonal changes during shock. Afferent stimuli travel up the spinal cord to the hypothalmus. Neurotransmitters secure the release of CRH, which in turn stimulates the pituitary to release ACTH, β-endorphine, growth hormone and prolactin. An increase in corticosteroids ensues.

The increase in catecholamines and corticosteroids leads to glycogenolysis, lipolysis and gluconeogenesis. Blood glucose rises. Furthermore, the effect of increased adrenaline and increased sympathetic activity leads to a fall in insulin and rise in blood glucose.

When the circulating adrenaline falls the plasma insulin begins to rise. However, insulin resistance develops and the blood glucose remains high. In spite of the high glucose, there is a switch to fat metabolism. The mechanism of this is as yet poorly understood.

Corticosteroid levels rise in proportion to the injury severity score until the highest value when it falls. This may reflect a failure of adrenal perfusion in the very severely injured.

A fall in capillary blood flow leads to tissue hypoxia. Platelet aggregates (microthrombi), electrolyte changes and tissue oedema develop. When reperfusion is established the return of these to the circulation is a factor in the development of 'shock lung'.

MANAGEMENT OF THE SHOCKED PATIENT

The management of the airway is the same, no matter what the underlying cause. The approach to fluid replacement will differ, however, depending on the underlying pathological process. In the absence of external signs of injury, always consider a ruptured aortic aneurysm, ectopic pregnancy or sepsis.

Haemodynamic monitoring

There are three phases in the treatment of shock:
1. Immediate resuscitation (airway control, oxygen therapy, fluid replacement and usually ventilation)
2. Early definitive surgery (where indicated)
3. Continued resuscitation, (on an adequately staffed and equipped intensive care unit).

The fundamental abnormality is failure of tissue oxygenation.

All phases of treatment are aimed at its restoration. The success of treatment can therefore only be assessed if oxygen delivery and consumption are measured. Furthermore the 'standard' measurements of pulse, blood pressure, CVP and urine output are known to correlate poorly both with oxygen utilisation and final outcome. The modern treatment of shock (i.e. the correct treatment) requires the insertion of a thermodilution pulmonary artery flotation catheter in the third phase of resuscitation. This will allow the measurement of pulmonary artery occlusion pressure (PAOP) — the equivalent of left ventricular end diastolic pressure, the cardiac output, the calculation of systemic vascular resistance, and sampling of blood from the pulmonary artery. Left ventricular and diastolic volume is a better measurement but requires radionucleide angiography and is therefore not available for routine bedside use.

Colloid is administered until the PAOP rises to about 18 mmHg and the cardiac index (cardiac output/surface area) is 4.5 $1/m^2$. A co-oximeter is used to analyse samples from the pulmonary artery (true mixed venous) and a systemic artery. Resuscitation must continue until the DO_2 (oxygen delivery) is greater than 650 ml/min/m^2 and the VO_2 (oxygen consumption) is greater than 150–170 ml/min/m^2. The shunt fraction should be less than 20% allowing for the 10% associated with intermittent positive pressure ventilation (IPPV). The administration of colloid and/or blood should be continued until the required levels of DO_2 and VO_2 are achieved or further fluid fails to increase the cardiac index. PEEP and then inotropic agents may be required to reach the target levels of oxygen utilisation. If these cannot be achieved, the patient will not survive. The acidosis associated with shock is a consequence of hypoperfusion. Its treatment lies in resuscitation as outlined above and not in the administration of bicarbonate.

There is no human evidence to support the use of corticosteroids in shock and they are not recommended.

THE SERIOUSLY INJURED PATIENT

The general management of the severely injured patient is dealt with in Ch. 14. This section deals only with the component of shock in relation to the injured.

Oxygen requirements

Always give 100% oxygen through face masks when treating seriously injured patients. The patient will not receive 100% oxygen, as only endotracheal intubation and ventilation through a circuit can actually deliver this concentration. Oxygen toxicity will not occur during the resuscitation of sick patients and inspired oxygen concentrations of 20–30% have no part in resuscitation. The caution about oxygen therapy in patients with chronic obstructive airways disease is inappropriate in seriously injured patients, who all require high levels of inspired oxygen.

Pulmonary hypoxic vasoconstriction is a protective mechanism that ensures that only well ventilated areas of the lung are perfused.

Oxygen therapy rapidly abolishes this reflex. The oxygen mask must not be removed if a profound fall in the arterial oxygen concentration is to be avoided. The reflex can also be abolished by movement. Oxygen therapy must be established before patients are examined.

Having enriched the supply of inspired gases with oxygen, it is essential to ensure that they can reach the lungs. Inspect the airway, with a laryngoscope if necessary and use a mechanical suction device to remove vomitus and blood from the oropharynx. Dentures must always be removed. Thrusting the mandible forward will lift the tongue from the pharynx and an oropharyngeal airway can then be inserted. A patient who will tolerate a laryngoscope will tolerate an endotracheal tube. A patient who will tolerate an endotracheal tube, NEEDS an endotracheal tube.

Apnoea is not the only indication for ventilation. A patient who is struggling to breathe or cannot maintain adequate arterial blood gases also needs ventilation. *Paradoxical breathing,* where the abdomen rises as the chest falls, is a sign of impending disaster. Apnoea will follow if ventilation is delayed. The patient must be ventilated immediately, with paralysing drugs and sedation if necessary, to reduce the hypoxic interval and avoid later complications. The adult respiratory distress syndrome (ARDS) and multiple organ failure are related to the degree and duration of hypoxia.

Cyanosis is not always a sign of significant hypoxia. It implies only that about 5 g/l of reduced haemoglobin is present in the circulation. Polycythaemic patients will cyanose when they have a large reserve of unreduced haemoglobin and anaemic patients will die without ever turning blue.

The commonest clinical signs of hypoxia are *restlessness* and *sweating.* Injured patients require oxygen and not sedation. Accessory muscles of respiration may be used. Hypoxia alone may be responsible for the tachycardia and hypotension.

Diagnosis and management can usually only be achieved with the patient in the supine position. This will add an additional threat to the airway, and the insertion of a cuffed endotracheal tube may be required to prevent aspiration.

Facial injuries involving the maxilla can bleed profusely into the oropharynx as can some basal fractures. A cuffed endotracheal tube is often required to prevent the aspiration of blood. Anaesthesia and paralysis are usually required.

Chest injuries should be ventilated sooner rather than later. Diffuse shadowing on a supine radiograph implies lung contusion. This alone, but certainly in the presence of altered blood gases and/or other injuries, is an indication for elective ventilation. The combination of lung contusion and long bone fracture is a harbinger of ARDS. Early ventilation may have a preventative role. In the presence of trauma and particularly in those patients who are to be transferred, surgical emphysema alone should be considered an indication for urgent chest tube thoracostomy. The development of a tension pneumothorax in transit is likely to be missed and, if recognised, treated with difficulty. Similarly, the combination of chest injury with intermittent positive pressure ventilation will substantially increase the risk of tension pneumothorax, and 'prophylactic' chest drains are usually required. The majority of serious injuries to the chest can be controlled by insertion of a chest tube and intermittent positive pressure ventilation. Hypoxia and hypercarbia will increase cerebral oedema in *head injured patients.*

Elective ventilation is required if normal blood gases cannot be maintained on 100% inspired oxygen. Any patient thought sick enough to warrant urgent transfer to a neurosurgical centre with a diagnosis of an expanding intracranial haematoma, must be first paralysed and ventilated. If the diagnosis is correct, then respiration will deteriorate and any compromise of the airway will profoundly and deleteriously compound the injury to the head. The neurological status of the patient must be recorded accurately by a senior doctor and other major injuries excluded or identified prior to transfer. This will often involve peritoneal lavage if the patient is paralysed.

Fluid requirements

Injured patients require fluid and when errors are made in trauma management it is usually because too little was given too late. 'Big drips' should be placed in 'big veins'. A 12–16 gauge cannula in each antecubital fossa will be required in the first instance, but additional lines should be placed below the diaphragm.

The central venous pressure will reflect compensatory vasoconstriction but is not a guide to fluid requirements. It may be difficult to access and attempts at cannulation may involve removal of the cervical collar for the internal jugular vein and pneumothorax for the subclavian vein. CVP catheters are narrow and will not permit an adequate rate of fluid administration. The central veins should therefore be cannulated only when peripheral access is impossible because of injury and then a wide-bore cannula should be used. This will involve a guide wire and Seldinger technique. These circumstances are rare and cut-downs on the long saphenous vein are a better alternative. 'Cut downs' also allow the connecting piece of the giving set itself to be inserted into the vein and sutured in place. This will allow a very rapid rate of fluid administration.

Before fluid is administered, obtain a specimen of blood for full blood count, biochemical profile, blood glucose and group and cross-match 6 units.

Fluid replacement

The amount of fluid required cannot accurately be assessed from clinical or biochemical parameters. The blood pressure will remain normal or even high if the sympatho-adrenal response is strong. This is often seen in young adults who, by the time they are hypotensive, are gravely ill and near to cardiorespiratory arrest. The haemoglobin level obtained on admission will reflect premorbid status but may be artificially high due to haemoconcentration. The need for fluid must be based on the *injuries observed* as well as the physiological status of the patient. More than 2 litres can be lost into the chest or abdomen with little in the way of physical signs. A similar amount can be lost from multiple rib fractures.

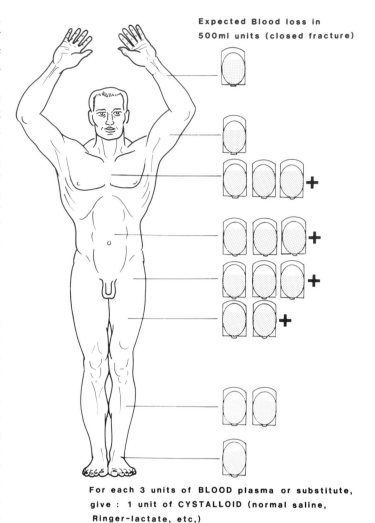

Expected Blood loss in 500ml units (closed fracture)

For each 3 units of BLOOD plasma or substitute, give : 1 unit of CYSTALLOID (normal saline, Ringer-lactate, etc,)

Fig. 13.1 Transfusion requirements for common injuries.

A fractured shaft of femur will lose 1–2 litres and injuries to the pelvis up to 3 litres or more. (see Fig. 13.1 and Table 13.1).

The optimal viscosity of the blood for tissue perfusion is a little below the normal haematocrit. A reduction in the haematocrit will increase tissue perfusion and oxygenation without an increase in the level of haemoglobin. The administration of both crystalloid and colloid in the early stages after injury will result in some degree of haemodilution. The reduction in viscosity this produces, plus the enrichment of the inspired gases with oxygen, will go some way to maintaining adequate tissue oxygenisation. Below a haematocrit of 25% any benefit gained from haemodilution is outweighed by the lack of haemoglobin and oxygen carrying capacity.

The choice of fluid

Crystalloid solutions, such as normal saline, can be stored 'run-through' in the resuscitation room for 12–24 h without risk of contamination and discarded if unused without risk of expense. They are poor expanders of the intravascular space. Large amounts

Table 13.1 Variation of physiological values with age, height and weight

Age (years)	Height/Weight (cm)	(kg)	Daily basic fluid requirements (ml)	Blood volume (ml)	Minute volume (litres)	Equal to: Tidal air × Rate (ml) (min)
½	–	10	250	800	1.2	60 ml × 20/min
1	–	12	1000	900	1.6	100 ml × 16/min
2½	75	15	1100	1200	2	130 ml × 15/min
4	100	18	1250	1400	2	150 ml × 14/min
7	125	25	2000	2000	3	240 ml × 13/min
10	140	30	2400	2400	3.5	290 ml × 12/min
12	150	40	2750	3200	4	360 ml × 11/min
Adult	175	70	3000	5600	6	600 ml × 10/min

Blood volume: 8% of body weight, extracellular fluid volume: 20% of body weight. Minimum urinary output in adult: 25 ml per hour.

are required to maintain the blood pressure as continuous leakage into the interstitial space occurs. There is a relationship between excessive crystalloid infusion and the adult respiratory distress syndrome. Their use is probably best limited to the immediate phase of resuscitation (500–1000 ml) after which a more effective agent should be employed.

Sugar solutions (e.g. 5% dextrose) cannot be stored 'run-through' without the risk of contamination and the sugar they contain will not be utilised in the switch to fat metabolism after injury.

Plasma expanders fall largely into two groups — the osmotically active group and the true expanders. The *dextrans* offer no advantages and have some specific disadvantages. They expand the circulation by drawing fluid in from the interstitial spaces. This tends to be less rapid than true exogenous expansion. Furthermore, the cross-matching of blood is very difficult in their presence and blood samples must be taken before their administration. Low molecular weight dextrans (m.w. 40 000) may sludge in the renal tubules and should not be used. Serious hypersensitivity reactions have been documented.

Hydroxrethyl starch is better, but hypersensitivity can still occur and it has no advantages over the gelatin solutions which have become the fluid of choice in many countries.

The gelatins do not affect the cross-matching of blood. Hypersensitivity reactions are rare, but more likely in patients with connective tissue disorders who may already have antibodies to collagen. They are excreted unchanged in the urine with a plasma half-life of about four hours. This may be prolonged in shock, when renal perfusion is poor. This relatively short half-life means that overtransfusion is unlikely but the patient will need to be continually 'topped up' and whole blood given as soon as possible.

Following 500–1000 ml of normal saline, 1000–2000 ml of gelatin can be given. Cross-matched *whole blood* should then be available and administered with further gelatin. It is usually possible to perform a rapid cross-match in about 20 minutes. At the very least, group- and type-specific blood can be given. If the need for replacement has been greater than the speed of cross-matching it will be necessary to give uncross-matched group O

(rhesus negative to women of child bearing years) blood after 3000 ml of gelatin have been given.

Whole blood is not ideal. The enzyme 2,3,DPG is essential for oxygen release from haemoglobin but is far less effective at lower temperatures. Blood is stored at 4°C and 2,3,DPG activity remains depressed for some time after transfusion. The low temperature of stored blood may render the patient hypothermic. There are many microaggregates in stored blood, which, if not filtered prior to transfusion, will be filtered by the lungs. All blood must therefore be warmed and filtered prior to administration. Whole blood stored for more than 24 hours has no effective platelets and no factor VIII after a further 24 hours. The citrate anticoagulant has been thought to decrease ionised calcium in the past, but recently this has been questioned. Routine replacement of calcium may not be indicated but symptoms and signs of hypocalcaemia should be looked for. Potassium leaks out of stored blood and must be monitored during transfusion. Although citrate is acid it does not produce a significant acidosis and any such changes must be considered to be the consequences of continued poor tissue perfusion. Fluid, not bicarbonate, is required. Platelets and clotting factors will eventually be required but not usually in the emergency room.

Plasma reduced whole blood in combination with a gelatin solution is an effective alternative to whole blood. Further components can be transfused as required.

Controlling pain

Patients must not be allowed to suffer pain. In addition to common compassion, it is essential to reduce the nociceptive afferent stimuli, which contribute to the size of the injury. Shocked patients are sensitive to small amounts of narcotic analgesia which can be diluted in saline and given in small boluses intravenously. Intramuscular and oral analgesia play no part in the management of the seriously injured patient. If analgesia cannot be achieved with intravenous narcotics, general anaesthesia is required.

Alcohol will lower the conscious level to varying degrees in different people. Its effects cannot be correlated accurately to conscious level, even at high blood concentrations. There is also a relationship between 'alcohol, minor injury and shock'. It is rare, and inappropriate transfusion is unlikely to be harmful before the absence of serious injury is recognised. Alcohol should therefore be ignored clinically, its measurements serving only to confuse rather than enlighten. If the symptoms are due solely to alcohol and the airway is protected the patient will recover over the course of the next few hours. If the patient is clearly injured then proceed as outlined in Ch. 14.

In the absence of external signs of injury and the presence of shock, always consider the possibility of a ruptured aneurysm or ectopic pregnancy. A nasogastric tube or rectal examination may confirm a gastrointestinal haemorrhage.

All the other aspects of dealing with the injured patient are dealt with in Ch. 14.

UPPER GI BLEEDING

About half the patients admitted with haematemesis have chronic peptic ulcers, duodenal outnumbering gastric ulcers by about 2 : 1. Other causes include gastric erosions, reflux oesophagitis, oesophageal mucosal tears (Mallory-Weiss syndrome), oesophageal varices, anastomotic ulcers, tumours and bleeding disorders.

History

The history may provide a clue to the source of the bleeding, although nearly half of these patients have had no relevant symptoms. Recurrent bouts of epigastric pain suggest a peptic ulcer, prolonged vomiting culminating in a haematemesis suggests the Mallory-Weiss syndrome, and haemorrhage from oesophageal varices usually occurs in patients known to have liver disease. Patients with cirrhosis, especially alcoholics, may also bleed from gastric erosions, peptic ulcers, or oesophageal mucosal tears. Initially, however, catastrophic haemorrhage should be assumed to be caused by a ruptured varix. Aspirin and corticosteroids can cause acute gastric erosions, but major bleeding from such lesions is probably rare.

Some idea of the amount of blood lost may also be gained from the history. The patient's estimate of the volume of the haematemesis, although often inaccurate, provides some guide. Accompanying melaena implies much more blood loss than haematemesis alone.

Examination

Peripheral signs of shock also provide some indication of the amount of blood lost but may be misleading. Some gastric tenderness may be found in patients with bleeding ulcers. A gastric carcinoma may be palpated. Stigmata of chronic liver disease may be obvious. The possibility of a generalised bleeding disorder should be actively considered.

Management

The resuscitation of the patient is carried out along similar lines to those outlined above. Bleeding oesophageal varices require additional specific measures. After a brief history and clinical assessment, an intravenous infusion is started and blood samples taken for grouping, prothrombin time, plasma electrolyte and glucose estimations. Six units of fresh blood (not more than 48 hours old) are cross-matched. Liver-damaged patients cannot metabolise citrate properly and, therefore, calcium gluconate (10 ml of 10% per litre of blood transfused) might be needed. In order to lower the portal venous pressure, vasopressin is infused intravenously (20 units diluted in 200 ml of 5% dextrose over 20 minutes). This measure alone controls bleeding varices in about 50% of patients; it will also control haemorrhage from the stomach and duodenum. The dose can be repeated several times if bleeding continues. A nasogastric tube should be passed, but powerful suction aspiration must be avoided because of the risk of causing further bleeding from the gastric muocsa. If sedation is necessary, small doses of intravenous diazepam (5 mg) are safest.

The skilful use of a Sengstaken-Blakemore tube can be a life-saving measure in the patient with severe continued bleeding. A diagram of the quadruple-lumen, double-balloon tube in position is shown in Figure 13.2.

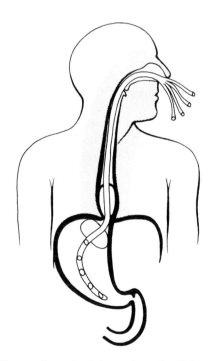

Fig. 13.2 Diagram of a quadruple-lumen Sengstaken-Blakemore tube in situ.

A new tube should be used for each patient. The bed-head is elevated and the balloons are tested for leaks. After removing gastric contents by gentle nasogastric aspiration, the well lubricated tube is passed into the stomach via the mouth. The gastric balloon is inflated with 80–100 ml of air and the tube retracted until the balloon is firmly lodged against the cardia. The oesophageal balloon is then inflated to about 40 mmHg and the tube strapped to the face. Blood can now be aspirated from the gastric tube. Copious saliva production can be troublesome with the tube in situ, and intramuscular atropine helps to minimise it. Once the tube is properly positioned, the patient can safely be moved to the operating theatre for injection of the varices.

All patients with chronic liver disease who have had a haematemesis, however small, must be admitted to hospital — a small leak may presage a torrential bleed. If the patient does not appear to have lost much blood, following the initial measures outlined above, direct endoscopic identification of the source of the bleeding may be attempted. This procedure is being carried out more and more at an early stage in the management of these patients. Intravenous cimetidine may be useful in controlling bleeding from gastric erosions (and possibly some peptic ulcers). The dose by intravenous infusion is normally 100 mg per hour for 2 hours, repeated at 4–6-hourly intervals.

Admit ALL patients to hospital after a gastrointestinal bleed, no matter how apparently trivial. Not to do so is dangerous. All patients with melaena or bleeding oesophageal varices should be admitted to the main hospital wards. Patients who have had a small haematemesis, often related to alcohol or aspirin ingestion, can be admitted to the observation ward, as can patients in whom there is some doubt about the history of bleeding.

The criteria for admission for observation are:
1. An isolated small haematemesis.
2. No signs of shock.
3. No anaemia to suggest long-term blood loss.

An intravenous line should be kept patent with normal saline in case of a further haemorrhage requiring transfusions. To begin with, the vital signs should be observed at 15–30 minute intervals, to enable the early recognition of continued occult bleeding. The next day the stools should be examined for melaena, and the patient endoscoped in an attempt to pinpoint the source of the haemorrhage.

CARDIOGENIC SHOCK

In cardiogenic shock there is a low cardiac output (cardiac index ≤ 1.8 l/min/m^2) secondary to disease of the left and/or right ventricles. Myocardial infarction is by far the commonest cause of cardiogenic shock. The disease is most often ischaemic heart disease causing damage to cardiac muscle, but cardiac output may fall when the heart rhythm is abnormal. Heart block, with a slow ventricular response will produce a reasonable blood pressure (filling time is prolonged and stroke volume maintained), but cardiac output will be low in spite of this because of the low heart rate (cardiac output = stroke volume × heart rate). A pacemaker will increase the cardiac output but ventilation and inotropic support may also be required. Very fast heart rates will not allow adequate ventricular filling to occur, stroke volume will be low and cardiac output will fall.

The use of positive inotropic agents will both improve cardiac contractility and tissue perfusion. Treatment can only be monitored safely by measurement of left ventricular end diastolic pressure cardiac output and pulmonary artery pressure. The systemic (and pulmonary) vascular resistance (SVR) must be calculated from the formula.

$$SVR = \frac{(\text{mean arterial pressure} - \text{right atrial pressure}) \times 80 \text{ dynes.sec.cm.}^{-5}}{\text{cardiac output}}$$

A pulmonary artery thermodilution flotation catheter is essential and transfer to a suitably equipped intensive care unit should be arranged as soon as possible.

If the preload i.e. left ventricular end diastolic pressure is low it can be raised by controlled volume expansion, titrated against PAOP and cardiac index. When fluid fails to increase the cardiac index, but DO_2 and VO_2 are still too low, inotropic support will be required. Vasodilators are used when the afterload is high (usually the case) or the preload is high.

Hypoxaemia in the presence of cardiogenic shock is an indication for elective ventilation.

Infarction of the left ventricle leading to shock is associated with large areas of muscle damage and a poor prognosis. The left ventricular end diastolic pressure is high as preload rises with loss of ventricular compliance. There is always some degree of pulmonary oedema.

Infarction of the right ventricle, often after inferior infarction, always involves some part of the left ventricle, but overall damage is less and the prognosis relatively good. The left ventricular and diastolic volume may be low, normal or a little high. Pulmonary oedema is not a feature.

Vasodilators such as sodium nitroprusside and intravenous nitrates have profound haemodynamic effects and can only be given safely when the haemodynamics are being measured. They are unlikely to be given in the emergency room as a pulmonary artery flotation catheter is a prerequisite for their use. The same applies to inotropic agents. If they are thought to be indicated then the haemodynamic status of the patient must first be recorded. The pulse, blood pressure and CVP reflect compensatory mechanisms but tell you little about cardiac output and systemic vascular resistance and nothing about oxygen utilisation. The haemodynamic status can as yet only be measured at the bedside by employing pulmonary artery flotation catheters.

Dopamine is thought to have dose-related effects ranging from renal vasodilation at 4 μg/kg per minute to vasoconstriction at 16 μg/kg per minute. This is rarely seen in practice and the responses can be unpredictable. Continuous monitoring is therefore required.

Dobutamine is not a profound vasoconstrictor. It is usually given at 2–15 μg/kg per minute, though higher doses are sometimes required. It is often used in combination with dopamine.

Inotropic agents will produce serious and potentially fatal dysrhythmias in patients who are hypoxic or hypovolaemic. These abnormalities must be corrected before their administration.

SHOCK WITH SEPSIS

If the cause of shock is not obvious, suspect septicaemia — overdiagnosis will do more good than harm. Table 13.2 lists some of the conditions which predispose patients to septic shock.

Table 13.2 Conditions associated with septic shock

Surgical
Genitourinary surgery or instrumentation
Gall bladder surgery
Extensive wounds or burns
Perforation of the gut
Tracheostomy

Medical
Chronic splenectomy patients (develop pneumococcal septicaemia)
Blood disorders
Diabetes mellitus
Rheumatoid arthritis
Ulcerative colitis
Chronic skin disease or ulcers
Arteriovenous shunts
Alcoholism
Drug addiction
Treatment with antibiotics or immunosuppressives
Neonates
The very elderly

Obstetric
Recent childbirth or miscarriage

Clinical features which should arouse suspicion in the individual patient are pyrexia accompanied by rigors and any unexplained tachycardia, tachypnoea or jaundice. Widespread peripheral vasodilatation occasionally occurs. Pyrexia, however, is often absent in the gravely ill.

Blood cultures should be taken while infusion and CVP lines are being set up. The result of the culture is critical for the later management. Colloid solution (polygelines are effective) can be used for initial volume expansion. All these patients should be given 100% oxygen. Urine and sputum samples should be obtained if there are appropriate clinical indications. Estimation of the haemoglobin concentration and white cell count should be routine. Many of these patients are anaemic and later will require a blood transfusion. An arterial sample, for blood gas and pH determination, is of particular importance. The modern management of this condition requires invasive haemodynamic monitoring and elective ventilation. Refer the patient to an intensive care unit capable of doing this. It is essential that the patient is adequately resuscitated before antibiotics are given. The release of endotoxin will produce widespread vasodilatation which must be anticipated.

The suspected origin of the bacteraemia gives a clue to the most likely infecting agent, e.g. urinary infection — *Escherichia coli*, burns — *Pseudomonas aeruginosa*. The most common organisms isolated are *Escherichia coli* and *Proteus*, occasionally *Staphylococcus* and *Pseudomonas*. The choice of antibiotic(s) depends on resistance patterns in the particular geographical area. Drugs should be given intravenously and combinations should be selected to provide wide cover. Haemodynamic monitoring will give an indication of the need for and effect of inotropic agents. Steroids are no longer prescribed in this condition.

ANAPHYLACTIC SHOCK

If no evidence of hypovolaemia can be found and cardiogenic or septic shock is thought unlikely, consider *anaphylactic shock*. The diagnosis is often suggested by collapse following a recognisable allergen. This history, however, is often not available. Most cases are caused by injections of antibiotics, vaccines, antisera, toxoids and corticotrophin. Occasionally insect stings, protein-containing foods (e.g. eggs, Brazil nuts, milk and fish) or orally administered drugs (e.g. aspirin and penicillin) are the culprits. The reaction starts within one or two minutes of exposure to the allergen. There is generalised itching, closely followed by intense bronchospasm, cyanosis and collapse. The patient has a rapid, thready pulse, becomes hypotensive and often develops oedema of the face, glottis and larynx, causing further respiratory difficulty (see Chapter 7). Death may ensue within minutes of the onset of symptoms Treatment must be started immediately in the following order.

1. Give 100% oxygen.
2. Adrenaline hydrochloride (0.5 ml of a 1 : 1000 solution) is injected intramuscularly. The same dose can be repeated in 10 minutes if there is no significant improvement.
3. This is followed by an intravenous injection of an antihistamine to neutralise excess circulating histamine. There is little to choose between diphenhydramine hydrochloride (10–20 mg), chlorpheniramine maleate (10 mg) or promethazine hydrochloride (50 mg).
4. In order to reduce further allergic manifestations an intravenous injection of hydrocortisone succinate (100–200 mg) is also given.

Many patients receive various types of injections in the A & E department every day. Anaphylaxis is, therefore, a potential daily risk. All such patients must be closely questioned regarding a past history of allergy. This will include previous reactions to drugs, asthma, hay fever and skin rashes. Therefore, all A & E departments must have at least one emergency treatment pack readily available in which the ampoules of adrenaline are regularly checked for signs of deterioration and routinely replaced every six months. Of equal importance, all medical and nursing staff must be shown its exact location.

SPINAL SHOCK

Loss of autonomic control may lead to widespread arterial and venous dilatation following injuries to the spinal cord. There will be no compensatory tachycardia for this relative hypovolaemia, and the heart rate may even be low. Tilting the patient head down is beneficial but careful volume expansion may be required. Autonomic tone returns in about 24 hours or perhaps a week if the cord has been totally transected.

ACUTE ADRENAL INSUFFICIENCY

Corticosteroids are used in the treatment of bronchial asthma, rheumatoid arthritis and a wide variety of other conditions. Such patients are susceptible to the development of acute adrenal insufficiency when stressed by intercurrent illness, either during prolonged treatment or within a year of the cessation of therapy. Acute adrenal insufficiency is also occasionally the presenting feature of Addison's disease, but more commonly is the result of failure to increase the dose of steroids during acute illness in a known case of Addison's disease.

The classic signs of an Addisonian crisis are severe generalised weakness, vomiting and hypotension. Abdominal pain is sometimes also a feature. There may be a prior history of anorexia, weight loss, a craving for salt and increasing pigmentation.

Successful treatment depends on the prompt administration of parenteral corticosteroids and intravenous fluids. Blood samples should be obtained for estimation of cortisol levels, electrolytes and sugar, but one should not wait for the results before starting treatment. An intravenous bolus of 100 mg of hydrocortisone should be given immediately, and an infusion of dextrose/saline, containing a further 50 mg hydrocortisone, started. This amount can safely be infused over an hour, unless the patient also has serious cardiovascular disease or renal failure. The more seriously ill patients should be managed in the intensive care unit, but the majority respond promptly to therapy and can be treated in a general medical ward.

FURTHER READING

The relation of oxygen transport patterns to the pathophysiology and therapy of shocked states Shoemaker W C 1987 Intensive Care Medicine 13: 230–243

The severely injured patient

THE ORGANISATION OF TRAUMA SERVICES

There is little doubt that trauma is one of the major problems facing medicine today. While it does not account for as many deaths as cardiovascular, respiratory, or neoplastic disease, in the United Kingdom it is the chief cause of death in people in their first 45 years. Between the ages of 10 and 24 years it accounts for 43.5% of all deaths and between 5 and 34 years it accounts for 33.4%

Usually in the 20th century when a problem of such substantial proportions has emerged, the response of doctors has been to treat it as a specialty with its own departments and a staff of specialised doctors who devote the whole of their time to its study and treatment. It was not surprising therefore that in 1940 William Gissane established a hospital to treat the victims of accidents. This was the Birmingham Accident Hospital. It accepted only patients with injuries and set itself to train accident surgeons. The research and teaching of the Birmingham Accident Hospital has had a profound influence on trauma care, not only in the United Kingdom but throughout the world. Yet its pattern of organisation has not been accepted in any other centre in Britain. It has been widely argued that it is better for a neurosurgeon to operate on severe brain injuries, an orthopaedic surgeon on fractures, a chest surgeon on lung injuries and that trauma care should be integrated into the whole work of hospitals with each surgical specialty making its contribution.

Another of the forces which might have led to a certain degree of specialisation was the Platt Report of 1962. This examined the whole trauma problem in Britain and concluded that hospitals should be categorised into three grades. The most severely injured would be cared for in regional centres specially organised for the purpose, the majority of injured patients with somewhat less severe injuries would be catered for in district general hospitals and major trauma patients would not be brought to hospitals smaller than a district hospital. While these ideas have received much lip service, and must to some extent have affected the pattern of work, there has been a great resistance to admit that only one hospital in a region is the recognised referral hospital. Clearcut categorisation has not taken place.

While a good case can be made for using the facilities of all the different specialties to treat injured patients, the effect has tended to be that what is everybody's business is also nobody's business. Especially in the case of patients with multiple injuries, if treatment is to be carried out by a number of different specialists, then there needs to be some agreement on general protocols of management which all concerned will follow. This can only come about if there is a corporate entity such as a trauma team or trauma syndicate which works out the protocols and obtains the necessary co-operation of all the different specialties. A & E doctors and intensive care specialists, both of whom are constantly relating to a wide spectrum of surgical specialists, are well placed to play an important role in such trauma syndicates.

In the USA there have emerged a number of centres with departments devoted entirely to trauma care. These are large departments staffed by many specialists — virtually hospitals within hospitals. However, American cities are large and the general level of trauma appears to be much higher than in Britain. In terms of potential years of life lost, trauma accounts for 40% in the United States, but only 5.4% in Britain. There is little doubt that more specialist organisation is simpler when the turnover especially of multiple injured patients is high. In Britain the incidence of such patients is relatively low. In this situation there is a danger that the problem may be tackled with less commitment. However our aim should surely be to press on with preventative measures and lower the incidence of trauma even further.

Achieving high standards of care in a situation where the turnover is low presents considerable difficulty. One valuable tool for this purpose is medical auditing. While this will be important in all hospitals treating injured patients, it is of paramount importance in regional referral centres.

Of the trauma patients who present at hospital, the vast majority present relatively few critical problems whereas a few will survive and make a good recovery only with skilled management by medical teams composed of several different specialties. The main potential for saving life appears to be not so much new therapeutic discoveries as ensuring that the correct patients are brought to hospitals with staff who have the necessary expertise and experience, and that when they arrive at such a hospital, doctors of adequate seniority and experience are mobilised.

This presents a great challenge to the A & E department. There are few departments in the United Kingdom with more than two consultants and one senior registrar. As trauma cases may arrive at any time of the day or night or any day of the week, it is not possible at present to ensure that one of these senior doctors will always be on duty and free from other responsibility. On many occasions the first doctor to examine injured patients is likely to be a relatively junior member of staff. The young doctor will find the great majority of his trauma patients well within his ability to sort out and treat. What he especially needs is help in spotting those few patients for whom he should immediately summon senior doctors within the A & E department and doctors from other units. It is the responsibility of the senior staff to ensure that someone is always available to be called.

Ambulancemen can also play an important role in ensuring that the right patient gets to the right hospital. They require training in the rapid assessment of severely injured patients. The regional boards and the various hospitals with the regions need to negotiate policies so that the ambulancemen can work to a well-known and mutually agreed system.

For medical audit within hospitals and between hospitals and for the rapid identification of patients who require the mobilisation of experienced staff, severity scoring can be of considerable help. There have been recently great developments in methods of scaling. New scaling systems are still emerging and old ones are undergoing revision. The four severity scoring systems described below are ones which have been widely accepted and evaluated in series with large numbers of patients.

INJURY SEVERITY SCORES

The Glasgow Coma Scale

This is possibly the most universally accepted and widely used

of all severity scales. It is concerned not with the totality of injury, but only the head injury component. Three different features of coma are examined — eye opening, best verbal response and motor response. The divisions and coding for each are as follows:

Eye opening	
spontaneous	4
to voice	3
to pain	2
no response	1
Verbal response	
orientated	5
confused	4
inappropriate words	3
incomprehensible sounds	2
none	1
Motor response	
obeys commands	6
purposeful movement (to pain)	5
withdrawal (pain)	4
flexion	3
extension	2
none	1

The total Glasgow Coma Scale is calculated by adding the scores of the three aspects. A patient whose level of consciousness has returned to normal will score 15. A person who is in coma will score 3. Some prefer to write the result in the form of an EMV score showing the 'eye opening' 'motor' and 'verbal' components. A fully responsive patient is stated to have a score of E4 M6 V5.

The Trauma Score (revised)

This severity scoring system devised by Champion and his colleagues in Washington DC is based on scales for the three main systems likely to show physiological response to severe injury — the respiratory system, the cardiovascular system and the central nervous system. In its original form the respiratory system was assessed on the basis of both respiratory rate and effort, the cardiovascular system on blood pressure and capillary refill and the central nervous system by the Glasgow Coma Scale, and the scale ran from 1 to 15. As a result of evaluation against a very large number of patients documented for the American College of Surgeons' Major Trauma Outcome Study, the respiratory effort and the capillary refill have been dropped, and the scale now has a crude form which runs from 0 to 12 and a weighted form which runs from 0 to 8.

The new values for the Revised Trauma Score in its crude form are shown in Table 14.1.

Table 14.1 New values for the Revised Trauma Score (crude form)

Glasgow Coma Scale	Systolic blood pressure	Respiratory rate	Coded value
13–15	>89	10–19	4
9–12	76–89	>29	3
6–8	50–75	6–9	2
4–5	1–49	1–5	1
3	0	0	0

For the purposes of immediate assessment, patients in good condition and unlikely to cause problems should score the full score of 12. Used in this way at the early stages of assessment, either prehospital or on arrival at hospital, it can be a useful tool in highlighting the serious cases. However it will be understood that in this very early stage the amount of blood-loss may still be relatively small and if the patient's homeostatic responses are working well, he may register a full score while still having a severe internal injury. In order to identify such patients Champion recommends that the history of the patient and the pattern of injury be scrutinised to show other factors indicating high risk. These are:

1. A penetrating injury to the chest, abdomen, head, neck or groin
2. Two or more proximal long bone fractures
3. Burns >15% combined with facial injury or airway problems
4. A flail chest
5. Evidence of a high energy impact
   a. Falls of 20 feet of more
   b. Change in velocity in crash of 20 m.p.h. or more estimated from outward deformity of car
   c. Rearward displacement of front axle
   d. Sideward intrusion of 15 inches or more on the patient's side of the car
   e. Ejection of patient
   f. Rollover
   g. Death of another person in the same car
   h. Pedestrian hit at more than 20 m.p.h.

It is obvious that information of this sort can be collected only where ambulancemen (of either sex!) are taught its significance, regularly examine the site of the accident to identify and record the evidence and regularly pass it on to doctors on arrival at hospital. It is of great importance than ambulancemen who attempt to do this get a sympathetic and encouraging reception at hospital. Should their efforts to report be met with indifference or hostility they will soon abandon them.

As well as its use in this crude form in association with other factors indicating high risk, the Revised Trauma Score can be used for late assessment for the purposes of medical audit. When used in this way the crude coding values are corrected with weighting factors. The code derived from the Glasgow Coma Scale is multiplied by 0.9368, the code for systolic blood pressure by 0.7326 and the code for the respiratory rate by 0.2908. After these weights are used, the Revised Trauma Score has a corrected value of between 0 and 8. This corrected value correlates very well with survival probability.

The Abbreviated Injury Scale/Injury Severity Score

The Abbreviated Injury Scale (usually referred to as the AIS) is a method of allotting agreed grading codes to specific lesions depending on the morphology of the lesion and its site. The Injury Severity Score (referred to as ISS) is an index of the combined severity of all the lesions, which correlates with the risk of death. Whereas the Trauma Score is physiologically orientated, the AIS and ISS are anatomically orientated.

The general principle of the AIS is that all lesions are graded between AIS 1 and AIS 6. AIS 1 is for very minor lesions, like small superficial wounds. AIS 2 is for lesions which are marginally more severe, such as a Colles fracture. AIS 3 indicates a moderately severe injury, like a fractured femur. AIS 4 is used for a severe injury, such as a ruptured spleen, and AIS 5 for a very severe injury, such as a major rupture of the liver or an extradural haemorrhage. Lesions like decapitation or total transections of the aorta which are incompatible with life are graded AIS 6.

The AIS system is supervised by the American Association of Automotive Medicine which produces a booklet in which the rules for grading all the different types of injury to each organ are set out. About every 5 years a revised edition is published. In the 1985 edition the severity grades are combined with specific coding numbers which may be used to indicate the nature and site of the lesion in place of either the International Classification of Disease or Snomed. (Snomed is an acronym for the systematised nomenclature of medicine. It is a classification system devised by the American College of Pathologists for use on computers).

In order to use the AIS numbers as a basis for a single patient severity number (the ISS), the body is first divided into a number of regions. These are:

1. External (for the skin and subcutaneous tissues all over the body)
2. The face
3. The head and neck (excluding the face)
4. The thorax
5. The abdominal and pelvic contents
6. The extremities (including pelvic bones, clavicle and scapula).

The Injury Severity Sore (ISS) is calculated by taking the three most severely injured regions (i.e. regions containing the highest AIS grades), selecting the AIS of the most severe injury in each of these regions, squaring it and adding the three together.

For example, a patient with a wound on his index finger has only one injured region. His wound is AIS 1. His ISS is $1^2 + 0^2 + 0^2 = 1$. A woman with a Colles fracture (AIS 2) has an ISS of $2^2 + 0^2 + 0^2 = 4$. A patient with an extradural haemorrhage (head and neck, AIS 5), a partial rupture of the aorta (thorax, AIS 5) and ruptured liver (abdominal contents) has an ISS of $5^2 + 5^2 + 5^2 = 75$. Even if there are other injuries in the same region or other regions, the ISS remains 75. The only exception to this rule is that a patient with any lesion graded AIS 6 is reckoned to have an ISS of 75 without further calculation.

Combination of Revised Trauma Score with Injury Severity Score (TRISS)

While both these scales correlate reasonably well with mortality, especially when used for groups of patients, if the two values are plotted against each other (see Fig. 14.1) the accuracy of prediction is enhanced. In such a diagram all patients whose co-ordinates fall below the oblique line are expected to live while those above are expected to die. The cases most requiring medical audit are those reasonably close to this line either below or above it. Using this method, the performance of a trauma unit is judged against the severity of the injuries of the presenting patients.

Apache II

This scale is probably more widely used in intensive care units than A & E departments. The acronym stands for Acute Physiology and Chronic Health Evaluation. The II indicates that like other scales, this one has been adjusted in the light of experience. The

form used for its calculation is shown in Figure 14.2. It will be seen that there are 11 physiological variables where the mean value scores 0, and deviations in either direction are scored as +1, +2, +3, or +4. To this is added 15 minus the Glasgow Coma Scale. Further numbers are added to indicate age and chronic health problems. When all these values are added together the result is the Apache II score. A young fit physiologically normal person will score 0. An elderly chronic invalid with maximal disturbance in all variables could score 71. The score correlates well with mortality. While this scale will not be used during immediate resuscitation in an A & E department, it may well be used by a trained group which is doing a medical audit on its most severely injured patients. (Apache II can also be used for assessing the severity of non-trauma cases who are gravely ill).

Conclusion

Trauma is one of the unresolved health problems of the 20th century. A & E doctors have a crucial role to play in improving trauma services. While it is possible that there may still be advances in diagnosis and treatment, the largest potential for immediate improvement is in organisation. A & E doctors have special responsibilities in ensuring that within their own departments patients needing special care and attention are seen by doctors of sufficient seniority. Within their hospitals they have a responsibility to promote a corporate body which will establish protocols and perform medical audit on the more severely injured patients. In their regions they should be involved in the categorisation of hospitals with the establishment of regional referral centres.

One essential tool for these tasks is the use of injury severity scoring. Many systems have been devised. Current scales are

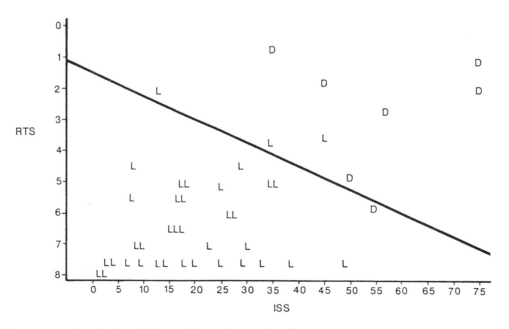

Fig. 14.1 The revised trauma score plotted against the lying severity score for a number of patients, showing outcome for each patient. L = lived, D = died.

PHYSIOLOGIC VARIABLE	HIGH ABNORMAL RANGE					LOW ABNORMAL RANGE			
	+4	+3	+2	+1	0	+1	+2	+3	+4
TEMPERATURE — rectal (°C)	≥41°	39°-40.9°		38.5°-38.9°	36°-38.4°	34°-35.9°	32°-33.9°	30°-31.9°	≤29.9°
MEAN ARTERIAL PRESSURE — mm Hg	≥160	130-159	110-129		70-109		50-69		≤49
HEART RATE (ventricular response)	≥180	140-179	110-139		70-109		55-69	40-54	≤39
RESPIRATORY RATE (non-ventilated or ventilated)	≥50	35-49		25-34	12-24	10-11	6-9		≤5
OXYGENATION: A-aDO₂ or PaO₂ (mm Hg) a. FIO₂ ≥0.5 record A-aDO₂	≥500	350-499	200-349		<200				
b. FIO₂ <0.5 record only PaO₂					PO₂ >70	PO₂ 61-70		PO₂ 55-60	PO₂ <55
ARTERIAL pH	≥7.7	7.6-7.69		7.5-7.59	7.33-7.49		7.25-7.32	7.15-7.24	<7.15
SERUM SODIUM (mMol/L)	≥180	160-179	155-159	150-154	130-149		120-129	111-119	≤110
SERUM POTASSIUM (mMol/L)	≥7	6-6.9		5.5-5.9	3.5-5.4	3-3.4	2.5-2.9		<2.5
SERUM CREATININE (mg/100 ml) (Double point score for acute renal failure)	≥3.5	2-3.4	1.5-1.9		0.6-1.4		<0.6		
HEMATOCRIT (%)	≥60		50-59.9	46-49.9	30-45.9		20-29.9		<20
WHITE BLOOD COUNT (total/mm3) (in 1,000s)	≥40		20-39.9	15-19.9	3-14.9		1-2.9		<1
GLASGOW COMA SCORE (GCS): Score = 15 minus actual GCS									
A Total ACUTE PHYSIOLOGY SCORE (APS): Sum of the 12 individual variable points									
Serum HCO₃ (venous-mMol/L) [Not preferred, use if no ABGs]	≥52	41-51.9		32-40.9	22-31.9		18-21.9	15-17.9	<15

B AGE POINTS:
Assign points to age as follows:

AGE(yrs)	Points
≤44	0
45-54	2
55-64	3
65-74	5
≥75	6

C CHRONIC HEALTH POINTS
If the patient has a history of severe organ system insufficiency or is immuno-compromised assign points as follows:
a. for nonoperative or emergency postoperative patients — 5 points
    or
b. for elective postoperative patients — 2 points

DEFINITIONS
Organ Insufficiency or immuno-compromised state must have been evident prior to this hospital admission and conform to the following criteria:

LIVER: Biopsy proven cirrhosis and documented portal hypertension; episodes of past upper GI bleeding attributed to portal hypertension; or prior episodes of hepatic failure/encephalopathy/coma.

CARDIOVASCULAR: New York Heart Association Class IV.

RESPIRATORY: Chronic restrictive, obstructive, or vascular disease resulting in severe exercise restriction, i.e. unable to climb stairs or perform household duties; or documented chronic hypoxia, hypercapnia, secondary polycythemia, severe pulmonary hypertension (>40mmHg), or respirator dependency.

RENAL: Receiving chronic dialysis.

IMMUNO-COMPROMISED: The patient has received therapy that suppresses resistance to infection, e.g. immuno-suppression, chemotherapy, radiation, long term or recent high-dose steroids, or has a disease that is sufficiently advanced to suppress resistance to infection, e.g., leukemia, lymphoma, AIDS.

APACHE II SCORE
Sum of A + B + C

A APS points _____
B Age points _____
C Chronic Health points _____

Total APACHE II _____

Fig. 14.2 Rules for calculating APACHE II severity of disease classification system.

subject to revision and new scales emerge. For help in patient assessment the Glasgow Coma Scale and the Revised Trauma Score are probably the most useful. For medical audit a combination of the Revised Trauma Score with the Injury Severity Score is valuable, as is also Apache II.

ARRIVAL OF THE PATIENT

The moment when the next accident will happen and the next injured patient will arrive is unknown. It may be at a time when many staff are on duty and there are few patients, or in a very busy period with staff already over-committed. Warning of even 2 or 3 minutes can be of great help in making preparations and the more serious the patient the more important the warning. A system where ambulancemen talk directly to the A & E staff has advantages in allowing them to ask for advice and ensuring that the real facts are being communicated. Potentially life-saving information can be relayed concerning the type of accident, the general condition of the patient and the nature of the injuries. A detailed description of the circumstances of the accident and the position of the injured person should alert the medical staff in the A & E department to suspect specific types of injury, e.g. head, neck, chest and leg injuries in front seat occupants of vehicles after involvement in head-on collisions. Accurate information will allow appropriate specialists (orthopaedic surgeon, neurosurgeon, anaesthetist, etc.) to be contacted. It is also good practice to warn the surgical staff of the ward receiving patients of the injured person's imminent arrival. They will often wish to be involved in the initial assessment and resuscitation, especially if they are responsible for late definitive surgical care. An anaesthetist may be of great assistance in the early stages.

Patients are usually transported in ambulances, lying on a low trolley. As the doctor gets his first glimpse of the patient, there should be a momentary hesitation to allow rapid assessment of the airway. This is done by looking at the lips to see of they are pink or cyanosed, putting the cheek down close to the face where breathing can be both felt and heard, at the same time looking along the chest wall to see of it is rising and falling. Unsatisfactory respiration will demand some remedial action even before lifting the patient across onto the hospital trolley.

Bleeding can usually be ignored for a few moments until the patient is transferred to the hospital trolley. Massive haemorrhage may be controlled with direct pressure of a thumb or a large gauze pad. Sometimes in a traumatic amputation one will see bleeding from the major vessels which may protrude beyond the end of the amputated bone. The immediate application of artery forceps or a temporary tourniquet will stop considerable unnecessary blood loss. However, in most situations attempts to apply artery forceps are dangerous and often lead to damage of peripheral nerves.

Transfer of patient from ambulance trolley to accident trolley

If possible, the patient will be lying on a lifting sheet or a scoop

stretcher on top of the ambulance trolley. Lifting them provides no problem — the lifting sheet will be kept as taut as possible in order to minimise any movement of the cervical, dorsal or lumbar spine. Poles and a spreader will help. Occasionally, a patient is brought in without a lifting sheet. A good lift then requires four people for the patient (three at the side and one at the head) and a fifth to pull away the ambulance trolley and to push in the accident trolley. None of the lifters should move his feet during this procedure. The patient is raised vertically well clear of the first trolley, and lowered down onto the second when it has been pushed into place (see Fig 14.3). Occasionally in a patient with leg fractures and no other injury, it may be preferable to apply splints first and then transfer the patient to the accident trolley.

Having placed the patient on the accident trolley, the airway is again quickly checked whilst proceeding with the next step — removal of all clothing.

Removal of clothes

In an accident and emergency department, stripping the severely injured patient nude never adds to the risks — failing to do so often may.

Removal of clothes should be rapid, should hurt the patient as little as possible and should not aggravate any injury. The most serious injuries which are in danger of aggravation are unstable fractures and dislocations of the spine. Before undressing the patient, the possibility of such an injury should be considered. In the conscious patient this will be indicated by severe pain and tenderness. In the unconscious, the patient must be handled as if he had a back injury until this has definitely been excluded.

If there is no back injury, heavy clothing will be found to come off most quickly by easing it off rather than attempting to cut it off. To remove coats and jackets, the patient's back is raised to 45° above the horizontal, one person supporting the head and neck, thus maintaining a straight line with the trunk. Coats and jackets are eased over the shoulder of whichever arm is less severely injured first, the elbow is bent and the forarm and hand extracted from the sleeve. The coat is passed across behind the patient, and the sleeve slipped off the more severely injured arm. If the manoeuvre is causing no distress, it may be quickest to pull much of the light clothing up over shoulders and head at the same moment. But, if any doubt, pullovers, shirts and vests should be cut off with heavy tailor's scissors (Fig. 14.4).

Trousers are usually best taken off. The pelvis is lifted, they are eased below the buttocks and the pelvis lowered. The less severely injured leg is extracted first. Underpants are cut away. Nitrous oxygen and oxygen anaesthesia (Entonox) may ease the discomfort of undressing.

Preliminary rapid assessment

This should take approximately 60 seconds.

1. *Check the airway*

Are the lips blue? Is air moving in and out of the mouth and nose?

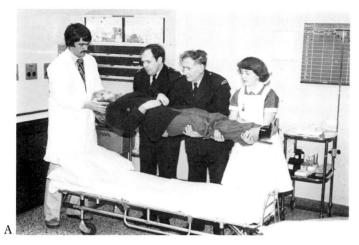

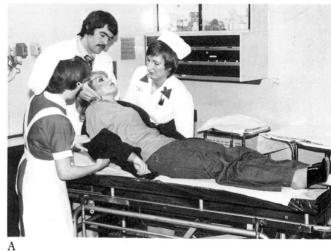

A

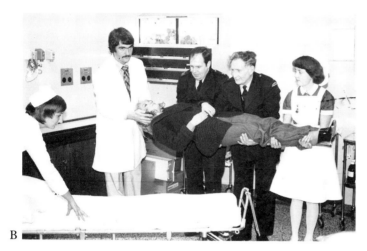

B

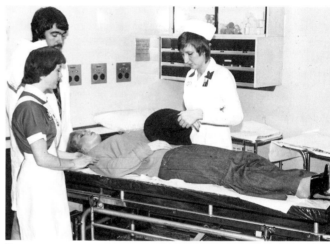

B

Fig. 14.4 A Removing heavy coats and jackets. Start by raising patient and removing sleeve from less injured arm. **B** Pass jacket behind body and remove sleeve from worse injured arm.

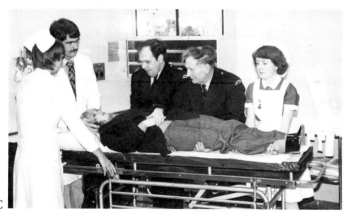

C

Fig. 14.3 A Lifting a patient without a lifting sheet. One person at head taking care of head and neck; three people at side. Patient lifted vertically upwards. **B** Lifters do not move. Fifth person removes one trolley and substitutes another. **C** Lifters lower patient onto second trolley.

Is the chest wall moving normally? If the patient is unconscious test the gag reflex to see whether the patient will tolerate an airway

2. *Assess the circulatory state*

Has the circulation already collapsed? Is the skin cold? Are the veins collapsed? Is a pulse palpable at wrist, groin or neck? Ask a nurse to check pulse rate and blood pressure.

3. *Level of response*

Is the patient fully conscious? Will he respond to commands, and speak? Will he respond to pain? Is he still alive? Are the pupils small or large? Are they equal? Do they react to light?

4. *Make first attempt at diagnosing injuries*

Examine from head to toe. A fuller examination will be repeated within 5 or 10 minutes; in the first rapid assessment, examination of the back, the anus and genitalia may be omitted, though they must never be omitted in the second, more thorough examination.

The extent of injury will make transfusion requirements clearer. Injuries needing instant attention (flail chest, sucking wound of chest, cardiac tamponade and massive bleeding) should be spotted and treated.

5. *Take the history*

For most medical conditions it is advisable to take the history before examining the patient. In severely injured patients the order is reversed. History-taking is the fifth section of the rapid assessment. The doctor should know at this stage what particular details of the history may help him in elucidating the injury. If the assessment is completed within 60 seconds, the ambulanceman and other people who were at the scene should still be available. If history-taking is omitted at this stage the opportunity to talk to witnesses may be lost.

Complexity of responsibilities in initial care of the severely injured

Much of the difficulty in caring for the severely injured patient arises from the complexity of the responsibilities involved. These have often to be discharged in an atmosphere of considerable emotional tension generated by the urgency of the task and the gruesome aspect of the patient. In theory five aspects of patient care can be identified, though in practice these have to be discharged concurrently rather than one after another.

> 1. Mobilise medical staff:
> a. to help with resuscitation in the A & E department
> b. to be ready to assume responsibility for treatment in the operating theatre and/or wards after leaving the A & E department.
> 2. Resuscitate.
> 3. Diagnose the injuries.
> 4. Monitor the injuries.
> 5. Make a good record.

MOBILISING MEDICAL STAFF

While each of the five elements is in its own way very important, this first step is crucial and is one where the inexperienced doctor can very easily fail. The condition of many injured patients brought to hospital by ambulance is not life threatening and it is easy, having seen a succession of such patients, to be lulled into a sense of false security and not to call for help quickly enough. Junior doctors in the A & E department looking for help from other units tend to call on colleagues who are at a similar stage of their career. For the life-threatening injuries it is often of great importance to involve more senior colleagues, and the easiest way for the young A & E doctor to do this is to contact a senior A & E colleague who will then involve senior colleagues from other specialties.

In a patient who has injuries which embrace several specialties, the resuscitation room may become flooded with a plethora of doctors. It is essential that someone should clearly be in charge. The A & E doctor should assume responsibility for co-ordinating all activity and decisions for as long as the patient remains in his department. This only works easily if he has the seniority to

assume this position. However, in circumstances where a junior A & E doctor cannot find a senior colleague within his department, he should still assume that he is in charge until the patient leaves his department. He should also make sure that of those who will continue to treat the patient, a clear leader has been appointed for the next stage of treatment.

In order to identify those cases in which it is necessary to call a senior colleague, the first stage is to perform the Revised Trauma Score in its crude form (see p. 155). This entails measuring the systolic blood pressure, the respiration rate and the Glasgow Coma Scale. (A nurse may make the first two measurements while the doctor makes the third.) The doctor should speak to the ambulanceman or anyone who can give information about the facts of the accident. He should also conduct a preliminary rapid examination to identify possible injuries. As explained on p. 155, he will use the history and examination to identify cases where the early arrival of the patient in hospital has not yet allowed enough physiological disturbance to upset the trauma score.

There will be cases where a call from the ambulance before it reaches hospital makes it quite clear that the patient's condition is life threatening. Where this is so, steps should be taken to mobilise the correct medical staff, or at least to warn them prior to the arrival of the patient. When the patient arrives, all the different aspects of resuscitation seem equally pressing, and it is all too easy to become totally absorbed in commencing infusions and passing intratracheal tubes. There may be cases where an urgent airway problem demands instant priority. However, even while dealing with this the doctor should already be thinking 'Are the right people here?' 'Has everyone that needs to be notified been notified?' 'Do I need help?' 'Is it clear who is in charge?' These questions must be faced and answered at the beginning rather than the end of resuscitation.

RESUSCITATION

It is impossible to overemphasise the importance of establishing and maintaining a good airway and good ventilation, and diagnosing and treating hypovolaemia. This is all fully described in Chs. 10, 11 and 13.

DIAGNOSIS OF INJURIES

Clinical examination

It is not always possible to diagnose accurately every injury during the brief period in which the patient is in the resuscitation room. However, this should always be the aim, for the more complete the diagnosis, the more effective the treatment will be. A careful systematic examination should reveal all serious injuries.

Where the patient is conscious, it is useful to obtain his description of exactly how the injury occurred. He should be asked to describe how he feels, in particular where he feels pain, then during the examination points of tenderness can be sought out and accurately localised.

In the unconscious patient, an ambulanceman, another victim of the accident or a witness may be able to supply the necessary details. Industrial accidents are often related in technical terms which need to be translated into simple English.

It is essential to use a systematic method for the physical examination. There is much to be said for starting with the scalp in the region of the vertex, moving down to the neck and trunk, examining the anterior surface and then the left and right lateral aspects. When the front and sides of head, neck and trunk have been fully examined, the four limbs are examined — it may be possible to examine them all from front and back as well as both sides. The patient then needs to be rolled onto one side to allow examination of the occipital region, the back of the neck and the back of the trunk. Special care must be taken not to miss injuries in the perineal region. During the examination, one may think that everything will remain clear in one's memory until it is written down, but when writing is started it is found that many details cannot accurately be recalled. It then becomes necessary to examine the patient a second or third time. It is therefore a great help if the examining doctor dictates what he sees, feels and hears during his examination.

The more specific points which the physical examination seeks to elicit will be elucidated in the sections of this chapter devoted to regional injuries.

Radiology

In some accidents the history will have made it quite clear that injuries are restricted to one specific area and that the rest of the body is uninjured. Then there will be few problems in deciding about radiological examination — only the injured parts need be so examined.

The place of radiology in examining injured patients is discussed in Ch. 8 and also in the sections of this chapter devoted to particular regional injuries.

Laboratory examinations

As with all specimens in A & E departments, great care should be taken with labelling. The time as well as the date of the specimen should be noted. The results of laboratory tests will usually be available only after the patient has left the accident and emergency department. However, the following tests may be valuable for establishing a baseline of the patient's state on arrival at hospital.

1. Blood group (plus cross-matching of blood for transfusion)
2. Haemoglobin concentration, haematocrit and, in Negro patients, tests for sickling
3. Electrolytes and urea
4. An appropriate battery of biochemical tests
5. Blood alcohol and osmolality
6. Arterial blood gas concentration and pH.

It is possible to omit some of these tests in some patients.

Monitoring

While the patient is being resuscitated, examined and investigated, time is passing and one wants to know whether the patient's state is improving, deteriorating or remaining unchanged. As already explained, trends in the patient's clinical condition and serial objective measurements are a much more meaningful guide to therapy than single observations. Baseline observations of pulse rate, blood pressure, level of consciousness, respiratory rate and the state of the peripheral circulation should be recorded as soon as possible after admission of the patient — the measurements should be repeated at 15-minute intervals while the patient is in the resuscitation area and while undergoing emergency investigations.

Accurate measurement of blood pressure is very important. An increase in diastolic pressure accompanied by a decrease in pulse pressure occur some time before there is any appreciable drop in systolic pressure. In the individual patient, changes in pulse pressure roughly parallel changes in the stroke volume of the heart. Unless the pulse rate increases, a fall in stroke volume results in a decreased cardiac output. In centres where the cardiac output is measured by dye dilution technique it has been found that the severity of shock correlates best with the decrease in cardiac output. An inflatable cuff attached to a sphygmomanometer is most commonly used to measure the blood pressure. As the stroke volume falls the Korotkoff sounds tend to become muffled. In the presence of severe vasoconstriction and marked reduction of stroke volume they may disappear altogether; in these cases the systolic blood pressure is usually less than 60 mmHg. On the other hand, a few patients who are vasoconstricted have a normal central arterial pressure, the auscultated blood pressure then being misleadingly low.

The best way of dealing with this in the A & E department is by the use of the 'Dinamap' machine. This is activated merely by the application of a sphygmomanometer type cuff. The machine gives readings of systolic, diastolic and mean blood pressure and pulse rates. It can be set to take these at regular intervals. As well as the visual display it is possible to have a printer attached which will give a permanent record. It is valuable in that the machine continues to make its regular recordings thus relieving one doctor or nurse from this duty. It is particularly valuable for low pressure values, which may be difficult to hear with a stethoscope when using a traditional sphygmomanometer, especially if there is competing noise from a lot of activity. The values are most reliable in the unconscious and unmoving patient. Arm movement can produce misleading results.

Where massive blood loss had occurred the haemodynamic effects of replacement with blood transfusion will require monitoring and for this the intensive care department may wish to have a Swann-Ganz catheter inserted. It will be a matter of local policy and co-operation whether this is inserted immediately in the A & E department, or later in the operating theatre or intensive care department.

Urine output should be measured by inserting a self-retaining catheter into the bladder and attaching it to a urinometer. This enables the urine output to be monitored. Volume recordings are usually made at hourly intervals, so occasionally the patient may still be in the A & E department when the first measurement is due.

The level of consciousness is best monitored by using the Glasgow Coma Scale. This is explained in the section on head injuries on pages 000 and 000. The ECG should be monitored in all severely injured patients, as changes of heart rate and dysrhythmias are common. The ECG may also reveal that the patient's accident has been caused by or resulted in a myocardial infarction.

Records

Making a good record is the fifth aspect of accident and emergency care during resuscitation in the department.

All the arguments for good records in the A & E department (see Ch. 3) apply with particular cogency to the record of the severely injured patient.

The exact format of the record will depend on the system of recording both for other types of cases in the department and for the recording system used in the main wards. A special record for the severely injured patient needs to be compatible with both these systems and easily understood and accepted by all who will use it.

A folder containing several types of case notes will be needed for each patient. This will usually include the following.

1. The basic form used for all accident and emergency patients. There are advantages to this being at least in duplicate on NCR paper. It makes this paper available as an X-ray request form, a communication sheet for theatre and ward and for the family doctor (GP).

2. An extra blank sheet — allowing a fuller description by A & E staff or comments by the other specialists called in to see the patient.

3. A sheet with a picture diagram of the body and agreed symbols for indicating a wound, a bruise, an abrasion, a fracture and a point of tenderness. This sheet may also contain a check list of items to tick or encircle. Often the original record can be made very quickly on this sheet, and subsequently a brief summary be transcribed onto forms 1. and 2. A system which includes both cursive description alongside drawings and encircled items is superior to one or the other.

4. A sheet of serial notation of those features which are being serially monitored.

5. A fluid balance chart. This should be the standard fluid balance chart used in the hospital. Special care is needed when two or three infusion lines are running simultaneously.

6. Laboratory request forms for the agreed tests (see p. 161). These may be kept in the same folder or on a nearby shelf with appropriate syringes and specimen bottles.

HEAD INJURIES

Introduction

In deaths caused by road traffic accidents, the brain is the most commonly damaged organ. In about 60% of cases the brain is damaged, compared with the lungs in about 50% and the liver in about 45% of cases (Mant 1978).

It has been estimated that approximately 100 000 patients are admitted annually to National Health Service beds because of head injuries. Of these patients, 1500 (many of whom are young) are returned to the community each year with severe residual disability. Not only does this present an enormous economic loss to the community, but it also results in fundamental changes to the pattern of life of the families involved. It is important, therefore, that the early management of these injuries should be well understood and facilities provided 24 hours a day and 7 days a week, since a high proportion of these injuries are sustained out of normal working hours.

For the purpose of this chapter a patient has incurred a severe head injury if he is brought into the department 'unconscious' or becomes unconscious shortly afterwards.

The term 'coma' is used here as defined by Jennett as a condition in which the patient does not obey commands, has no intelligible speech and no spontaneous opening of the eyes. Details of the Glasgow Coma Scale are given on p. 154.

Mechanism and associated pathology

At the time of impact, the head may be at rest (static injury), or may be submitted to sudden acceleration, deceleration, shearing or rotational forces. The consequent pathological changes in the brain are different in the two groups, although there may be considerable overlap. In either group the injuries may be open or closed.

Static injuries to the head

Sometimes the head, at the moment of injury, does not move significantly, either because the side opposite to the injury is resting against a firm surface, or because the inertia of the head and neck is relatively great compared with the momentum of the object which strikes the head. Such objects may be relatively sharp. (Blunt objects are more likely to cause acceleration, deceleration injuries.) These are called 'static injuries' and the result is likely to be localised damage to the scalp, skull or brain and is often accompanied by fissured, stellate or depressed fracture of the vault of the skull (Fig. 14.5). This is the 'primary injury'. A short period of unconsciousness is usually followed by early recovery, but if *secondary* deterioration occurs it is likely to be due to an intracranial haematoma, rather than to cerebral oedema. It may also be due to hypoxia and/or hypovolaemia from associated injuries. The intracranial haematoma is commonly extradural and such a patient should recover completely if treatment is carried out promptly. Failure to do so may result in death or permanent disability. These constitute a large proportion of the patients who 'talk and die' (Reilly et at 1975). The time between the injury and clinical deterioration (latent interval) may vary from a few minutes to two days, but is usually a few hours. The earlier the deterioration the more rapidly does cerebral compression, and tentorial herniation, take

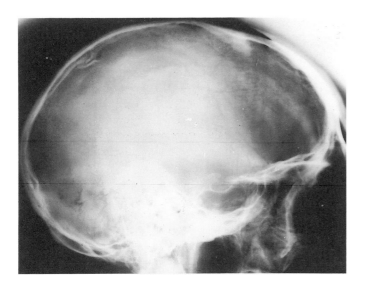

Fig. 14.5 Depressed fracture seen in lateral radiograph of skull.

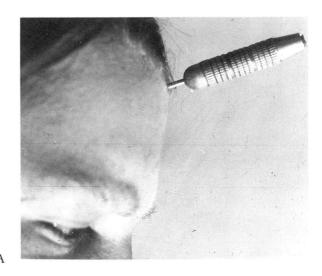

A

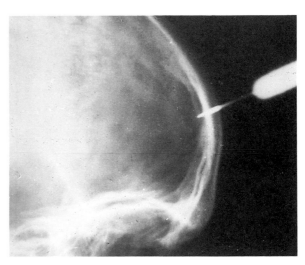

B

Fig. 14.6 A Static injury of head. Skull pierced by dart; minimal brain damage. **B** Radiograph of same patient.

place. This is closely followed by irreversible changes in the brain stem and death.

Penetrating injuries, such as those caused by a dart, seldom cause prolonged loss of consciousness but carry a high risk of infection to the brain or meninges — as do all open fractures (Fig. 14.6).

Deceleration/acceleration injuries

When the patient's moving head is suddenly decelerated on coming into contact with a static object, or if the head is suddenly accelerated or rotated violently by contact with a rapidly moving object, shearing and rotational forces are applied to the brain causing *diffuse injury*. Most of these patients will have obvious external injuries to the head or neck (Fig. 14.7). Some patients (often helmeted motor cyclists) may have little or no external evidence of injury to the head — and no fracture of the vault of the skull (Fig. 14.8). They may, however, have a fracture of the base of the skull, as indicated by bleeding from the nose or the ears (or blood visible behind the ear-drum). Such fractures may have serious consequences when a pathway for infection is opened between the paranasal sinuses and the cerebrospinal fluid. At autopsy there may be little macroscopic evidence of injury to the brain, the major part of the damage being at a cellular level. These changes constitute the primary injury which may result in death or permanent disability.

This early primary diffuse brain damage may then be followed by *secondary* changes, which may be grouped as follows.

Intracranial haematoma — which may be extradural, subdural or intracerebral and may, under these circumstances (particularly with the subdural and intracerebral haematomata) be accompanied by a localised or diffuse cerebral oedema (see below) (Fig. 14.9).

Cerebral oedema (Fig. 14.10) — which is the consequence of the primary brain damage and may be maximal in one or other hemisphere (producing a midline shift) (Fig. 14.11) or may be diffuse. In either case, compensatory shifts of fluid within the skull will take place, but vasoparesis occurs and eventually the intracranial pressure rises. Tentorial herniation follows, producing brain stem compression and death — as in the untreated extradural haematoma.

Gunshot wounds of the head — see p. 190.

Differential diagnosis

Unconscious patients brought to the A & E department may sometimes be thought to have sustained a head injury when the coma results from another condition such as hypoglycaemia or stroke (see Ch. 12). Nevertheless, a fall precipitated by one of these conditions may still be complicated by an intracranial haematoma and caution must be exercised before attributing all the clinical signs to such a condition.

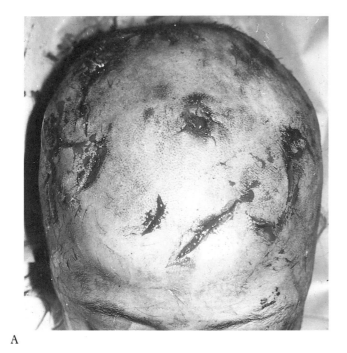

A

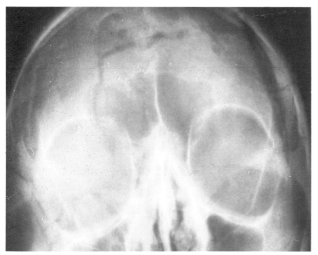

B

Fig. 14.7 A Multiple hammer blows to head. **B** Radiograph of same patient showing severe fractures.

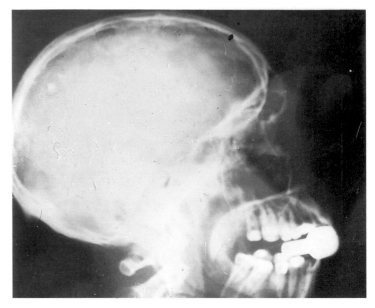

Fig. 14.8 Acceleration/deceleration injury from motor car accident. No skull fracture, brain injury so severe that patient died.

Alcohol (or other drugs of addiction)

Severely injured patients have frequently consumed alcohol before their accident. If the level of blood or breath alcohol is not measured the doctor will usually make a guess at the level of intoxication. Such clinical estimates have been shown to be wildly inaccurate, sometimes indicating gross intoxication in patients with zero blood alcohol and sometimes indicating that no alcohol has been drunk where a blood estimation shows 300 mg/100 ml. It seems preferable to know the true level, especially as this can be done quickly and simply with a breath alcohol estimator. However, there are dangers in this also, for even a blood alcohol above 300 mg/100 ml does not prove that an extradural haematoma is not present. The test is most helpful in those cases where a high level

was suspected and a low reading is found. One should always be very cautious of attributing the clinical condition solely to alcohol, even when the blood level is very high.

Hypoglycaemia

This may be caused by alcoholic excess, especially in children, and the blood glucose level should always be checked.

Cerebrovascular accidents (stroke)

The presence of a hemiparesis and coma shortly after the accident suggests that either a cerebral contusion occurred at the time of impact or a cerebrovascular accident occurred immediately prior to the accident. In neither case will an immediate operation be indicated, unless there is clear evidence from the history of a rapid progression of symptoms and signs in between the accident and arrival at hospital. There may also be a history of hypertension or previous stroke.

Occasionally (as with the 'developing stroke') a dense hemiparesis may develop without a deterioration in the coma score. The possibility of injury to the internal carotid artery (followed by progressive distal thrombosis) should be considered (Fig. 14.12). In the history there may be evidence of the head being forced to the opposite side or examination may reveal bruising on one side of the head and neck. Auscultation may reveal a bruit.

Subarachnoid haemorrhage

There may be a history of a preceding severe headache of sudden onset and the level of response and the neurological signs may

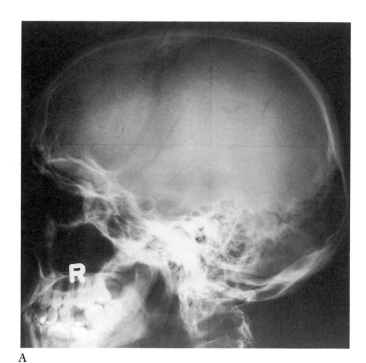

A

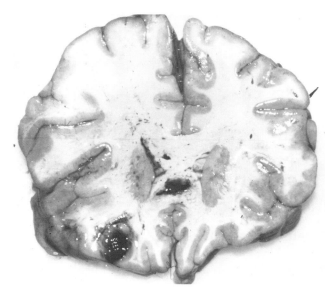

Fig. 14.10 Cerebral oedema causing tentorial herniation. There were no lateralising signs.

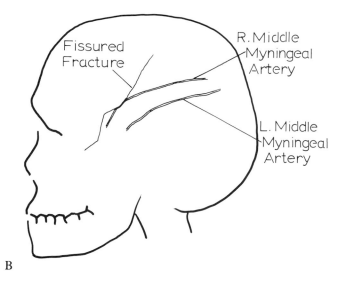

B

Fig. 14.9 A Lateral radiograph of skull showing fissured fracture crossing middle meningeal artery. **B** Line drawing of same radiograph. There is a danger of an extradural haemorrhage complicating such an injury.

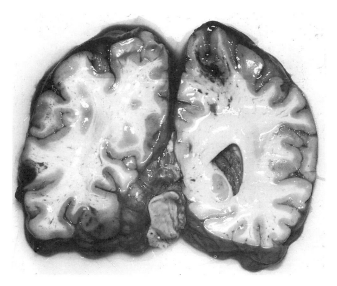

Fig. 14.11 Cerebral oedema affecting mainly one side and causing midline shift.

Other conditions complicating the head injury

Hypothermia (see Ch. 28)

Patients who have been injured outside in cold weather may rapidly become hypothermic and comatose. This may be attributed to head injury, or to hypovolaemic shock since the patient will be drowsy and hypotensive. The rectal temperature should be monitored if the initial reading is below 35°C.

Hypoxia

Often this may not be immediately obvious on clinical examination. It may be combined with a severe degree of metabolic acidosis.

change rapidly and independently. There may be localising signs. Neck stiffness may not become apparent for some hours following the onset. In the absence of a clear history of injury, the diagnosis must therefore depend on careful repeated recording of the symptoms and signs.

Diabetes

Evidence of this may be obtained from the patient's belongings and from a blood sugar stick (Dextrostix test), which should be carried out on all unconscious patients (see Ch. 12).

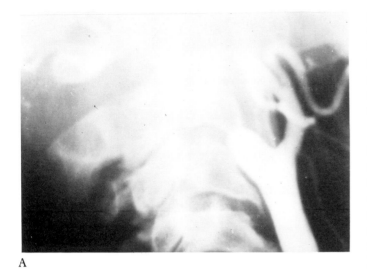

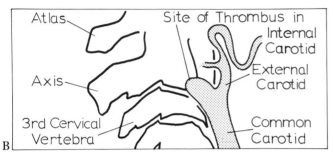

Fig. 14.12 A Angiogram of patient with thrombosis in internal carotid artery following a blow to the side of the head causing lateral stretching of the neck. **B** Line drawing of angiogram.

Hypoxia may result from *respiratory obstruction*, injury to the *chest* or from the advanced stages of *hypovolaemia*. It is mandatory, therefore, to measure the arterial blood gases and pH at an early stage. High cervical cord injury, accompanied by quadriplegia, may also reduce respiratory exchange and be a major cause of hypoxia.

Caution must always be exercised in manipulating the head and neck. Radiological examination of the cervical spine is necessary but in some hyperextension injuries the radiographs may be normal.

Overwhelming fat embolism

This may contribute to early onset coma — and also to hypoxia — but rarely in the A & E department

Clinical presentation

From the practical point of view, patients with severe closed head injury may be divided into three groups, as follows.

Improving group. In these patients, symptoms and signs continue to improve following arrival at the hospital. In such patients (usually following a static injury) the diffuse primary damage is not severe and close observation in the ward is all that is required. (The indications for admission of minor head injuries, the interpretation of radiographs and subsequent management are described in Ch. 40.) Any secondary deterioration is likely to be due to an intracranial hematoma for which urgent surgical treatment will be required, as described below.

Stable or slowly deteriorating group. In these patients the symptoms and signs remain the same or deteriorate only slowly over the course of hours or days. Such patients may be slowly developing an intracranial haematoma, cerebral oedema or infection and should be discussed with a neurosurgeon to make a decision as to whether the patient should be transferred for further investigations (such as computerised tomography, angiography or EMI scan) or for surgery.

Rapidly deteriorating group. The pathology may be either a rapidly developing haematoma or cerebral oedema. Immediate action is required in both these conditions — but the clinical picture and the treatment is different.

Haematoma

A rapidly developing intracranial haematoma results in a deteriorating level of response followed by the development of *lateralising signs* in the limbs (such as slight reluctance to move one arm or leg) and of pupillary changes (inequality and failure to react to light). In 80% of cases the pupil on the same side as the lesion dilates. The prognosis of extradural haematoma is better than that of a subdural or intracerebral haematoma, because it is seldom accompanied by diffuse primary brain damage. However, the time available for successful surgical intervention is short and is least when the lucid interval has been shortest. A & E doctors and nurses should therefore be aware of the necessity for urgent operation at the earliest signs of deterioration, which may have already begun when the patient is first seen in the A & E department. As the laterising signs are late, it is a deterioration in the level of consciousness which must be most rigorously sought. Any such deterioration is an indication for immediate consultation with neurosurgical colleagues.

Cerebral oedema

The term 'cerebral oedema' is used as a convenient clinical label. But pure cerebral oedema, e.g. in benign intracranial hypertension, may be extreme without causing any of the signs described below. The exact pathophysiology in these cases is often unknown. Most of these patients have signs of brain-stem involvement on initial examination. The intracranial pressure is not invariably raised. The clinical picture (which is similar in its later stages to that which follows untreated intracranial haematoma) is as follows.

1. The level of response deteriorates.
2. The limbs become increasingly *spastic*. Usually this is symmetrical but it may be asymmetrical, or may affect the legs more than the arms, or the arms may be flexed and the legs extended.
3. Both pupils become small.
4. The body temperature rises.
5. The blood pressure often rises, the pulse pressure widens and the pulse rate falls.
6. The respirations may become rapid.

If this syndrome is left untreated, the pupils will suddenly dilate, and pulse rate will rise, the blood pressure will fall and breathing will cease.

Management

Management will be considered in two main sections: first, those steps which are necessary immediately in the resuscitation room; and, second, subsequent management in which the A & E doctor may be involved to a greater or lesser degree.

First steps

The cervical spine

Assume this is injured until proved otherwise.

The airway

In head injuries it is of particular importance to ensure a clear airway and to administer 100% oxygen. In an unconscious patient, especially if he is vomiting or there is blood in the throat, this may only be possible by passing an endotracheal tube. The details of airway care and intubation are the same as for all severely injured patients (see p. 160). If a patient warrants referral to a neurosurgeon then they warrant an endotracheal tube. It is essential to maintain both a high oxygen level and a low carbon dioxide level. Where there is difficulty in passing an endotracheal tube, the patient should be anaesthetised.

History

Attempts should be made to get a good account of the accident and the previous medical history of the patient.

General examination

This is the same as for all severely injured patients (see p. 160). It is very important to establish or exclude associated injuries which might contribute to hypoxia, hypovolaemia or metabolic acidosis. In examining the central nervous system as well as establishing the level of responsiveness (see below), special attention should be given to the size of the pupils and whether they react to light. If it is possible, the presence of absence of sensation should be noted. Examination of motor function will include both movement and tone in upper and lower limbs. Special notice is taken of any differences between the left and right side of the body.

Intravenous fluids

In closed head injury unaccompanied by injuries elsewhere in the body intravenous fluids may not be required. Intravenous fluids should be given for head injuries with bleeding from scalp and or brain, or those accompanied by injuries elsewhere in the body. The details of fluid replacement are the same as with other injuries (see p. 146).

Radiological examination

Where this can be performed in the resuscitation room, it is helpful to do so while resuscitation is proceeding. If the patient has to be removed to a radiological department, it should be postponed until resuscitation is complete. The most valuable examination is probably a radiograph of the chest, this should be followed by a lateral view of cervical spine, and this by a lateral view of the skull. A good lateral radiograph of the whole of the cervical spine can be obtained if the doctor stands at the foot end of the couch or trolley and pulls firmly down on the patient's arms.

The presence of a vault fracture crossing a vascular groove warns of a possible extradural haemorrhage and indicates the side and site for the first burr hole should operation become necessary. A radiograph may demonstrate the presence of depressed fragments of bone or of intracranial foreign bodies. These may require operative intervention and will greatly increase the risk of infection and of subsequent epilepsy.

If a basal skull fracture is suspected, a brow-up lateral view should be obtained — a fluid level in the sphenoid sinus or an aerocoele in the frontal region may be seen and is diagnostic. More often, the diagnosis of such a fracture is made on clinical grounds. The relevance of incidental abnormalities in the skull radiographs may need to be considered.

Detailed radiographs of the facial bones can usually be postponed until later. The importance of fractures of the mandible or facial bones lies in the threat that they pose to the patient's airway — and this should be rapidly corrected without recourse to radiology. Patients suspected of brain haemorrhages may be referred for CT scanning where this is available. Some centres find midline ultrasound valuable. A & E departments should consult with their local neurosurgeon to establish protocols for these examinations.

Further action

This depends on the correct diagnosis of the pathological conditions referred to above.

The improving group

A patient in this group will require admission to a ward for continued monitoring until he is fully conscious and fit for discharge.

The stable or slowly deteriorating group

These will be admitted either to a neurosurgical or possibly to an intensive care ward. A neurosurgeon will decide about further treatment.

The rapidly deteriorating group with lateralising signs

These are in urgent need of exploration with burr holes to see if there is an extradural or subdural haemorrhage. The technique for this procedure is given in the books suggested for further reading.

The rapidly deteriorating group without lateralising signs

Early treatment for this condition is just as important as is operation for an extradural haematoma — but the treatment is basically medical rather than surgical. It should be initiated, if necessary, in the resuscitation room, in consultation with the responsible admitting surgeon or neurosurgeon. The aims of treatment are as follows:

1. The patient should be anaesthetised, intubated and ventilated.

2. Correction of *hypoxia* or *hypercarbia* if these exist. Oxygen alone may be sufficient to correct hypoxia, but intermittent positive pressure ventilation may be required if there has been inhalation of vomitus or if there is an associated injury to the chest.

3. Specific measures to *reduce cerebral oedema*. Controlled ventilation is likely to be the most effective in the long term, but dehydrating agents such as mannitol may be used in the short term.

If it is decided to ventilate such a patient, the detection of an expanding intracranial haematoma will become more difficult. It is very important to have the Glasgow Coma Scale carefully assessed and recorded before anaesthetising. Under these circumstances other methods of excluding a haematoma will need to be considered in consultation with the admitting surgeon or the neurosurgeon. Such measures may include CT scanning, angiography, midliner ultrasound scan or the making of burr holes.

Management of open fractures

Most open fractures encountered in civilian life are the result of static injuries and produce only localised brain damage. The problems therefore are those of *infection,* rather than diffuse brain damage or cerebral oedema. Like any other compound fracture, they should be treated within six hours of injury. If possible, the patient should be transferred to a neurosurgical unit within this time. The wound is covered with a sterile dressing and the patient given an intramuscular injection of a broad spectrum antibiotic such as ampicillin or flucloxacillin and tetanus toxoid.

Three types of open fracture may be easily missed.

1. Fine penetrating wounds such as may be caused by a needle or a dart. Although the entry wound may be small, the meningeal barrier may have been breached and the patient should be admitted to hospital and given ampicillin or flucloxacillin. Failure to do this may result in meningitis or a brain abscess.

2. Apparently trivial injuries (e.g. a brick thrown at a child's head) may cause a small wound which conceals a depressed fracture. This may not be noted if a radiograph has not be requested and meningitis or a brain abscess may result. Thus all scalp wounds should be carefully explored. In a patient who has had no unconsciousness or amnesia, if a fracture is found and there is no depression of the fragments, antibiotics should be given and the patient carefully followed up at an outpatient clinic. If radiological examination or wound exploration reveal depressed fragments, a neurosurgical opinion should be requested.

3. Patients who develop cerebrospinal rhinorrhoea following a fall on the nose may not regard this symptom as significant. Sometimes they may notice that they cannot smell. Such patients may never have lost consciousness and may show no signs of injury to the head other than a broken nose. Radiological examination is unlikely to be helpful unless air has entered the cranial cavity through the fracture in the anterior fossa. Such patients should be instructed not to blow the nose, should be given antibiotics and referred to the neurosurgeons. It follows that all patients who have a severe blow to the nose should not only be examined for the present of a septal haematoma and for associated fascial fractures, but should also be questioned about leakage of fluid (often blood-stained) from the nose. Where there is any doubt, the patient should be admitted. Meningitis can develop in under 48 hours.

Penetrating wounds.   Penetration by fine instruments has already been mentioned. Bullet wounds are dealt with on p. 190.

Associated conditions (which may influence early management)

Epilepsy

Epilepsy is commoner in children but may also occur in adults. It is alarming, not only because of the sudden onset, but also because it may precipitate a further episode of hypoxia and may be followed by a period of diminished responsiveness which may suggest the development of an intracranial haematoma. In practice, however, epilepsy is seldom a herald of intracranial haematoma. The airway should be maintained and the convulsions brought under control by an intravenous dose of diazepam. Careful observation for any further change in signs should be continued.

Bleeding from the ears

Bleeding which does not come from the external ear or auditory meatus must come from a rupture of the drum associated with a fracture of the petrous temporal bone (see Ch. 44). Sometimes bleeding is accompanied by cerebrospinal otorrhoea. Further examination with an auroscope is contraindicated under these circumstances. The hair around the ear should be shaved immediately and a dressing secured over the ear with elastic strapping and a cap, made from elastic tubular gauze bandage, fastening under the chin. If this is not done and the patient vomits, the ear may become soiled, increasing the risk of intracranial infection. All these patients should be given antibiotics. Where there is no bleeding from the ears, the drum should be inspected with an auroscope. This may reveal blood behind the intact drum, which is evidence of a fracture of the base of the skull. Such fractures seldom show in the initial radiographs but may be confirmed a day or two later when a bruise appears behind the ear over the mastoid process, or by subsequent tomography.

Bleeding from the nose

Expistaxis may be due to a fracture of the nose, but is often due to bleeding from a fracture at the base of the skull involving the nasopharynx or the roof of the nose (the cribriform plate). Bleeding may be so profuse as to require a rapid transfusion of blood. Postnasal packing may be a life-saving procedure and antibiotics should be given. Fractures involving the cribriform plate usually result in anosmia, which in most patients does not recover.

Bleeding from the scalp

This can be very profuse (especially in elderly people) and may necessitate transfusion. The scalp should be rapidly sutured in the resuscitation room as part of the first steps in management. Scalp wounds are otherwise better left unsutured and merely dressed until radiographs have been taken. Open depressed fractures should then be referred to a neurosurgeon. All other scalp wounds, however, should be carefully shaved and cleaned and the edges excised and sutured to minimize the risk of infection. At the same time, the underlying bone is inspected or palpated with an index finger or forceps to detect the presence of a fissured fracture line.

Hypotension

If a head-injured patient becomes hypovolaemic a source of *internal* bleeding should be sought in the abdomen (most frequently a rupture of the spleen), in the pelvis or in the chest. Peritoneal lavage and erect chest X-ray film may confirm or exclude bleeding in these sites.

Abnormalities in the eyes

The well-known changes in the size and reaction of the pupils may be of value in defining changing neurological status, but the relevance of a dilated pupil may not be as obvious as it seems; the following alternative explanations need to be considered before jumping to the conclusion that an intracranial haematoma is developing.

Bilateral dilated pupils may be due to severe hypoxia or to drugs (including alcohol).

A unilateral dilated pupil may be the result of a direct blow to the eye ('traumatic mydriasis'), a severed oculomotor or optic nerve, a previous injury or operation, an artificial eye, previously administered mydriatics, or a small pupil in the other eye due to pilocarpine. It should be remembered that pupillary changes are often late in head injuries.

The eyes must be examined for injury to the cornea or globe. Papilloedema or fundal haemorrhages are seldom present initially unless the patient has suffered an overwhelming head injury which is likely to be ultimately fatal, or unless there was a pre-existing intracranial space-occupying lesion.

In the more severe head injuries it is worth listening with a stethoscope over the forehead for the presence of a bruit due to a major vessel injury within the skull, and also over the neck to detect injury to the internal carotid artery outside the skull.

Summary

Urgent treatment of the severely head-injured patient can and should be initiated in the resuscitation room. The information required to make these early decisions which are vital to recovery depends in the first instance, not on radiological examination, but on the following.

1. A knowledge of the mechanism and the circumstances of the accident
2. Careful clinical examination of the patient
3. Careful recording of the vital signs and levels of response on a suitably designed chart
4. An awareness of the necessity for urgent action at the first signs of deterioration, and a readiness to act

Prevention of the secondary effects following severe head injury should begin outside the hospital with efficient first aid and ambulance care. Medical staff capable of establishing an adequate airway rapidly must be available 7 days a week and 24 hours a day on site in every A & E department. Clear lines of communication must be established, not only with the ambulance service to provide warning of the imminent arrival of such patients, but also with the anaesthetists, admitting surgeons and neurosurgeons, so that the management of these difficult patients can be carried out quickly and efficiently.

FRACTURES OF THE FACIAL BONES

From the point of view of the doctor in the A & E department, facial fractures can be divided into two types.

1. Those with gross disruption where it is virtually impossible to overlook the diagnosis. Immediate treatment of the airway is urgent and the disposal is to specialists in maxillofacial surgery. This category includes all explosive wounds of the face and severe impact injuries, where swelling will be gross and progressive.

2. Those cases where the patient may at first be thought to have

suffered only soft tissue injuries (e.g. a black eye, abrasions over the cheek or a swollen lip) and whose presence in the major injuries area has been dictated by serious injuries elsewhere.

Gross facial fractures

The patient will be bleeding from the mouth and nose, often profusely. Airway problems are almost inevitable, due to blood clots, to backward displacement of the palate in fractures of the middle third of the face, or of the tongue in multiple fractures of the mandible. The diagnosis is suspected from the patient's appearance. There is often gross deformity of the face with a crooked nose, a dished, elongated face or a grossly deformed lower jaw. In gross fractures of the mandible, the lower teeth are out of alignment and do not match with the upper teeth — the deformity is so obvious that it is hardly necessary to palpate. In fractures of the middle third of the face, if the upper teeth and adjoining gums are gripped, movement of the bones may be detected. Diagnosis is considered in more detail in the section on orofacial problems (Ch. 42).

The patient with gross facial injury will be in a much safer position once a cuffed endotracheal tube is in situ. Inserting a tube is not easy — manipulation of the laryngoscope may be very painful and profuse bleeding easily obscures the light source. An anaesthetic with a muscle relaxant may be required. When the facial fracture is only one of several injuries, the maximum use should be made of the time prior to anaesthetising the patient to carry out as full an examination as possible and, especially, to establish whether or not there is any lesion in the abdomen.

Where the airway is obstructed and there is difficulty with, or contraindication to, muscle relaxation and endotracheal intubation then an emergency laryngotomy through the cricothyroid membrane may be necessary (see section on airway obstruction, Ch. 11). This procedure precedes a formal tracheostomy.

Facial injuries may bleed profusely and transfusion may be required, but where there is significant hypovolaemia other serious injuries should be looked for.

The patient should be treated by maxillofacial specialists. It is common for other injuries to co-exist — injuries to the eyes, brain or throat in particular. All who will be involved in definitive treatment should be assembled as soon as possible so that operating priorities may be established and the best place for postoperative treatment agreed.

Facial fractures in danger of being overlooked

These fractures most often present in the walking area in patients thought to have minor injuries. On occasion a patient in the resuscitation room has minor facial fractures accompanying serious injury elsewhere. The routine for examination of such patients is described in Chapter 42. Unless such a routine is followed, preoccupation with the more severe injuries may lead to the facial fractures being overlooked — with possible permanent disfigurement.

NECK INJURIES

Injuries involving the cervical spine and spinal cord

By far the most common serious injury in the neck is that to the cervical spine. Rarely, stab wounds may pierce the ligamentum flavum and the cord, and bullet wounds may pass through cervical vertebrae producing compound fractures. The great majority of spinal injuries in the neck, however, are closed injuries.

Serious injuries of the cervical spine result from blows to the head or upper part of the neck. Most injuries can be classified as flexion or extension injuries, although the force may contain also a lateral or rotatory element or some vertical compression. Sprains of the neck ('whiplash' injuries) are dealt with in Ch. 41.

Stable and unstable injuries to the spine

A vertebra can be thought of as containing four sections: 1. a vertebral body, 2. the upper and lower articular processes and pedicle on the left side, 3. the upper and lower articular processes and pedicle on the right side, and 4. a spinous process with its adjoining laminae. The spine is made up of a column of vertebrae piled on top of another. One can think of the spinal column as consisting of four columns corresponding to the four sections of a single vertebra. Where a fracture or dislocation causes discontinuity in a single column, the spine as a whole will stay stable. But where two or more columns are discontinuous, the lesion will be unstable. From this point of view, the ligaments which join the sections of a vertebra to the vertebra above or below are counted as part of the four columns. Thus tearing of the interspinous ligament or the annular ligament of the intervertebral disc will cause discontinuity of a column.

Spinal cord injuries

With displacement of the cervical vertebrae, damage to the cord is very likely because the size of the cord corresponds closely to the size of the bony foramen. This injury may be a concussive injury, which proceeds within a few days to total recovery, a partial lesion of the spinal cord with partial recovery, or a total transection with no recovery. Shortly after the patient's arrival in hospital, one cannot tell with certainty whether recovery is possible. Therefore, in every case, efforts must be made to prevent possible aggravation to what may at that point be only a temporary lesion.

The height of the lesion in the neck is of the greatest importance. A patient with a major cord injury above C3 will rarely remain alive long enough to reach hospital. Injury at this level causes both intercostal and diaphragmatic movement to cease, and only instantaneous and continued inflation of the lungs by mouth-to-mouth respiration or mechanical ventilation can keep a patient alive.

Injuries to the lower four cervical vertebrae may leave sufficient innervation through the phrenic nerve to maintain diaphragmatic respiration. There will be no intercostal movement and, as abdominal muscles are paralysed, abdominal wall movement secondary to diaphragmatic movement is much more obvious than in a person with normal muscular tone. The result is that the abdomen moves in a paradoxical manner.

In some patients there may have been only very slight injury to the cord causing minimal paraesthesia or weakness, but it is much more common to see an almost complete quadriplegia. Where the patient is conscious this is very obvious and there is no difficulty in diagnosis. Where the trauma was transmitted to the neck through the head the patient may be unconscious because of the head injury. In an unconscious patient one has to consider the possibility firstly of an injury to the spine and secondly to the cord. If such a patient is not moving his arms or legs, the possibility that this may be due to an injury of the spinal cord complicating a head injury should always be seriously considered. In testing whether such a patient responds to painful stimuli, the stimuli should be applied to the face or scalp.

In severe cord damage, the lower part of the cord quite quickly begins to take over some reflex function. One effect of this in male patients is that the penis becomes erect, obvious when removing the patient's clothes.

The effect of cord damage on the peripheral circulation should be remembered. The vascular dilatation is very similar to that caused by a high spinal anaesthetic. Blood pressure falls due to poor venous return and this can be corrected by tilting the foot of the trolley upwards to 30°.

Special points in the history

Where the type of accident is such that a neck injury may have occurred, the patient should be specifically asked about sensations in the neck, arms, trunk and legs.

Examination

Great care should be taken during all movements if there is any suspicion of injury to the neck. However, it is as important in these patients as in all severely injured patients to examine the back of the patient as well as the front. One way of handling the situation is to attach traction calipers immediately to the skull, and to use these to apply manual traction as the patient is rolled over onto his side, while gentle counter-traction is applied to both head and feet. If calipers are not being used, a doctor should grasp the head with two or three fingers below the angle of the jaw on each side and apply gentle traction while turning the head in line with the trunk. The procedure is known as log roll (Fig. 14.13).

Once the patient is on his side, the spines of the vertebra are palpated, and points of tenderness, gaps in the deep tissues and malalignments are sought. The rest of the back is examined for accompanying injuries.

The patient with cord damage at C6/7 is often obvious from his posture. His paralysed legs are extended. His extensors of the elbow are paralysed, but there is still some power in his elbow flexors and in his pectoral muscles. His flexed forearms lie across his upper chest.

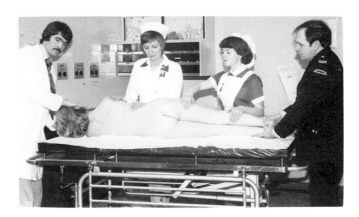

Fig. 14.13 Patient with suspected neck fracture being rolled 'like a log'.

Radiological examination

Good radiographs are of prime importance in deciding further treatment and disposal. A doctor should remain with the patient while radiological examination is taking place to maintain traction to the head and to provide downward traction of the arms (Fig. 14.14), as it is most important to attempt to visualise the seventh cervical vertebra fully in the lateral view. Sometimes this proves impossible and tomography may be necessary. If there is considerable spasm, it may be necessary to repeat flexion/extension views after a few days when the pain has settled. AP views will include one view through the mouth to show the atlas and axis vertebrae. Any doubt about the interpretation of these three basic views may be resolved by taking right and left oblique views to show the foramina and neural arches. When examining the radiographs particular attention should be given to the articular facets and to the distance between the spinous process. Dislocation, or otherwise, of the vertebral bodies can accurately be assessed by following the curvature of the posterior margins of the vertebra.

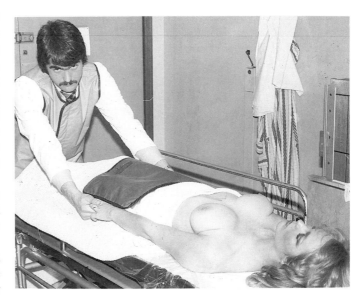

Fig. 14.14 Applying traction to arms to get adequate lateral view of cervical spine.

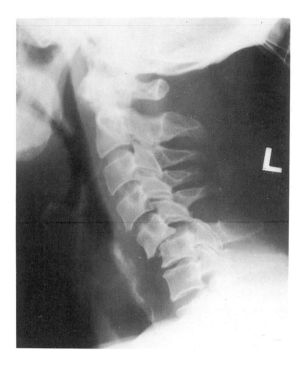

Fig. 14.15 Lateral view of cervical spine. Dislocation of C5 on C6 with interlocking of facets.

After a severe blow, if the neck is very tender but the lateral view is normal, radiographs may be taken with neck flexed and extended. These movements should be made very slowly and gently while applying traction and stopped immediately if paraesthesiae are caused. They should never be attempted if the patient is unconscious (Fig. 14.15).

Treatment in the department and disposal

Severe neck injuries with neurological damage are best treated in special centres. The accident and emergency department in such a centre should inform the surgeons at an early stage and involve them in decisions about where and when to apply traction calipers to the skull. This may be done either in the accident and emergency department or in an operating theatre.

Where a patient with a damaged spinal cord is to be transferred to another hospital, calipers should be inserted in the A & E department and traction maintained during transit, preferably through a spring-loaded device attached to the stretcher.

In patients with a cervical dislocation but no cord damage, a collar should be applied which incorporates braces to support the chin and occiput, and the patient's trunk and head supported by a spinal board.

OPEN INJURIES TO THE NECK

Larynx and trachea

In contrast to spinal injuries in the neck, which are mostly closed, severe injuries to other neck structures are mostly open. An exception is rupture of the larynx or trachea, most commonly caused in a road accident by a blow against the dashboard, following which air escapes into the subcutaneous tissues. On inspection the neck is very swollen and on palpation surgical emphysema is felt. Before it becomes clinically manifest, rupture of the larynx and trachea may be suspected by the finding of mediastinal air on the chest radiograph. These patients often die before reaching hospital, but if still alive constitute one of the rare indications for emergency tracheotomy in the A & E department (see p. 119). If they survive the first half hour after laryngeal trauma, the outlook is much better.

Some wounds of the neck, if pulled open from opposite sides, can be clearly seen to be superficial. If this cannot be established, the wound must be treated with great suspicion. Gunshot wounds will have either two holes (entry and exit) or one hole and a foreign body seen on the radiograph. From this the track can be deduced and the injured organs predicted. The likelihood, especially with high velocity missiles, of damage beyond the immediate track should be remembered (see p. 189).

With stab wounds and gunshot wounds the possibility of injury to the thorax should be remembered.

A suicidal cut-throat wound is usually a clean linear incision running obliquely across the front of the neck. In right-handed people the left end of the wound is higher, and vice-versa in left-handed people. Not uncommonly there are one or two small tentative superficial wounds parallel to the main one. The patient may also have wrist wounds or may have taken an overdose of drugs. In over half the cases the wound is superficial, injuring only the skin, subcutaneous tissues and, possibly, muscles. The most commonly divided blood vessels are the anterior and external jugular veins. With most severe injuries the wound may enter the floor of the mouth, the larynx or the trachea but the patient may be able to breathe satisfactorily through the wound.

Superficial wounds may be repaired in the A & E department and the patient admitted to the observation ward and referred to a psychiatrist. Patients with wounds involving the air passages or major blood vessels should be admitted to a surgical ward. Usually respiration is unaffected and the patient can be taken to theatre for repair. In a few cases tracheostomy in the A & E department may be necessary (see p. 119).

Vessel injuries

Most of these will be open and accompanied by profuse bleeding. The bleeding may be obviously arterial or venous. A minor arterial injury may have stopped bleeding. On auscultation a systolic murmur may be heard. A large haematoma will rapidly develop if there is no external wound. Bleeding from wounds of the external or internal carotid arteries or their main branches will usually decrease markedly when the common carotid artery is compressed against the transverse process of C6. If this does not reduce the bleeding, the possibility of its originating from the vertebral artery should be considered. This is especially likely where a transverse process is fractured.

Major vessel injuries in the neck are often easier to repair if they have been demonstrated before operation by arteriography. Where radiological expertise is available, four vessel angiography should be carried out.

Admission is mandatory if a major vessel injury is suspected.

Nerve injuries in the neck

Wounds in the neck may involve the glossopharyngeal, vagus, spinal accessory or hypoglossal nerves, the cervical sympathetic ganglia or the cervical or brachial plexus.

Division of the glossopharyngeal nerve affects taste and movements of the palate and pharynx. Injuries of the vagus or recurrent laryngeal nerves cause paralysis of one vocal cord, which can be seen on laryngoscopy. Division of the spinal accessory nerve results in weakness of the trapezius and sternomastoid, and division of the hypoglossal nerve causes a paralysis of one side of the tongue. Division of the cervical sympathetic cord or severe bruising close to it may cause Horner's syndrome — a constricted pupil, drooping eyelid and lack of sweating on the affected side of the face. The most important cervical nerve is the phrenic — division causes paralysis of that side of the diaphragm. The brachial plexus may be divided or occasionally avulsed. There will then be areas of anaesthesia, weakness of certain muscle groups and absent reflexes in the arm.

The only way to diagnose these injuries is to bear in mind the possibility that they may have occurred and deliberately test for and record the presence or absence of the relevant signs.

INJURIES TO THE THORACOLUMBAR SPINE

Introduction

The spinal cord ends at the level of the second lumbar vertebra. Below this level is the cauda equina. Major injuries to the back may produce fractures or fracture dislocations of the spine with or without accompanying damage to the spinal cord or the cauda equina.

Stab and gunshot wounds of the back involving the spinal cord are rare. The diagnosis is unlikely to be missed, provided the back is carefully examined in all patients; what is said below about the management of the more common closed injuries applies in principle to the open injuries.

As in the neck one should think of the vertebral column as a composite of four columns: 1. the vertebral bodies, 2. the upper and lower articular processes and pedicles on the left side, 3. the upper and lower articular processes and pedicles on the right side, and 4. the spinous processes with the adjoining laminae. A fracture or dislocation in one of these columns does not cause any instability of the spine. But if two or more columns are discontinuous, the spine becomes unstable, and the spinal cord or cauda equina are more likely to be injured.

There are two common mechanisms of injury: 1. severe flexion of the spine from a downwards and forwards thrust on head and shoulders or an upwards and forwards thrust on the pelvis; 2. direct anteroposterior forces applied nearer the centre of the back. The

former is inclined to produce a compression fracture of the body of the vertebra (Fig. 14.16) and the latter a fracture dislocation involving pedicles and articular processes (Fig. 14.17). Asymmetrical forces cause rotation, which greatly increases the damage, so almost all flexion rotation injuries have neurological complications.

The most common levels of injury are T12/L1 and L4/5. All patients with spinal injuries should be carefully examined for neurological abnormality. This includes testing sensation in the perineum and testing the anal and bulbocavernous reflexes. If the patient is conscious, he should be asked to pass urine.

If interruption of spinal cord function is complete from the outset, recovery is very unlikely. If there is any sparing at all of sensory or motor function below the level of the lesion, then some degree of recovery can be expected — provided that further cord damage is prevented by careful protection of the spine during the early stages of management.

History and examination

A good description of exactly how the injury occurred is helpful for the prediction of likely damage. The patient will always

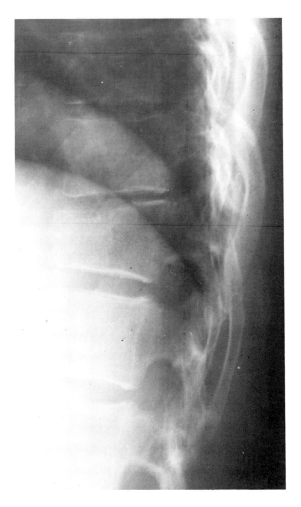

Fig. 14.16 Wedge compression fracture of T12.

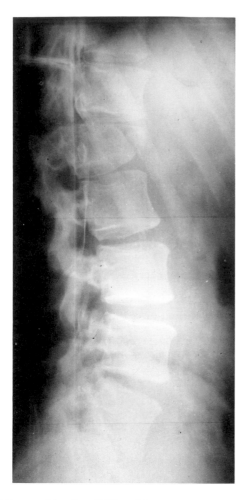

Fig. 14.17 Fracture dislocation of T12 on L1.

to examine the back. Even in their absence, if the history suggests the possibility of an unstable fracture equal care must be taken. If an orthopaedic surgeon is expected shortly the examination of the back may be postponed until his arrival. The patient will then only need to be rolled over once, but the examination is never complete until the back has been inspected and palpated.

To turn a patient with a suspected unstable spine, one person should apply traction upwards at the axillae, one downwards by gripping the ankles, while three people roll the patient over on his side 'like a log' (Fig.14.18).

The most dangerous injuries are inclined to cause considerable trauma to the back as a whole, and abrasions, bruises and wounds may be seen. On palpation, subcutaneous damage may be felt, and the finger may sink into a gap in a torn interspinous ligament. The spinous processes should be palpated and tender spots localised as accurately as possible.

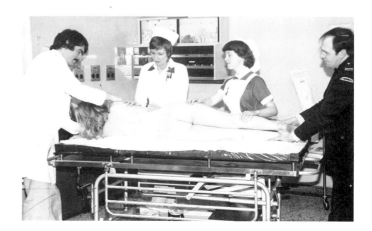

Fig. 14.18 Patient with suspected thoracolumbar spinal injury being rolled over for examination of back while traction is applied.

complain of pain in the back. It is to be hoped that he is already on a lifting sheet and can be transferred to an accident trolley without further deformity of the injured area. When removing clothes, it is probably best to start with shoes and socks, and immediately test sensation in the feet and movement of the toes. Any signs of nerve damage are an indication to cut off all clothes — even coats, jackets and trousers.

After the patient has been stripped, a fuller examination of the nervous system is undertaken. In fractures at L4/5 anaesthesia will be limited to the foot, back of the leg and thigh and near the anus. The knee jerk will be normal but the ankle jerk will be absent. The patient will in time develop a full bladder, but this is not often evident on arrival in hospital.

If there is cord damage from a fracture in the T12/L1 region, the legs will be anaesthetic and the patient unable to move his feet, legs or thighs. The knee and ankle jerks will be absent, as will the lower abdominal, cremasteric and plantar reflexes. An erect penis will commonly be present and in time the bladder will distend.

It is possible to determine the presence or absence of these neurological signs while the patient is still supine. If they are present very great care must be taken in rolling the patient over

Radiological examination

The site of any fracture should have been identified clinically and radiographs of the spine centred on this part. A doctor should remain with the patient during the radiological examination, both to ensure that no further damage occurs and also to reassure the radiographers. The dangers of these injuries are often so stressed to radiographers that fear inhibits them from making those small preparations which help to ensure a good quality radiograph.

The severely injured patient may also require radiographs of the chest, abdomen and pelvis.

Treatment in the department

Pain should be controlled with opiates given intravenously. If there is going to be any delay before transfer to a unit caring for spinal injuries, then a urinary cather should be inserted. It is important to prevent bladder distension. Many patients have a high urine output due to alcohol. Some paraplegic units prefer intermittent catheterisation and others suprapubic cystostomy, and their advice should be sought. Where a catheter is going to be passed in such a patient (and indeed in all patients), very great care should be taken to maintain a strict aseptic technique.

Disposal

All patients with spinal injuries require admission to hospital. Those with unstable fractures and those with neurological damage require treatment in a specialised spinal unit. The doctors from the unit should be contacted as soon as the diagnosis has been made in the A & E department.

CHEST INJURIES

Closed injuries

Pain following a blow on the chest, which is worse on deep breathing or coughing and is accompanied by localised tenderness or pain on 'springing' of the chest wall, is diagnostic of a fractured rib or costal cartilage (Fig. 14.19). A radiograph (which may or may not show the fracture) is needed only to confirm or exclude injury to the structures within the chest. Thus it may suggest a haemo- or pneumothorax, intrapulmonary bleeding or damage to mediastinal structures. Radiological examination may also bring to light unexpected incidental disease in the heart or lungs.

The pain from a fracture of a costal cartilage is often more severe and more prolonged than that from a fracture of a rib, but in both conditions the pain usually starts to improve after four or five days, when stabilisation of the fracture occurs.

The importance of fractures of one or two ribs lies not so much in the discomfort which they undoubtedly cause, but in the danger that the patient with pre-existing lung disease may develop a serious chest infection due to suppression of his cough. For the elderly bronchitic, even one or two fractured ribs may constitute a threat to life. Such patients must be admitted and given adequate analgesia (either by mouth or by intercostal injection of bupivacaine) in order that they may expectorate retained sputum. They must also be given a prophylactic broad-spectrum antibiotic.

The functional disturbance caused by a blow on the chest bears little relation to the radiological appearances (see also Gunshot wounds of the chest, p. 191). On the one hand, compression of a child's chest following a fall from a roof may cause no fractured ribs (because the ribs are so elastic) but may cause sufficient disturbance of lung function to require oxygen therapy or even ventilation. Similarly, a steering column injury to the front of the chest in an adult may fracture the costal cartilages on each side of the sternum and produce a flail anterior segment. The functional disturbance may again be sufficiently severe to require IPPV — yet the chest radiograph may fail to demonstrate any abnormality. On the other hand, a radiograph may show multiple posterior fractures of the ribs in a patient who has little disability other than pain.

The *functional* assessment of the consequences of a chest injury therefore depends on a careful clinical examination, supplemented by estimation of the blood gases. *Radiographs* are required to confirm gross anatomical lesions such as a haemopneumothorax

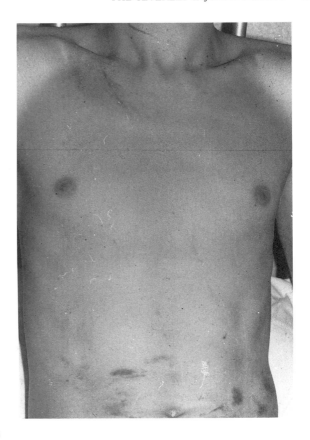

A

B

Fig. 14.19 A Bruising of chest wall and abdominal wall from seat belt. No serious internal injuries. **B** Car in which patient was travelling.

or a widening of the mediastinum. For chest radiographs to be adequately assessed, an erect (or semierect) film is essential. Only if this is impossible should a lateral decubitus radiograph be accepted.

A patient who is brought in with a history of severe blunt injury to the chest and who is short of breath, should be rapidly undressed and examined specifically to detect the following lesions which may require urgent intervention.

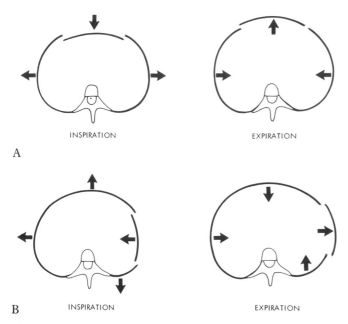

INSPIRATION   EXPIRATION

A

INSPIRATION   EXPIRATION

B

Fig. 14.20 A Flail chest, anterior section. **B** Flail chest, lateral section.

Flail segment of chest wall (Fig. 14.20).

An anterior flail segment (which may be sternum and costal cartilages only) is likely to cause more functional disturbance than a posterior flail segment, but the latter must be sought by sitting the patient forwards or turning him onto his side (Fig. 14.21).

If the patient is *in extremis,* preliminary oxygenation followed by intubation (under suxamethonium) and positive pressure ventilation must be initiated without delay. This is immediately followed by the insertion of an intercostal drain on one or both sides because of the risk of a tension pneumothorax developing as a result of the positive pressure applied within the injured lung.

In the less acutely ill patient, there are advantages in not proceeding too quickly to mechanical ventilation. The assessment

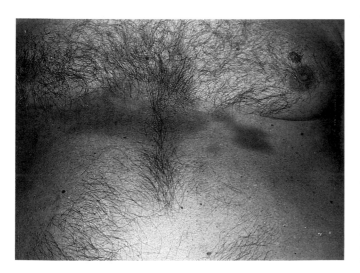

Fig. 14.21 Anterior flail chest injury sustained in head-on high speed road traffic accident. Patient elderly and bronchitic; died two days after injury.

of the severely injured patient is often considerably easier if the patient is conscious and can co-operate in his examination. Oxygen should be administered and the blood gases measured. Efforts should be made to reduce the restlessness, though this is often caused by hypoxia and settles when this is treated. If the PCO_2 is greater than 45 mmHg (6 kPa) or the PO less than 60 mmHg (8 kPa) when the patient is receiving oxygen, mechanical ventilation will probably be required. However, there are also dangers in postponing ventilation until the patient is tired and hypoxic. The decision will be made jointly by the A & E doctor, the anaesthetist and the surgeon.

Pneumothorax

This is more often unilateral than bilateral and may be detectable by diminished air entry and movement on the affected side. A resonant percussion note and shift of the mediastinum may help to confirm the diagnosis

A pneumothorax should always be suspected in the presence of a flail chest or surgical emphysema of the chest wall. There should be no hesitation in inserting a chest drain if the patient is short of breath. Radiological examination may be performed after drainage to ensure that re-expansion of the lung is proceeding satisfactorily. If positive pressure ventilation has to be initiated, drainage of both pleural sacs is usually indicated as stated above. Sometimes one-way valves are recommended during transport of the patient to the radiology department or operating theatre, but underwater seal drains are more efficient and provide a better visual indication of what is happening. The bottles can be carried on a shelf below the trolley. The tubes should never be clamped.

Surgical emphysema appearing first in the neck may be the result of injury to air-containing structures in the neck itself (such as the trachea or oesophagus), or to tracking of air up through the mediastinum. The latter is most commonly due to injury to one of the large bronchi.

Haemorrhage within the chest

If a patient with an injury to the chest is also pale and hypotensive, internal bleeding must be suspected. However, a haemothorax may not become evident clinically until more than 500 ml of blood has collected. In addition to the chest, the abdomen and pelvic region must also be carefully examined; in selected cases, peritoneal lavage may be indicated (see p. 182).

It is in those with suspected intrapleural bleeding that good chest radiographs (at 1.5 m distance, with the patient upright) are so essential and yet are so often not done for fear of moving such a sick individual. Radiographs, however, can be obtained safely if the manoeuvre is carefully planned and executed on a properly designed trolley. The film is placed beneath the chest of the supine patient. The back rest is then elevated whilst the patient's pelvis is supported in order to prevent any sliding. The exposure is completed and the backrest lowered — the whole procedure taking less than a minute. One good film should give reliable evidence of the presence or absence of haemothorax or wide mediastinum

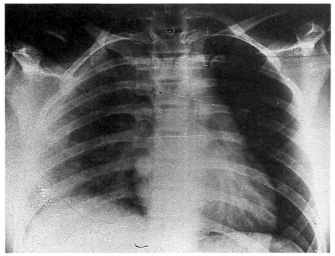

A

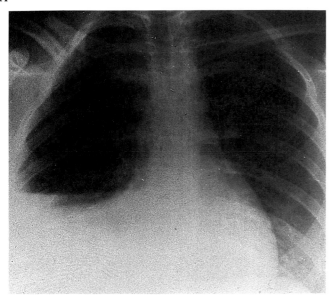

B

Fig. 14.22 A Haemopneumothorax in right chest, difficult to see because radiograph has been taken with patient supine. **B** Same patient, radiograph taken with patient erect showing fluid level between blood and air.

(discussed below), neither of which may be unequivocally diagnosed from a supine film taken at a short tube-to-chest distance (Fig. 14.22).

Pulmonary contusion and alveolar haemorrhage. This may result from a severe blunt injury to the chest. Sometimes the patient will cough up frothy blood-stained sputum. The blood-oxygen level may fall and the carbon dioxide level rise. The diagnosis is confirmed with a chest radiograph. The condition is particularly important when combined with long bone fractures and severe blood loss, when there is a danger of progressing to the adult respiratory distress syndrome (ARDS). The patient will require ventilation and admission to the intensive care unit.

Haemothorax. This often occurs in association with a pneumothorax and may have already been diagnosed following insertion of a chest drain. A small haemothorax may be left without aspiration or drainage but repeat radiographs should be taken some hours later.

Drainage of a haemothorax is best carried out using an intercostal tube and an underwater seal — and not with a needle. The fourth intercostal space in the mid-axillary line is a good site. It is not necessary for the tube to be at the lowest part of the pleural cavity. The technique of inserting a chest drain is given in Ch. 11, p. 133. If bleeding is more than 1 litre in an hour, then thoracotomy may be required and this should be discussed with a surgeon.

Wide mediastinum.   A wide mediastinum may be caused by one of the following:

1. Short tube-film distance in a supine chest radiograph.

2. Rounding of the cardiac outline ('water bottle' heart), caused by a haemopericardium. Under certain circumstances this may require emergency intervention (see below).

3. Widening of the upper mediastinum, which may indicate either bleeding from relatively small vessels or impending rupture of the aorta (Fig. 14.23). Rupture of the aorta commonly occurs just distal to the origin of the left subclavian artery and initially involves all the layers except the adventitia, which surprisingly may hold back the flood for a period which may vary from minutes to days, months or even years (by which time a false aneurysm has formed). Rupture into the pleural cavity may occur.

4. Fracture of the sternum with retrosternal haematoma. This can cause an apparently widened mediastinum. The diagnosis can be made with a lateral view.

As soon as suspicion is aroused by the appearance of the mediastinum in the radiograph (even if the patient is otherwise well and showing little or no sign of bleeding), an experienced radiologist should be contacted and the clinical problem discussed with the staff of the nearest cardiothoracic centre. The circumference of the neck should be measured — it may increase due to mediastinal bleeding (Powley's signs). The pulses and blood pressure in both arms should be checked and recorded and the patient monitored with an ECG. A decision may be made to repeat radiological examination of the chest in two hours. If a CT scan or an aortogram is required, this will necessitate transfer to a special investigation unit, often at some distance from the A & E department. A variable-height trolley equipped with suction, oxygen and, if necessary, a small ventilator mounted on a rail on the trolley, minimizes the risk to the patient.

Rupture of the diaphragm (Fig. 14.24)

This injury often accompanies severe trauma to the pelvis, to the femur or to the liver and spleen. Clinical signs in the chest are usually minimal or absent. Making a diagnosis at an early stage depends on maintaining a high degree of suspicion, taking good radiographs and carefully scrutinizing the area of the diaphragm in the radiographs (Fig. 14.25). Screening of the diaphragmatic movements by fluoroscopy may be helpful and also CT scanning.

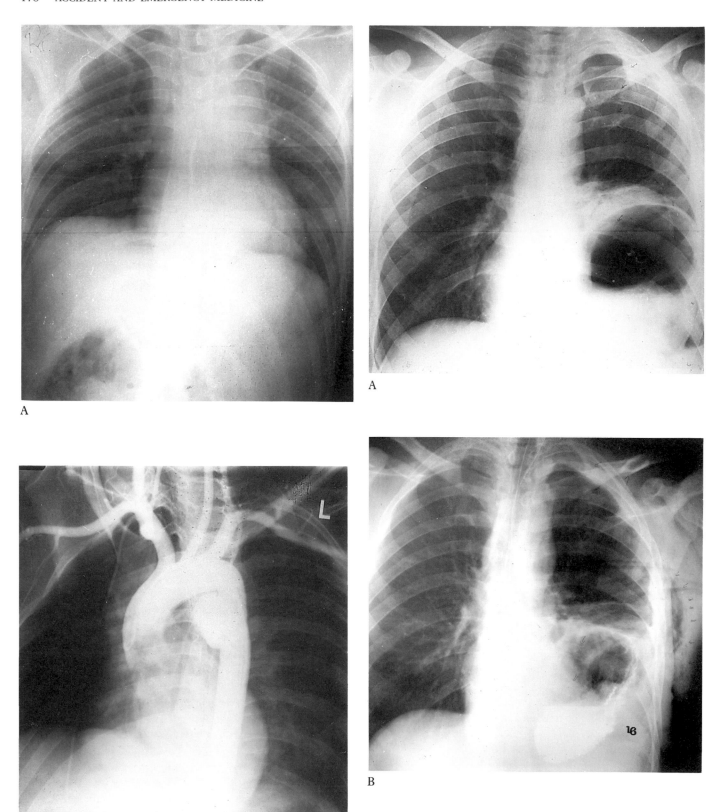

Fig. 14.23 A Wide mediastinum which was seen in repeat radiograph to be increasing in width. **B** Angiogram in same case showing rupture of arch of aorta.

Fig. 14.24 A Rupture of diaphragm. **B** Same patient. Position of stomach outlined with contrast medium. Note also fractures of posterior ends of third to seventh left ribs, and surgical emphysema on lateral aspect of left chest wall.

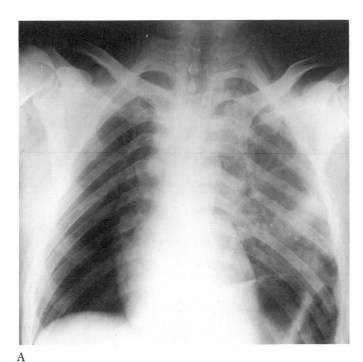

A

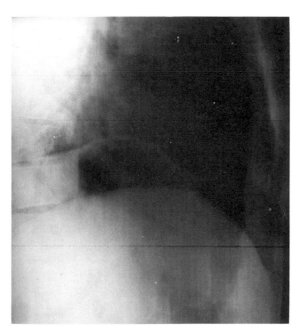

B

Fig. 14.25 A Suspected left diaphragmatic rupture. **B** Confirmed with lateral shoot-through film outlining stomach above diaphragm with fluid level in stomach. The anterior chest wall is seen at the top of the picture.

Later management of closed chest injuries in the observation ward

As with all injured patients, repeated clinical and, in this case, radiological examination are necessary in order to detect delayed development of a haemo- or pneumothorax or parenchymal lung damage.

For those patients in the observation ward who have difficulty in coughing, repeated small intramuscular doses of an analgesic

should be timed to precede the visit of the physiotherapist. A mixture of equal volumes of nitrous oxide and oxygen (Entonox) may also be of value; in some patients intercostal nerve block or epidural analgesia may also be considered. A sputum sample should be cultured and the result used as a guide to the appropriate antibiotic.

The blood gases and the haemoglobin should be estimated daily or more often because functional damage to the lung may not be at its maximum for one, two or three days following the injury, and continued blood loss may only be recognised from a falling haemoglobin.

Open injuries

Impaling injuries

If the patient has been removed from the impaling object, the immediate management will be to close the resulting sucking wound by means of a large airtight dressing and to insert a chest drain.

If the impaling object is still present in the patient on his arrival at hospital, it is best left in situ until he is in theatre and everything is prepared for a thoracotomy. An intercostal drain should be inserted immediately, even before X-rays are taken.

Stab wounds

The patient's front and back must be examined carefully for wounds, which may vary in size from that due to a broad-bladed knife to a minute puncture wound caused by a hairpin. The direction taken by the piercing implement may be guessed from the description of the assault (including the nature and size of the weapon) and from the appearance of the edges of the wound itself (size, obliquity and undermining of its edge). This should be recorded for medicolegal or forensic purposes before the entry wound itself is excised. The site and direction of the wound or wounds will lead to suspicion concerning which organs above or below the diaphragm may have been injured. A blood transfusion may be required, a haemopneumothorax may need draining or, more urgently, cardiac tamponade may need evacuation.

Cardiac tamponade

Cardiac tamponade results from bleeding within the fibrous non-distensible pericardial sac. It may come from an injured coronary vessel, from a puncture of one of the ventricles (usually the left) or, less often, from one of the atria. Clinically, the patient prefers to sit upright, is short of breath and becomes increasingly cyanosed and restless. The jugular veins become distended and (if this is being measured) the central venous pressure rises. The pulse pressure is narrowed and the cardiac impulse cannot be felt. The heart sounds are difficult to hear. Time should not be wasted with radiography. The theatre and the appropriate surgeons should be notified at once, whilst a no. 14 needle is inserted as high as possible between the xiphisternum and the left costal margin (Fig. 14.26). The needle is angled at 45° to the mid-plane and 45° to

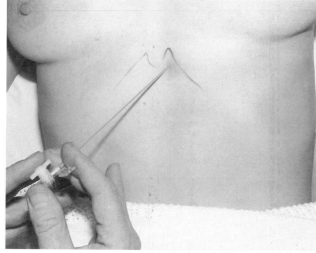

A

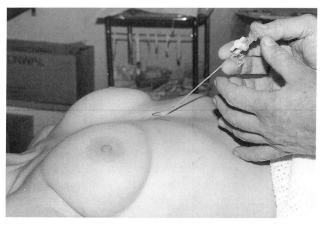

B

Fig. 14.26 Position of canula in tapping cardiac tamponade, **A** seen from the front, **B** seen from the side.

the plane of the anterior abdominal wall. The resistance of the diaphragm can usually be felt. If suction is maintained on the plunger, as the needle is felt to pass into the pericardium blood will be aspirated. If there is no blood in the pericardium, a small amount of straw-coloured fluid may be withdrawn. If the needle has passed into the left ventricle, it will pulsate and electrical aids using an EGC electrode should not be necessary. This manoeuvre may allow sufficient time for transfer to the operating theatre — but it if is unsuccessful the chest and pericardium should be opened through the fifth left intercostal space and a finger placed in the hole in the ventricle until the thoracotomy pack is opened and the surgical team arrives.

Bullet wounds of the chest

These are dealt with on p. 191.

ABDOMINAL INJURIES

Wounds

All gunshot wounds and most other penetrating wounds require surgical exploration. The patient may be very ill and require urgent resuscitation, but decisions about admission and operation rarely present difficulties in the accident and emergency department.

As with other trunk wounds, one should think upwards and downwards. Is an abdominal wound also affecting the chest, or a chest wound also affecting the abdomen? Is a wound of the buttock, the thigh or the perineum running through to the abdomen? Evisceration may occur through a fairly small wound such as that caused by goring by the horn of an animal. A weak operation wound may burst days or years after the operation. In both these types the prognosis is relatively good. Evisceration following severe road traffic accidents or bomb blasts is likely to be part of a fatal injury.

Radiological examination

Many abdominal wounds can be treated satisfactorily without abdominal radiographs. Radiographs are of most help when damage to the renal tract is suspected, when intravenous urography (i.v.u.) is essential. With a gunshot wound and a single entry wound, it is helpful to find the location of the bullet before laparotomy. It may be in the abdomen, chest or a limb. Two wounds may be due to a single through-and-through shot or to injury from the bullets which have remained in the patient's body.

Treatment in the A & E department

The wounds should be covered with sterile dressings and an intramuscular injection of a broad-spectrum antibiotic given. Pain may require relief using a small dose of narcotic intravenously.

Blunt injuries

Blunt injuries are among the most difficult to diagnose accurately of any injury in the body. It is quite possible that the only abnormal physical sign may be tenderness of the abdominal wall. Such tenderness may also be due to bruising of the abdominal wall alone. If the patient raises his feet off the trolley, thereby tensing the abdominal wall, and this abolishes any tenderness, then it is likely that the source is intra-abdominal. Continuing tendernesss while the abdominal muscles are tensed, though consistent with bruising of the abdominal wall, does not rule out intra-abdominal injury.

Assessing the state of the abdomen at this stage is particularly difficult because of the phenomenon of pain insensibility immediately after a major accident. Even patients with very severe injuries may, for a while, feel little or no pain.

It is true that if one waits and repeatedly examines the patient, eventually signs will manifest themselves. But the aim of the accident and emergency specialist must be to diagnose as high a proportion of injuries as possible during the first hour after the patient's arrival; this will lead to earlier operative care and a better prognosis.

By careful examination, by carrying out the most appropriate radiological investigations, by examining a sample of urine for blood and by the judicious use of peritoneal lavage, the majority of patients who require a laparotomy should be identified.

Clinical examination

Any bruising or swelling should be noted and, in particular, the presence sought of a clear clothes imprint on the skin of the abdominal wall (Fig. 14.27). Pressure hard enough to cause such an imprint is sufficiently severe to rupture any viscera lying between the object which applied the pressure and the bodies of the lumbar vertebrae.

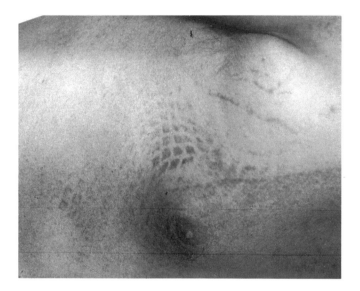

Fig. 14.27 Clothes imprint seen on chest wall. When seen on abdomen is suggestive of damage to internal organs.

On palpation, if there is any tenderness, every effort should be made to locate it as accurately as possible. Pain may be referred (e.g. pain in the shoulder tip suggests that the diaphragm is being irritated by blood or gut contents). But tenderness locates damaged tissue and, where it is present, indicates the precise point of injury.

The degree of cardiovascular collapse gives some indication of the severity of the injury, though this effect may be confused by major injuries in other parts of the body. The most spectacular haemorrhages occur from injuries to the aorta, inferior vena cava or their main branches, or from rupture of the liver or spleen. Urgent laparotomy is required if any of these injuries is suspected.

Radiological examination

These patients should have radiographs taken of their chest, abdomen and pelvis even if the clinical signs only suggest an injury in one of these areas. It is not unusual to find major chest and pelvic injuries where clinical examination had raised no suspicion of their presence.

Fractures of the lower right ribs should raise suspicion of liver damage, and of the lower left ribs of splenic injury. Following kidney injuries, there may be scoliosis with concavity towards the injured kidney. Fractures of the vertebral pedicles and transverse processes may accompany injuries to the duodenum or kidney. Retroperitoneal tears may be manifested by gas in the perinephric tissues, which may track down the psoas sheath (Fig. 14.28). Free gas in the peritoneal cavity may be seen on a lateral shoot-through film, lateral decubitus or below the diaphragm if the patient is fit to sit up. The lateral decubitus position is preferably right side up; where possible, the patient should be positioned in this way for 15 minutes before taking the film. Using this technique, very small amounts of gas may become apparent. Obliteration of the psoas shadows may indicate retroperitoneal haemorrhage in that area.

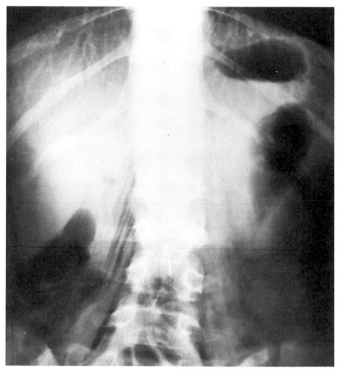

Fig. 14.28 Retroperitoneal gas in right psoas region due to retroperitoneal rupture of duodenum.

Indication for special radiological procedures. Suspicion of a duodenal injury may be raised following a road traffic accident where the seat-belt seems to have bruised the upper abdomen, especially if there is also a fracture of the pedicles of a lumbar vertebra or gas near the right crus of the diaphragm. In such cases a study of the upper gastrointestinal tract using sodium and meglumine diatrizoates (Gastrografin) is indicated. This occasionally reveals the site of the tear. It is worth taking a delayed film after an hour when an obvious leak is not seen on the first film. A 'picket fence' appearance of the duodenal mucosa and/or an intramural filling defect may indicate the presence of an intramural haematoma of the duodenum.

An intravenous urogram (i.v.u.) is indicated if there is blood in the urine accompanied either by obvious tenderness and swelling in the renal area, or by signs in the straight X-ray film of injury

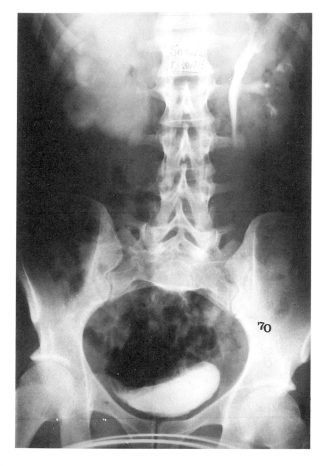

A

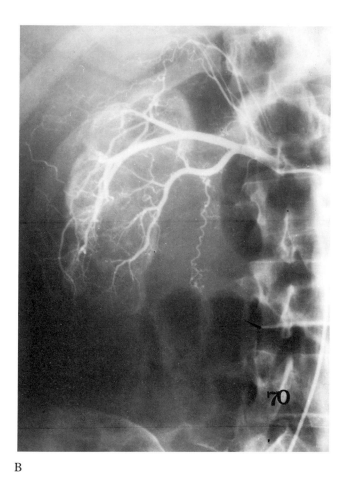

B

Fig. 14.29 I.v.u. in patient with trauma to right loin and haematuria. Obstruction at right pelviureteral junction with marked back pressure changes are due to pathology present prior to trauma. Scoliosis and absence of right psoas shadow suggest rupture of right kidney. **B** Angiogram in same patient. Splaying of vessels from old back pressure changes. Defect in cortex on lateral border of kidney suggests rupture at this point, which was confirmed at operation.

near the kidney area (Fig. 14.29). For intravenous urography in a severely injured patient, 100 ml of 45% sodium diatrizoate should be used routinely. Tomograms may reveal abnormalities that cannot otherwise be seen, such as splitting of the renal substance and even shattering of the kidney. One looks for spilling of contrast medium outside the normal renal limits, or an area of kidney where there is no excretion. (If there is no excretion, or impaired excretion, an arteriogram should be carried out.) In the urogram the ureters should be carefully inspected and delayed films taken, if necessary, up to 24 hours. This may reveal tearing of a ureter, or deviation or compression by retroperitoneal haematoma. CT scanning shows retroperitoneal bleeding well and may be helpful in many intra-abdominal injuries. Ultrasound is good for displaying injuries to liver and spleen.

Blood tests

In addition to those tests carried out on all seriously injured patients (see p. 161), the serum amylase should be measured in suspected injuries of the pancreas.

Peritoneal lavage

This procedure is a reliable test of an intraperitoneal injury. False positive and false negative results are rare. It is of particular value in those patients who are unconscious or paralysed.

Technique.   Catheterise the bladder, and test the urine for blood. The skin is infiltrated with local anaesthesia just below the umbilicus. Through a midline incision 1–2 cm long, a dialysis catheter is introduced into the abdominal cavity. If blood appears, no more need to be done. Otherwise, 1 litre of normal saline is run into the abdomen. The patient may be gently rolled onto one side and then the other. Two or three minutes after running the fluid in, it is siphoned back out. Where the returning fluid is red and bloody, a strongly positive result is immediately obvious. Where there is only a small amount of blood, the fluid will appear somewhat opaque. A rough test is to try to read newsprint through the fluid. If this is not legible the test is positive, indicating sufficient haemorrhage to require laparotomy. The fluid can be analysed more scientifically in the laboratory. A red cell count greater than 1 000 000/mm^3 or a white cell count over 500/mm^3 is abnormal.

Where CT scanning is available, it may prove an acceptable alternative to peritoneal lavage in the diagnosis of intraperitoneal haemorrhage.

Disposal.   When a suspected injury to the abdomen is but one of a number of other injuries, admission will usually be indicated for the treatment of these other injuries. However, where there is no injury elsewhere and the clinical examination, radiographs and other investigations are all negative, admission is still advisable if there is the slightest doubt about a possible intra-abdominal injury. The following points may help to decide in favour of admission.

> 1. A history of severe impact (such as a fall from 2.5 m or more, a head-on collision at 30 m.p.h., or a blow under the left costal margin from, for example, a cricket ball, which may rupture the spleen).
> 2. Pressure marks on the skin of the abdomen (particularly from a safety-belt).
> 3. Vomiting, persistent pain in the abdomen (sometimes referred to the shoulder) or haematuria all merit further hospital observation. The pulse and blood pressure should be measured and recorded frequently, a drip inserted with a large bore cannula and blood should be cross matched.
> 4. Any constant localised tenderness or any instability of the pulse or blood pressure will also merit admission. These findings imply the need for at least two or more examinations separated by an hour.

Thus the slightest suspicion of injury to the abdomen, loin, or lower chest should at least be followed by a period of observation, since it is well recognised that blood in the peritoneum may initially cause very little reaction, and insidious bleeding from the spleen or liver may pass unnoticed by the patient or doctor until sudden circulatory collapse occurs some hours later. If this should happen at home, where the patient may be unattended, the outcome can be fatal.

PELVIC INJURIES

Wounds

The problems raised by most pelvic and perineal wounds are very similar to those of abdominal wounds. In men, wounds of the penis and scrotum will be obvious, and they will usually require admission for operative repair. Women and girls who fall on stakes or spikes may sustain vaginal wounds. Such wounds may also result from coitus, particularly rape. A gynaecologist should be consulted in these cases. Often the examination should be performed under anaesthesia, enabling the surgeon to proceed to immediate operation where necessary.

Radiographic examination may reveal free gas in the abdomen or a foreign body.

Patients with perforating wounds through the anus require immediate admission for operation.

Closed injuries of the pelvis

These are closely related to closed injuries in the abdomen. Pelvic injuries are frequently associated with fractures. In addition, there may be injuries to the pelvic arteries and veins, and blood loss of 3–5 litres is common.

The organs most often damaged in closed pelvic injuries are the bladder, either intra- or extraperitoneally, and the urethra. Intraperitoneal rupture usually only occurs if the bladder is full at the time of injury. A car accident or assault after a heavy night's drinking is a common cause. Extraperitoneal injury is usually associated with fractures of the pelvic bones, as is rupture of the membranous urethra in the male.

Examination

Bladder injuries are associated with suprapubic tenderness. There may also be tenderness in the pouch of Douglas. Rupture of the urethra often causes a drop of blood to appear at the urethral meatus. This should be carefully looked for. Digital examination per rectum may reveal that the prostate is displaced or impalpable.

Although oedema of the lower abdominal wall may be caused by extravasation of urine, this sign is not often present when the patient arrives in hospital.

Radiological examination

Radiographs of the pelvis should be obtained in all patients with major injuries involving the trunk, and also in all unconscious patients who have evidence of injuries above and below the abdomen (e.g. to the chest and legs). Where a fractured neck of femur is suspected but not found, the pelvic rami should be carefully scrutinised. Pain from a fracture of a pubic ramus may be referred along the sensory distribution of the obturator nerve (i.e. to the inner side of the thigh). The sacroiliac joints must be closely scrutinised in order to assess the degree to which the pelvis has been 'opened up'. It is the posterior damage which causes severe haemorrhage. In doubtful cases CT scanning is helpful.

When a clinical examination raises the suspicion of a urethral rupture, an ascending urethrogram should be performed using 30 ml of 25% sodium diatrizoate. No attempt should be made to pass a catheter. If the bladder is filling up and needs to be drained, this should be done by a suprapubic cystostomy.

A cystogram may be performed by instilling 300–400 ml of sodium diatrizoate into the bladder (Fig. 14.30). This may be done through a urethral or suprapubic catheter. Compression or deformity of the bladder outline may indicate an unsuspected pelvic haematoma, in addition to other intrinsic bladder injuries.

Disposal

An undisplaced fracture of a pubic ramus in an otherwise healthy

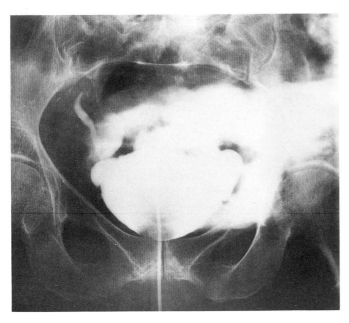

Fig. 14.30 Cystogram showing ruptured bladder.

and uninjured patient does not necessarily warrant admission. If there is displacement, if the acetabulum (one or both sides) is involved, or if there are other associated injuries admission to hospital will be necessary. Unsuspected severe disruption of the pelvis in an unconscious patient may be the cause of death due to uncontrollable extraperitoneal bleeding. A G-suit (shock pants) may be helpful to control haemorrhage in these patients.

LIMB INJURIES

We are considering in this section only the immediate care of patients with major limb injuries, which may or may not be associated with injuries to the trunk and head. Less severe limb injuries are described in Chapter 35.

Immediate management

The presence of multiple injuries may affect the immediate management of injured limbs in one of two ways.

1. If the patient's airway is at risk or if, in the absence of an obvious external source of bleeding, the patient is clearly hypovolaemic, the definitive management of the limb injuries must be postponed until the patient's general condition has been stabilised.

2. On the other hand, if the patient has adequate cardiorespiratory function, but is nevertheless restless and confused (e.g. from an associated head injury), or if there is exsanguinating bleeding from one or more of the limbs, detailed examination of the rest of the patient may have to take second place to:

    a. arrest of the bleeding,
    b. urgent transfusion and
    c. temporary splinting of the limbs

in order that further damage to the muscles, arteries and nerves may be prevented. In some cases a small intravenous dose of an analgesic combined with the administration of 50% nitrous oxide/50% oxygen (Entonox) may be appropriate before transfer from the ambulance stretcher trolley to the hospital trolley.

Arrest of bleeding can usually be achieved by direct pressure with sterile pads soaked in povidone-iodine, firm bandaging and elevation of the limb. Copious arterial bleeding is rare and is best dealt with by proximal application of an automatically inflatable (Kidde's) tourniquet. The time of application of the tourniquet must be recorded and the tourniquet must not be left inflated for more than one hour. Avulsion of a limb is often surprisingly bloodless.

In all long bone fractures, steady traction in the long axis of the limb will reduce movement at the fracture site, and thus relieve pain. This in turn will allow the application of dressings, bandages and splints. The question of splintage is dealt with in Ch. 38.

The initial rapid assessment of the patient may now be supplemented by a more thorough and complete examination. At this stage the patient may require further small doses of intravenous analgesia or Entonox.

A careful assessment of the peripheral circulation and peripheral nerves must be carried out (see below). 'Glove and stocking' anaesthesia is much more likely to represent vascular impairment than is nerve root or peripheral nerve damage — even in the presence of a relatively normal-looking skin circulation. Comparison of skin temperatures in the two limbs may be helpful. Instruments for measuring arterial pulsation or flow can be dangerously misleading. The presence of a wound or a fracture at a site adjacent to a major vessel (see below), together with diminished peripheral sensation or muscle power and pallor of the skin, should be sufficient to make a provisional diagnosis of an arterial injury. The surgeon who will be responsible for dealing with this should be contacted forthwith, since delay in restoring the circulation may result in loss or permanent disability of the affected limb. The decision as to whether or not arteriography is indicated before exploration of the wound will rest with the surgeon. Any necessary radiographs should be taken at this stage.

Less urgent management

In describing the immediate management, some diagnostic assumptions have been made, but many fractures will be clinically obvious and will not require radiographs for their diagnosis at this early stage. Indeed, careful examination (e.g. by pressure above and below a fulcrum applied to the injured segment of a limb) may clearly indicate the integrity or otherwise of a long bone. However, even a careful examination of hip, knee, ankle, shoulder or elbow may not be sufficient to distinguish dislocations or ligamentous injuries from fractures. High quality radiographs will be easier to obtain if they are taken when the patient's general condition has been stabilised.

Special circumstances

Vascular injuries (Fig. 14.31)

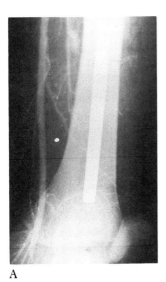
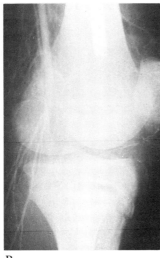

A   B

Fig. 14.31 Angiogram in patient with fracture of femur and through tibial epiphyseal plate. Femoral fracture has been pinned. **A** Shows that vascular injury is not at level of femoral fracture. **B** Shows vascular injury opposite epiphyseal plate of tibia.

The diagnosis of a vascular injury has already been discussed in general terms. The injuries commonly associated with arterial damage are listed below.

1. Severely displaced fractures of the clavicle or a posterior dislocation of the sternoclavicular joint involving the subclavian or innominate arteries.
2. A fracture dislocation of the humeral head involving the axillary artery.
3. A supracondylar fracture of the humerus in children, involving the brachial artery.
4. A fracture of the lower third of the femur, supracondylar fracture or disruption of the knee joint involving the femoral artery.
5. Dislocation of the knee with damage to the popliteal artery.
6. Injury to the upper tibial epiphysis in children or to the upper tibia in adults, injuring the bifurcation of the popliteal artery or posterior tibial vessels.

Peripheral nerve injury

Nerve injury is uncommon and, not surprisingly therefore, is often missed because the symptoms are masked by the pain of the associated soft tissue or bony injuries. The following are some examples.

1. Injury to the top of the shoulder, accompanied by forced lateral flexion of the head in the opposite direction, may result in a brachial plexus injury — commonly to the upper or lower trunk, rarely to the whole plexus. There may be associated fractures of the first or second ribs. Incomplete lesions usually recover without active treatment. The more severe lesions, however, may require special investigations, including myelography (and early repair). Such patients should be referred early to an orthopaedic surgeon or neurosurgeon.

2. Circumflex and radial nerve damage are well-known complications of fracture dislocations of the shoulder and of fracture of the shaft of the humerus respectively. It is important that these nerve lesions should be diagnosed early — both because special treatment may be required and because their detection before treatment (by reduction of the fracture or dislocation) must be recorded for medicolegal purposes. These patients should, therefore, be carefully examined both before and after treatment and the results of both examinations recorded in the notes.

3. Acute median nerve symptoms are fortunately rare, even after a severely displaced Colles' fracture. But about one-half of patients who have sustained one of the varieties of perilunar or lunate dislocations present with median nerve paraesthesia. The lesion itself is most readily spotted in the lateral radiograph, and should be reduced without delay if permanent median nerve damage is to be avoided.

4. Posterior dislocation of the hip occurs most commonly following head-on car collisions and motor-cycle accidents, when the femur is driven backwards out of the acetabulum or through its fractured posterior wall, impinging on the closely subjacent sciatic nerve. This is a very painful lesion and the posture is characteristic: the hip is flexed and adducted. Early reduction is important not only to relieve the pressure on the sciatic nerve, but because the risk of avascular necrosis of the head of the femur increases the longer reduction is delayed. General anaesthesia with muscle relaxation is required and the reduction is greatly facilitated if the patient is anaesthetised on a carrying sheet or a variable height trolley which can be lowered to a convenient height for the appropriate manoeuvres.

Degloving injuries

'Degloving' implies detachment of the skin from the underlying tissues, with concomitant loss of the nerve and blood supply. This injury is usually produced by a rolling/crushing injury, such as is caused by a wheel passing over a limb. Sometimes the skin surface is torn and the 'degloving' may be obvious. Sometimes, however, the skin remains intact, but (if carefully examined) is found to be anaesthetic and pale or bruised in appearance. It is important that the death of this skin should be appreciated early, so that appropriate surgical treatment can be carried out (usually by a plastic surgeon).

Traumatic amputation

This may be by avulsion or by a sharp instrument — and may be anywhere from the proximal to the distal part of the limb. Reattachment of a proximal amputation of the leg is seldom likely to result in more useful function than a good prosthesis. However, reattachment of an arm or a hand is worthwhile if the operation can be carried out by a skilled team within six hours of the amputation and provided there has not been serious injury to the distal part of the limb or severe crushing close to the site of amputation.

At the site of the accident, the limb should be surrounded by ice if available and wrapped in a clean plastic sheet until its arrival in hospital. The surgical team should have been warned of the patient's arrival. They may elect to perfuse the vessels of the detached limb. However, no harm will result from failure to irrigate the limb, provided the operation can be arranged speedily, and the limb is kept clean and cool in the interim. Radiographs should be taken of the injured limb and the severed part. Meanwhile, the patient will often need to be transfused and have more blood cross-matched. He should be given tetanus toxoid and a broad spectrum antibiotic and be prepared for what will probably be a long operation.

Amputated thumbs or fingers may sometimes be dealt with similarly when a suitably skilled surgeon and an operating microscope are available.

BURNS

This section deals with the management of major burns in the A & E Department. (The care of other thermal injuries is described in Ch. 36.) The role of the accident department is to receive and assess patients with serious burns and to prepare them for transport to the burns centre. A burn should be considered 'major' if there is involvement of one of the following:

1. More than 25% body surface area in an adult
2. More than 10% body surface area in a child
3. More than 5% body surface area in an infant
4. Burns to face, head, neck or perineum
5. Circumferential burns
6. Thermal or smoke injury to the respiratory tract.

The following scheme should be adopted on reception of the serious burn injury.

Priorities

1. The first medical priority is control of the airway and breathing. The patient should be given 100% oxygen by mask. If there are any signs of respiratory distress proceed immediately as indicated in 2–5 below.
2. Remove all clothing. Remember that chemical burning due to mineral acids and caustic sodas may still be continuing. Decontamination should be effected by copious lavage with water.
3. A rapid assessment of the extent of burning may be made employing Wallace's Rule of Nine (Fig. 14.32). One side of the *patient's* hand covers 1% of the body surface area at all ages.
4. Assess the circulatory state (pulse, BP, capillary filling) and the conscious level (Glasgow Coma Scale).
5. Briefly check for evidence of other trauma or underlying medical condition.

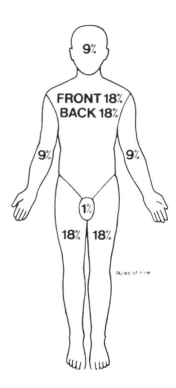

Fig. 14.32 Wallace's Rule of Nine for calculating extent of burn.

Ensure that the airway is clear and that the breathing is adequate

Fires are responsible for more deaths from asphyxia than from the effect of burning. Poisoning from carbon monoxide (see Ch. 28) or other respiratory irritant may complicate the burning. This should be anticipated and carboxyhaemoglobin measured. Where this is suspected 100% oxygen should be given.

Upper airway obstruction

With deep burns to the face and neck oedema invariably develops, though it may not be evident at the time of admission. Direct thermal injury to the upper airway may be caused by the inhalation of flame, hot gases or steam or may follow the aspiration of hot liquids during scalding of the face.

In such cases there is a real risk of laryngeal oedema and the airway should be protected before the onset of sudden, complete upper airway obstruction leading to respiratory and cardiac arrest.

The warning signs are:

1. Soot on the nose and mouth
2. Singeing of nasal hairs
3. Erythema, or even burning of the tongue and oropharynx (Fig. 14.33).

If hoarseness of the voice or stridor develops endotracheal intubation should be performed without delay. Endotracheal intubation should be carried out by the most senior anaesthetist available as often the procedure is tricky and hazardous.

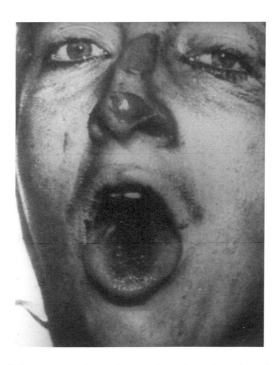

Fig. 14.33 Burn on nose, lips and tongue. In such a patient, airway is in danger.

Pulmonary damage

Smoke inhalation injury is being increasingly recognised as a major problem leading to deaths following burning. Burning polyvinyl chloride products liberate phosgene and a dense vapour of hydrochloric acid which can produce a severe corrosive burn injury of the lungs. From burning acrylic fabrics comes ammonia whilst blazing modern wall coverings release acetaldehyde, paraldehyde, acetic acid and the oxides of nitrogen. The smoke from burning polyurethane foam — found in many varieties of domestic furniture — contains compounds of cyanide, a lethal agent in its own right. Smoke inhalation without upper airway damage will rarely require treatment in the A & E department other than the administration of high concentrations of humified oxygen. Rarely bronchospasm will be present and this can be relieved by the administration of nebulised salbutamol. The pulmonary damage that occurs as a result of smoke inhalation may not develop for several hours and the decision to ventilate will rarely need to be made in the A & E department. The use of high-dose corticosteroids as prophylaxis against smoke inhalation pneumonitis is controversial and recent evidence does not appear to support their use.

Embarrassment of ventilation

Areas of full thickness burns circumferentially surrounding the chest may restrict the movement of the chest wall and hinder ventilation. Relief may be obtained by the performance of the operation of grid-iron escharotomy employing longitudinal incisions through and along the full length of the burned skin. Accident officers should caution against a hasty desire to perform this procedure, however, for quite substantial haemorrhage may occur

from the incision and this is often difficult to control. As the tourniquet effect upon the chest takes some time to develop — at least an hour — then perhaps escharotomies should be left to the plastic surgical experts who are in a better position to apply skin grafts to the defects as required.

Ascertain details of the accident

Question the ambulancemen about the *time* and nature of the accident. Remember that the plan of fluid replacement is based on the time the accident occurred and NOT the time of admission.

Provide analgesia

In theory full thickness burns should be painless as the sensory nerve ending will have been divided. Nevertheless analgesia is necessary to allay the fear, anxiety and discomfort which a major burn produces and to relieve much of the restlessness interfering with treatment. The patient may be using the inhalational analgesic Entonox offered by the ambulance attendants. The use of this agent should be encouraged until other, stronger, analgesia can be provided. One analgesic for burned patients is *morphine sulphate*, 0.1–0.2 mg/kg injected intravenously together with *chlorpromazine* 0.5 mg/kg. These agents are complementary and potentiating and may provide all the immediate analgesia necessary. Subsequent 'invasive' procedures then become all the more easy.

Set up a reliable intravenous drip

It is essential to secure an adequate route for fluid replacement before the advent of irreversible burns shock. Do not compromise with a poor drip — the patient's life depends on it. Look for a good arm vein cutting down through burned skin if necessary. Insert as large a bore cannula as possible and secure it firmly. Central lines are not recommended in cases of uncomplicated burning because of the high risk of secondary septicaemia. The femoral vein can be very useful.

The choice of fluid is according to local preference although the Mount Vernon formula (see p. 188) is based on colloid administration (usually plasma). When burns are very extensive (60% plus), very deep (e.g. electrical burns), or there has been a delay of an hour or more in fluid resuscitation then a low molecular weight colloid, e.g. dextran 40 or 'Haemaccel' may be useful as the initial fluid because its rapid renal excretion prompts a solute diuresis that may be beneficial when degraded haem pigmenta are present in the glomerular filtrate.

Take blood samples

You will need venous blood for haemoglobin and haematocrit, electrolytes and urea and blood grouping and cross-matching. An arterial specimen will be required for blood gas analysis. A venous sample should be taken in a blood gas syringe.

Catheterise the bladder

This is an important task in major burns in order that hourly analysis of the volume and composition of the urine can take place. A self-retaining catheter should be used, the tube between the catheter and drainage bag being as short as possible. The first urine sample should be tested for blood and retained for measurement of osmolality, etc.

Assess the burn

A more detailed description of the burned area can be recorded on a Lund and Browder chart (Fig. 14.34) and the total surface area of the burn calculated. Ignore simple erythema. The convention is for full thickness burns to be expressed as a cross-hatch and partial thickness burns as a single-hatch.

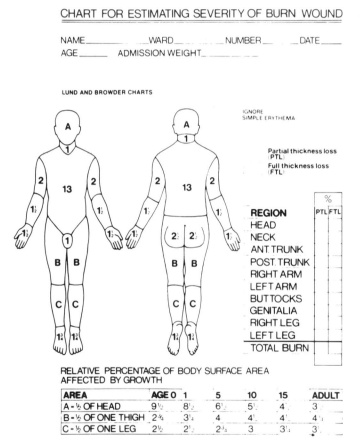

Fig. 14.34 Lund and Browder chart.

Calculate the rate of fluid replacement

The standard British practice is to resuscitate burned patients with plasma according to the Mount Vernon formula (Muir & Barclay 1974); the expected fluid replacement in ml, for the first four hours after injury is given by:

$$\frac{total\ \%\ area\ burn\ \times\ weight\ in\ kg}{2}$$

Each subsequent treatment block utilises this same volume of fluid. If plasma is not immediately to hand, a gelatin may be used. The A & E department's aim should be to deliver the patient to the burns centre suitably hydrated and neither under nor overtransfused.

Examine the patient carefully for the presence of other injuries or diseases

Some problems concomitant with burning may include epilepsy, accidental or deliberate poisoning or other forms of self harm, metabolic coma, cerebrovascular accident and alcoholic intoxication. Look for a head injury if the patient has fallen either prior to or as a result of the burning. Radiographs of the skull and chest should be considered.

Arrange transfer to the burns centre

Give the centre adequate warning. Referrals should be made doctor-to-doctor and not through an intermediary. The admission criteria vary from centre to centre and according to circumstances, although the guidelines listed at the beginning of this section are a reasonably accurate guide to criteria for acceptance. Don't put on Flamazine or a burns dressing before transfer: cover the burns with 'cling film', a polythene sheet or surgical drapes.

INJURIES FROM GUNS AND BOMBS

Gunshot wounds

The capacity of any missile to injure depends firstly on the amount of energy which it contains, and secondly on its capacity to transfer that energy to a person. This is as true of motor cars or falling bricks as of bullets.

To calculate the energy in a moving object, the following formula is applied:

Energy = ½ mass × square of the velocity

$$\left(E = \frac{mv^2}{2} \right)$$

From the formula it is clear that one may increase the energy by increasing either the mass or the velocity. Doubling the mass will double the energy. Doubling the speed will quadruple the energy and a 10-fold increase in speed will multiply the energy a 100-fold. Using this principle, modern weapons now fire bullets at very great speeds; although relatively light, these bullets carry enormous amounts of energy. By convention the speed of sound divides low from high velocity missiles. Low velocity missiles mainly consist of bullets fired from hand-guns. These bullets are short and thick, and are usually fired at close range. A rifle bullet is a typical high velocity missile. It is thinner, lighter and, because of the rifling of the gun barrel, spins on its long axis which keeps it travelling in a straight line. Its slight tendency to yaw increases as it travels — especially when it enters the tissues, which are 800 times more dense than air.

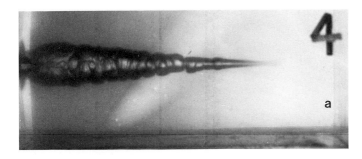

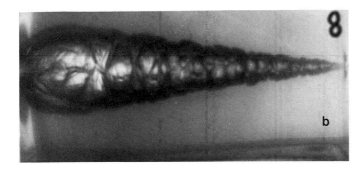

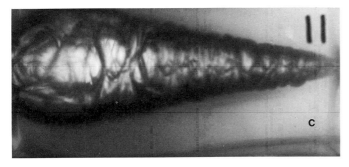

Fig. 14.35 Steel sphere 0.25 inch diameter fired through a block of gelatine: **A** at 400 metres per second, **B** at 800 metres per second, **C** at 1100 metres per second. (Crown copyright reserved).

The way that bullets injure tissues can be understood by watching the effect of firing bullets through blocks of gelatin (Fig. 14.35). Low velocity missiles cause a small cavity which quickly collapses, leaving a track roughly the size of the missile. In passing through tissues, any cavitation effect is minimal or absent. Only a small amount of tissue close to the track is destroyed. Contamination may be caused by infected material carried in by the bullet. High velocity missiles cause a relatively enormous cavity in human or animal tissues. Cavitation may be demonstrated in a gelatin block. As the cavity collapses, it sucks in contaminated particles from either end of the track through the entry and exit wounds. Shock waves travelling out from the missile damage the tissues directly. Clotting in small blood vessels following epithelial damage results in further tissue death. The combination of dead tissue and contamination produces ideal conditions for clostridial infection, with a high risk of gas gangrene.

While the behaviour of bullets passing through gelatin gives a general picture of how they injure tissues, there is obviously considerable difference between muscle, lung, brain and bone, and the nature of the injury varies depending on the precise tissue injured and its relationship to other tissues.

Gunshot wounds of the limbs

Skin, fat, fascia and muscle in limbs act more like a gelatin block than almost any other tissue. A low velocity bullet which passes deeply through a muscle mass (e.g. in the buttock, thigh, calf or shoulder) will leave a track surrounded by some dead muscle, contaminated near the entry and exit wounds with bacteria (Fig. 14.36). High velocity wounds in these regions always cause considerable destruction. With more superficial wounds and wounds through places without much muscle bulk (e.g. the first interosseous space in the hand) there is much less damage. It must be remembered that the amount of damage done is proportional to the amount of energy left in the body. Where a rifle bullet cuts neatly through a thin piece of tissue leaving it almost as rapidly as it entered, it will only have given up a very small proportion of its potential energy in the body.

Where the bullet strikes a bone, the conditions immediately alter (Fig. 14.37). The bone will probably shatter as the bullet gives up all or most of its energy. The bullet may also start to tumble, offering a far higher resistance as it passes through the remaining

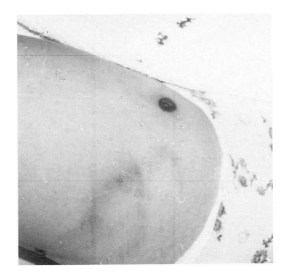

Fig. 14.36 Low velocity gunshot wound through soft tissue of thigh. Note bruising beyond track of wound.

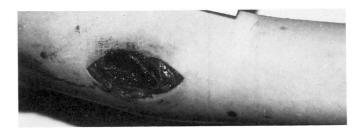

Fig. 14.37 Low velocity exit wound where bullet hit bone.

tissues. The pieces of bone may travel through the muscle as secondary missiles. A low velocity bullet hitting bone or yawing badly may give rise to a large exit wound. With high velocity bullets large exit wounds are common, especially if a bone is struck (Fig. 14.38). Yet occasionally one will see such an injury with a small exit wound.

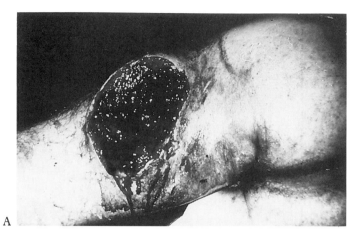

A

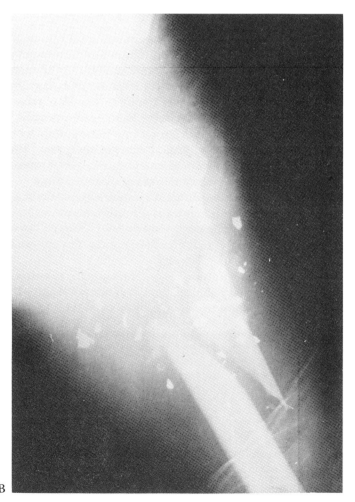

B

Fig. 14.38 A High velocity exit wound in back of thigh where bullet hit bone. **B** Radiograph of same patient showing shattered femur and fragments of bullet.

Damage may also occur to major vessels or nerves. Vessels seem more vulnerable and often if a major artery is divided its accompanying vein is also divided. A section of several centimetres may be missing. Nerves are not severed nearly so often. With low velocity missiles, they sometimes appear to slip out of the pathway of the bullet. Conduction may be interrupted without division. This is more common with the blast forces caused by high velocity wounds.

Examination

Clinical examination should reveal an entry wound and, if the shot has passed through the patient's body, an exit wound. Multiple wounds may be difficult to interpret — separate wounds may both prove to be entry wounds from one missile. Low velocity missiles often remain in the body. High velocity bullets almost always pass through the body. It is not usually difficult to diagnose accompanying fractures. One should attempt to diagnose damage to vessels and nerves, as the results of operation will be better if everyone is fully prepared for a vascular repair.

Radiological examination

This is useful to locate retained bullets, and to show the nature of any fractures. A thick short bullet indicates a low velocity missile. High velocity bullets are slimmer, longer and only rarely remain in the body. Be prepared to look for bullets which have taken unusual paths within the body and ended up in unexpected places.

Disposal

Some patients with superficial low velocity wounds can be treated as outpatients following an overnight stay in the observation ward. However, most will require admission for immediate excision and later delayed primary suture.

Treatment in the A & E department

It is usual to give broad-spectrum antibiotics to these patients; the first dose may be given while the patient is still in the A & E department.

If a patient with a gunshot wound is treated in the department, one should lay open the whole track, excise all dead tissue and dress the wound. It is quite safe to allow such a patient to go home and to perform delayed primary suture as an outpatient five days later.

Very superficial wounds can be treated by excision of the entry and exit wounds and cleaning of the track by pulling gauze through it. The two wounds are closed on the fifth or sixth day by delayed primary suture.

Gunshot wounds of the head

A bullet fired through an empty skull will make two small neat holes in it. But a high velocity bullet passing through a person's head causes the whole skull to shatter. The entry wound is small, the exit large. The disparity illustrates the way in which the brain tissue transmits the blast waves outwards from the track of the bullet. In doing so, much brain tissue is pulped. The resulting wound is a bloody affair, with torn vessels in the scalp, skull, meninges and brain. The pulped brain tissue produces oedema and a rising intracranial pressure. The torn vessels cause dramatic haemorrhage.

A low velocity missile will act in a similar way, but the blast wave is very much less (Fig. 14.39). This leads to brain damage localised much more closely to the track of the bullet. There is still a rise in intracranial tension and some bleeding, but not on such a dangerous scale.

While the general features of high and low velocity missiles have been described in clinical situations and even at autopsy, it may not be possible to distinguish one from the other (Fig. 14.40).

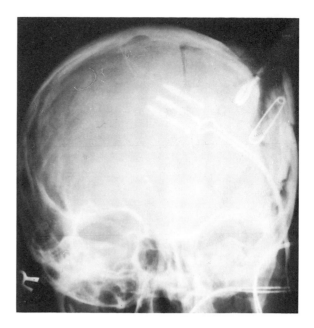

Fig. 14.40 Tangential high velocity wound to head.

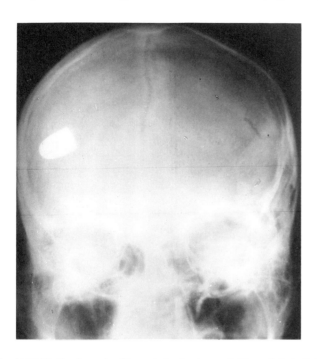

Fig. 14.39 Skull radiograph of low velocity head wound. Note relatively little skull damage and short fat bullet.

Examination and treatment

A glance will establish the presence of a gunshot wound of the head. It now becomes a matter of extreme urgency to pass an endotracheal tube and commence ventilation. Respiratory obstruction is the most likely cause of further deterioration. Lowering the carbon dioxide tension helps to prevent a rise in intracranial tension and a high oxygen tension provides the optimum conditions for brain recovery.

While preparing to pass the endotracheal tube, the reaction of the pupils to light and the patient's response to pain should be noted. If the pupils are widely dilated and there is no reaction to pain, the prognosis is virtually hopeless.

Where efforts to resuscitate are felt to be worthwhile, the means for rapid intravenous infusion should be set up — two infusion lines with no. 14 gauge cannulae and a central venous line. The bladder should also be catheterised.

The patient should be completely undressed and a search made for other wounds and injuries.

Radiological examination

This is not absolutely essential, but if two views of the skull can be taken without more than a few minutes delay this should be done.

Disposal

A neurosurgeon should be consulted. He may decide that immediate surgery is necessary or, alternatively, that a period of mechanical hyperventilation in the intensive care unit is indicated.

Gunshot wounds of the chest (Fig. 14.41)

The chest consists of two very spongy distensile lungs separated by a central column which consists, at the front, of the mediastinal organs and vessels and, at the back, the spinal column, spinal cord and surrounding muscles. Missiles travelling through lungs alone do much less damage than through muscle, for the resistance to the shock wave is much less. Missiles travelling through the mediastinum are quite likely to cause fatal haemorrhage, though low velocity missiles do on occasion pass right across from one lung, through the mediastinum and out through the second lung (Fig. 14.42). High velocity missiles travelling through vertebrae or paravertebral muscles transmit shock waves with such efficiency that, even when the track is well away from the spinal cord, a permanent paraplegia is likely to result.

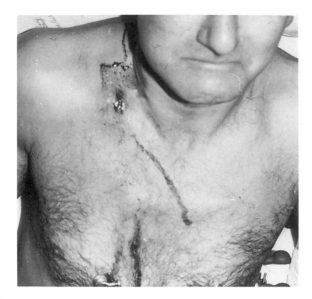

A

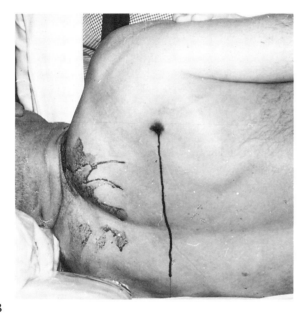

B

Fig. 14.41 A Entry gunshot wound below right clavicle. **B** Exit wound through right scapula.

Examination

The location of wounds is accurately noted. A quick examination of heart and lungs is made. A paraplegia is confirmed or excluded.

Treatment

A gunshot wound of the chest is an indication for inserting a chest drain (see p. 133). This should be done prior to radiological examination.

Radiological examination

Once the drain is in position, an anteroposterior chest radiograph

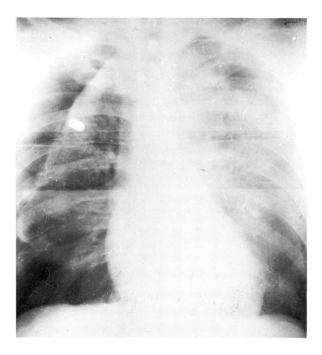

Fig. 14.42 Low velocity gunshot wound of chest. Entry through left side, passed through mediastinum without major injury. Severe contusion of left lung and haemopneumothorax in right chest.

is obtained, preferably with the patient erect. For accurate localisation of the retained missile, two views are essential: anteroposterior and lateral. The possibility of a missile entering the chest and ending up in the neck, head, abdomen or limbs should be remembered.

Disposal

All these patients must be admitted to hospital. Many will be transferred direct to the operating theatre.

Gunshot wounds of the abdomen (Fig. 14.43)

Low velocity bullets cause damage by penetrating organs. When high velocity bullets pass through solid organs they cause massive shattering of the tissues. The mortality is much greater with high velocity wounds, but all wounds, from both low and high velocity, will need surgical exploration.

Examination

This consists of noting the location of the entry and exit wounds and considering which organs might have been damaged. If the track runs near to the vertebrae, paraplegia should be confirmed or excluded.

Radiological examination

Retained missiles are located using anteroposterior and lateral views.

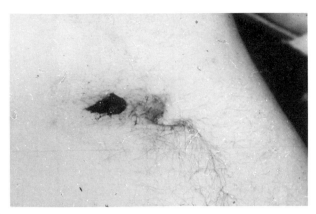

A

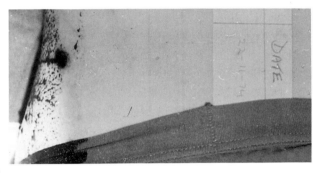

B

Fig. 14.43 Gunshot wound of abdomen. **A** Entry to right of umbilicus.
B Exit wound in posterior aspect of left flank. At operation several wounds
found in intestine.

Treatment

Dressings are placed on the wounds. A broad-spectrum antibiotic
is given and an intravenous infusion started.

Disposal

All these patients require immediate surgical exploration.

Shotgun injuries

A cartridge fired from a shotgun behaves somewhat differently from
a bullet. It consists of an outer casing containing many small
particles of lead shot. Very close to the gun they almost act as
a single mass, with considerable power to wound. Very rapidly
the particles spread out and decelerate; when fired beyond a
distance of 20–30 metres, most of them will penetrate only as deep
as the subcutaneous tissues. The criminal's sawn-off shotgun is
a lethal weapon since, at close quarters, shot can penetrate the
thorax or abdomen. From greater distances, severe damage is only
likely if a pellet strikes an eye or divides a major artery or vein.

Examination

Examination will reveal the peppering of the body with small
missiles. There may be a central region where they are more closely
gathered (Fig. 14.44).

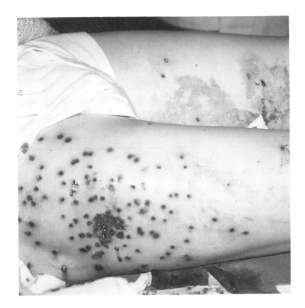

Fig. 14.44 Shotgun injury to lateral aspect of the thigh.

Radiological examination

Radiographs in two planes will help to show the depth of
penetration.

Disposal

Where the shot is in the subcutaneous tissues, the patient may
be treated either as an outpatient or in the observation ward. Where
there is injury to an eye or to deep structures, admission for
operation will be necessary.

Treatment in the A & E department

Large masses of pellets must be excised. This will usually require
admission to a surgical ward. There may be an area of non-viable
skin which must be excised at the same time. Repair with a skin
graft performed a week or so later, either as an outpatient or on
an overnight basis.

Scattered pellets do not all need to be removed. Many will do
no harm if left alone. However, some patients are very inclined
to be upset and fearful about such foreign bodies and it is
sometimes necessary to remove most of the easily accessible ones.
If there are only a few pellets, local anaesthesia is sufficient.

INJURIES CAUSED BY BOMBS

A bomb consists of an explosive substance in some form of
container, a detonator to set off the explosion and a timing device.
Some bombs are deliberately made with the intention of injuring
one victim or a small group of victims, e.g. letter bombs, booby
traps and antipersonnel bombs. When a bomb explodes, energy
is dissipated outwards from the centre of a sphere, along its radii.
If the explosion occurs in a crowded area, the possibility of many

people being wounded and arriving simultaneously at hospital for treatment is high. Management of bomb explosions therefore involves disaster drill as well as clinical management (see Ch. 7).

Bomb injuries are classified as direct and indirect. Direct injuries are caused by the bomb itself or the atmosphere. Indirect injuries are those mediated by other objects in the environment, such as broken glass or falling debris.

Direct injuries

Blast pressure waves

The explosion creates enormous volumes of gaseous products. These compress the surrounding air and a very high pressure pulse travels radially at high velocity. When this pulse strikes the body, it is transmitted through the tissues without much damage; however, when it reaches an interface between tissues and gas, it creates a tremendous disruptive force in the wall of the gas-containing viscus. Thus the middle ear, the lungs and the gas-containing portions of the gastrointestinal tract are affected in that order of susceptibility.

Blast damage to the ears may affect the drum, causing perforation, or the inner ear, causing tinnitus and sensorineural deafness. This effect is common and immediate. At the time, patients who are distressed and confused may not realise that they have gone totally deaf, nor may those who are looking after them.

The lungs may be damaged with small, multiple areas of alveolar disruption and haemorrhage, causing hypoxia. Such injuries are uncommon in survivors of home-made bombs with limited blast pressure waves. Massive lung haemorrhage and oedema are common findings in those killed by bombs.

Blast wind

The expanding gases from the explosion displace an equal volume of air and this travels radially at high speed. It is this blast wind which literally blows pieces off the body and, in extreme cases, causes disruption or total destruction.

Fragments of the bomb casing (Fig 14.45)

These are missiles just like bullets. Close to the bomb they may have the effect of high velocity missiles, but their irregularity slows them down quickly, both in the air and during passage through clothing and the patient's tissues. They are often multiple and injure tissues exactly as bullets do.

Burns

The chemical reaction of the explosion releases a lot of heat. The high temperature lasts only a short time. The result is a flash burn of exposed skin, often with burning of the eyebrows and hair.

Radioactivity

The immediate damage following nuclear explosions is from blast, wind and heat. The effects of irradiation become evident over the

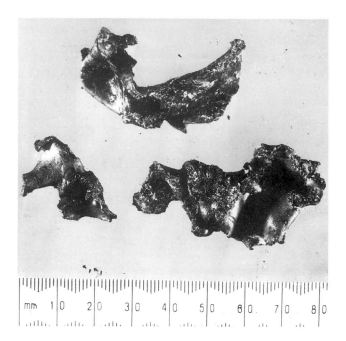

Fig. 14.45 Fragments of bomb casing which were removed at operation.

ensuing hours, days, weeks and years depending upon the dose received. Explosions at nuclear powered electricity stations such as occurred at Chernobyl seem to harm mainly through the effects of irradiation. These affects are discussed in the chapter on environmental emergencies (Ch. 28).

Fear

This is much the most common way in which a bomb injures. It causes an immediate acute distress reaction, especially in women and in those just beyond the region where physicial injuries are taking place. The badly injured are very calm whilst the physically uninjured are very distressed. Weeping, shaking and hysterical aphasia will pass off in a few hours, but may be followed by a milder anxiety state which can last for years.

Indirect effects

Multiple small foreign bodies (Fig. 14.46)

Explosions generate an immense amount of dust and grit. These may merely coat the patient, but often penetrate exposed skin and may even pass through clothing and underlying skin.

Larger foreign bodies from the environment (Fig. 14.47)

These may consist of pieces of metal or wood, stones and every conceivable and inconceivable type of object picked up from the environment by the blast. The patient may be transfixed.

Wounds from flying glass

These are very common where bombs have exploded in city streets.

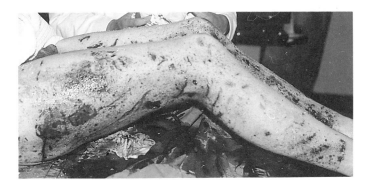

Fig. 14.46 Injuries from multiple small foreign bodies due to bomb.

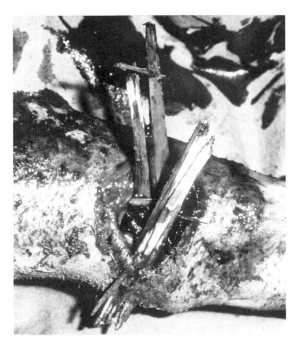

Fig. 14.47 Larger foreign bodies from environment.

The wounds are no different from any other laceration. They are most common in parts unprotected by clothes.

Fire

Burns caused by a fire following an explosion are likely to be much worse than direct flash burns. Some bombs are deliberately made with a very small amount of explosive but containing an inflammatory liquid. The burns caused are no different from other burns. The effect of smoke inhalation on the lungs should not be forgotten (see Burns, p. 187).

Collapse of building (Fig. 14.48)

This may cause major crush injuries.

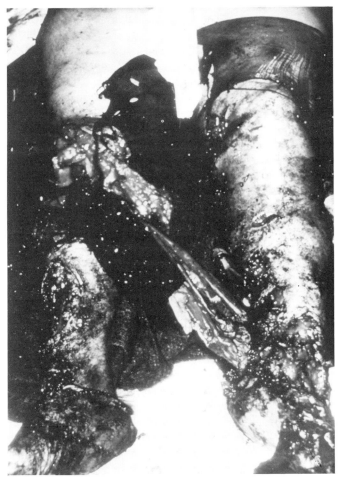

Fig. 14.48 Crush injuries from collapse of building.

Wind effects

These mainly occur with very large bombs. People may be blown against other objects (Figs 14.49, 14.50).

Examination of bomb victims

This is similar to the examination of any injured patient. Multiple injuries are common and are often difficult to describe well. It is helpful to dictate notes while observing the injuries. A photographic record may be helpful. Arrangements should be made to have the ears examined by an ENT surgeon either immediately or on the following day.

Radiological examination

Unexpected foreign bodies are common. All seriously injured patients should have the appropriate radiological examination.

Treatment

Patients with nervous shock should be taken to a large room somewhat removed from the main treatment area. Friendly

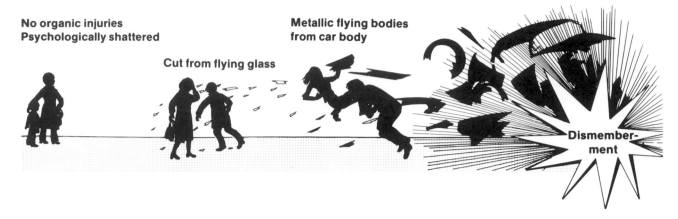

Fig. 14.49 Typical injuries from bomb exploding in street.

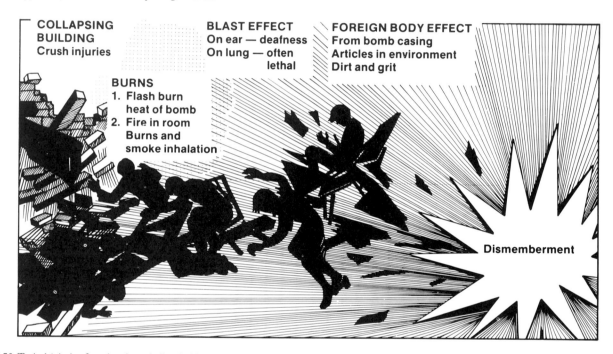

Fig. 14.50 Typical injuries from bomb exploding inside room.

volunteers should administer tea. Tranquillisers are often given, but it may well be better to assist the patient to express and discharge grief without damping the reaction down with drugs.

Patients with small wounds can have them sutured.

Some patients with grit embedded in the skin can have it scrubbed out under anaesthetic in the A & E department, but most with embedded foreign bodies require admission.

In very badly injured patients, the possibility of blast lung should be remembered. In these circumstances overtransfusion is as dangerous as undertransfusion. A CVP line and monitoring of urine output are therefore essential.

Disposal

There is not usually much difficulty in separating patients into those who are fit to go home and those who must be admitted.

REFERENCES

Mant A K 1977 Natural death while in charge of transportation. Legal Medicine (Annual) pp 111–126

Muir I F K, Barclay T I 1974 Burns and their treatment. 2nd end. Lloyd Luke, London

Reilly P L, Graham D I, Adams J et al 1975 Patients with head injury who talk and die. Lancet II: 375–377

FURTHER READING

Hospital trauma index American College of Surgeons 1980 American College of Surgeons Bulletin 2: 32

The injury severity score: a method for describing patients with multiple injuries and evaluating emergency care Baker S P, O'Neill B, Haddon W, Long W B 1974 Journal of Trauma 14: 187–196

The injury severity score: an update Baker S P, O'Neill B 1976 Journal of Trauma 16: 882–885

Evaluating trauma care: the TRISS method Boyd, Carl R, Tilson M A, Copes W A 1987 Journal of Trauma 27: 4 370–378

The injury severity score of road traffic casualties in relation to mortality, time of death, hospital treatment time and disability Bull J P 1975 Accident Analysis and Prevention 7: 249–255

Severity indices and their implications for emergency medical services research and evaluation Cayten C G, Evans W 1979 Journal of Trauma 19: 98–102

An anatomical injury scale in multiple trauma victims Champion H R, Sacco W, Ahman W, Long W B, Gill W 1975 Proceeedings 19th Conference American Association Automotive Medicine 375–382

An anatomic index of injury severity Champion H R, Sacco W J, Lepper R L, Atzinger E M et al 1980 Journal of Trauma 20: 3, 197–202

Assessment of injury severity: the triage index Champion H R, Sacco W J, Hannan D S et al 1980 Critical Care Medicine 8: 201–208

Trauma score Champion H R, Sacco W J, Carnazzo A J et al 1981 Critical Care Medicine 9: 672–676

Shock trauma/critical care manual: initial assessment and management Cowley R A, Dunham C M 1982 University Park Press, Baltimore

Gunshot wounds. Practical aspects of firearms, ballistics and forensic techniques Di Maio Vincent J M 1985 Elsevier, New York

Indices of severity for emergency medical evaluative studies: reliability, validity and data requirements Gibson G 1981 International Journal Health Services 11: 597–622

CRAMS scale: Field triage of trauma victims Gormican S P 1982 Annals of Emergency Medicine 11: 132–135

A decision theory approach to measuring severity in illness Gustafson D H, Holloway D C 1975 Health Services Research 10: 97–106

Management of head injuries Jennett B, Teasdale G 1981 Davis Philadelphia

Trauma index, an aide in the evaluatio of injury victims Kirkpatrick J R, Youmans R L 1971 Journal of Trauma 11: 711–714

APACHE II: A severity of disease classification system Knaus W A, Draper E A, Wagner D P, Zimmerman J E 1985 Critical Care Medicine 13: 818–829

Indices of severity: underlying concepts Krischer J P 1976 Health Services Research 11: 143–157

Indices of severity: conceptual development Krischer J P 1979 Health Services Research 14: 56–67

Severity measurement in multiple trauma by use of ICDA conditions Levy P S, Goldberg J, Hui S, Rothrock J et al 1982 Statistics in Medicine 1: 145–152

Clinical orthopedic examination 2nd edn. McRae R 1983 Churchill Livingstone, Edinburgh

Practical fracture treatment McRae R 1981 Churchill Livingstone, Edinburgh

Advances in trauma Maull K 1986 Year Book Medical, Chicago, Vol I

Hormone substrates inter-relationships following trauma Meguid M M, Brennan M F, Aoki T T et al 1974 Archives of Surgery 109: 776–783

Development and prospective study of an anatomical index and an acute index Mulholland A V, Cowley R A, Sacco W J 1979 American Surgeon 4: 246–254

Trauma care Odling-Smee W, Crockard A 1984 Academic Press, London

Trauma Management for Civilian and Military Physicians Wiener S L, Barrett J 1986 WB Saunders, Philadelphia

Peter G. Nelson

Other life-threatening conditions

The conditions described in this chapter are all rare (apart from tetanus in developing countries) but they must be recognised early if death is to be prevented. Each has characteristic clinical features and each requires specific therapy.

TETANUS

Tetanus is still a significant cause of death in countries without an effective immunisation programme. The classic causative wound is deep, soiled and contains necrotic tissue, but many cases are associated with trivial injuries. The illness may also arise from burns, compound fractures, septic abortions and puerperal sepsis, bowel operations, circumcision, ear-piercing, intramuscular injections, skin diseases (e.g. 'shingles') and infection of the raw umbilical stump (neonatal tetanus). The incubation period is usually one to two weeks but may range from two days to several months. In general, if it is less than 10 days the illness is likely to be severe.

Painful muscle stiffness is usually the first symptom, commonly starting in the masseters and neck extensors and later spreading to the trunk and limbs. Difficulty opening the mouth (trismus) is the classic presentation and the corollary is that any patient who can open his mouth normally is unlikely to have tetanus. Difficulty with speaking, swallowing and breathing is also common. Part of the difficulty is due to muscular rigidity and incoordination and part due to fear of inducing the painful muscular spasms which characterise fully developed tetanus. The time taken for the disease to progress from the first symptom to the establishment of spasms, known as the period of onset, provides a better prognostic guide than the incubation period. If it is less than 24 hours severe disease is likely. Occasionally patients with partial or passive immunity develop symptoms and signs in muscles close to the site of injury (local tetanus), but eventually they usually progress to generalised muscle involvement.

Tetanus is a clinical diagnosis and it is best made by observing the patient carefully, for 10–20 minutes if necessary, while causing the minimum of physical disturbance. Even the most trivial external stimulus can provoke a painful spasm, as may internal stimuli such as coughing or a full bladder. The most difficult cases to diagnose are those presenting with a little pain and stiffness in the back or very slight trismus. Then long periods of observation may be necessary. Evidence of tonic muscular rigidity and spasms are the cardinal diagnostic signs. Muscular rigidity produces trismus, alteration of the patient's normal facial expression ('risus sardonicus') and stiffness of the neck, trunks and limbs. An early sign of the rigidity of the jaw muscles can be elicited by pressing the patient's tongue with a spatula. Patients developing tetanus respond by contraction of the muscles of the face and neck and closure of the mouth. Resuscitation facilities should be ready before doing this test as it may cause a severe spasm. It is often impossible for the patient to put his chin on his chest. Sometimes excessive contraction of the long spinal extensors leads to alarming opisthotonus. The abdomen may become intermittently board-like causing the patient to lie like a ramrod. The simultaneous rigidity of agonists and antagonists, which is so characteristic of the disease, may be detected by *gently* palpating the erector spinae and abdominal muscles bimanually. The tendon reflexes are usually increased. Involvement of the bulbar muscles may cause the patient to speak with a peculiar high-pitched voice and to complain of dysphagia. The latter is of serious import as it may lead to inhalation of saliva or drinks, causing laryngeal spasm. If taking a drink of water makes the patient cough, then his airway needs protection initially by endotracheal intubation and often later by tracheostomy. Inability to swallow a mouthful of water in one gulp indicates bulbar muscle dysfunction. Shallow, jerky respirations are also common.

Reflex spasms are abrupt in onset and very painful. They may occur spontaneously, or in response to touch, noise, movement, swallowing or merely talking. These patients not unnaturally tend to be very agitated and anxious between spasms and this lowers the threshold for their recurrence. The spasms may be fleeting (e.g. a mere twitch of the limbs) or result in prolonged muscular contractions in which the patient stops breathing and becomes cyanosed. Sometimes a series occurs in rapid succession. Death from hypoxia can take place very rapidly and is not unknown during a patient's first spasm. The accelerated hypoxia is due to a combination of incoordinate activity of the respiratory muscles, laryngeal spasm and the greatly increased metabolic demands of the patient's hypertonic muscles. The duration, frequency and intensity of muscle spasms should be carefully recorded. Other clinical features include fever, which may progress to hyperpyrexia and autonomic imbalance. The latter most commonly produces a hyperadrenergic syndrome characterised by profuse sweating, tachycardia and hypertension. Excessive production of salivary and bronchial secretions can add to the patient's respiratory difficulties.

Neonatal tetanus usually occurs within two weeks of birth. The infant sucks poorly and the cry tends to be stifled. The arms and legs are held slightly flexed, the arms being partly crossed over the abdomen and the hands clenched. Often the tip of the thumb may be seen protruding between the index and middle fingers.

Management

The initial treatment of tetanus *must* be carried out in circumstances in which the patient can be instantly paralysed, intubated and mechanically ventilated, should a spasm cause respiratory arrest. A syringe containing a muscle relaxant (e.g. suxamethonium) should be kept at hand and an anaesthetist should be standing by. Emergency tracheostomy in the resuscitation area should never be necessary.

The three aims of treatment are:

> 1. To control the symptoms caused by the tetanus toxin already bound to the central nervous system.
> 2. To attempt to neutralise toxins still circulating in the blood.
> 3. To eliminate the *Clostridium tetani bacillus* itself.

The painful and very frightening symptoms of tetanus all take place in a state of clear consciousness. Therefore the first essential is sedation and pain relief. Diazepam (initially 0.15 mg/kg i.v.) plus pethidine (50–100 mg i.v.) are a useful combination. Much larger doses of diazepam may be required to relieve the muscle spasms.

Both physical and mental disturbances should be minimised and oxygen administered by mask. Loading doses of cloxacillin (500 mg) and human antitoxin (30 i.u./kg bodyweight) should be given intramuscularly. Cloxacillin is better than crystalline penicillin where the wound may contain a mixed infection. It can be combined with metronidazole. Contaminated wounds and wounds containing a lot of dead tissue should be thoroughly cleaned and debrided. Autonomic circulatory disturbances will rarely be encountered in the A & E department, as they are usually late manifestations of the disease. Labetalol, which has both α- and β-adrenergic blocking properties, is the most useful drug for these complications.

Once the primary care is complete the patient should be transferred to a respiratory intensive care unit for further management.

The prophylaxis of tetanus is discussed in Ch. 32.

Differential diagnosis

Dyskinetic states associated with phenothiazines, butyrophenones and metoclopramide may superficially resemble tetanus and are much commoner than tetanus in the British Isles. A history of recent drug exposure (the idiosyncrasy can occur after one dose), involuntary opening as well as closing of the mouth, flexing of the limbs and oculogyric crises should give the clues to the diagnosis. Dysphagia does not occur. A therapeutic trial of intravenous procyclidine (10 mg) can help if the diagnosis is in doubt.

The clinical picture following strychnine poisoning also resembles tetanus. General awareness is heightened and fierce spinal convulsions triggered. Unlike tetanus, however, muscular relaxation between the spasms is complete. In rabies there is usually a history of an animal bite and there is no trismus. Hyperventilation can induce tetany (see Ch. 31). In this condition the spasms begin in the extremities. Complex partial epileptic fits may also occasionally mimic tetanus.

Trismus alone may be caused by painful lesions near the jaw, such as dental abscesses or quinsy, and by temporomandibular dislocation, but beware of making a diagnosis of a 'sore throat' in a patient who cannot open his mouth. Encephalitis may also cause trismus but there are always other neurological abnormalities.

Finally if the clinical picture is not typical of any particular disorder the possibility of hysteria should be considered.

THYROID CRISIS OR STORM

This rare condition occurs only in thyrotoxic individuals, although in some the hyperthyroidism may have gone unrecognised. The onset is usually abrupt and is due to the liberation of large amounts of thyroid hormones into the circulation. Infections, surgical procedures and accidental trauma are the common precipitants. Occasionally it occurs during radio-iodine treatment. The physical signs are largely accentuations of those found in uncomplicated thyrotoxicosis. The individual usually has a goitre and 'eye signs'. Fever and sweating are almost invariable and the main clinical features are:

1. *Cardiovascular:* marked tachycardia (often due to atrial fibrillation), heart failure and shock.

2. *Central nervous system:* agitation, tremor, confusion, acute psychosis, and stupor progressing to convulsions and coma.

3. *Gastrointestinal:* abdominal pain, vomiting, diarrhoea, dehydration and jaundice due to hepatocellular failure.

The following is an outline of the management. Tablets can be crushed and given via a nasogastric tube if necessary.

1. Set up an intravenous line, monitor the ECG and administer 100% oxygen to combat hypoxia due to increased metabolic demands. (Blood samples for later analysis for T4 and T3 may be obtained.)

2. Start appropriate measures to counteract hyperpyrexia (see Ch. 28).

3. Give propranolol (1–5 mg intravenously or 40 mg orally) to antagonise sympathetic overactivity. Propranolol should be used with extreme caution if the patient is shocked, is in heart failure or has obstructive airways disease.

4. Give initial oral doses of propylthiouracil (150–300 mg) or carbimazole (15–30 mg) to inhibit hormonal synthesis.

5. Give intravenous hydrocortisone (500 mg) to correct the relative adrenal insufficiency and reduce conversion of T_4 to T_3.

6. Infuse 5% dextrose and B vitamin complex to correct dehydration and provide an energy source.

7. Treat heart failure and atrial fibrillation with digitalis and diuretics.

8. Give a broad-spectrum antibiotic if an infection is suspected.

9. Occasionally chlorpromazine may be required for sedation.

Oral potassium iodide (100 mg) or Lugol's iodine (20 drops), which block the release of stored thyroid hormones, should be given 2 hours after the administration of propylthiouracil or carbimazole. Earlier administration can be danagerous. This treatment will normally be the responsibility of the admitting medical team. Sodium iopodate (3 g) is possibly a safer and better alternative.

Occasionally these patients fail to improve with the conventional treatment outlined. Then plasma exchange, peritoneal dialysis or exchange transfusion can be used to reduce the amounts of circulating thyroxine. Death is usually related to severe hyperpyrexia and/or pulmonary oedema associated with cardiac dysrhythmias and shock. Differential diagnoses include severe infections, paroxysms associated with phaeochromocytomas and acute manias. The absence of a goitre and exophthalmos in these conditions should point the way to the correct diagnosis.

MYASTHENIC AND CHOLINERGIC CRISES

It is important to distinguish between these two conditions, both characterised by an increase in weakness particularly affecting the respiratory and bulbar muscles, as inappropriate treatment may cause worsening of symptoms. A myasthenic crisis may occur spontaneously or in response to physical or emotional stress and

certain drugs (e.g. aminoglycoside and polypeptide antibiotics, procainamide, quinidine and quinine). Warning of a cholinergic crisis is often given by parasympathomimetic side effects (miosis, salivation, abdominal colic and bradycardia) indicating that anticholinesterase drug overdose is being approached. Intravenous edrophonium (2 mg) may help differentiate between the two conditions. Following injection, strength is transiently increased in a myasthenic crisis, in contrast to an increase of weakness in a cholinergic crisis, which is often associated with an exacerbation of parasympathomimetic effects. Acute respiratory difficulties may necessitate endotracheal intubation and artificial ventilation in either case. A myasthenic crisis is treated by an appropriate increase in anticholinesterase medication (neostigmine or pyridostigmine). Occasionally a resistant crisis may only be conquered by withdrawal of drugs for a few days, during which artificial ventilation is required, followed by their gradual reintroduction. In a cholinergic crisis anticholinesterase drugs are withdrawn and atropine (2 mg) given intravenously. This dose should be repeated until the patient is fully atropinised. Intravenous pralidoxime (50–100 mg) may occasionally be required, but should only be used under the direction of a poison's expert.

In either case the advice of a neurologist should be sought as early as possible. If necessary the patient can be mechanically ventilated until such advice is obtained.

ACUTE PORPHYRIA

Alarming attacks of acute porphyria are most common, as the name suggests, in the acute intermittent type, but also occur in two rare varieties — hereditary coproporphyria and variegate porphyria. The inherited enzyme defects (autosomal dominant transmission) render affected individuals sensitive to various drugs (Table 15.1) which, if ingested, may precipitate an acute attack. Attacks may also occur in relation to menstruation, starvation and intercurrent infections. Onset is rapid and the most prominent clinical features are:

1. Abdominal, back and limb pain
2. Vomiting
3. Muscular weakness and paralysis
4. Autonomic dysfunction causing tachycardia, hypertension, urinary retention and constipation
5. Neuropsychiatric disturbances ranging from mild confusion through acute psychotic states to grand mal convulsions
6. The passing of wine-coloured urine.

Fatalities are now rare and are usually caused by respiratory failure.

When the patient or other members of the family have had previous acute attacks the diagnosis is fairly straightforward; however, latent disease is frequent. Confirmation of the diagnosis depends on the demonstration of porphobilinogen in the patient's

Table 15.1 Potential precipitants of acute porphyria

Alcohol	Methyldopa
Amitriptyline	Oestrogens
Barbiturates	Pentazocine
Carbamazepine	Phenylbutazone
Chloroquine	Phenytoin
Chlorpropamide	Progesterone
Dichloralphenazone	Sulphonamides
Ergotamine	Tetracyclines
Griseofulvin	Theophylline
Halothane	Thiopentone
	Fasting
	Infection
	Menstruation
	Pregnancy

urine; 2 ml of fresh urine is added to a tube containing 2 ml of Ehrlich's reagent (2% p-dimethylaminobenzaldehyde in 50% hydrochloric acid). After mixing well, 4 ml of chloroform are added. The mixture is then shaken vigorously and allowed to settle. Any colour remaining in the upper aqueous layer indicates excess porphobilinogen.

To prevent permanent neurological damage it is important to terminate a porphyric attack as quickly as possible. Carbohydrate loading remains the mainstay of treatment. While the patient is in the A & E department a large vein should be cannulated and an infusion of 10% fructose (laevulose) or glucose begun. In addition, a freshly prepared haematin infusion may be used in the treatment of this condition (4.8 mg/kg given over 30 minutes). Instability in solution, thrombophlebitis and coagulation disturbances have all caused problems and more stable preparations have been developed (e.g. haem arginate). The patient may also require symptomatic treatment for pain (morphine, pethidine or dihydrocodeine), vomiting and behavioural disturbances (promazine or chlorpromazine), tachycardia and hypertension (propranolol) and convulsions (diazepam, chlormethiazole or sodium valproate). Aspirin, paracetamol, chlorpheniramine and penicillin are also safe drugs to use if indicated.

All these patients must be admitted to hospital and treatment continued until there is clinical and biochemical evidence of improvement. Many weeks may elapse before they are well enough to leave hospital. Occasionally paralysis of the respiratory muscles may necessitate tracheostomy and mechanical ventilation.

ACUTE RHABDOMYOLYSIS

Severe crush injuries are the most common cause of acute rhabdomyolysis. The diagnosis of non-traumatic rhabdomyolysis is easily missed. It has been reported after prolonged coma, usually due to drugs or alcohol (occasionally prolonged immobility in the elderly following a fall or a 'stroke'); intense exercise; heat stroke; sustained bouts of heavy drinking in chronic alcoholics; abuse of amphetamines, LSD, barbiturates, phencyclidine and opiates; carbon monoxide poisoning; muscle ischaemia; inflammatory disorders such as polymyositis and viral myositis; severe infections, e.g. legionnaires' disease and toxic shock syndrome; grand mal fits

and cataleptic trances. Severe muscle pain, tenderness and swelling are usual but not invariable. Proximal muscle weakness may progress to flaccid areflexic quadriparesis. The diagnostic feature is massive myoglobinuria. The urine is dark brown and strongly positive on testing for blood but contains no erythrocytes. Haemoglobin in the urine produces similar findings, but the patient's serum will be red due to haemolysis. Blood samples should be obtained for estimation of serum electrolytes, creatinine, myoglobin, creatine phosphokinase and acid/base analysis. Muscle swelling may be severe enough to necessitate fasciotomy.

The two principal complications of acute rhabdomyolysis are hyperkalaemia and acute renal failure (50% of patients). The development of acute tubular necrosis is indicated by a falling urine output and the presence of cells and granular casts in the urine. Early treatment with a forced alkaline diuresis may prevent renal failure. However, if it is already established, the patient will require fluid restriction and admission to a renal unit for dialysis.

Hyperkalaemia may cause serious cardiac dysrhythmias culminating in cardiac arrest. A plasma potassium concentration exceeding 6.5 mmol/l or, more importantly, the following ECG changes indicate the need for urgent action (Fig. 15.1):

Tall peaked T waves
Prolonged PR interval
Disappearance of P waves
Widened QRS complexes
Slurred ST segments
Sine wave preceding cardiac arrest.

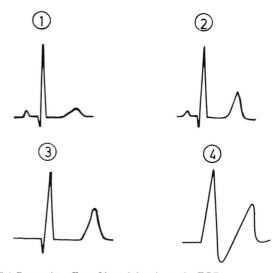

Fig. 15.1 Progressive effect of hyperkalaemia on the ECG:-
1) normal; 2) tall tented T wave; 3) loss of P wave and 4) widening of the QRS complex with terminal sine wave pattern.

An intravenous injection of 50 g of glucose covered by 15 units of soluble (short-acting) insulin will reduce the plasma potassium by about 1 mmol/l and the effect will last up to 2 hours. If there is widening of the QRS complexes and slurring of the ST segments intravenous calcium must be given *immediately* and continued until the ECG returns to normal. The initial dose is 10 ml of

10% calcium gluconate given over 3 minutes which can be repeated up to a total of 50 ml. If the patient is also acidotic, 50–100 ml of 4.2% sodium bicarbonate should be infused over 10 minutes. These patients should all be referred for dialysis.

NEUROLEPTIC MALIGNANT SYNDROME

This rare disorder is a potentially lethal idiosyncratic reaction to neuroleptic drugs. It has been described in association with administration of phenothiazines, thioxanthenes, antidepressants and tetrabenazine, but haloperidol and depot fluphenazines are most commonly implicated. It has also been reported after treatment with laevodopa has been stopped. The onset is unpredictable and occurs at normal therapeutic dosages. It can arise early in the course of treatment or after many months or years of maintenance therapy. In some cases exhaustion and dehydration appear to be predisposing factors.

The syndrome shows some striking clinical similarities with malignant hyperpyrexia (see Ch. 9). The cardinal features are hyperthermia, muscular rigidity, a fluctuating level of consciousness and autonomic dysfunction with tachycardia, pallor, a labile blood pressure, sweating, excessive salivation and urinary incontinence. Tremor, choreiform movements and oculogyric crises also occur. The full blown syndrome takes about 24–72 hours to develop. Often the first signs are hypoactivity developing into akinesia and mutism and eventually stupor and coma. The patient's mental state often fluctuates between alertness and clouding of consciousness. Muscular rigidity may cause dysphagia, dysarthria and dyspnoea. Hyperthermia usually develops after the motor symptoms. Complications include aspiration pneumonia, thromboembolism, renal failure and cardiovascular collapse. The mortality is about 20% and the commonest cause of death is respiratory failure.

Treatment consists of withdrawal of the offending drug, active cooling, rehydration and management of complications as they arise. Mechanical ventilation may be necessary. Hyperthermia and rigidity may respond to intravenous dantrolene (cf. malignant hyperpyrexia, Ch. 9). Benzodiazepines, amantadine and bromocriptine have also been used. Recovery normally takes between 5 and 10 days, but may be longer after depot preparations.

Differential diagnoses include catatonic states, meningoencephalitis, heat stroke and tetanus.

HYPERCALCAEMIC CRISIS

A rising serum calcium can lead to a vicious cycle of increasing nausea, vomiting, dehydration, confusion and renal failure. The most common cause is malignant disease of the lung, breast or reticuloendothelial system. Bone involvement is present in 75% of these patients and treatment with oestrogens, androgens or tamoxifen increases the risk. Other causes include hyperparathyroidism, chronic vitamin D intoxication (cod liver oil tablets from health shops), milk alkali syndrome, sarcoidosis, thiazide diuretics and prolonged immobility in such conditions as Paget's disease and thyrotoxicosis in which there is increased bone turnover. The only clue to the condition in a semiconscious patient may be a shortened QT interval on the ECG.

When hypercalcaemia is suspected a venous blood sample should be obtained for serum calcium, electrolyte and urea and albumin estimation *without* using a tourniquet. The height of the hypercalcaemia determines the urgency of the case. Levels above 3.5 mmol/l require immediate treatment. The value may require correction to a serum albumin of 40 g/l. Starting simple rehydration with intravenous saline is the only measure required in the A & E department. Care should be taken in patients with very low serum albumin levels, or impaired cardiac or renal function. Decisions regarding the use of frusemide, calcitonin, diphosphonates, corticosteroids and mithramycin can be left to the medical staff of the admitting unit.

PHAEOCHROMOCYTOMA

Phaeochromocytomas are tumours derived from chromaffin cells of neuroectodermal origin. Ninety per cent arise in the adrenal medullae. The second most common site is the organ of Zuckerkandl adjacent to the aortic bifurcation. They are very rare outside the abdomen and pelvis. Some cases are familial and there may be an associated thyroid medullary carcinoma and parathyroid tumours. Von Recklinghausen's neurofibromatosis is another well-known association. Symptoms and signs are due to sustained or spasmodic overproduction of catecholamines. The most ominous clinical effects are on the cardiovascular system. An acute rise in blood pressure can precipitate a cerebral haemorrhage or severe heart failure and dangerous cardiac dysrhythmias may also occur. The clinical manifestations are protean. Symptoms include:

1. Sudden pounding headaches
2. Sweating
3. Palpitations
4. Apprehension and tremulousness
5. Chest and abdominal pain
6. Nausea, vomiting and diarrhoea
7. Dizziness and fainting
8. Generalised weakness
9. Paraesthesiae
10. Weight loss.

The following clinical signs may be found:

1. Hypertension which may be paroxysmal or sustained
2. Hypotension after an attack
3. Postural hypotension
4. Cardiac dysrhythmias
5. Warm clammy skin
6. Facial pallor followed by flushing
7. Tremor
8. Fever
9. Pupillary dilatation.

In addition to the above, the patient may have signs of a coexisting syndrome (e.g. café au lait spots, neurofibromas, a Marfanoid habitus or thyroid tumour), or have suffered a complication such as a 'stroke', myocardial infarction, dissecting aneurysm or heart failure. Some tumours are large enough to be felt in the abdomen.

The course of the disease is often punctuated by alarming and life-threatening crises. A variety of precipitating events have been described. Most have in common an increase in pressure on the tumour, for instance, alteration of body posture, abdominal palpation, straining at stool, micturition or external trauma. Exercise, sympathomimetic drugs, certain foodstuffs (e.g. cheese), mental stress and laughter can also provoke attacks. They usually last less than an hour and are followed by a feeling of total exhaustion. During a classical paroxysm the patient is hypertensive, pale, sweating, tremulous and has a rapid pulse. Headache is the predominant symptom. Severe abdominal pain may mimic a surgical emergency. The blood sugar and haematocrit are often raised. Hypotension frequently follows an attack, which may be misleading.

In an acute pressor crisis the head of the bed should be elevated and a bolus of phentolamine (2–5 mg) given intravenously. If the diagnosis is in doubt, a fall in the systolic blood pressure of greater than 35 mmHg is suggestive of a phaeochromocytoma, although the test is not specific. The action of phentolamine, an α-adrenergic blocking agent, is short-lived and if necessary the dose can be repeated at 5-minute intervals. The patient's blood pressure must be monitored closely as it can fall precipitously. In a prolonged crisis phentolamine can be infused intravenously starting at a dose of 1 mg/minute. Sodium nitroprusside is an alternative vasodilator but it should only be administered under conditions of full haemodynamic monitoring (see Ch. 11). The patient's ECG should be monitored throughout treatment. If cardiac tachydysrhythmias occur practolol (5–10 mg) or propranolol (1 mg/min up to a maximum dose of 10 mg) should be given intravenously. β-adrenergic blocking agents should not be administered before the patient has had an adequate dose of an α-blocker as they may cause a paradoxical rise in blood pressure.

The dramatic acute presentation of a phaeochromocytoma can be mimicked by the malignant phase of idiopathic or other secondary forms of hypertension, acute anxiety, a subarachnoid haemorrhage, a thyrotoxic crisis or a pressor response to tyramine containing foods in a patient taking a monoamine oxidase inhibitor.

HEREDITARY ANGIO-OEDEMA

This rare condition is inherited as an autosomal dominant trait. There is a deficiency of the inhibitor of the enzyme C_1 esterase, one of the components of complement. The submucosal and subcutaneous swellings that occur are *not* accompanied by urticaria. Skin trauma produces transient erythema followed by oedema. A history of recurrent colicky abdominal pain is common. Death from acute upper respiratory obstruction often occurs in early adult life. Treatment entails:

1. Prompt relief of the respiratory obstruction by endotracheal intubation or, in extremis, tracheostomy
2. Administration of oxygen
3. Correction of the enzyme deficiency by transfusion of fresh, fresh frozen or freeze dried plasma.

Adrenaline 0.5 ml subcutaneously and hydrocortisone 100 mg intravenously are usually also given although, unlike in other acute urticarias, their beneficial effect is minimal. Tranexamic acid and ϵ-aminocaproic acid have also been used to control spontaneous attacks. Attacks may be aborted by the use of oral methyltestosterone (10 mg) or danazol (200 mg).

FURTHER READING

Myasthenia gravis Albuquerque E X, Eldefrawi A T 1983 Chapman and Hall, London

The porphyrias: clinical chemistry, diagnosis and methodology Elder G H 1980 Clinical Haematology 9: 371–398

Emergencies in clinical medicine Kennedy H J 1985 Blackwell Scientific, Oxford

Thyroid emergencies McLellan A R, Alexander W D 1987 Hospital Update 13: 375–393

The porphyrias Moore M R, Brodie M J 1985 Medicine International 2: 604–608

Myasthenia gravis Newsom-Davis J 1983 Medicine International 1: 1490–1492

Endocrine and metabolic emergencies Sonksen P H, Lowy C 1980 (Clinics in Endocrinology and Metabolism 9: 435–643) W B Saunders, London

Williams textbook of endocrinology Wilson J D, Foster D W 1985 W B Saunders, Philadelphia, 7th edn

Major Conditions

INTRODUCTION

Area for patients with major conditions

Most departments reserve certain of their cubicles or examination rooms specifically for this group of patients. In large departments where all patients are assessed before admission to the hospital wards the proportion of medical to surgical conditions is roughly 50:50. About half the surgical complaints are the result of trauma and the commonest symptom dealt with is pain. Where general practitioners admit patients directly to the hospital wards there will be fewer patients with major conditions and relatively more with either life-threatening or minor conditions.

Some patients are referred by their family doctors with an explanatory letter, or following a warning telephone call. Others are brought to the hospital by ambulance or private car following the sudden onset of an acute illness either at home or in a public place. The remainder make up some of the so-called casual attenders who, for one of several reasons, decide to consult a hospital doctor rather than their family doctor.

The most important decision to be made by the A & E doctor is whether or not the patient requires admission to hospital. This decision is primarily a clinical one, but other factors such as home circumstances or the bed occupancy in the hospital at the time may have to be taken into account. In some patients the timing of an operation may also have to be considered and, under these circumstances the surgeon who will be performing the operation should be consulted early and given the option of assessing the patient in the A & E department.

Whilst some simple investigations may be necessary to confirm the diagnosis and provide a baseline, admission should not be delayed by performing investigations in the A & E department which could equally well be carried out in the ward.

Urgent treatment may be required before the patient is transferred to the appropriate ward, or to a specialised unit in another hospital. Interhospital transfer of patients who are suffering from chest pain, peritonitis or any other critical illness, should be avoided if possible, and should be allowed only when special arrangements have been made for their transfer and reception.

The decision not to admit a patient to hospital (perhaps influenced by the lack of beds) may present difficulties to a junior doctor, because he will be aware that there are a number of lethal conditions which are easily missed or mistakenly diagnosed in the early stages. A senior opinion should always be available in this area of the department; in particular, no patient who has been referred for admission by a general practitioner should be discharged without the advice of a more senior doctor.

Should it be decided that a patient presenting with a major condition does not require admission, the following arrangements should be considered.

1. The patient may be allowed home following a telephone call to the family doctor (or with an accompanying letter). This will communicate recommendations for treatment, or a change of present therapy, or may request follow-up during the ensuing few days. Advice may also be given to the general practitioner as to the line of action if the patient's response to this treatment is unsatisfactory. The results of simple investigations can be forwarded as soon as they are known.

2. Various community services may be mobilised in an attempt to maintain the patient in the community. The help of medical social workers is invaluable.

3. Geriatric domiciliary assessment may be suggested.

4. Some patients will be referred for outpatient investigation and consultation in a specialist clinic.

Observation ward

Many A & E departments have a small ward attached. The variety and complexity of the problems which can be dealt with efficiently depends on the number of beds in the unit, the available investigative facilities, the relationships with other specialties and the interests of the head of the department. In most A & E departments, however, it is a short-stay ward and the main function is to provide facilities for serial observations of the patient in well regulated surroundings. The nature and timing of observations should be clearly specified by the doctor and carefully recorded by the nurse. Minor changes in the observations must be reported immediately to the doctor, as treatment decisions will often depend on these changes. 'Observation' refers not only to the regular recording of vital signs, but also to the general attitude of the patient while in the ward. This will include appetite, mobility and reactions to relatives and friends.

These wards usually have a rapid turnover of patients, a high bed occupancy, and often a higher percentage of psychiatrically disturbed or difficult patients than is found in other medical or surgical wards. The nursing staff must be able to communicate with patients from a wide range of backgrounds, who may be suffering from injury or from medical, surgical or psychiatric illness. In such a ward, therefore, a senior nurse must always be available throughout the 24 hours. Arrangements should be made for the continuation of regular medication, prescribed on standard drug sheets in the same manner as for any other patient in the hospital. Similarly, clinical records should be made with care, and it is important to follow hospital rules concerning admission and discharge, documentation and diagnosis, and communication with general practitioners.

The essential qualification for admission to such a short-stay observation ward should be that the patient is not initially considered to have a condition requiring intensive medical or major operative treatment. The following groups of patients may be considered suitable.

1. Patients who seem unwell but in whom a provisional diagnosis cannot be readily made. Often the extra information obtained during 24 hours observation, added to that obtained from previous hospital notes and from consultation with their relatives, may enable a specific diagnosis to be made and a definitive plan of management agreed.

2. Minor illnesses of limited duration, such as epilepsy, hypoglycaemia, minor self-poisoning, headaches, syncopal attacks and renal colic.

3. Minor surgical conditions, including sepsis and minor trauma.

4. A patient in whom serious disease seems unlikely but whose presenting symptom (such as mild chest pain or abdominal pain) may be a warning of a more serious illness.

5. In some hospitals these beds may serve a variety of functions not directly connected with the A & E department. These include day surgery, chemotherapy for malignant disease, treatment for haematological disorders (such as haemophilia) and investigations such as myelography, arteriography and other imaging investigations.

6. In other hospitals such a ward may also serve as a night admissions unit, and may contain a room specially designed for disturbed, drunk or violent patients. This arrangement minimises the disturbance of patients in the general wards of the hospital at night.

After 24 or 48 hours in this ward, the patient's main problem should have become clear and a plan of management agreed. The majority will be fit for discharge, but a small number will be found to be more seriously ill than was at first thought and will be transferred to other wards in the hospital, or to other hospitals. Clear rules should be laid down about transfer procedures and these must be rigorously applied. An observation ward can only work when there is proper understanding and co-operation from those in charge of other wards. It is particularly important that the elderly patient with chronic physical ailments, whose main problem is inability to cope in the community, should not remain in such a ward. Regular review of the disposal of patients helps to guard against misuse.

In the chapters in this section we have tried to cover the major conditions encountered in the A & E department. The list is by no means exhaustive. A problem-orientated approach has been used whenever possible.

The poisoned patient

Acute poisoning is a common medical emergency and may occur in patients of any age. Accidental poisoning usually occurs in small children who often swallow household products, tablets or plant material. Deliberate self-poisoning sometimes occurs in children as young as 6 years. Small children may also be poisoned by their parents in a form of 'non-accidental injury'. In adults deliberate self-poisoning is much more common than accidental poisoning and some episodes claimed to be accidental are in fact deliberate. Few episodes of self-poisoning are really suicide attempts: most are impulsive acts at a moment of crisis and involve overdoses of drugs, especially psychotropic drugs or analgesics. Alcohol is often taken with or before the overdose and more than one drug is taken in about a third of cases. Homicidal poisoning is fortunately uncommon.

Most episodes of poisoning present no threat to life but many patients require admission for observation and assessment. Some patients need resuscitation and intensive care.

INITIAL MANAGEMENT

It is essential to ensure that the patient's airway, breathing and circulation are adequate. Most deaths from poisoning result from respiratory obstruction or respiratory depression. Convulsions require immediate treatment. The pulse, blood pressure, temperature, respiratory rate and level of consciousness should be assessed and recorded. Information about the poison involved should be obtained as soon as possible, while the patient is being resuscitated.

HISTORY

Most patients remain conscious after an overdose and it is usually possible to elicit some history of the episode of poisoning. It is important to determine and record the drug or drugs involved, the quantity taken and the time of ingestion. The time of ingestion may not be known, especially if the patient is unconscious. In such cases it is useful to determine when the patient was last seen before the overdose.

Many patients are able to identify the drugs which they have taken and the tablet containers may be available. Some patients, however, do not know what drugs they took and a few patients give deliberately misleading information. The patient's relatives and general practitioner may know what drugs were available. Tablets may be identified by the size, shape, colour and markings with the aid of colour charts or the Tablident drug identification system (Edwin Burgess Ltd, Longwick Road, Princes Risborough, Aylesbury, Buckinghamshire). The quantity of drugs or poisons taken is often not clear. Many patients do not count the tablets but take them by the handful. Some patients deliberately exaggerate or understate the quantity taken. Small children are often found with open bottles of tablets or household products with no definite history of ingestion. In many cases the maximum quantity available can be determined from the containers.

Symptoms caused by poisoning should be elicited. For example, tinnitus is an important symptom of aspirin poisoning and also occurs in quinine poisoning, which is rare. If the patient vomited after taking the overdose this should be recorded.

EXAMINATION AND TREATMENT

Conscious level

The level of consciousness must be assessed and recorded in all poisoned patients. The Glasgow Coma Scale (Ch. 14) designed for head-injured patients can be used. However, a simpler but useful scale in poisoned patients is the *Edinburgh coma grading system*, in which the depth of coma is assessed by the response to commands and pain:

Grade 0	Fully conscious
Grade 1	Drowsy but obeys commands
Grade 2	No response to commands but good response to pain
Grade 3	Minimal response to pain
Grade 4	No response to pain

Squeezing the ear lobe is an adequate painful stimulus. Patients in grades 2, 3 and 4 are unconscious.

Airway and breathing

The important physical signs are cyanosis (usually indicating hypoxia), noisy snoring respiration (upper airway obstruction), diminished chest movement with shallow respiration (evidence of respiratory depression) and respiratory rate. A raised respiratory rate may be caused by respiratory obstruction, pneumonia, metabolic acidosis or aspirin poisoning. Slow respiration occurs in poisoning by opiates and other CNS depressants: a therapeutic trial of naloxone (1.2 mg i.v. in an adult) may help in the diagnosis and management. It is essential to clear the airway of any vomit or other obstructing matter. The airway should be maintained by extending the head and pulling the jaw forward. If the patient has no gag reflex a cuffed endotracheal tube is needed to protect the airway. If an endotracheal tube is not tolerated an oral or nasopharyngeal airway is often helpful to prevent obstruction of the airway by the tongue. The patient should be positioned on his front and left side in the 'recovery' position (Ch. 12). If the airway is clear but respiration appears inadequate ventilation is needed. The patient should initially be ventilated with a bag and mask, or if necessary by mouth-to-mouth or mouth-to-mask breathing, and then intubated as soon as possible with a cuffed endotracheal tube and ventilated on oxygen. If a patient is deeply unconscious but respiration appears to be adequate, the arterial blood gases should be checked, since severe hypoxia may occur before cyanosis is apparent. When measuring blood gases it is important to be sure that the sample is arterial. The inspired oxygen concentration should be recorded, with details of whether respiration was spontaneous or ventilated. The blood gas results must be corrected for temperature if the patient is hypothermic or pyrexial. Many unconscious poisoned patients have a mixed metabolic and respiratory acidosis. Ventilation is necessary if there is carbon dioxide retention, or hypoxia despite treatment with oxygen.

Circulation

The circulation is assessed by measurement of the pulse and blood pressure and assessment of tissue perfusion by mental state (if conscious), skin temperature and urine output (if catheterised). A systolic blood pressure of 80 mmHg in young adults or 90 mmHg in patients aged over 40 is usually adequate. If hypotension occurs one should first check for and treat hypoxia and hypothermia. Elevation of the foot of the trolley increases venous return to the heart and often raises the blood pressure. If hypotension persists it can usually be reversed by infusing 500 ml of a plasma expander such as polygeline (Haemaccel). Occasionally it is necessary to measure the central venous pressure and infuse further fluid or dopamine.

The heart rhythm should be monitored in patients who are unconscious or hypothermic, or who have taken overdoses of digoxin, β-blockers, antiarrhythmic drugs, potassium or bronchodilators. If dysrhythmias occur one should check for and correct hypoxia, acidaemia and hypo- or hyperkalaemia. Bradycardia may be caused by hypoxia or hypothermia or by poisoning with digoxin, β-blockers or clonidine. Tachycardia may be caused by anxiety or distress, airway obstruction, hypoglycaemia or by many drugs, especially antidepressants, sympathomimetics and amphetamine derivatives. Antiarrhythmic drugs are rarely needed in poisoned patients and may cause hypotension.

Hypothermia

Hypothermia is common in severe poisoning, especially poisoning with barbiturates, phenothiazines or chlormethiazole. The rectal temperature should be recorded with a low reading thermometer. The patient should be wrapped in extra blankets and will usually rewarm spontaneously. Hypothermia is discussed in Ch. 28.

General examination

It is important to examine the patient thoroughly to look for evidence of toxicity and to assess whether the clinical features suggest any particular poison or another illness or injury. One should also look for signs of complications of poisoning, especially aspiration pneumonia in unconscious patients. Excessive sweating is often caused by aspirin poisoning but can also result from hypoglycaemia or fever. Injection marks over veins suggest drug addiction (and thus a risk of hepatitis and AIDS), or possibly recent hospital treatment. Erythema or blistering over pressure areas show only that the patient has been immobile for some hours: such blisters were once thought to be diagnostic of barbiturate poisoning but can occur with any drug which causes prolonged coma.

Small pupils suggest poisoning with an opiate or (rarely) a cholinesterase inhibitor. Dilated pupils may be caused by hypoxia or by poisoning with anticholinergic drugs (e.g. tricyclic antidepressants, antihistamines, orphenadrine or benztropine), or by sympathomimetic drugs such as ephedrine or amphetamines.

Dystonic reactions and muscle spasm are commonly caused by metoclopramide or by phenothiazines and related tranquillisers. Neurological signs in poisoned patients are often due to anticholinergic drugs, especially tricyclic antidepressants.

Analysis of drugs and poisons

Emergency drug analysis is only indicated if the result will affect the management of the patient. This is so in poisoning due to paracetamol, aspirin (or other salicylates), iron, lithium and paraquat. Screening for paracetamol and salicylate is needed if it is not clear what drug has been taken. All unconscious poisoned patients should be screened for paracetamol in case it has been taken with a sedative drug.

Screening for sedative drugs is never necessary in an A & E department. If the cause of coma is not clear one should:

> Examine the patient carefully
> Discover what drugs or poisons were available
> Exclude hypoglycaemia
> Consider giving naloxone (see section on opiates, p. 212)
> Look at the ECG for anticholinergic changes (see section on tricyclic antidepressants, p. 211).

Blood should be kept for later analysis if necessary in any patient who is unconscious or severely poisoned, or in whom there is any likelihood of later legal proceedings (e.g. suspicion of deliberate poisoning by another person). Gastric contents and urine (50 ml) should also be kept in such circumstances, with all samples carefully labelled with the patient's identity, date and time. Ten millilitres of blood in a lithium heparin tube is usually adequate for drug analysis, but a plain tube must be used if measurement of lithium is needed.

Antidotes

The administration of antidotes can occasionally produce dramatic and life-saving improvements in poisoned patients, but antidotes are only available for a few poisons. The antidotes most commonly needed are listed in Table 16.1. Further information about antidotes for opiates, paracetamol and β-blocking drugs is given in the relevant sections.

Emptying the stomach

Emptying the stomach, by inducing vomiting or by gastric lavage, may reduce the amount of poison which is absorbed, but it is certainly not necessary in every poisoned patient. It is indicated if the patient has taken a potentially dangerous overdose in the previous four hours. This time limit may be extended to six hours for opiates, anticholinergic drugs and salicylates, which may delay gastric emptying. Coma is associated with reduced gut motility and so gastric lavage should be performed (if this can be done safely) in every unconscious poisoned patient. Emptying the stomach is contraindicated after poisoning by strong acids or alkalis because of the risk of perforation of the oesophagus. It is usual to avoid gastric emptying after ingestion of petroleum products, which can cause severe pneumonia, but in fact there is no evidence that emptying the stomach increases the risk of pneumonia.

Saline must never be used as an emetic since it is often ineffective and may cause fatal poisoning from hypernatraemia. Ipecacuanha is an effective emetic in both adults and children, but must only be used if the patient is fully conscious. It is greatly preferable to gastric lavage in children. Ipecacuanha is given as a syrup (Paediatric Ipecacuanha Emetic Mixture, BP) in a dose of 10 ml

Table 16.1 Antidotes

Poison	Antidote	Adult dose/notes
β-blockers	Glucagon	See section on β-blockers
Digoxin	Digoxin antibodies (Digibind) &/or atropine	Discuss with Poisons Unit
Insulin Hypoglycaemic drugs	Dextrose	50 ml of 50% solution then infusions of dextrose, with potassium if necessary. Diazoxide might help in chlorpropamide poisoning: discuss with Poisons Unit
Iron salts	Desferrioxamine (Desferal)	See section on iron
Metoclopramide	Procyclidine (Kemadrin)	5–10 mg i.v. for dystonic reaction. Diazepam may be used instead
Opiates	Naloxone (Narcan)	See section on opiates
Paracetamol	Acetylcysteine (Parvolex)	See section on paracetamol
Potassium	Calcium gluconate. Glucose and insulin	20 ml of 10% solution. 50 g glucose + 20 units soluble insulin
	Calcium Resonium	Ion exchange resin
Warfarin	Vitamin K	10 mg i.v. Do not give this if patient must remain anticoagulated: use fresh frozen plasma instead
Cyanide	Dicobalt edetate (Kelocyanor)	600 mg (40 ml) i.v. Use only if patient is *unconscious*. Give oxygen
Ethylene glycol Methanol	Ethanol	Loading dose 50 g orally (125 ml of whisky or gin). Discuss with Poisons Unit
Organophosphorus insecticides	Atropine + pralidoxime	Discuss with Poisons Unit
Paraquat	Fuller's earth Bentonite	See section on paraquat
Adder bite	Zagreb antivenom	See Chapter 28 (p. 306)

Antidotes are also available for some other drugs and poisons but are rarely needed. Information is available from the Poisons Information Services.

for a child aged 6–18 months, 15 ml for an older child and 30 ml for an adult, followed by 200 ml of water or orange juice. Ipecacuanha may be repeated after 20 minutes if vomiting has not occurred.

Gastric lavage must never be used as a punitive measure and must always be authorised by a doctor. Careful attention to technique is essential to minimise the risk of aspiration of fluid into the lungs or perforation of the oesophagus. If the patient does not have a good cough reflex a cuffed endotracheal tube must be inserted to protect the airway. The patient should lie on the left side with the foot of the trolley raised about 20 cm. Powerful suction apparatus with a large suction catheter must be immediately available. In an adult the stomach tube should be of size 30 English gauge (external diameter about 14 mm). The appropriate length of tube from mouth to stomach should be measured against the patient and the tube lubricated with water-soluble jelly before insertion. Force must not be used to pass the tube. The position

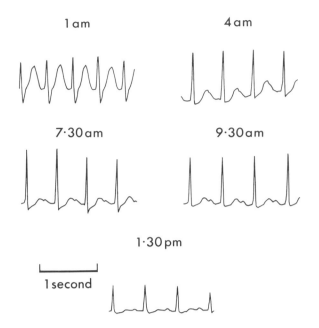

1 am   4 am

7·30 am   9·30 am

1·30 pm

|—————|
1 second

Fig. 16.2 ECG changes in tricyclic antidepressant poisoning showing improvement over 12 hours without specific treatment.

diuresis, haemodialysis and haemoperfusion are useless in tricyclic antidepressant poisoning.

Tetracyclic antidepressants

The tetracyclic antidepressant maprotiline has the same effects in overdose as the tricyclic antidepressant drugs. However, mianserin, another tetracyclic antidepressant, seems relatively non-toxic in overdose, although it may cause drowsiness and occasionally heart block.

Barbiturates

Poisoning with the barbiturate hypnotics such as Tuinal (quinalbarbitone and amylobarbitone) is becoming less common, since these drugs have been largely replaced by the benzodiazepines. Barbiturates are often injected by drug addicts. Barbiturate poisoning causes coma with respiratory obstruction, respiratory depression and often hypotension and hypothermia. Emergency measurement of plasma barbiturate concentrations is seldom required since the result rarely alters the management. Intensive supportive therapy is adequate in the great majority of patients. A few patients who deteriorate or fail to improve despite intensive care require haemoperfusion to remove the barbiturate.

Phenobarbitone causes similar features to the barbiturate hypnotics but the effects are more prolonged and deep coma is less common. Forced alkaline diuresis may be needed, or occasionally haemoperfusion.

Chlormethiazole

Chlormethiazole (Heminevrin) is a hypnotic and sedative drug.

It can be used in the management of alcohol withdrawal but unfortunately it is often prescribed, incorrectly, to chronic alcoholics who continue to drink and also become dependent on the drug. Overdosage causes similar features to the barbiturates, with coma, respiratory obstruction, respiratory depression, hypotension and hypothermia. Increased salivation occurs in some patients and may predispose to aspiration pneumonia. Treatment is supportive, with frequent pharyngeal suction and ventilation if necessary.

Opiates

The opiate group of drugs includes morphine, codeine and related drugs and derivatives which are used as analgesics, cough suppressants and antidiarrhoeal agents. Many analgesic tablets contain combinations of codeine, dihydrocodeine or dextropropoxyphene with paracetamol or aspirin. Lomotil tablets contain the opiate diphenoxylate and also atropine. Morphine, heroin and other opiates are often injected by addicts. The clinical features of poisoning with an opiate drug are coma, respiratory depression and pin-point pupils. Respiratory arrest, hypotension, vomiting, convulsions and pulmonary oedema may occur. Death from hypoxia may occur within one hour of an oral overdose of an opiate drug.

The initial treatment for opiate poisoning is to clear and maintain the airway and support respiration if necessary. The specific antagonist naloxone (Narcan) reverses the toxic effects of the opiates and often produces dramatic recovery of consciousness. Naloxone can be used as a therapeutic trial if there is suspicion of opiate poisoning. The initial dose of naloxone is 1.2 mg intravenously for an adult (0.4 mg for a child) and this can be repeated as often as necessary. The duration of action of naloxone is less than that of most opiates and so the patient must be observed carefully in case coma and respiratory depression recur. Further injections of naloxone are often needed, or alternatively an intravenous infusion of naloxone in 5% dextrose.

Venous access may be difficult in drug addicts who have injected heroin or other drugs frequently. Naloxone can be given down the endotracheal tube if a patient has been intubated. Naloxone may precipitate an acute withdrawal syndrome in opiate addicts, with abdominal pain, nausea, diarrhoea and vasoconstriction. This syndrome may be distressing but it is seldom very severe and is not a contraindication to the use of naloxone in serious poisoning in addicts. Drug addicts are often carriers of hepatitis B virus and human immunodeficiency virus (HIV), which is associated with AIDS (see Ch. 25). Care is needed to avoid contamination of staff with blood or secretions from known or suspected addicts.

Paracetamol (acetaminophen)

Severe liver damage may occur in adults after an overdose of more than 7.5 g (15 tablets) of paracetamol, although it is uncommon unless more than 15 g are taken. Alcoholics and patients taking barbiturates are at particular risk. Urgent treatment is needed to prevent liver damage, which is caused by a toxic metabolite of paracetamol. Liver damage is rare in children since the metabolism of paracetamol is different from adults and usually little of the drug is taken. There is, however, no information about toxic levels in children and so they should be managed in the same way as adults.

Many patients who take overdoses of paracetamol do not take enough to cause liver damage and develop no symptoms. However, nausea and vomiting are common within a few hours of a serious overdose. If untreated the patient develops pain and tenderness around the liver and jaundice occurs after about three days. Liver failure may occur about four or five days after the overdose, with hypoglycaemia, lack of clotting factors and hepatic encephalopathy.

Renal failure due to acute tubular necrosis occurs occasionally. Liver and renal damage are preventable by early treatment with acetylcysteine or methionine.

Gastric lavage should be performed if it is less than 4 hours since the overdose. Blood should be taken immediately, or at 4 hours if the patient is seen before then, for measurement of the plasma paracetamol concentration. The precise time of the sample must be recorded. The result should be plotted on the treatment graph (Fig. 16.3). Serious liver damage is likely if the plasma level is above the line joining 200 mg/l at 4 hours with 50 mg/l at 12 hours. Specific treatment is needed in such patients. The most effective treatment in severe paracetamol poisoning is intravenous acetylcysteine (Parvolex). The loading dose of acetylcysteine is 150 mg/kg in 200 ml of 5% dextrose over 15 minutes, followed by 50 mg/kg in 500 ml of 5% dextrose over 4 hours and then 100 mg/kg over the next 16 hours. The alternative treatment is methionine, which is given orally in a dose of 2.5 g 4-hourly for four doses. This is much cheaper than acetylcysteine, but oral treatment is unreliable if vomiting or severe nausea occur, as in most patients with serious paracetamol poisoning. Treatment with acetylcysteine or methionine is very effective in preventing liver and renal damage if started within 8 hours of the overdose. These antidotes are less effective if started at between 8 and 12 hours and treatment started at more than 15 hours is ineffective. It is therefore important to start treatment within 8 hours of the overdose if possible. If the result of a paracetamol assay will not be available by that time treatment should be started at once: oral methionine is satisfactory if the patient is not vomiting, but intravenous acetylcysteine is needed if vomiting occurs, or if the patient is unconscious as a result of taking another drug in addition to paracetamol. Acetylcysteine usually causes no side-effects but a few patients develop an allergic rash or bronchospasm.

Patients who present more than 15 hours after a paracetamol overdose tend to be severely poisoned and at high risk of liver damage. Supportive treatment is needed, with daily measurement of liver and renal function for at least four days. Prolongation of the prothrombin time is usually the first evidence of serious liver damage. Many patients who develop liver damage make a complete recovery, but some deteriorate and die from liver failure despite intensive treatment.

Salicylates (aspirin)

Salicylate poisoning causes tinnitus, deafness, nausea and vomiting, hyperventilation, vasodilatation, sweating and tachycardia. Fever may occur in children. These features of salicylism are associated with plasma salicylate concentrations above 400 mg/l. Most patients remain fully conscious, but confusion and coma can occur in children and occasionally in adults, especially at salicylate concentrations above 800 mg/l. Unconscious patients may develop convulsions or cardiac arrest. Other rare complications include pulmonary and cerebral oedema and renal failure. Salicylate intoxication causes complex metabolic disturbances with a mixed metabolic acidosis and respiratory alkalosis. The respiratory alkalosis predominates in most patients but in some small children and a few adults acidaemia develops, often in association with confusion or coma. Hypoglycaemia occasionally occurs in children but is very rare in adults. However, animal studies suggest that in very severe salicylate poisoning brain glucose levels may be low despite a normal blood glucose concentration.

The stomach should be emptied in patients presenting within 6 hours of an overdose. The plasma salicylate concentration should be measured. It may be necessary to repeat the measurement after three or four hours if symptoms of salicylism develop or become worse, or if a slow-release preparation has been taken.

Adult patients with salicylate concentrations below 450 mg/l (3.3 mmol/l) and children below 350 mg/l usually require only an increase in oral fluid intake. Occasional patients with these salicylate concentrations require intravenous fluids because of vomiting. Patients with higher concentrations who are fully conscious should

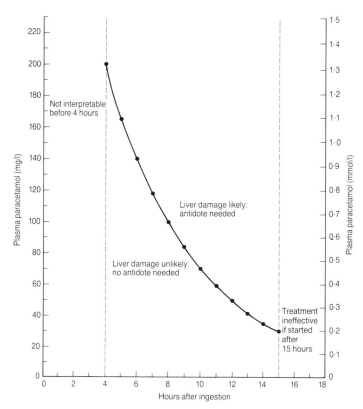

Fig. 16.3 Paracetamol treatment graph.

be treated with a forced alkaline diuresis, unless they have cardiac or renal failure when haemodialysis may be needed. A suitable regimen for forced diuresis in an adult is 5% dextrose (1 litre, with potassium chloride 40 mmol), 0.9% saline (500 ml) and 1.26% sodium bicarbonate (500 ml) given intravenously in rotation at 2 litres per hour for 3 hours. The plasma electrolytes and arterial gases should be measured. The symptoms of salicylism improve as the plasma concentration falls due to haemodilution and excretion of salicylate in the urine. Alkalinisation of the urine is much more important than diuresis in eliminating salicylate and the urine pH should preferably be about 8.

The real problems occur in the rare patients with aspirin poisoning who are confused or unconscious (unless due to a sedative drug taken in addition). Such patients may suddenly deteriorate with convulsions and irreversible cardiac arrest. The electrolytes and arterial gases must be measured and acidaemia corrected. Forced diuresis is liable to precipitate fatal pulmonary oedema in these patients. Immediate haemodialysis is required to remove salicylate and correct the fluid, electrolyte and acid-base disturbances. Intravenous glucose should be given. Curarisation and mechanical ventilation might be helpful since the work of breathing may contribute to the acidaemia. The mortality is high in patients unconscious due to aspirin poisoning but fortunately such cases are rare.

Iron

Ferrous sulphate and other iron salts may cause fatal poisoning. The early features of iron poisoning are nausea, vomiting, abdominal pain and diarrhoea. The vomit and stools may be dark grey or black. In most patients these symptoms settle within about 8 hours. Severely poisoned patients develop coma, metabolic acidosis and shock, usually 1 or 2 days after overdose but occasionally in the first few hours. Gastric strictures may cause obstruction after about 2–5 weeks. Gastric lavage is necessary. Five grams of desferrioxamine dissolved in 100 ml of 5% sodium bicarbonate should be left in the stomach after lavage. A plain abdominal radiograph taken within 2 hours of the overdose will show any remaining iron tablets, but after this time the tablets may have disintegrated. Whole gut lavage should be considered if capsules or a slow-release iron preparation remain in the bowel. The serum iron concentration must be measured urgently. Intravenous infusion of desferrioxamine is needed if the patient is shocked or unconscious or if the serum iron is higher than the total iron binding capacity: the dose is 15 mg/kg per hour to a maximum of 80 mg/kg in 24 hours. Desferrioxamine may cause hypotension if infused too rapidly. If the serum iron cannot be measured at once, but the patient has symptoms of iron poisoning, treatment with intramuscular desferrioxamine should be started (initial dose 1 g for a child or 2 g for an adult) after a blood sample has been taken. The urine colour should be observed — the urine becomes pink if there is free iron in the plasma and this shows that further desferrioxamine is needed. Patients with severe iron poisoning should be discussed with a poisons unit.

β-blockers

Poisoning with β-adrenergic blocking drugs such as propranolol or oxprenolol is uncommon, but may be rapidly fatal. Severe hypotension and bradycardia occur, sometimes with coma and convulsions. There may be electromechanical dissociation with sinus rhythm on the electrocardiogram but no palpable pulse. Sometimes the ECG shows a severe bradycardia with wide irregular QRS complexes.

The cardiac rhythm and blood pressure must be monitored. Atropine (0.6–1.2 mg i.v.) should be given before gastric lavage and further doses may be needed if bradycardia occurs. External cardiac massage is needed if no pulse is palpable. Cardiac pacing and infusions of adrenaline or isoprenaline are usually ineffective. The treatment of choice is glucagon (10 mg i.v. as a bolus), which causes dramatic recovery of cardiac output. Further injections, or an infusion of glucagon may be needed to maintain cardiac output and some patients have needed a total dose of 50 mg of glucagon. Glucagon often causes vomiting. The preservative for the Lilly brand of glucagon contains phenol and so if more than 10 mg of glucagon is needed it should be dissolved in 5% dextrose instead of the diluent provided. Glucagon activates myocardial adenylcyclase by a mechanism that is not blocked by β-blocking drugs.

Aminophylline and theophylline

Overdosage of the bronchodilators aminophylline and theophylline can cause severe toxicity. Vomiting, tachycardia, agitation and hyperventilation are common. In severe poisoning, gastrointestinal bleeding, coma, convulsions, cardiac dysrhythmias and cardiac arrest may occur. There are complex metabolic disturbances with hypokalaemia and acid-base changes.

The heart rhythm should be monitored. The stomach should be emptied and activated charcoal given. Whole-gut lavage may be considered if slow-release tablets have been taken. Blood should be taken for measurement of electrolytes, drug concentrations and blood gases. Intensive care and removal of the drug by charcoal haemoperfusion may be needed. Severely poisoned patients should be discussed with a poisons unit.

Ethanol

Hypoglycaemia may occur in alcohol poisoning, especially in children and when poisoning follows exercise, fasting or malnutrition. Hypoglycaemia should be corrected with intravenous glucose. Most patients with alcohol intoxication recover uneventfully with supportive care. The patient should be in the coma position to reduce the risk of aspiration of vomit. Rarely patients develop lactic acidosis or ketoacidosis and require intensive care. Blood ethanol concentrations can be measured directly or estimated using a breath alcohol analyser. This can be helpful in the assessment of coma, but the results may be difficult to interpret since some patients become unconscious at ethanol concentrations of 3 g/l whereas others are still conscious at 5 g/l.

Paraquat

The weedkiller paraquat is available in granules containing 2.5% paraquat (Weedol, Pathclear and other products) and as liquid concentrates containing 100 or 200 g/l (the commonest being Gramoxone, which contains 200 g/l). The fatal dose may be as little as 1.5 g, i.e. one sachet of Weedol granules or 10 ml of Gramoxone. Ingestion of 1.5–6 g of paraquat causes nausea, vomiting, abdominal pain and diarrhoea. Painful burns in the mouth and throat develop after about one day and renal failure after one or two days. Pulmonary oedema and fibrosis cause progressive hypoxia. Death from paraquat lung usually occurs 7–10 days after the poisoning but may be delayed for as long as 1 month. If more than 6 g of paraquat is ingested shock, metabolic acidosis and coma develop with death within 1 or 2 days from shock and pulmonary oedema.

Treatment must be started immediately. Fuller's earth (200 ml of 30% suspension) or bentonite (200 ml of 7% bentonite in glycerine and water) should be given to absorb paraquat in the stomach. Activated charcoal 50 g can be used if neither Fuller's earth nor bentonite is immediately available. Gastric lavage is needed if it is less than 6 hours since ingestion. Fuller's earth or bentonite should be left in the stomach. Urine should be tested for paraquat. A knife-point of sodium bicarbonate and the same amount of sodium dithionite are added to 5 ml of urine in a test-tube. If paraquat is present a blue colour appears immediately. If this occurs blood should be taken for paraquat assay and the case discussed with the local renal unit and a poisons unit. Haemodialysis and haemoperfusion are sometimes used but are unlikely to alter the outcome after paraquat poisoning. Analgesics, antiemetics and intravenous fluids may be needed. Oxygen should not be given since it increases the pulmonary toxicity of paraquat.

The dithionite screening test can be performed on gastric contents as well as on urine and is helpful in confirming or excluding paraquat poisoning rapidly. A negative urine test 4 hours after exposure excludes significant absorption of paraquat.

Non-poisons

Numerous household products and some drugs which are often ingested by small children are non-toxic in the quantities usually taken and require no treatment. The non-toxic drugs include oral contraceptives, antacids, vitamins (unless combined with iron) and antibiotics (unless allergy occurs). Cosmetics, many skin creams, crayons and water-based paints and glues are non-toxic. Information is available from the Poisons Information Service.

Many children eat laburnum and other berries or plant leaves but serious poisoning is very rare. Unless the plant is identified and known to be non-toxic it is advisable to give ipecacuanha and observe the child for a few hours.

FURTHER READING

Poisonous plants in Britain and their effects on animals and man Cooper M R, Johnson A W 1984 HMSO, London

ABC of poisoning: part I: drugs Henry J, Volans G 1984 British Medical Journal, London

Diagnosis and management of acute poisoning Proudfoot A T 1982 Blackwell Scientific, Oxford

Poisoning: diagnosis and treatment Vale J A, Meredith T J (eds) 1981 Update Books, London

A colour atlas of poisonous plants Frohne D, Pfander H J 1984 Wolfe Medical, London

Head and neck pain

HEADACHE

Although only two or three patients a week may present in the A & E department complaining primarily of headache they are often a disproportionate source of concern. This is because, while the majority of the causative lesions are relatively trivial and the patient can be managed at home, in a few patients the headache heralds a life-threatening emergency necessitating urgent admission to hospital. The causes of headache presenting at the A & E department are shown in Table 17.1, the more common being listed first.

Table 17.1 Causes of headache (Modified from Lance J W 1982 Mechanism and management of headache. 4th edn. Butterworth Scientific, London).

Post-traumatic headaches (see Ch. 40)

Migraine and cluster headaches (migrainous neuralgia)

Tension

Combined tension-vascular headache

Other psychogenic causes
Depressive, conversion and hypochondriacal states

Intracranial vasodilatation
Fever, postalcoholic excess, hypoxia, hypercapnia, hypoglycaemia, carbon monoxide poisoning, certain foodstuffs (e.g. monosodium glutamate — the 'Chinese restaurant syndrome') and various drugs (e.g. nitrates)

Meningeal irrigation due to subarachnoid haemorrhage or meningoencephalitis

Postictal headache

Referred pain from the eyes, ears, sinuses, throat, teeth, neck and temporomandibular joints

Intracranial space occupying lesions — tumours, haematomata or abscesses

Cranial arteritis

Cranial nerve pain due to compression or inflammation — tumours, aneurysms, trigeminal and postherpetic neuralgia. Atypical facial pain

Miscellaneous
Hypertension
Exertional and cough headache
Hydrocephalus
Cerebral oedema, e.g. acute nephritis
Local scalp and skull lesions

History

In the majority of patients with headache the history is much more important than the physical examination, which is often completely normal. This may even be so in the early stages of conditions such as meningitis, encephalitis and subarachnoid haemorrhage. The history must therefore be recorded in a systematic fashion, asking each patient the same set of questions in the same sequence. Patterns of headache will then often emerge enabling a diagnosis to be made. The following information should be recorded in every case.

1. Age and sex
2. Presentation
3. Age of onset of headaches
4. Frequency and duration
5. Site, radiation, quality and severity
6. Time and mode of onset
7. Premonitory and prodromal symptoms
8. Associated symptoms
9. Precipitating, aggravating and relieving factors
10. Medication, present and past
11. General health (system review)
12. Past medical history
13. Family history
14. Social and personal history.

It is also worth asking patients:

1. Their ideas of the cause of the pain — headache often provokes intense fear of serious disease.

2. What made them visit hospital at that particular time? The latter question is specially relevant to patients who have had headaches for many years. For instance, there may have been a recent change of pattern or a bout of intercurrent depression.

Young children often pose a difficult diagnostic problem because they may not complain of headache but just cry.

Examination

Although the examination of a patient complaining of headaches is often unhelpful, it is important to establish this fact. While the examination is concentrated on the head and neck, a careful general examination, including the vital signs, must never be omitted. There are a few points in this examination worth emphasising.

The general appearance and demeanour of the patient should be noted. Restless movements and rhythmic contractions of facial musculature betray the tense, anxious individual. Hysterical patients may describe severe headaches with a winning smile on their faces, although hysteria is an exceedingly unsafe diagnosis to make on first meeting a patient in the A & E department. The patient with migraine is often pale with suffused conjunctivae and cranial arterial pulsation may be greater on the affected side. With cluster headaches the forehead may be flushed and the conjunctival vessels dilated only on the side of the headache. The affected eye is often streaming with tears and may exhibit a partial Horner's syndrome. The pain of muscle contraction headache is accentuated by movement of the muscle and often relieved by heat, cold or analgesics.

Palpation and auscultation of the skull and eyelids should not be overlooked. It may reveal tumours, infection, bruits or, in the elderly, the thickened, tender arteries of giant cell arteritis. In infants, the fontanelles should be palpated and the head circumference measured and compared to the normal range for children of the same age and height.

The patient's mental state should be assessed and each cranial nerve examined in turn, paying particular attention to the special senses. Many patients with brain tumours, especially children, have neurological signs at the time of diagnosis (e.g. ataxia, head tilt, pupillary abnormalities, oculomotor pareses and papilloedema). The optic fundi and ear-drums must be examined and the cervical spine tested for tenderness and mobility. Since the signs of meningeal irritation may not appear for several hours after a subarachnoid haemorrhage, this diagnosis should not be dismissed even if neck stiffness is absent. Finally, after a full general examination, the patient should be asked to stand and then walk a few steps so that his balance and gait may be observed. The motor ability of children should be related to their age and previous performance.

The duration and periodicity of a headache provide the most important clues as to the seriousness or otherwise of their nature and may be discussed under three headings.

Severe headaches of sudden onset

Severe headaches of sudden onset suggest either a subarachnoid haemorrhage, meningitis or encephalitis. Meningitis can be just as dramatic in its onset as a subarachnoid haemorrhage. Focal neurological signs may occur with either condition but many patients remain ambulant and this should not deceive the doctor.

1. *Subarachnoid haemorrhage*

Eighty per cent of these patients are over 40. There may be a history of hypertension, polycystic kidneys or coarctation of the aorta. Forewarning localised headaches or episodes of diplopia may

have occurred. The classical onset is characterised by a sudden, violent headache described as like 'a blow to the head', 'a terrible bursting sensation' or 'the worst headache I've ever experienced'. Some patients, however, describe their headache as mild. Initially the pain may be frontal or occipital but soon becomes generalised. Consciousness may be unimpaired or the patient may be rendered instantly comatose. More usually there is a short period of unconsciousness. Vomiting is common in the early stages. Patients may also complain of pain on moving their head, pain and stiffness in their neck, dizziness, diplopia and photophobia. Atypical manifestations such as chest pain, back pain, leg pain, blindness or sudden hearing loss may also occur.

The patient is often fully conscious but is resentful of being questioned or disturbed in any way. There may or may not be neck stiffness, impairment of consciousness or focal cranial nerve pareses, most commonly of the oculomotor nerves. Subhyaloid haemorrhages may be seen in the fundi.

Management.   If a subarachnoid haemorrhage is suspected, the regional neurosurgical unit should be contacted immediately and many centres will admit such patients directly. In ideal circumstances computed tomography should be the primary investigation. While the patient is in the A & E department the vital signs and neurological status should be monitored frequently, paying particular attention to the blood pressure. Short periods of hypertension may herald recurrent haemorrhage and should be controlled by elevating the head of the trolley. The neurologist may also advise the use of oral propranolol or nifedipine to control the blood pressure. The aim should be to keep the systolic pressure between 120–160 mmHg and the diastolic pressure under 100 mmHg. The ECG should be monitored and 100% oxygen administered by mask or nasal cannulae. Codeine phosphate can be given for pain and intravenous diazepam may be required for fits. Patients with impaired consciousness in whom cerebral oedema is likely should be given intravenous dexamethasone (adult dose 10 mg). The use of antifibrinolytic agents and the newer calcium channel blocking agents should be left to the specialists undertaking the patient's definitive management.

2. *Meningitis* (see also Ch. 25).

Often there is a prodrome of general malaise, perhaps associated with an upper respiratory tract or middle ear infection. Meningeal invasion is signified by severe generalised headache, a high fever, vomiting and drowsiness. The patient is often confused and delirious. Photophobia and neck stiffness are common but will not be evident if the patient is comatose or very young. Fits and cranial nerve palsies may occur. In very young children the signs are non-specific and include irritability, general lethargy, feeding difficulties and vomiting. A bulging fontanelle is a late occurrence. Meningococcal meningitis may be epidemic and the presence of a generalised purpuric rash indicates septicaemia.

Management.   Immediate hospital admission should be arranged. Lumbar puncture never needs to be carried out in the

A & E department. Patients with meningitis, especially those with septicaemia, should not be transferred from one hospital to another as they may die in the ambulance.

3. *Miscellaneous*

A severe headache may be a first attack of migraine. A bout of coughing can also produce severe headache. Patients with obstruction to the CSF pathways can also present with acute bilateral headache. All patients with severe headache of sudden onset should be admitted to hospital.

Intermediate

1. *Intracranial space-occupying lesions*

In this category are those patients who complain of progressively more painful headaches. The first priority in such cases is to identify the individual with an expanding intracranial mass. The characteristics of the headache associated with raised or rising intracranial pressure should be familiar to all doctors. The important points, in summary, are as follows:

> 1. Worse in the early morning and/or wakening the patient.
> 2. Increasing in frequency and severity and/or changing in character.
> 3. Exacerbated by stooping, coughing, sneezing or straining at stool.
> 4. Accompanied by vomiting without preceding nausea.
> 5. May be associated with other neurological features: for example, visual disturbances, unsteadiness, paraesthesiae, altered consciousness, drop attacks, convulsions, cranial nerve palsies, hemiparesis, papilloedema and personality or behavioural changes (in children a change in school performance).

The site of the headache may help in the location of the brain lesion. Unilateral headaches are usually on the side of the pathology. Tumours of the posterior fossa cause occipital headaches and local tenderness. In contradistinction, supratentorial tumours cause frontoparietal headaches, but only before intracranial pressure rises, after which the headaches become generalised.

Management.   All should be referred for urgent neurological investigation.

2. *Cranial (giant-cell or temporal) arteritis*

This is an important cause of headaches in the older patient. It is a diagnosis which must not be missed because early treatment with corticosteroids may prevent blindness in one or both eyes. The headaches have a severe aching, boring or throbbing quality, may be generalised or restricted to the frontal, temporal or occipital regions and are often worse at night. The scalp arteries are often tender and swollen and may have reduced or absent pulses.

Claudication of the jaw muscles is virtually pathognomonic, but uncommon. Diplopia may also occur but sudden visual loss due to ischaemia of the optic nerve is the most dramatic presentation. About a quarter of patients with giant-cell arteritis have polymyalgia rheumatica which causes general malaise, loss of weight, night sweats and aching and stiffness in the proximal muscles of the limbs. The ESR is usually above 40 mm per hour.

Immediate hospital admission is indicated. Oral prednisolone (20 mg) should be given in the A & E department while waiting for the ESR result. Treatment is particularly urgent if the sight in one eye has been lost. Occasionally, treatment will reverse near blindness but total loss of vision is invariably permanent.

3. *Chronic subdural haematomata*

In the elderly this may be easily missed because the headache is masked by other non-specific symptoms such as personality changes or drowsiness. The initiating injury can be very trivial. The relevant investigations are discussed on p. 221.

4. *Tuberculous meningitis*

Tuberculous meningitis is suggested by an indolent illness with headache, fever, malaise and eventual cranial nerve involvement. The patient may have miliary tuberculosis (see Ch. 25).

A history of many years duration

This suggests a benign cause ('A headache of more than one year's duration without physical signs is not due to a structural lesion' — Sir Charles Symonds). In a considerable number of patients with longstanding headache the consultation is precipitated by underlying depression and/or anxiety. Beware of the patient whose headaches have changed in quality, frequency or pattern. Most chronic headaches are either migraine, tension headache, muscle contraction headache, or a combination of these. Headaches with a vascular component have a throbbing quality made worse by sudden jolts, coughing, sneezing or straining. The majority of these patients should be referred back to their general practitioners for their initial management. The family doctor is usually in the best position to decide if specialist advice should be sought. It is virtually never appropriate to start investigations in the A & E department.

Migraine

Migraine sufferers tend to have premonitory symptoms, prodromes (auras) and periodicity which are constant for that individual (classic migraine). However, isolated and first attacks can cause diagnostic difficulties. Premonitory symptoms which may precede the headache by up to 24 hours include an elevated or depressed mood, overactivity or drowsiness and unnatural thirst or hunger. The aura immediately preceding the headache may include visual hallucinations (e.g. scintillating lights, fortification spectra or object distortion), scotomata, hemianopias, paraesthesiae and, rarely, pareses or dysphasia. The headaches often occur in the period of relaxation following intense stress and in women the bouts may be linked to menstruation or associated with starting the contraceptive pill. A variety of other trigger factors are also thought capable of precipitating migraine in susceptible subjects, e.g. fatigue, exercise, head injury, changes in the weather, bright lights, irregular meals, certain foodstuffs and alcohol. Attacks are usually over in a few hours but may last several days. In three-quarters of cases the throbbing headaches are unilateral and photophobia, phonophobia, nausea, vomiting, shivering and facial pallor are common accompaniments. Typical headache without an aura is the commonest type (common migraine). Hemiplegic migraine is inherited in an autosomal dominant mode. Vertebrobasilar migraine occurs mainly in adolescent girls in whom visual disturbance, ataxia, dysarthria, vertigo, tinnitus and peripheral dysaesthesiae are followed by occipital headache. Occasionally a focal neurological deficit lasts for more than 24 hours after the headache (complicated migraine). Once the headache is past most people just want to sleep and many awaken totally refreshed. About 40% of migraine sufferers are also subject to sudden jabbing pains ('icepick pains') in the head, whether or not they have their characteristic headache at the time. It is rare for patients to experience a first attack of migraine over the age of 45 unless they are hypertensive. In this context it should be remembered that migraine may be secondary to an underlying structural cause such as a cerebral tumour (symptomatic migraine). Migraine is quite a common condition in children, sometimes associated with cyclical vomiting. Many migraine sufferers also have a history of hay fever, asthma or skin rashes, and a family history of the disorder is often found.

Some patients with classic migraine complain that their headaches have persisted for several days or weeks and are getting worse. In such cases ergotamine toxicity should be considered.

Cluster headaches (migrainous neuralgia)

These have a different periodicity from migraine and are considerably less common. More than three-quarters of patients are male and the peak age of onset is in the twenties. The headaches recur in bouts lasting from a fortnight to three months with intervals of total freedom maintained for several months or years. The attacks often wake the patient at night and may return up to three times in 24 hours, lasting from 10 minutes to 2 hours on each occasion. Pain felt deeply in and around the eye is typical and the symptoms and signs are unilateral. The pain is particularly distressing and accompanying nausea occurs in about half of those affected. Physical signs include facial flushing and hyperalgesia, prominence and tenderness of the temporal artery, conjunctival injection, streaming eye, drooping eyelid (which may progress to a complete Horner's syndrome) and nasal irritation or blockage. Alcoholic drinks may precipitate the headache during clusters and some relief may be obtained by the application of heat or pressure to the affected eye and temple. The pain can be so severe that the patient faints. Facial migraine is easily differentiated because, in these patients, the attacks last several hours and other features of classic migraine are usually present.

Management. Most of these patients can be referred back to their family practitioners after appropriate symptomatic treatment. Only when the diagnosis is unclear do they need referral to a specialist. They should be reassured that they do not have a life-threatening disease and advised to avoid recognisable precipitants as far as possible. Women taking the contraceptive pill should stop it. Often simple analgesics such as aspirin or paracetamol are all that are necessary, combined with oral or intramuscular metoclopramide if nausea and vomiting is a problem. Prochlorperazime suppositories should be substituted for metoclopramide in children. If a stronger analgesic is required mefenamic acid is worth trying. For particularly severe attacks of migraine or cluster headaches ergotamine tartrate is the drug of choice. It can be given as a tablet, by aerosol or by suppository and the dose should not exceed 1–2 mg per attack. It is most effective when used prophylactically. Occasionally rebreathing from a paper bag will abort an attack. Patients with mixed tension-vascular headaches may require both a tranquilliser or an antidepressant, and an antimigraine preparation.

Tension and 'psychogenic' headaches

Typical tension headaches may be episodic at first when related to particular stressful events, but they often become chronic, the sufferer being rarely free from background headache. The ache is symmetrical, bitemporal, frontal and/or occipital and often likened to a tightness, a band or a vice gripping the head, or a pressure, like a weight on top of the head. There is no vomiting, blurring of vision or focal neurological symptoms and the pain rarely interferes with daily work, although children frequently miss school. Sufferers tend to be anxious individuals and the headaches are exacerbated during periods of mental stress. Many have signs of 'primary' muscle overcontraction with excessive frowning, clenching or grinding of the teeth and restless hand movements. Additional symptoms, such as pain in the abdomen or limbs, are common. Tension headaches are commonly improved by taking alcohol whereas chronic vascular headaches are almost always made worse.

Headaches are a common symptom of depression. In general, unusual descriptions and exaggerated similes suggest a psychogenic origin (see Ch. 31). In children there may be other evidence of psychiatric disturbance, such as disruptive behaviour or destruction of property.

Muscle-contraction headaches

These are due to muscle spasm adjacent to a painful site, such as an impacted wisdom tooth or dysfunctional temporomandibular joint.

Mixed types

Tension, 'psychogenic' and muscle-contraction headaches tend to form a continuum with a variable aetiological input in each patient. For instance, there may be a background tension headache punctuated by migrainous exacerbations. It is important to recognise both aspects because each requires separate treatment.

Management.   The background information available to the general practitioner is invaluable in the management of these patients. For example, he may be aware that a friend or relative of the patient has recently had a brain tumour diagnosed which has aroused fears in the patient's mind. Tension headaches respond poorly, if at all, to analgesics but may be helped by relaxation therapy. Underlying anxiety and depression may require specific treatment. Muscle-contraction headaches are usually relieved by treating the underlying cause.

Trigeminal neuralgia ('tic doloureux')

Trigeminal neuralgia typically occurs in the older patient and is characterised by repetitive, fleeting jabs of severe pain, usually affecting the sensory distribution of the mandibular or maxillary branches of the fifth cranial nerve. Women are affected twice as often as men and again the pain is unilateral. Initially the attacks are self-limiting and occur in clusters lasting days or weeks. There may be years of freedom between attacks but there is a tendency for the episodes to become progressively worse in frequency and severity. The pain may be precipitated by talking, eating, drinking, extremes of temperature or touching the face or gums (trigger points) when shaving or cleaning the teeth. When tic doloureux occurs in a young person, or there is sensory loss over the face, an underlying condition such as multiple sclerosis should be suspected.

Management.   The patient can be started on carbamazepine 100 mg twice or three times daily and referred to a neurologist.

Finally, one of the commonest causes of chronic recurrent headache is injury to the head. This and other aspects of the postconcussional syndrome are fully described in Ch. 40.

Investigations

Very few patients with headache require any investigation in the A & E department beyond a careful history and physical examination. The longer the headaches have been present without change in character or the development of abnormal physical signs, the less likely a serious intracranial disorder becomes. Referral for specialist neurological investigation mainly arises when there is diagnostic difficulty or the suggestion of a serious disorder. Specialist referral should usually be arranged by the patient's general practitioner.

Plain radiographs of the skull

Among groups of patients with headaches the yield of abnormal skull films is less than 5%. However, skull radiographs should be obtained in patients with clinical evidence of raised intracranial pressure or progressive neurological signs. A cerebral tumour or subdural haematoma are the likely causes. A chest X-ray should be taken at the same time to identify any primary pulmonary pathology. Abnormalities that may be seen on plain skull films include pathological calcification (Fig. 17.1), displacement of the pineal gland (Fig. 17.2), bony erosion (Fig. 17.3) or sclerosis (Fig. 17.4), pressure changes in the sella turcica (Fig. 17.5) or separation of the sutures in children (see Fig. 26.1, p. 282). If the lateral view shows a calcified pineal gland, a straight anteroposterior projection will show whether there is significant displacement of midline structures (i.e. 2–3 mm).

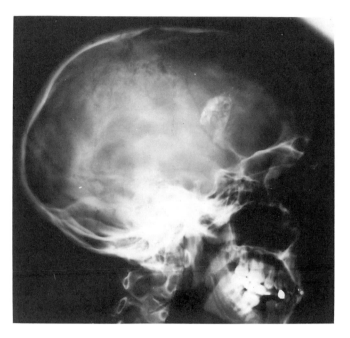

Fig. 17.1 A calcified tumour.

Apparently trivial head injuries may cause subdural haematomata, especially among the elderly. If there is any suspicion of trauma, both right and left lateral, anteroposterior and posteroanterior skull views must be taken and the films examined minutely for hairline fractures. 'Midline shift' may not occur with bilateral haematomata. Chronic subdural haematomata sometimes calcify. Aneurysms and arteriovenous malformations, which are potentially remediable causes of intracranial bleeding, may also calcify or cause abnormal bony vascular channels. Additional views (which will include Towne's view) should be requested if pathology in the nasal sinuses or facial bones is suspected.

Although negative radiographic findings may be as important as positive ones, progression to more specialised investigations should be based mainly on clinical judgement. A normal skull film in no way rules out the presence of raised intracranial pressure, a tumour or an aneurysm.

The taking of skull radiographs should never be used solely for reassurance of the patient.

Blood tests

Patients over 50 with headaches should always have their erythrocyte sedimentation rate (ESR) estimated. Significant

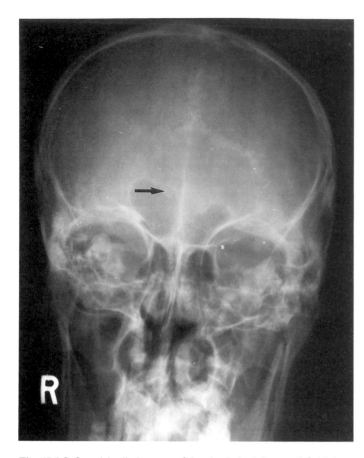

Fig. 17.2 Left to right displacement of the pineal gland due to a left-sided subdural haematoma.

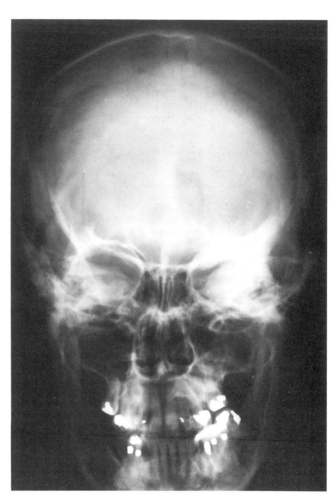

Fig. 17.4 Bony sclerosis associated with a sphenoidal ridge meningioma.

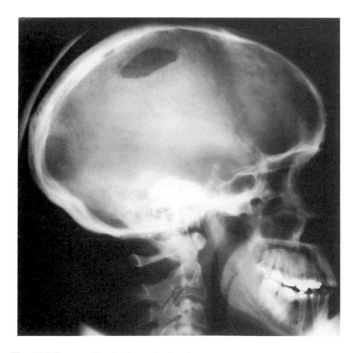

Fig. 17.3 Bony erosion in the parietal region.

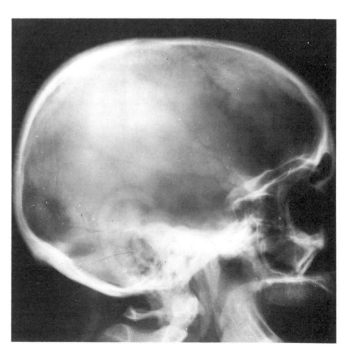

Fig. 17.5 Erosion of the floor of the pituitary fossa and the posterior clinoids caused by increased intracranial pressure.

elevation (greater than 40 mm per hour) indicates the need for hospital admission for further investigation. Apart from cranial arteritis, such elevation may draw attention to occult malignancy (e.g. multiple myeloma), a hidden focus of infection, or autoimmune disease.

All patients with significant headache should also have a full blood count. Leukaemia may present with intracranial deposits and anaemia may indicate neoplasia or other generalised disease. If septicaemia is suspected blood cultures are essential.

Echoencephalography

This is of value in the display of 'midline shift' and is also useful for the rapid assessment of patients with suspected intracranial haematomata. It is not an investigation for the occasional user: regular practice is necessary in order to obtain reliable information.

Lumbar puncture, electroencephalography, angiography, isotope, CT and MR imaging.

Apart from CT scanning, these investigations are inappropriate to the A & E department. The selection of the most suitable specialised investigation is normally the prerogative of a neurologist or neurosurgeon.

Summary

The following groups of patients should be admitted to hospital immediately:

> 1. Those complaining of severe headache of sudden onset especially if there is no past history of similar attacks.
> 2. Any patient who complains of headache in whom abnormal neurological signs, including drowsiness, or evidence of meningeal irritation are found, however minimal.
> 3. Patients suspected of having cranial arteritis.

The groups of patients listed below should be referred to a neurologist or paediatrician either directly or via the patient's general practitioner.

> 1. Those whose longstanding headache has changed its pattern and increased in frequency or severity.
> 2. Nocturnal or early morning headache especially if the history is less than 6 months.
> 3. Very severe headaches.
> 4. Fits or other neurological abnormalities with or after the headache.
> 5. Recent behavioural change or school failure.
> 6. Age less than 5 years.

NECK PAIN

Acute infective conditions of the throat (viz. tonsillitis, quinsy and retropharyngeal abscess) are described in Chapter 44, 'whip lash' injuries in Chapter 41 and the pain and stiffness accompanying meningitis and subarachnoid haemorrhage have already been dealt with in this chapter.

Wry neck

Wry neck is a benign, self-limiting condition of unknown aetiology. It should not be confused with the chronic recurrent disorder known as spasmodic torticollis which is a focal dystonia (see Ch. 26), nor with the acute dystonic reaction which may be precipitated by phenothiazines, butyrophenones or metoclopramide. The classical patient with wry neck awakes with pain, often severe, down one side of his/her neck, having been totally pain free going to bed the previous evening. On examination the chin points to one or other shoulder and is slightly uptilted. The muscles on one side of the neck are in spasm and any movement of the head to the opposite side causes more severe pain. An identifiable underlying cause is unusual. Immediate physiotherapy, with or without heat, and massage should be arranged. The patient should be encouraged to move his head actively, gradually increasing the range of movement, within the limits of bearable pain. Many patients are relieved by a single session of this treatment. If severe pain persists they can be given a soft surgical collar and the procedure repeated in 2–3 days time.

Torticollis occasionally develops secondary to an acute cervical disc prolapse, inflamed cervical lymph nodes, vertebral tuberculosis, ocular disorders or injuries of the cervical spine (see Ch. 41).

Cervical spondylosis

This is the commonest disorder of the cervical spine and most patients are over 50. The onset of pain may be spontaneous or initiated by an accident. Usually the onset is gradual and the pain is often worse at night and on first getting up. The area of pain referral is rarely limited to one dermatome and can be surprisingly wide. It may include the shoulders, arms, upper chest and back, occiput and even the face. Often the patient only complains of the referred pain. Burning and tingling sensations are also common but muscle weakness is rare.

The range of movements of the neck should be recorded and a full neurological examination carried out, paying particular attention to the arms. Some diminution of appreciation of light touch and pin prick may be found in the dermatomes of the affected radicular nerves.

Plain radiographs of the cervical spine may show narrowing and irregularity of the intervertebral spaces, sclerosis and/or cystic changes in the adjoining vertebral bodies and osteophyte formation (Fig. 17.6). However, radiographs are often unhelpful as many asymptomatic patients in this age group have spondylotic changes and patients with severe symptoms can have remarkably normal-looking films. Therefore, initially, the diagnosis should be clinically

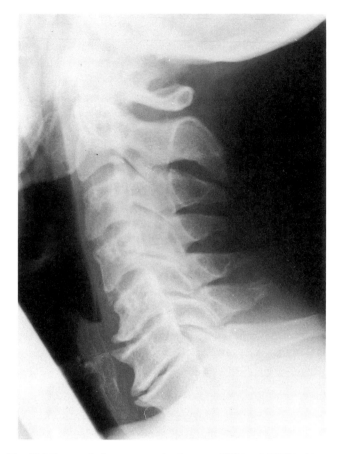

Fig. 17.6 Intervertebral space narrowing between C5/C6 and C6/C7 with prominent degenerative changes.

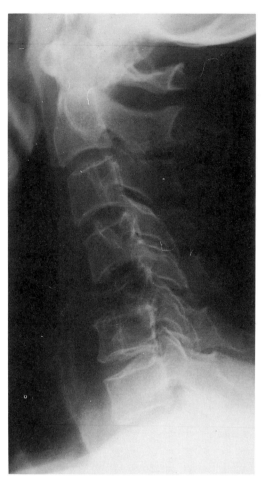

Fig. 17.7 Destruction of the body of C5 due to a secondary tumour.

based. Two to three weeks rest in a soft surgical collar plus appropriate analgesia helps the majority of sufferers. A non-steroidal anti-inflammatory agent is often the best drug. Then they can wean themselves off the collar and start neck exercises. If there has been no improvement, referral to an orthopaedic, neurological or physical medicine clinic should be arranged. In some instances persistent root pain is caused by a *prolapsed cervical disc* which can be the consequence of a relatively trivial event, e.g. the patient stretching on waking. It is totally inappropriate to follow up these patients in an A & E department.

Radiology of the cervical spine should always be carried out if neck pain has been constant and of increasing severity, especially if there are severe root pains which may indicate vertebral collapse. Marked neurological abnormalities in the arms, legs or cranial nerves are other indications. Such symptoms and signs may be produced by very rare primary tumours of the vertebrae (e.g. sarcomas, myelomas and osteomas) or by secondary deposits, the most common primary sites being the breast, thyroid, prostate or lung. Tumours produce either osteolytic (Fig. 17.7) or, more rarely, osteosclerotic changes in the vertebral bodies. Other rare causes of severe neck pain are tuberculous osteitis (Pott's disease), osteitis deformans (Paget's disease), intramedullary and extramedullary spinal tumours. Spinal compression causes considerable pain in the neck and occiput which is intensified by any movement of the cervical spine. Pain, paraesthesiae and weakness in the arms occur early. There may be muscle wasting. If the tumour extends upwards through the foramen magnum the lower cranial nerves may be affected. Sensation is often impaired in the arms and there may be signs of corticospinal tract compression in both upper and lower limbs.

These patients all require admission to hospital for urgent neurological investigation.

Glossopharyngeal neuralgia (see also Ch. 44)

This condition is much rarer than trigeminal neuralgia but shares similar general characteristics. The brief attacks of severe unilateral pain usually begin in the side of the throat and radiate in front of the ear and behind the mandible. They are often precipitated by swallowing or by protruding the tongue, and the ear may be hyperaesthetic. Similar pain may be caused by nasopharyngeal tumours. These patients should be referred to a neurologist. Carbamazepine can be prescribed as for tic doloureux.

Carotidynia

Carotidynia is a syndrome of neck pain associated with tenderness over the carotid artery. In one type, affecting youngish adults, the pain is of acute onset and lasts about two weeks. The patient may complain of other symptoms suggestive of a viral infection. Treatment is symptomatic. Another type is recurrent and may be related to migraine as it responds to ergotamine or migraine prophylactics. Occasionally pain along the artery is caused by cranial arteritis or a dissecting aneurysm.

Rheumatoid arthritis

Atlantoaxial subluxation can occur in rheumatoid arthritis, especially in those patients with severe peripheral joint disease. Suggestive symptoms are high cervical pain made worse by neck movements, which may radiate to the occiput, temples or behind the eyes. Some patients complain of a 'clunking' sensation when they nod their heads. Compression of the spinal cord may produce shooting pains in the arms and legs, limb weakness, sphincter

disturbances or, in the worst cases, complete quadriplegia. Patients are at special risk during general anaesthesia when normal protective reflexes are lost. Therefore any patient with severe rheumatoid disease who requires a general anaesthetic should have radiographs of the cervical spine taken in flexion and extension and the anaesthetist warned if there is any instability.

Similar atlantoaxial instability may also occur in patients with Down's syndrome.

Other referred neck pain

Pain in the throat and lower jaw brought on by exertion suggests angina and the necessity for an ECG recording. There may be no accompanying chest pain.

Occasionally disease processes in contact with central parts of the diaphragm cause pain referred to the neck.

FURTHER READING

Migraine: clinical, therapeutic, conceptual and research aspects Blau J N 1987 Chapman and Hall, London

Neck and arm pain 2nd edn. Cailliet R 1981 Davis, Philadelphia

Wolff's headache and other head pain Dalessio D J 1980 Oxford University Press, New York

Mechanism and management of headache 4th edn. Lance J W 1982 Butterworth Scientific, London

Migraine and its variants Selby G 1983 ADIS Health Science Press, Sydney

18

Anthony D. Redmond

Chest pain

INTRODUCTION

Dr Asher once asked an audience of eminent physicians whether they had ever experienced sharp shooting pains over the heart. The majority of his listeners confessed to this experience but no-one could offer a diagnosis. There was little concern about this, however, because the absence of a diagnosis did not preclude the possibility of a prognosis — which was excellent. In assessing any patient in the A & E department, but particularly those complaining of chest pain, it is this immediate short-term prognosis or element of risk which is important to establish. This can be determined firstly from the history and then from the clinical examination. Investigations in the A & E department may be used to support these findings but not to refute them.

'Chest pain' is often synonymous with ischaemic heart disease in the minds of A & E department staff. Conversely a patient who is described as having a 'pain in the chest' may be thought to have a more benign condition. This is an inherent danger of labels.

The reason of course why 'chest pain' assumes such a degree of significance is its close relationship to ischaemic heart disease and the prevalence of this disease. Approximately 1 in 4 of *all* deaths in the United Kingdom are due to ischaemic heart disease. It is a bigger killer than cancer. Furthermore, the majority of deaths from cancer occur in the older age groups whereas deaths from IHD often affect younger people. These statistics are shared with other western countries, although many have achieved a greater success in reducing this horrendous mortality. In addition to the knowledge that ischaemic heart disease is common, the fact that death is often sudden and unforeseen places the isolated casualty officer in a position of insecurity. This can be relieved to some extent if all cases of 'chest pain' are assessed according to a protocol and allowed home only if 'positive' discharge criteria are fulfilled. Although ischaemic heart disease is common, it is not the only cause of chest pain and other diagnoses must always be considered.

ISCHAEMIC HEART DISEASE

The present epidemic of ischaemic heart disease in the western world appears to have peaked and even fallen in some countries, though noticeably not in the UK. The disease is thought to be largely preventable although any measures taken now will be for the benefit of future generations as the disease appears to be established in early adult life. The risk factors are listed below:
1. Family history/ageing/male
2. Smoking
3. Hypertension
4. Diet (serum cholesterol)
5. 'Stress'
6. Lack of exercise/obesity
7. Diabetes
8. Hyperlipidaemia

It can be seen that the greatest — family history, ageing and gender — cannot be changed. The remainder can be controlled and in countries where this has been done the mortality from IHD has been reduced. The exact relationship between some risk factors and IHD is not clear. Obesity may place a person at risk because of its association with hypertension and lack of exercise. The relationship between the disease and the patient's general lifestyle is more clear. Personality and, in particular, the ambitious restless 'type A' person is thought to have an increased risk of the disease. 'Stress' is often quoted but it is important to appreciate what is truly stress.

It is not merely the presence of a problem which is stressful — this may in fact be stimulating, — it is the inability to solve it that is stressful. Problems occur at all levels in society but it is the most socially disadvantaged that are least likely to solve them. This is reflected in the changing social pattern of disease. Moreover, other risk factors are also class-related, smoking and poor diet for example, and IHD is now tending towards being a disease of the poor people of rich countries.

Smoking is the most obvious avoidable risk factor and is absolutely preventable. Members of the medical and nursing professions who smoke must question the effect this positive advertising has on their patients.

Hypertension — the 'silent killer' — is all too often undiagnosed.

The A & E department has a large part to play in informing its patients of their blood pressure and the family doctor of any abnormal readings.

Regular moderate exercise can serve to protect the heart. It is true that, while exercising, the risk of sudden death is increased. However, the overall risk of sudden death is far greater in those who never exercise.

Assessment

It is a wise precaution to ensure that a patient complaining of chest pain is assessed in an area that contains all the facilities for resuscitation. If the patient is clearly distressed and obviously ill then administer 100% oxygen and establish venous access prior to a full assessment. Give analgesia early and ensure the patient is continuously monitored.

Establish the site of the pain and if it is referred anywhere. Ask the patient to describe it in his own words. Is it continuous or intermittent? Is it affected by respiration? Has he experienced this pain before? Are there any associated symptoms? The duration of the pain is very important, as is the effect of any medication.

An examination of the patient must include the abdomen as pain in the chest can sometimes be a referred pain. When feeling the pulses ensure that they are synchronous and all peripheral pulses are present. A dissecting aneurysm has first to be considered before it can be diagnosed.

Investigations must always include an ECG, chest X-ray and blood glucose. If the patient is breathless then measure the blood gases. 'Clinical' parameters of improvement do not accurately reflect true physiological status. The efficacy of treatment should be measured and a demonstrable improvement in blood gases is one such measurement.

A patient with chest pain can only be allowed home if he fulfills *all* of the following criteria:

1. The pain is not of an ischaemic nature.
2. He is no longer in pain and feels well.
3. The pain lasted for less than 20 minutes.
4. Physical examination is normal.
5. The ECG is normal, or any changes thought to be 'old' have been confirmed as such by reference to a previous ECG.
6. The chest radiograph is normal.

The conditions giving rise to chest pain which may commonly present to western A & E departments are outlined below. The most important task for the A & E department is usually to distinguish cardiac from non-cardiac pain.

Myocardial infarction can also present without pain. 'Silent' or painless infarction may precipitate dyspnoea, dysrhythmias, syncope and emboli. Occasionally it is an incidental ECG finding. Painless infarction is more common in diabetics and hypertensives and in the presence of atrial fibrillation. Negroes and elderly patients are also more susceptible, as is anyone in the perioperative period. Clearly in some cases, diseases of the autonomic nervous system can be implicated (e.g. diabetes) but generally the reasons for painless infarction are not clearly understood.

Cardiac pain

Myocardial ischaemia produces a characteristic pain in the chest. It is central and retrosternal. It is often described as gripping in nature and the patient may clench his fist over his sternum as he describes it. The pain can be referred to the neck, the jaw and down either arm. It is sometimes associated with tingling in the fingers. Many variations occur and sometimes the site of referral is the dominant pain, e.g. severe pain in the arm as the sole feature of myocardial ischaemia.

When ischaemic pain is not associated with muscle damage then the term *angina* is used. Great care must be exercised in making this diagnosis in the A & E department. It is wise only to confirm the diagnosis in those already known to suffer with the condition rather than make the original diagnosis in the emergency setting. *Stable angina* is predictable and therefore avoidable. It is relieved by nitrates. Occasionally a patient may present to the A & E department following an attack of his 'usual' angina. However, even if the quality of the pain was the same as previous attacks if the duration of pain was more than 20 minutes then the angina must be assumed to be *unstable*. Similarly if the quality of the pain has altered, or it has been precipitated by an unusual event, or come on spontaneously then consider a diagnosis of *unstable angina*. Refer such patients for a medical opinion.

The ECG may show ST segment depression and T wave inversion during an attack of angina. However, such 'ischaemic' changes may also occur during the early stages of a myocardial infarction. Any decision about patient management must be based on the history and physical examination and not solely on the ECG tracing. Similarly, although the patient may have 'old' changes on the ECG they may be in the prodromal phase of a new ischaemic episode which has not yet registered on the ECG.

Ischaemic pain can occur with spasm of the coronary arteries and in these circumstances may be associated with ST elevation — Prinzmetal's variant angina. The diagnosis is never made in the A & E department, but on the coronary care unit.

Central crushing chest pain, 'ischaemic' in nature, lasting 20 minutes or more must be considered to be a *myocardial infarction* until proven otherwise. This proof should be sought as an inpatient. Of those patients who suffer a myocardial infarction, 50% may die within three weeks of the attack. However, of those deaths, 50% will have occurred within the first one or two hours of pain. Many of these deaths will have followed an episode of ventricular fibrillation — a potentially reversible condition. The use of defibrillators by ambulance personnel and family doctors can prevent many of these deaths. Furthermore, the patient may still be in an unstable condition on arrival in the emergency department. There are some measures available to reduce the risk of cardiac arrest, but equally important the patient should be in a place where all the relevant treatment facilities and staff are available.

When the diagnosis of myocardial infarction is suspected then the patient should be placed in the resuscitation room with a doctor and senior nurse in attendance. The pain is very often accompanied by sweating and dyspnoea and the patient is usually very frightened.

The patient should be sat up, if this makes breathing easier, and given 100% oxygen through a face mask. There is some evidence that the early administration of oxygen may limit the degree of tissue damage. Venous access should be established and adequate analgesia given. Diamorphine 5 mg intravenously over two minutes is a good start but some patients may require more. It is usually necessary to give an antiemetic as well. The relief of pain and anxiety by the administration of adequate amounts of opiates may reduce the level of circulating catecholamines and thereby reduce the risk of ventricular fibrillation. It is also much appreciated by the patient. If too much narcotic is given it can always be reversed by naloxone 0.4–0.8 mg i.v. Oral or intramuscular analgesia has no place in the early management of myocardial infarction in the A & E department. A mixture of nitrous oxide and oxygen (Entonox) is a useful analgesic agent for use by ambulance personnel and the nitrous oxide may even promote coronary artery dilatation.

The presence of physical signs of heart failure is an important prognostic indicator and should be looked for as soon as possible. The patient may already have experienced dyspnoea, increasing fatigue and episodes of paroxysmal nocturnal dyspnoea. When chest pain is associated with left-sided heart failure sitting the patient up may relieve their orthopnoea. Pulmonary oedema may complicate myocardial infarction and should be rapidly recognised and treated. The jugular venous pulse rises as the

right heart fails. The normal slight fall in venous pressure on inspiration may be reversed and is known as Kussmaul's sign. Additional heart sounds and, in particular, a IVth heart sound are associated with heart failure and produce a 'gallop rhythm'. Bilateral fine basal crepitations are a feature of pulmonary oedema. They do not clear on coughing.

Congestive cardiac failure of some standing is associated with peripheral oedema. If the patient has been bedfast for a time then the oedema will be in the sacral area. The peripheral pitting oedema of heart failure is a late manifestation of sodium retention and not the result of increased venous pressure. Effusion into all the serous cavities can also occur.

One should look for signs of heart failure on a radiograph of the chest. The heart size may be enlarged on the PA view. On the erect film there may be features of increased pulmonary venous pressure with prominence of the upper lobe veins. Septal lines appear and a prominent 'bat's wing' hilum and parietal as well as pleural effusions may be seen.

The electrocardiograph must be recorded. The earliest signs of injury are inverted, symmetrically enlarged ('arrow-head') T waves. If the damage is confined to the subendocardial region then ST segment depression in those overlying leads will be seen. If subepicardial or transmural injury has occurred then ST segment elevation will be seen.

It may take several hours for a pathological 'Q' wave to form. Although the definitive electrocardiographic diagnosis of myocardial infarction rests on the demonstration of pathological 'Q' waves in limb leads other than III and aVR, the diagnosis cannot be excluded by their absence. Caution must always be

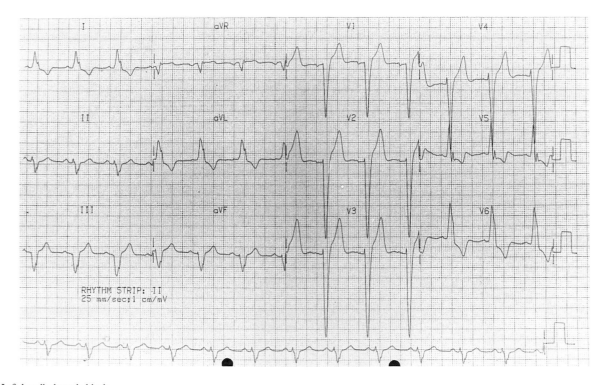

Fig. 18.1 Left bundle branch block.

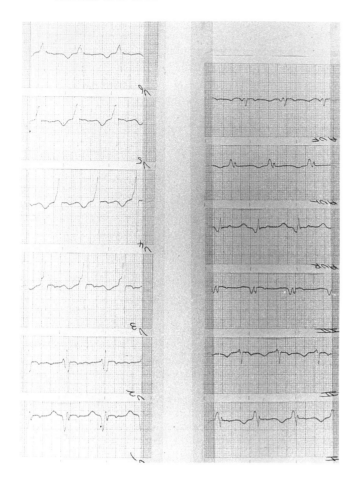

Fig. 18.2 Right bundle branch block.

exercised in a patient with left bundle branch block (LBBB). This can occur acutely in myocardial infarction and is associated with the absence of any 'Q' wave in leads I, aVL and V_4–V_6 (Figs. 18.1, 18.2). Hence the presence of LBBB precludes an ECG diagnosis of myocardial ischaemia, infarction or even ventricular hypertrophy.

The ECG in the A & E department may be of some help however to locate the site of the infarct and identify arrhythmias. Table 18.1 outlines relationships between changes described above in certain leads and the site of the injury. A true posterior infarction is recognised by reversed changes in V_1 and V_2. A tall 'R' wave and ST segment depression is a reversed image of a Q wave with

Table 18.1 Locating the infarct

Anterior (Fig. 18.3)	'V' leads	anteroseptal	V_1 – V_3
		anterior	V_2 – V_4
		anterolateral	V_4 – V_6 I, aVL
		extensive anterior	V_1 – V_6 I, aVL
Inferior (Fig. 18.4)	Limb leads II, III, aVF		
Posterior	V_1 – V_2		

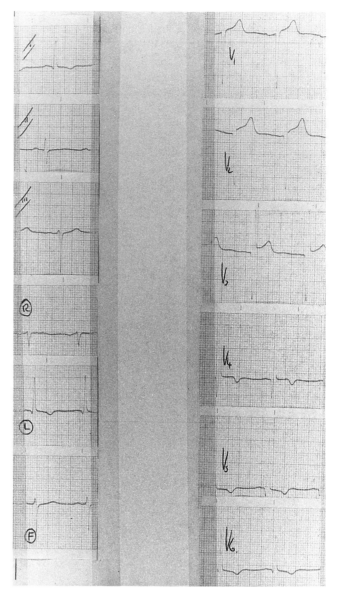

Fig. 18.3 Anteroseptal infarction.

ST segment elevation. A subendocardial infarction may occur at any site and be manifest in any lead. Changes in the anterior leads are reciprocated in the inferior leads and vice versa. For example, an anterior infarction with ST elevation in the 'V' leads may be associated with reciprocal ST depression in leads II, III and aVF.

Cardiogenic shock is said to occur when the cardiac output is low but the left ventricular filling pressure is normal. The disease process can involve left, right or both ventricles. Systemic arterial pressure falls and pulmonary arterial pressure rises. The management of such patients requires invasive monitoring, the insertion of pulmonary flotation catheters and the measurement of cardiac output.

Elective ventilation will secure optimal oxygenation and is an essential precursor of later therapeutic manoeuvres. Inotropic

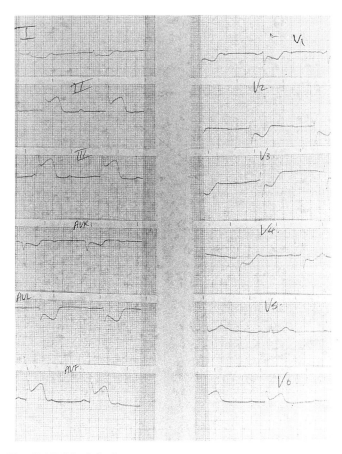

Fig. 18.4 Inferior infarction.

support and manipulation of the circulation with vasodilators, or fluid administration in some cases of right ventricular infarction, can improve survival, but invasive monitoring of the effects of such manoeuvres is mandatory. Rapid transfer to an appropriately staffed intensive care environment is therefore essential.

Right ventricular infarction. This condition is increasingly diagnosed as invasive haemodynamic monitoring becomes more widespread. It occurs most commonly after acute inferior infarction when disease of the right coronary artery produces significant right ventricular dysfunction with relative preservation of the left ventricle. The differential diagnosis includes massive pulmonary embolus, cardiac tamponade, constrictive pericarditis and septicaemia. The diagnosis is confirmed following the insertion of a pulmonary artery flotation catheter. The right atrial and right ventricular end diastolic pressures are high but the pulmonary capillary wedge pressure and cardiac output is normal or low.

Complications of acute myocardial infarction

An episode of ischaemia may be complicated by several phenomena which are listed below:

1. Dysrhythmias
2. Cardiac failure
3. Cardiogenic shock
4. Thromboembolism
5. Aneurysm
6. Pericarditis
7. Dressler's syndrome
8. Mitral regurgitation
9. Ventricular septal defect

These may also occur in the absence of ischaemic heart disease. Some of the more common conditions are discussed below.

ARRHYTHMIAS

The heart can be beating either too quickly, too slowly or at a normal rate. The condition of the patient will tell you how effective their heart rate is. The normal heart rate varies but usually lies within the range of 60–110 b.p.m. The mere presence of a condition is not an indication to treat it. The effect the condition is having on the patient now and any it might have, must first be assessed.

It is not only the heart rate that may be abnormal but the impulse generation and conduction may be disturbed. It is essential to locate the origin of the dysrhythmia anatomically if treatment is to be both effective and safe.

Too fast

A rapid heart rate (> 110 b.p.m.) is too fast if it produces signs or symptoms. 'Palpitations' may not require immediate intervention, but chest pain or hypotension will. It is rare for intervention in the emergency room to be more desirable than transfer to a specialised unit. However, if transfer cannot be arranged (unlikely) or transfer might be hazardous (more likely) then intervention should be considered if:

1. The patient is rapidly deteriorating (blood pressure falling, rhythm becoming more unstable, pain more severe).
2. Deterioration is likely.

Supraventricular tachycardias (SVT)

SVT can occur when an abnormally fast heart rate is produced by an abnormality within the atrium.

The commonest is *atrial fibrillation* (AF) and occurs when the atrium contracts at between 350–600 b.p.m. Such rapid shallow activity does not produce a 'P' wave but irregular 'fibrillation' waves may be seen, particularly in V_1. The A-V node can only conduct a proportion of this activity to the ventricles. The ventricular response is variable and random and determines the degree (if any) of circulatory impairment (Fig. 18.5). Atrial fibrillation can occur during an episode of ischaemia but is a feature of many other conditions, e.g. thyrotoxicosis. Any lesion within the chest can precipitate AF. Alcohol intoxication with or without an underlying

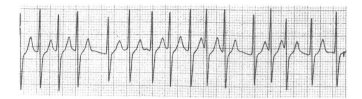

Fig. 18.5 Atrial fibrillation with rapid ventricular response.

cardiomyopathy can be associated with this dysrhythmia. Digitalis will slow the ventricular rate.

A rapid ventricular response may fail to produce an adequate cardiac output. Rapid transfer to a specialised unit is essential and definitive treatment is usually administered there. DC synchronous cardioversion is usually effective but relapse is common. Anaesthesia is essential, but in an emergency 10 mg of Diazepam intravenously can be used. In principle, the lowest effective voltage should be employed and most clinicians would start at 50 J, (proceeding with 50 J increments). Digitoxicity necessitates very low voltages (start at 5–10 J) if asystole is to be avoided. Intravenous Verapamil (5–10 mg over 30–60 s) can be given to slow the ventricular response. It is contraindicated if the patient has received an intravenous or oral beta blocker or is digitoxic, as profound bradycardia or asystole may ensue. Intravenous digoxin (0.5 mg) is often advocated but can precipitate serious bradyarrythmias.

It may of course be necessary to terminate the rhythm in the emergency department if the patient is deeply shocked and safe rapid transfer to a specialised unit cannot be effected.

If the atrial rate is slower at 250–350 b.p.m. then recognisable 'P' waves may be seen. The 'saw-tooth' pattern of *atrial flutter* is characteristic and such rates are usually associated with a regular ventricular response (Fig. 18.6). There is still a degree of block through the AV node and only a proportion of 'P' waves terminate in a QRS complex. Cardioversion at low voltages (25–50 J) is usually effective.

Atrial tachycardias of 120–250 b.p.m. can be associated with a normal ventricular response. However, there is usually some degree of AV block. Digitoxicity is often the precipitating factor. Cardioversion may be required.

Digitoxicity may be precipitated by overadministration but also by hypokalaemia and renal impairment. Quinidine, Verapamil and Amiodarone also reduce the threshold for toxicity. Nausea and vomiting occur, but more importantly acute arrythmias can be precipitated. Both tachycardias and heart blocks occur and pacing may be indicated.

Paroxysmal supraventricular tachycardia occurs when re-entry of the impulse through the AV node stimulates the atria. Accessory pathways outwith the AV node can lead to overexcitation of the ventricles. A pathway from atria to myocardium occurs in the Wolff-Parkinson-White syndrome (Fig. 18.7) and from atria to bundle of His in the Lown-Ganong-Levine syndrome. The former is characterised by a delta wave and short PR interval.

If the abnormal focus is low in the atria then retrograde depolarisation of the atria may result in reversed 'P' waves on the ECG.

Supraventricular tachycardia responds well to Verapamil and this

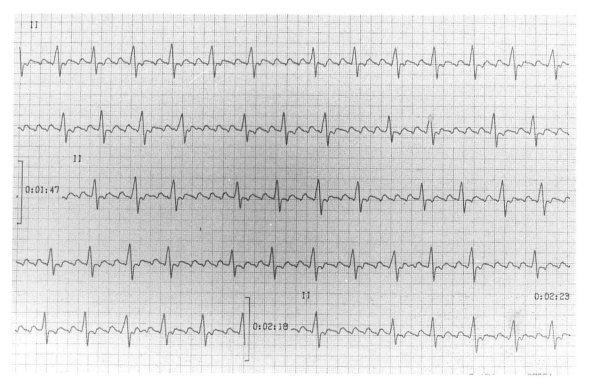

Fig. 18.6 Atrial flutter.

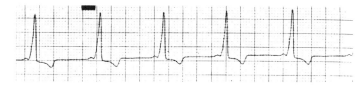

Fig. 18.7 Wolff-Parkinson-White syndrome.

is the drug of choice in the A & E department. This calcium antagonist will slow conduction through the AV node and slow the ventricular response. It is absolutely contraindicated in any patient who has recently received any β-blocker. It is also potentially hazardous to patients who may be digitoxic. Indeed digixitoxicity may precipitate supraventricular dysrhythmias and the administration of Verapamil in these circumstances may induce asystole.

The dose of Verapamil is 5–10 mg administered intravenously over 30–60 seconds. Vagal stimulation with carotid sinus massage, valsalva manoeuvre or eyeball pressure can sometimes be effective. It often isn't and sometimes precipitates asystole.

Ventricular tachycardias (Fig. 18.8)

These runs of ventricular ectopics are more often associated with ischaemic episodes than SVTs and are potentially life-threatening. A broad complex tachycardia of 120–250 b.p.m. should be assumed to be a VT, particularly when the patient is elderly and this is the first episode. In acute myocardial infarction an 'SVT with block' is very uncommon and in these circumstances the rhythm must always be assumed to be a VT. The inappropriate use of Verapamil may be harmful if an erroneous diagnosis of SVT is made.

There are essentially four ECG features which distinguish a supraventricular tachycardia with aberrant conduction from ventricular tachycardia.

1. Atrioventricular dissociation — the presence of atrial activity unrelated to ventricular activity is a feature of ventricular tachycardia.

2. A QRS duration of > 140 ms indicates ventricular tachycardia.

3. Left axis deviation (≥ −30°) is strongly suggestive of VT.

4. Variations in QRS shape during tachycardia and a different QRS shape during sinus rhythm suggest VT.

The first line treatment of ventricular tachycardia in the absence of circulatory arrest is lignocaine. A bolus of 100 mg i.v. is given followed by an infusion of 1–4 mg/min. If circulatory arrest occurs then defibrillation is indicated. Disopyramide, 1.5–2.0 mg/kg (max. 150 mg), is an alternative to lignocaine. It is effective

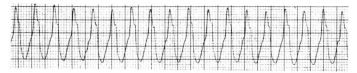

Fig. 18.8 Ventricular tachycardia.

against most ventricular dysrhythmias and some supraventricular dysrhythmias. It should be given intravenously over at least 5 minutes. A shorter infusion period may induce profound circulatory collapse. Lignocaine is a negative inotrope and should be used with caution when the blood pressure is low.

Warning dysrhythmias — runs of ventricular ectopics, (Fig. 18.9), frequent VEs and 'R' on 'T' VEs — have been described. In fact ventricular fibrillation occurs just as often in the absence of such disturbances. It is still probably worthwhile, however, to institute prophylactic lignocaine therapy when these abnormalities are recorded.

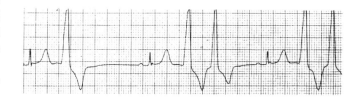

Fig. 18.9 Ventricular ectopics.

Torsade de Pointes is a ventricular tachycardia where the axis is continuously changing. The rapid broad complexes regularly change in amplitude and direction. It is rare, but the condition may be aggravated by antiarrhythmic drugs. Causes include tricyclic overdosage and hypocalcaemia.

Sinus tachycardia often occurs during myocardial infarction. It is associated with pain, fear, high circulating catecholamines, increased sympathetic activity and hypoxia. Treatment with oxygen and an analgesic may reduce the heart rate. The effectiveness of β-blockers in the early stages to reduce the size of the infarct has not been conclusively demonstrated and so routine administration in the emergency department is not indicated.

Too slow

Sinus bradycardia may be the normal heart rate for athletes, but is also a feature of ill health. Hypothyroidism and hypothermia are associated with bradycardia, as is treatment with β-blockers and digoxin. Inferior myocardial infarction and increased parasympathetic activity are also causes of bradycardia. The bradyarrhythmias associated with inferior infarction may carry a better prognosis than those of an anterior infarction as they may be the result of autonomic overactivity rather than damage to cardiac tissue.

Bradycardia in the setting of myocardial infarction may be associated with AV block. Syncope or reduced conscious level are indications for immediate pacing. Slow heart rates may maintain a deceptively high blood pressure due to the long ventricular filling time. Cardiac output (stroke volume × heart rate), however, is usually reduced. Atropine (0.6 mg i.v.) may be effective if parasympathetic stimulation is a feature and isoprenaline infusions are sometimes of temporary assistance. However, cardiac pacing is often necessary. The decision to insert a transvenous pacing wire and the operation itself are usually undertaken by the specialist medical team on-call. However, local circumstances and sometimes the urgency of the situation may require that pacing is undertaken in the accident and emergency department.

External cardiac pacing has returned as a therapeutic tool. The needles in the chest have been replaced by large self-adhesive pads. The procedure is relatively painless and can be tolerated in the conscious patient. Its most useful application is increasing the heart rate prior to insertion of a transvenous lead. The increase in heart rate will improve the patient's condition and make insertion of the wire itself a little easier.

1st degree heart block with delayed conduction through the AV node results in a prolonged PR interval of 0.2 s but every impulse is conducted.

In *2nd degree heart block* the delay through the AV node results in intermittent failure of ventricular capture and 'block'. If the block occurs at regular intervals then it is described as 'Mobitz type II' (Fig. 18.10). If there is a progressive delay through the AV node then progressive lengthening of the PR interval occurs until ventricular capture fails. This is Wenkebach's phenomenon or 'Mobitz type I' (Fig. 18.11).

In *3rd degree heart block* or complete heart block, there is dissociated activity of atria and ventricles (Fig. 18.12). The pulse rate is usually between 30 and 50 b.p.m. i.e. the idioventricular rate. 'P' waves and 'QRS' complexes occur but they are independent of each other. Complete heart block may be complicated by asystole and sometimes ventricular fibrillation. Syncope as a result of such loss of ventricular atrophy is a Stokes-Adams attack. The patient characteristically falls down, pale and pulseless. Recovery is usually spontaneous and, within a minute or two, their face becomes deeply flushed. Sometimes they may need a thump on the chest or a short

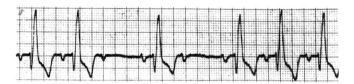

Fig. 18.10 Intermittent Mobitz type II.

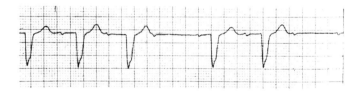

Fig. 18.11 Wenkebach's phenomenon.

period of external cardiac massage before spontaneous cardiac output returns.

Delays in conduction can occur below the AV node and affect any or all of the three fascicles beyond the bundle of His. The right bundle and anterior and posterior fascicles of the left bundle can be individually or totally affected.

Left anterior fascicular block results in an initial 'R' wave in lead III and aVF and a left axis deviation.

Left posterior fascicular block results in an initial 'Q' wave in lead III and aVF and a right axis deviation.

Bifascicular block refers to a right bundle branch block with either a posterior or most commonly an anterior fascicular block.

Cardiac pain may, of course, not be due to myocardial infarction.

Pericarditis

Sharp, retrosternal chest pain, exacerbated by movement is a feature of pericarditis. Inflammation of the pericardium can occur in many conditions, both local and general. It is most often seen during infection with coxsackie B virus. Other than chest pain, the patient may be remarkably well. The ECG may show widespread ST elevation but, unlike infarction, the segment is concave downwards. There may be a widespread scratchy friction rub. If, however, fluid collects in the pericardium, the murmur may disappear and the heart sounds become faint.

If the pericardial effusion restricts venous filling then cardiac tamponade ensues. The JVP rises, the BP falls and pulsus paradoxus is measurable. Pericardiocentesis can be immediately life-saving in these circumstances. The restrictive effect of fluid in the pericardial sac is not always proportional to the amount of fluid or the size of the cardiac shadow on a chest X-ray. If cardiac tamponade is suspected and supported by a fall in blood pressure and rise in venous pressure then one should proceed with pericardiocentesis.

Delayed sequelae of myocardial infarction can include pericarditis, pleurisy and pneumonitis. These symptoms and signs may occur singly or as a syndrome (Dressler's, or postmyocardial infarction syndrome). This syndrome occurs 1–6 weeks after infarction and may sometimes present to the A & E department. When the syndrome occurs soon after infarction pericardial pain can be confused with ischaemia. It is not usually possible to make the definitive diagnosis in the emergency department and the patient should be admitted.

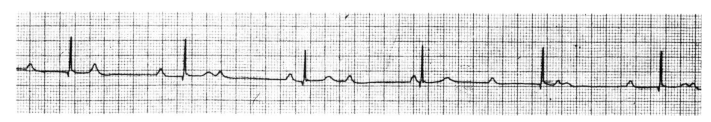

Fig. 18.12 Complete heart block.

NON-CARDIAC CHEST PAIN

Having established that the patient is not describing cardiac pain then non-cardiac conditions should be considered. Although oesophageal pain is probably the commonest cause of non-cardiac pain that presents to an A & E department, other life-threatening causes should be considered first.

> The main causes of non-cardiac chest pain are as follows:
> Aortic dissection
> Oesophageal pathology, including perforation
> Perforated peptic ulcer
> Pancreatitis
> Cholecystitis
> Pleuritic pain

Aortic dissection

Necrosis of the media will allow a tear in the intima to provide a parallel path for blood, which rapidly, and often fatally, ends in this new channel splitting its way into the pericardium or elsewhere. The pain is sudden, severe, within the chest but radiating through to the back. Depending on the direction of the dissection it can be felt in the neck, abdomen or legs. *The pain is characteristically unrelieved by morphine.*

If the coronary arteries become involved, ECG changes, suggestive of infarction may be seen. Involvement of spinal arteries may produce neurological signs and symptoms. Peripheral pulses may be lost. A chest X-ray may show widening of the mediastinum. Referral to a specialised unit is indicated.

Pleuritic pain

Perhaps the commonest cause of pleuritic chest pain encountered in the A & E department is 'pleurisy'. Viral chest infection and pneumonia may have chest pain as the dominant feature. Other features of the underlying condition will give the diagnosis.

Pulmonary embolus

This is an important cause of pleuritic chest pain. Diagnostic features are often not demonstrable in the early stages and the diagnosis often has to be assumed without confirmation (see p. 131). Remember that the commonest ECG change is a tachycardia and that the 'classic' $S_1Q_3T_3$ pattern merely reflects right ventricular strain and therefore takes time to develop. Haemoptysis is not a constant feature.

Pneumothorax

A spontaneous pneumothorax can present as chest pain (see p. 132). 'Hyper-resonance' of the affected side is in reality only a demonstrable difference in quality of percussion notes between the affected and unaffected sides. Always establish the position of the mediastinum by identifying both the apex beat and trachea and confirm that the pneumothroax is not under tension.

Intercostal myalgia (Bornholm's disease)

This can mimic 'pleuritic' chest pain. It is associated with infection by the coxsackie B virus. The patient is usually young and there are associated features of an upper respiratory tract infection.

Oesophageal pain

Oesophageal pain is commonly confused with cardiac pain, particularly when the pain is the result of motor dysfunction rather than reflux. As manometric studies of the oesophagus become more commonplace it is increasingly apparent that many cases of 'angina' are in fact oesophageal dysfunction. Moreover, the symptoms can be associated with ECG abnormalities and relieved by nitrates. However, it cannot be emphasised enough that this is a diagnosis made in retrospect. The rules outlined at the beginning of the chapter always apply.

The differentiation from cardiac pain may be clear however. Pain related to eating and posture, burning in character and relieved by antacids is likely to be reflux oesophagitis. 'Waterbrash' associated with 'heartburn' is not a common complaint but is a well recognised associated feature.

Prolonged vomiting may lead to tearing of the oesophageal mucosa. The pain is usually severe, lower retrosternal in position and vomitus may contain variable amounts of fresh blood (Mallory-Weiss syndrome).

Musculo-skeletal pain

This is usually associated with specific areas of tenderness and is aggravated by certain movements. Prolonged or severe coughing can result in stress fractures of the ribs. Very rarely a stress fracture of the first rib may cause 'pleuritic' chest pain. This unusual injury can occur when lifting with the shoulder in abduction and external rotation.

The pain of *shingles* precedes the rash usually by several days. The distribution along a nerve route may suggest the diagnosis.

Upper abdominal pathology may be perceived as chest pain. *Pancreatitis* and *gall bladder disease* (sometimes with ECG changes) can be confusing at times and, as with oesophageal disease, the diagnosis may only be made when cardiac disease has been excluded.

SUMMARY

> 1. The ECG will not exclude the diagnosis of acute myocardial infarction and changes can only be assumed to be 'old' after inspection of an 'old' ECG.
> 2. In the A & E department, chest pain of an ischaemic nature, lasting 20 minutes or more is a myocardial infarction until proven otherwise.

FURTHER READING

Cardiac arrhythmias. Practical notes on interpretation and treatment, 2nd edn. Bennet D 1985 Wright, Bristol

Breathlessness and cough

The management of life-threatening respiratory emergencies has already been described in Chapters 10 and 11. Many patients also arrive in the A & E department less critically short of breath. Decisions concerning treatment, admission and referral must be made.

Patients and many doctors are quite unaware of the fine distinctions between dyspnoea, tachypnoea and hyperpnoea. Uncomfortable awareness of breathing constitutes breathlessness and the degree of breathing difficulty which different people are prepared to tolerate varies greatly. Cough, chest pain, wheeze and stridor are common accompaniments.

HISTORY

Breathlessness

The severity should be recorded. A simple description of the amount of exertion which brings on the shortness of breath is all that is needed. Primary lung disorders are by far the commonest cause, followed by left heart failure. There are many other possible causes including pleural effusions, neuromuscular disorders, thoracic cage abnormalities, metabolic acidotic states (e.g. diabetic ketosis, uraemia or septicaemia), anaemia, thyrotoxicosis, obesity, ascites, pregnancy and psychogenic problems. Knowledge of the rate of onset helps to determine the cause. A sudden onset over a matter of minutes suggests a pneumothorax, pulmonary embolus, pulmonary oedema (see Ch. 11) or psychogenic hyperventilation (see Ch. 31). A less dramatic onset over several hours is more typical of bronchial asthma, moderate left heart failure, pneumonias and allergic alveolitis. Increasing breathlessness over days or weeks suggests an exacerbation of chronic bronchitis, a pleural effusion

or pulmonary neoplasia, while chronic dyspnoea over months or years occurs in chronic bronchitis, pneumoconiosis, pulmonary hypertension and non-pulmonary conditions. Recurrent attacks of breathlessness are most often due to bronchial asthma, heart failure and anxiety states.

The second most important aspect of the history are the circumstances in which the breathlessness occurs. Orthopnoea usually occurring at night is classically caused by left heart failure but may also be a symptom of severe chronic lung disorders and, rarely, bilateral diaphragmatic paralysis. Early morning deterioration in the respiratory function of bronchial asthmatics is also common. Acute asthmatic attacks may be precipitated by exercise or exposure to identifiable allergens (e.g. animal dander and pollens). The patient's occupation(s)*, present and past, and hobbies must be ascertained. In occupational asthmas (e.g. baker's asthma) the breathlessness, at least initially, occurs only in the working environment. Extrinsic allergic alveolitis (e.g. farmer's lung and pigeon fancier's lung) is similar but is less acute in onset (e.g. 4–6 hours). In pneumoconiosis (e.g. coal worker's lung, asbestosis or silicosis), as a consequence of repeated dust exposure progressive pulmonary fibrosis develops over several years.

Most breathless patients improve with rest or removal from trigger factors. Exceptions are patients with psychogenic dyspnoea whose breathing difficulty may only occur at rest and may be worse in crowded areas. A complaint of 'difficulty in getting enough air in' is often erroneously regarded as being pathognomonic of psychogenic dyspnoea. In fact it is also a complaint of patients with neuromuscular disorders which produce weakness of the respiratory muscles, such as poliomyelitis, ascending polyneuritis, myasthenia gravis and motor neurone disease (see Ch. 26).

Cough

The most important features of a cough are its chronicity, sound and the presence or absence of expectoration of sputum. Inflammation of the pharynx and upper airways, bronchial neoplasms and early pneumonias produce a dry cough. A dry

*Occupational Disease Reporting: Information for doctors on the new arrangements 1986. Health and Safety Executive (HSE 18).

cough, especially at night, may also be the predominant symptom of bronchial or cardiac asthma. A habit cough is characterised by spasms of non-productive barking present for many years. Laryngitis produces a harsh sound (croup). A productive cough suggests chronic bronchitis, bronchiectasis or pulmonary tuberculosis. Yellow, green or brown coloured sputum indicates infection. Paralysis of the vocal cords due to pressure on the recurrent laryngeal nerves by bronchial or mediastinal tumours, occasionally by aortic aneurysms, produces a prolonged low-pitched bovine cough. Coughing after food, especially when lying down after food, suggests oesophageal or neuromuscular disease causing aspiration of stomach contents into the lungs. A change of posture may also stimulate bouts of coughing in bronchiectasis. A chronic postnasal drip is another common cause of coughing and history taking should always include careful enquiry about catarrh, sinusitis, sneezing, a need to clear the throat frequently and an actual sensation of postnasal drip.

In children a cough which is worse at night and is accompanied by vomiting should be labelled whooping cough until proven otherwise. The characteristic whoop may not be produced. Children who have a choking episode while playing with small objects must always be assumed to have inhaled something. The choking and coughing can pass off quite quickly and give a false sense of security (see Ch. 44).

The presence of blood in the sputum always worries both the patient and the doctor, even though in about 50% of cases no cause is ever found. It can sometimes be difficult to determine if the blood has originated from the gastrointestinal tract or the airways. In haemoptysis the blood is bright red as distinct from brown in a haematemesis. Postnasal dripping of blood from an epistaxis can also cause confusion. The most important conditions causing frank haemoptysis are bronchial tumours, pulmonary embolism with infarction, mitral stenosis and tuberculosis. Pulmonary oedema may be associated with pink, frothy sputum and early pneumonia with rusty coloured sputum. Rarer causes of haemoptysis include blunt thoracic trauma, endometriosis and coagulation disorders. Recurrent haemoptysis over many years is seen with healed cavitating tuberculosis and bronchiectasis.

Persistent *hiccoughs* are usually associated with pathology immediately above or below the diaphragm. If there are no other symptoms the possibility of uraemia should be excluded. Continual hiccoughing can exhaust the patient and occasional deaths have been recorded.

Chest pain (see also Ch. 18)

Pain in the chest is the third cardinal symptom of intrathoracic disease. Typical pleuritic pain is sharp and well localised and exacerbated by movement, breathing and coughing. Bacterial and viral infections are the commonest causes, followed by pneumothoraces and pulmonary emboli. Persistent coughing can cause localised tears in thoracic muscles or a more generalised muscular ache around the lower rib cage. Bornholm disease, herpes zoster and secondary deposits in ribs can all cause pain indistinguishable from pleurisy. The pain of ischaemic heart disease, a common cause of left ventricular failure, is discussed in Chapter 18. Tumours in the major bronchi and mediastinum and various oesophageal disorders can cause deep aching retrosternal pain. Sharp transitory left inframammary pain causing a momentary catching of the breath is common in young people. Its cause is unknown but it seems to be benign. Similar pain may accompany the hyperventilation syndrome (see Ch. 31).

Other symptoms

Wheeze is the term that patients or their relatives use for harsh noisy breathing. It occurs classically in bronchial asthma and obstructive bronchitis and is often accompanied by a sensation of tightness in the chest. Sneezing, lacrimation and a history of eczema is also common in younger asthmatics. Contrary to popular belief asthmatics find it more difficult to breath in than out. Among patients with irritable bronchi wheeze, cough and breathlessness tend to get worse during cold weather and in response to inhalation of dust and fumes. Partial obstruction of the larynx or major airways causes a harsh inspiratory sound called *stridor*. *Fever* and *malaise* accompany infections and extrinsic allergic alveolitis. *Weight loss* may be the main feature of pulmonary tumours and tuberculosis. Abnormal *fatigue*, usually associated with breathlessness, may precede the onset of angina or myocardial infarction. Complaints of *palpitations*, *faintness* and *tingling* in the extremities are common in the hyperventilation syndrome. Of course, young children cannot explain any of these symptoms and they are brought to hospital because someone has noticed their breathing difficulties.

General points in the history

Past medical history

Inquiry should always be made concerning previous 'chest trouble', even many years previously. Patients readily forget that they were treated for pulmonary tuberculosis 20 or 30 years ago. Persistent early morning cough and mild exertional dyspnoea are typical of chronic bronchitis. Past operations may have significance if they were for malignancy or as a potential cause of venous thrombosis. Previous psychiatric illness may suggest a non-organic cause for breathlessness. All patients should be asked if they have had previous chest radiography as the films may still be available.

Social history

Smoking habits should be recorded. Remember that patients usually minimise the number of cigarettes smoked daily. The importance of the patient's occupation has already been mentioned.

Family history

A family history of lung disease may be obtained from patients with bronchial asthma, pulmonary tuberculosis and the rare early-onset emphysema associated with inherited α_1-antitrypsin deficiency.

Drug history

Current drug therapy may be relevant in one of three ways:

1. Diseases which affect respiration may be evidenced.

2. Some drugs reduce host resistance to infection, e.g. corticosteroids and immunosuppressives.

3. Some drugs can cause bronchospasm (e.g. β-adrenergic blocking agents, aspirin and non-steroidal anti-inflammatory drugs) or, more rarely, pulmonary fibrosis (e.g. busulphan).

PHYSICAL EXAMINATION

Points to be noted on *inspection* include:

1. The presence or absence of central cyanosis; hypercapnia produces peripheral vasodilatation.

2. Clubbing and nicotine staining of the fingers.

3. The pattern of breathing; a rate of more than 20 breaths/minute in an adult is abnormal. Is it laboured and are the accessory muscles of respiration being used? Is there indrawing of the intercostal muscles indicating airflow obstruction? Is there wheeze or stridor or the bubbly noisy breathing characteristic of pulmonary oedema? Psychogenic problems are suggested by frequent deep sighs and a generally irregular pattern.

4. The configuration of the chest; is it barrel-shaped due to hyperinflation? A pigeon chest may indicate severe bronchial asthma beginning in childhood. Scoliosis can be a cause of progressive respiratory failure.

5. Elevation of the jugular venous pressure caused either by obstruction of the venous return to the heart (e.g. cardiac tamponade, tension pneumothorax or upper mediastinal tumours) or right heart failure (e.g. cor pulmonale secondary to chronic bronchitis).

6. Poor expansion of the chest on one side due to underlying disease.

7. Contamination of the mouth and pharynx if there has been exposure to smoke or other fumes.

8. Scars from previous surgery.

The patient's temperature must be recorded. The location of the mediastinum and size of the heart should be determined by *palpation* of the trachea and the apex beat. The pulse will often be rapid due to hypoxaemia and hypercapnia. A slow rate suggests either that the patient is in heart block, or is taking digoxin or β-blockers. Liver enlargement is an important sign of heart failure in small children.

Bronchial breathing over airless lung (i.e. consolidation, atelectasis or dense fibrosis) may be heard on *auscultation*. Polyphonic rhonchi occurring randomly throughout the respiratory cycle are typically heard in asthmatics and chronic bronchitics. The loud coarse sound of a pleural rub usually indicates either an infection or pulmonary infarction.

Sputum should be examined for signs of infection or blood. If a cardiorespiratory cause for the breathlessness is not obvious a quick general examination may reveal a neuromuscular or metabolic cause.

INVESTIGATIONS

The following patients should have a posteroanterior film of the chest taken in inspiration while in the A & E department; those with:

1. Recent onset of breathlessness, especially if accompanied by chest pain or productive cough

2. Recent deterioration in their chronic chest symptoms which have failed to respond to simple therapeutic measures

3. Acute bronchial asthma

4. Haemoptysis

5. Cough persisting for more than 3 weeks

6. Other indicators leading to suspicion of intrathoracic malignancy or pulmonary tuberculosis.

If the patient is very distressed an anteroposterior film may be all that can be managed. Lateral chest films rarely influence decisions concerning treatment or the necessity for hospital admission. Occasionally a small pneumothorax may only be seen on a straight film taken in full expiration. Its recognition may be critical in patients with chronic obstructive pulmonary disease and poor respiratory reserve. When possible previous chest films should be obtained for comparison.

If heart disease or pulmonary embolism is suspected an ECG should be recorded. Arterial blood gases should be measured in the more severely breathless especially if there are signs of hypoxia and/or hypercapnia (see Ch. 11). It is useful to keep an instrument in the department for recording peak expiratory flow rates (e.g. a mini-peak flow meter). The PEFR is reduced in all conditions which reduce ventilatory capacity and its measurement provides a useful baseline against which to judge the effects of therapy. Occasional patients who are being referred back to their family doctors for treatment may have sputum samples sent for bacteriological analysis.

MANAGEMENT DECISIONS

The options available for the management of breathless patients are similar to those available for patients with other major health problems who attend the A & E department. Do they require admission to hospital, or is referral back to their family doctors or on to a specialist outpatient department appropriate? Abnormalities on the chest X-ray and less often, the ECG, can influence the decision as much as the patient's clinical state.

In general, the severity of a person's breathlessness is the major determinant of the necessity for admission to hospital. Shortness of breath at rest or with minimal exertion usually indicates the need for inpatient treatment. This simple yardstick does not apply to patients suffering from chronic respiratory disease who are continuously short of breath. Unless there has been a dramatic worsening of their state, they are better managed at home, away from the danger of infection with the antibiotic-resistant organisms characteristically found in hospitals. Patients in heart failure and those suspected of having had a pulmonary embolus should all be admitted. A person who has coughed up a little blood but otherwise appears well and has a normal chest X-ray can be given an urgent outpatient appointment for further investigation. Patients who, on X-ray examination, are discovered to have a single, small, well demarcated lung opacity ('coin' lesion) should be referred immediately to a thoracic clinic. If the lesion is spiculated, urgent needle biopsy is indicated.

These examples have been given in order to illustrate the spectrum of urgency involved in the clinical management decisions. Some points in the specific management of *bronchial asthma, lower respiratory tract infections, pulmonary embolism* and *pneumothorax* are now discussed.

BRONCHIAL ASTHMA (see also Ch. 11)

Bronchial asthma is characterised by reversibility of airflow obstruction over short periods of time, usually either bronchoconstriction in response to specific stimuli or bronchodilatation in response to treatment. Older patients who are labelled as having chronic bronchitis often have a degree of reversibility of their airways narrowing ('wheezy bronchitis').

Most of the dangers and deaths from acute asthma arise from a failure to appreciate the severity of an attack. Increasing frequency in the use of bronchodilators without relief is an important indication of loss of control. Some people, especially children, deteriorate very quickly and a knowledge of the pattern of previous attacks can be extremely helpful. Increasing breathlessness during the night is part of a well known pattern of diurnal variation in ventilatory capacity. The doctor should not be lulled into a false sense of security when the patient arrives in the department in the afternoon and pleads great improvement in his breathing. Loss of a night's sleep is an indication for hospital admission. In childhood severe asthma is commoner among boys than girls and recurrent attacks may retard growth and produce chest deformities. Such children often have a family history of atopy and are more likely to also suffer from eczema and rhinitis. In general, the threshold for admitting young children to hospital should be low.

The severity of the breathlessness is the most important factor influencing the decision whether to bring an asthmatic into hospital or not. If the patient is short of breath at rest or on very minimal exertion, unless chronically so, he needs to be in a hospital bed. A respiratory rate above 25 breaths per minute at rest in a wheezing adult is a rough guide. The other clinical features of severe asthma are detailed in Ch. 11.

Most wheezing infants should be brought into hospital, especially if they are not feeding properly. Some go on to have several similar, usually mild, attacks during infancy which do not return after they start school ('fat happy wheezers'). Others later develop recurrent asthmatic attacks.

When possible a baseline measurement of the PEFR should be obtained before any treatment is given. This value provides an objective assessment of the degree of respiratory obstruction and

if it is less than 25% of the expected value this is another absolute indication for hospital admission. All patients must have arterial blood gases measured.

The treatment of acute bronchial asthma is described in Ch. 11. Asthmatic attacks are very frightening and the patient should be constantly reassured.

When the patient's breathing is satisfactory a chest X-ray can be obtained. All these patients must be examined radiographically otherwise small pneumothoraces, mediastinal emphysema or evidence of bacterial infection may be overlooked.

Immediate improvement after treatment in the A & E department may provide false reassurance, as severe asthma may quickly return. In a mild attack if the initial response is adequate, as evidenced by improvement in the clinical signs and PEFR, and supervision is available, it may be possible to manage the patient at home. The PEFR must be at least 75% of the predicted value for that patient before he/she is allowed home. The plan should be discussed with the family doctor. Partial responders may be admitted to the observation ward and treatment continued with oral bronchodilators. In either case the patient's condition must be assessed regularly and often. Serial reading of the PEFR should be used as an objective indicator of relief of airways obstruction because clinical signs can be misleading. When there is any doubt vigorous treatment and admission to hospital are advocated. Never start oral prednisolone and send the patient home.

One should always pose the question, 'Why did the patient get so ill in the first place?'. Most attacks are brought on by viral infections or allergies. Some are the consequence of the patient not taking medication properly or running out of the drugs. Ideally, asthmatic patients should be given simple written instructions on how to take their medication and what to do and who to contact if they become ill. A few develop wheeze as a side effect of β-blockers, aspirin, or non-steroidal anti-inflammatory drugs and must be warned not to take them again.

Wheezing is not necessarily due to bronchial asthma. The differential diagnoses in children include bronchiolitis, inhaled foreign bodies, cystic fibrosis, pulmonary tuberculosis (especially in immigrants) and intrathoracic masses compressing the large airways. Among adults wheeze may be due to left heart failure, bronchopulmonary aspergillosis, carcinoid syndrome or polyarteritis nodosa.

A final reiteration:

Virtually all patients complaining of increasing shortness of breath and wheeze deserve at least an overnight stay in hospital.

LOWER RESPIRATORY TRACT INFECTIONS (see also Ch. 11)

This section is limited to bronchitis and the pneumonias. Among children acute bronchitis is often a sequel to a viral upper respiratory tract infection. There is always a cough which may be accompanied by wheezing, but pyrexia is unusual. Symptoms usually resolve within a week. If they last longer bacterial superinfection is likely to have occurred and the child should be admitted to hospital for treatment with antibiotics. Children who suffer recurrent bronchitis should be referred to a paediatrician. They will require a chest X-ray, a Mantoux test for tuberculosis, a sweat test to exclude cystic fibrosis and perhaps plasma immunoglobulin studies. Pneumonia is suggested by a rapid respiratory rate, pyrexia and flaring of the alae nasi. Over the affected area breath sounds are typically reduced and there are crepitations. A chest X-ray will confirm the diagnosis and all such children require admission to hospital. The radiographic findings are frequently much more extensive then the clinical signs suggest and many of these children will need oxygen.

In adults, lower respiratory tract infections are more common in men, in the elderly and in those who are debilitated or live in poor housing conditions. The clinical features of pneumonia vary widely and depend on such factors as the age of the patient, the particular organism, the severity of the infection and the presence of pre-existing lung or systemic disease. In a previously healthy person the onset is usually abrupt with fever, headache, rigors, cough and pleuritic pain. Tachycardia and tachypnoea are usually present and herpetic cold sores are also common. In the elderly, the presentation may be much more non-specific with a general deterioration in health and development of confusion. Lower lobe pneumonias associated with diaphragmatic pleurisy may present with abdominal pain and guarding. Jaundice can also occur with severe infections. The unwary may then mistakenly diagnose cholecystitis or cholangitis. When pneumonia is slow to resolve an underlying cause should be suspected, e.g. tuberculosis (Fig. 19.1), a bronchial carcinoma or the possibility of defective immunity as can occur in leukaemia, myeloma and AIDS.

Many patients with mild pneumonia or acute bronchitis can be managed at home. For patients who are not seriously ill, trimethoprim or a broad-spectrum penicillin (e.g. amoxycillin) are the drugs of choice for adults of all ages and children under 5 years. These antimicrobials are active against *Streptococcus pneumoniae* and *Haemophilus influenzae*, the organisms causing the vast majority of pneumonias and acute exacerbations of chronic bronchitis seen in the community. Erythromycin is the treatment of choice for children over the age of 5 years and teenagers because *Streptococcus pneumoniae* and *Mycoplasma pneumoniae* are the commoner causes. It can also be used in adults failing to respond to initial therapy.

The *atypical pneumonias* (psittacosis, Q fever, mycoplasmal pneumonia and legionnaires' disease) cannot reliably be diagnosed clinically. About half the cases of psittacosis give a history of contact with various types of birds. It is not only exotic cage birds which transmit this disease but also turkeys, ducks and pigeons. Q fever is contracted from infected sheep and cattle, especially in the lambing and calving seasons. Mycoplasmal pneumonia is prone to occur in epidemics among children and young adults every three to four years. Headache is prominent and pleuritic chest pain very unusual. Legionnaires' disease is most often reported in patients returning from holidays in Mediterranean resorts, but there are

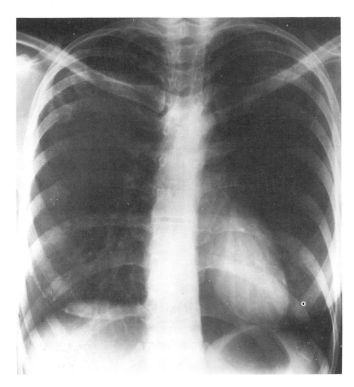

Fig. 19.1 Soft shadowing in the right upper lobe due to active pulmonary tuberculosis.

many sporadic cases. The organisms are found in showers and cooling systems and the illness can be very severe or quite mild. Antibody titres are required for confirmation of the diagnosis in these conditions. The first three respond to tetracyclines but legionnaires' disease must be treated with erythromycin. All patients with suspected atypical pneumonias must be admitted to hospital.

In patients recovering satisfactorily the initial antibiotic should be continued for ten days. If recovery is delayed and chest signs persistent a change may be made. This change should seldom be made earlier than the fourth day. If possible, the second antimicrobial should be chosen on the basis of bacteriological results. Chronic bronchitic patients unresponsive to first-line therapy but not ill enough to be hospitalised should therefore have a sputum sample for bacteriological examination. Where bacteriology has proved unhelpful and the initial choice was trimethoprim or amoxycillin, tetracycline (except in children under 10 and uraemic patients) or erythromycin are reasonable second choices. Erythromycin does not, however, cover psittacosis adequately. As a general rule, if a patient is recovering the antimicrobial agent should not be changed. The three stages of recovery are:

1. the patient feels better;
2. the chest signs disappear;
3. radiological evidence of pneumonia disappears.

Chest signs may persist for several days after clinical recovery and radiological evidence of pneumonia can persist for several weeks. All patients who have had pneumonia require a follow-up chest X-ray at 4–6 weeks.The importance of the X-ray examination is to see that the pneumonia has cleared completely and exclude as far as possible an underlying lung problem such as a bronchial carcinoma.

Patients with pneumonia who are being returned to the care of their family doctors should also have a white cell count. A normal count or leucopenia suggests a viral or atypical pneumonia and leucocytosis a bacterial cause. Chronic lymphatic leukaemia, which not uncommonly presents with pneumonia, may be brought to light.

When deciding which patients to admit to hospital, both medical and social factors need to be weighed up. The main reasons for admission are:

1. Severe illness, indicated by cyanosis, hypotension, drowsiness and confusion; remember that staphylococcal pneumonia frequently occurs when there is an outbreak of influenza. Also, recent instrumentation (e.g. cystoscopy or bowel surgery) may lead to Gram negative pneumonias.

2. Where there is pre-existing lung or heart disease, when a mild infection may have a serious effect on cardiorespiratory function.

3. Where the patient has a significant general medical problem, e.g. diabetes mellitus, AIDS, is on immunosuppressives following transplant surgery, or is taking long-term antibiotic therapy; pneumonia in these patients is often caused by Gram-negative bacilli, fungi, *Pneumocystis carinii* or *Mycobacterium tuberculosis*.

4. Where a complication such as a pleural effusion (Fig. 19.2) or lung abscess is suspected.

5. Where the diagnosis is uncertain, e.g. a pulmonary embolus cannot be excluded.

6. Where the home facilities are unsuitable for proper care; for instance the elderly patient living alone.

PULMONARY THROMBOEMBOLISM (see also Ch. 11)

The typical case is sudden in onset with pleuritic pain and sometimes haemoptysis. It is likely to occur after periods of immobilisation (e.g. after aeroplane flights and postoperatively). Other risk factors are the presence of varicose veins, malignancy, cardiac failure, the use of oral contraceptives, pregnancy and a history of a previous deep venous thrombosis. These risks are cumulative. The chest X-ray may show subpleural shadows, areas of linear atelectasis or a small basal effusion, but is frequently normal. The ECG may show signs of right heart strain. In more than 50% of cases there is no evidence of a deep venous thrombosis in the legs. Such patients require immediate admission to hospital for anticoagulation. Unfortunately, less typical cases occur. The patients are often young women who suffer multiple emboli most typically following pregnancy. They may complain only of increasing tiredness and breathlessness and have no acute symptoms. An urgent ventilation/perfusion lung scan should be arranged for this type of patient along with an immediate medical opinion.

PNEUMOTHORAX (see also Ch. 11)

Breathlessness caused by a spontaneous pneumothorax rarely causes any initial diagnostic difficulty. As a rule of thumb, patients with collapse of more than 25% of their single lung volume should be admitted to hospital. Most will require the insertion of a chest drain with attachment to an underwater seal. An alternative is to aspirate the air using a 50 ml syringe and three-way tap. If the leak is smaller and the patient comfortable, he can be allowed home to rest and brought back to the A & E department after a few days for repeat X-ray examination. He should be told to return immediately if increasing breathlessness or pain are a problem. Small pneumothoraces occurring secondary to underlying lung disease may be clinically less obvious. Doctors must be aware of the increased incidence of pneumothorax complicating asthma, chronic bronchitis and emphysema, carcinoma and tuberculosis. In these patients sudden worsening of symptoms, even to the point of respiratory failure, is more likely to be due to a pneumothorax than infection. A shallow apical pneumothorax is easily missed unless the chest X-ray is scrutinised closely and even then may only be seen on a film taken in expiration. All patients who have had a pneumothorax should eventually be seen by a chest physician or surgeon, especially if the problem is recurrent or has complicated other pulmonary disease.

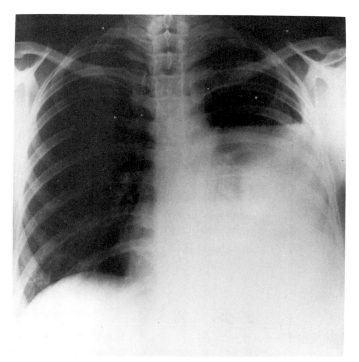

Fig. 19.2 A massive left-sided pleural effusion.

Back pain

Pain the back is an extremely common complaint. Patients may come to the A & E department complaining of pain which was precipitated by a traumatic incident (either external violence or their own physical effort) or they may come complaining of a pain which developed spontaneously.

The pathology of these two types of complaint ('traumatic' and 'non-traumatic') is so distinct that, although the symptoms may seem to be similar and the radiological investigation identical, they will be dealt with separately.

TRAUMATIC BACK PAIN

Major injuries to the neck and back

These have been described in Ch. 14 (see pp. 170 and 173).

Pain resulting from physical effort

History

The symptoms are usually caused by straining the back, in such actions as the lifting of heavy objects. Sometimes the pain is precipitated by a single movement, such as bending forwards or twisting. The onset is usually sudden and the pain often severe. Ask the patient the following questions:

Have there been previous episodes of back pain?

Does the pain radiate to the legs and is there any tingling, numbness or weakness in the legs?

Is the pain made worse by coughing or sneezing?

Have they had difficulty in passing urine?

Physical examination

In a comprehensive examination of the back, all clothes except underpants should be removed and the patient should stand facing away from the examiner. Observe the build and posture and the ease or difficulty with which the patient moves. Ask him to indicate the site and any radiation of the pain. Palpate the back for local tenderness, then instruct the patient to perform the six standard spinal movements of flexion, extension, lateral flexion to right and left, and rotation to right and left.

The patient should next lie supine on the examination couch. Palpate the abdomen. Examine straight leg raising and hip movements. Test the reflexes at knees and ankles and the plantar responses. Test for weakness of dorsiflexion and plantar flexion of the toes and for areas of diminished sensation in the legs and feet.

Finally, ask the patient to roll over and lie prone. Again observe the ease or difficulty with which he moves. If initially he had been unable to stand up, this part of the examination is used for inspection and palpation of the back, and palpation along the line of the sciatic nerve. It is also used to see if the patient can raise his head and shoulders from the couch without using his hands), i.e. spinal extension, and also to test hip extension by raising a leg from the couch.

Radiological examination

Radiological examination of the lumbar spine and pelvis subjects the patient to a relatively large dose of radiation. It should not be undertaken lightly and must be avoided during pregnancy. When there is no urgency, all women of child-bearing years should be asked if they are, or may be pregnant before lumbar spine, pelvic or abdominal radiographs are taken. If the answer is 'no' then it is safe to proceed. If the answer is 'yes' then the examination should be deferred until any time after the onset of menstruation, or when pregnancy testing is negative. The examination may (1) establish the diagnosis, (2) bring anomalies to light which may or may not be relevant to the present complaint, or (3) show that there is no radiological abnormality. The interpretation of these films requires experience, and their relevance must be correlated with the history and physical findings (Fig. 20.1). There should always be a good clinical reason for exposing a patient to this expensive and potentially dangerous investigation.

Diagnosis and management

Pain following back strain may arise from damage at one of three sites:
1. The muscles of the back
2. The intervertebral facetal joints
3. A prolapsed intervertebral disc.

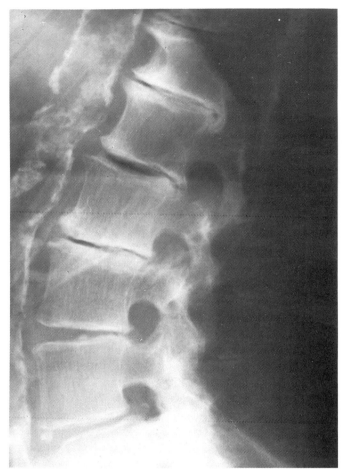

Fig. 20.1 This patient with lumbar spondylosis, disc degeneration and advanced aortic calcification did not complain of backache.

Muscles of the back. A muscle strain produces immediate pain and stiffness, with tenderness to palpation over the paravertebral muscles, but with no neurological signs. Radiological examination may show a scoliosis due to muscle spasm but any other abnormalities will not be directly related to the symptoms. Therefore, radiological examination should be requested only when the diagnosis is in doubt. Ethyl chloride spray may relieve the pain and muscle spasm. This diagnostic manoeuvre then makes radiological examination unnecessary. In the more severe cases, recovery will follow bed rest at home on a mattress supported on boards, analgesics and local warmth, and will be complete within a week to 10 days. Admission to hospital is rarely necessary, and the patient can be referred to the care of their general practitioner.

Intervertebral facetal joints. Damage to the intervertebral facetal joints often produces a low grade backache which may be present intermittently for months or years. Sudden extra physical effort will then produce an acute exacerbation. The patient complains of pain in the back, which may radiate into the thigh but usually not as far as the knee. Movements of the back and straight leg raising are limited but a neurological deficit in the legs is unlikely. There is tenderness to deep pressure over the affected joints.

The patient can be treated at home by rest on a firm mattress, analgesics and local warmth. For the first few days the patient should get out of bed only to go to the toilet or to eat. Sitting up for a quick meal is probably less damaging than twisting in bed. At this stage crutches will make the patient's life more comfortable. Without them, walking may be almost impossible, but with them it is possible to get to the toilet or the table. Pain will usually begin to diminish markedly in three or four days and at this point the patient should begin spinal extension exercises. Over the next few days the crutches can gradually be discarded and the patient start to sit up a few more hours each day.

The patient should be reviewed at the end of two weeks. In the great majority of cases there will be good improvement. The patient should continue spinal extension exercises and be instructed about posture and the correct way of lifting heavy weights. Those cases which are not improving with this treatment should be referred to an orthopaedic surgeon for possible admission to hospital.

Prolapsed intervertebral disc. The popular diagnosis of a 'slipped disc' is a fashionable one applied to many forms of backache — usually incorrectly. When an acute disc prolapse does occur, the symptoms are often quite dramatic. There is a sudden onset of severe pain in the back, radiating down the line of the sciatic nerve, often as far as the heel. Straight leg raising is limited to 30° or less and there will be diminished reflexes at the knee or the ankle, weakness of dorsiflexion or plantar flexion of the big toe and diminished sensation in the appropriate dermatome depending on whether the L4, L5 or S1 nerve root is principally involved. Clinically, if the patient can stand, there is a loss of the normal lumbar lordosis and development of a scoliosis which will be confirmed by radiographs. A diminished disc space is sometimes apparent.

Some mild cases can be treated conservatively with bed rest at home, as described for intervertebral facetal joint derangements. Severe cases should be referred immediately to an orthopaedic or neurosurgeon, for admission to hospital and possibly operation. Rarely, central prolapse of the disc will produce urinary retention and paraparesis, and is an indication for urgent surgery. It is therefore essential to *ask a patient to attempt to pass urine* after an acute disc prolapse.

NON-TRAUMATIC BACK PAIN

History

Patients who come to the A & E department complaining of pain in the back without any obvious cause may nevertheless have a serious condition. If the pain has been present for several weeks, the patient should be advised to consult his general practitioner, but if the pain is acute and of recent onset, a careful history, physical examination and investigations must be undertaken. This will follow the steps already outlined for a patient with back pain of traumatic origin, but the doctor is now concerned not only with the site and extent of the lesion but also with elucidating its cause and its relationship to other body systems. Consequently when taking the history, questioning will be more searching, the physical examination will be wider and investigations will probably need to be more extensive. Malignancy within the spine should always be considered a possible cause but it must be appreciated from the outset that the cause of the pain may not be in the vertebral column. Upper abdominal disease such as a posterior peptic ulcer, gall bladder disease or pancreatitis can present as pain in the back, as can urinary tract disease, gynaecological disorders and aortic aneurysm. Features which become important in the history are as follows.

1. Weight loss, cough, a previous mastectomy, difficulty in micturition or painless haematuria which, respectively, may indicate secondary carcinoma from primaries in the bronchus, breast, prostate or kidney.

2. Dyspepsia and the chronic use of antacids or aspirin.

3. An aversion for fatty foods, a history of jaundice or chronic alcoholism.

4. Urinary tract disorders such as frequency, dysuria, or haematuria.

5. Gynaecological disorders — vaginal discharge or menstrual irregularity.

6. In an elderly patient sudden severe pain in the back may come from a dissecting or a ruptured aortic aneurysm and the patient should be questioned about other circulatory problems.

Physical examination

A general inspection of the patient will quickly indicate the presence of a severe illness such as pancreatitis, a ruptured aneurysm or an acute osteomyelitis of the spine; otherwise, physical examination will follow the lines described for a traumatic back injury, but will include a rectal examination or, in the female, a vaginal examination and examination of the breasts. The temperature, pulse and blood pressure must be taken in all patients.

Investigations

Examination of the urine. This may indicate the presence of a urinary tract infection which may be the cause of the pain. Painless haematuria may indicate the presence of a tumour of the kidney, and secondary deposits in the spine are a more likely cause of pain than is the primary growth in the kidney.

A urethral smear may reveal evidence of gonorrhoea or a non-specific urethritis which may be present, respectively, in gonococcal arthritis and Reiter's disease.

Examination of the blood. Erythrocyte sedimentation rate and red and white cell counts will help to differentiate many conditions, such as acute osteomyelitis, myelomatosis and tuberculosis, from chronic degenerative diseases. Also, the ESR is raised in ankylosing spondylitis and various types of malignant disease.

A raised *alkaline* phosphatase accompanies active osteolysis from whatever cause. A raised *acid* phosphatase is found when carcinoma of the prostate has produced secondary deposits in the spine.

Radiological investigation. Mention has already been made of the potential hazard of this investigation, particularly in women of child-bearing age. The investigation may help to establish a diagnosis, bring anomalies to light which may or may not be relevant to the present complaint, or exclude any significant radiological abnormality (Fig. 20.2). The interpretation of the films requires experience and their relevance must be correlated with the history and physical findings. For example, congenital anomalies of the lower lumbar spine are common and may not necessarily be the cause of symptoms. Such anomalies will include spina bifida, spinal dysraphism, hemivertebra, sacralisation of the L5 vertebra or lumbarisation of the first element of the sacrum. Spondylolisthesis may be a congenital anomaly or the result of stress fractures in the regions of the pars interarticularis (usually of the L5 vertebra, but occasionally of the L4 or, more rarely, the L3 vertebra). The effect is best shown in the right and left oblique views. The condition may be symptomless until a sporting accident in the teenager or increasing weight in middle age causes the affected vertebra to slip forwards on the vertebra below. The condition is then described as spondylolysis and orthopaedic treatment will be required.

Ankylosing spondylitis is another condition in which the definitive diagnosis is made by radiological examination. Classically the disease first causes erosion of the sacroiliac joints and the anterior aspects of the vertebral bodies. This is followed by loss of the normal anterior concavity of the vertebrae, which becomes

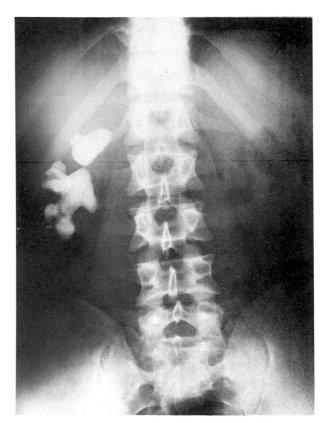

Fig. 20.2 A staghorn calculus in the right kidney was the cause of this patient's back pain.

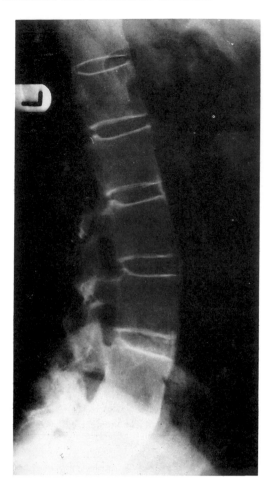

Fig. 20.3 Ankylosing spondylitis produces a bamboo-like spine and can be a cause of chronic, low grade backache.

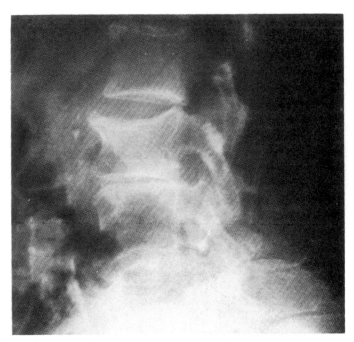

Fig. 20.4 Partial collapse of a vertebral body, due to senile osteoporosis, causes backache in some patients but is symptomless in others.

'squared' in outline on the lateral view. Finally, fusion of the sacroiliac joints and ankylosis of the intravertebral ligaments gives the spine a 'bamboo rod' appearance (Fig. 20.3). The patient should be referred for orthopaedic advice.

In acute osteomyelitis the patient may present with severe pain, fever and an acutely tender vertebra before radiological changes have developed. When they do appear, there will be destruction of the vertebral body starting in the *centre* of the body. Conversely, the bony destruction which is seen in tuberculous (Pott's) disease of the spine is typically located *adjacent to the intervertebral disc.* This form of bony tuberculosis often affects two adjacent vertebrae so that the spine angulates forwards with the intervening disc at the apex of the angle. This causes the gibbus deformity of a 'hunchback'. In the early evolution of tuberculosis, pus forms and creates a spindle-shaped paravertebral abscess which will be clearly seen on the AP view. In the later stages when there is resolution of the disease, adjacent affected vertebrae will fuse together so that two or three bodies will be joined as one mass of bone.

Osteoporosis from whatever cause often results in compression fractures of vertebral bodies. With an ageing population it is not uncommon to find one or more compression fractures in the dorsal

or lumbar spine due to senile osteoporosis in an elderly patient. Such fractures are a contributing factor to the small stature of many 'little old ladies'. They may or may not complain of pain in the back and often a compression fracture is an incidental radiological finding (Fig. 20.4). No specific local treatment is required and nothing will make the vertebra re-expand to its former volume. However, a diffuse form of myeloma can occasionally produce a similar appearance.

The most common degenerative change in the spine is the formation of osteophytes which grow like beaks of bone above and below the intervertebral discs. Described as lumbar spondylosis, the condition is so common as to be almost normal beyond the age of 60. It is very doubtful if it is responsible for any significant backache. The range of movement in the spine often diminishes with age as osteophytes appear, but they should not be regarded as the likely explanation for back pain.

Paget's disease (osteitis deformans) is another condition which may affect the lumbar spine, causing bony hypertrophy. One or more vertebral bodies will increase in size (Fig. 20.5). There may be aching in the back but the more serious symptoms are those of spinal cord compression, paresis in the legs and loss of bladder control as the diameter of the spinal canal is reduced.

Malignant changes in the spine are commonly due to secondary metastatic carcinoma, occasionally due to the widespread malignant changes of multiple myeloma and rarely due to bone sarcoma. As has been mentioned, the discovery of an isolated metastatic deposit is sometimes the first sign of malignant disease and its discovery provokes the search for the primary growth.

Finally, an X-ray examination of the spine may incidentally reveal evidence of a relevant disease process outside the vertebral column.

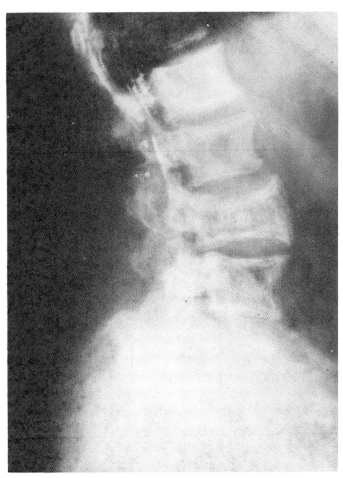

Fig. 20.5 Enlargement of a lumbar vertebra due to Paget's disease (osteitis deformans) caused backache and symptoms of spinal cord compression in this patient.

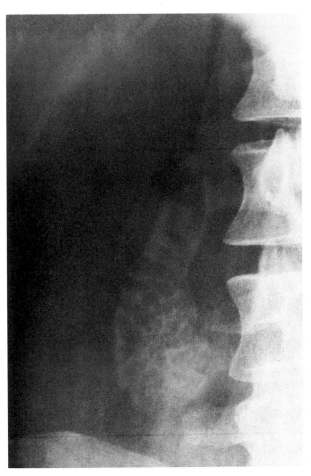

Fig. 20.6 Radiological investigation of back pain may reveal a cause outside the vertebral column. In this patient it was a gallbladder full of stones.

Gall-stones, pancreatic calcification, renal calculi, bladder stones or a calcified aortic aneurysm may be evident on the film and any of these conditions may sometimes be the underlying cause of the pain in the back (Fig. 20.6).

All these conditions may be demonstrated radiologically, but there should always be a good clinical reason for exposing a patient to the potential danger of radiological investigation of the abdomen, lumbar spine and pelvis.

Abdominal pain and bowel problems

INTRODUCTION

When patients with acute abdominal pain present to the emergency department, the examining doctor must decide:

1. Does the patient need resuscitation?
2. Does the patient require admission?
3. What is the diagnosis?
4. Can I give pain relief?
5. Can the patient go home?

The order of the questions is deliberate. Like so many conditions, the definitive diagnosis may not be established in the A & E department but this will not prevent appropriate resuscitation or referral. Discharge home without a firm diagnosis is undesirable but permissable if the patient is clearly well, examination is normal and he can be referred to a general practitioner.

The pain in the abdomen is usually a symptom of a pathological process within the abdominal cavity, but may be a symptom of a more generalised condition. Diabetic hyperglycaemia can present with abdominal pain when the patient is dehydrated and in impending coma. The association of abdominal pain and peripheral neuropathy is uncommon but is a feature of diabetes, porphyria and lead poisoning.

Pain in the shoulder can be referred from the diaphragm and epigastric pain referred from a myocardial infarction, oesophageal rupture, or basal pneumonia. Pain in the loin or lumbar region and abdominal pain in general may have its origin in the testes and renal or ureteric pain may be referred to the scrotum. Pain in the abdomen may be referred from the spine or nerve root pathology. Shingles produces unilateral pain across a dermatome and this pain is present before the rash. An obstructed femoral hernia may produce central abdominal pain. In someone below the age of 20, a tender swollen testis must always be assumed to be a torsion until proven otherwise. Even in young adults the

diagnosis of torsion must be excluded before the patient is discharged.

ASSSESSMENT

The following points will need to be established in the history.

1. The site of the pain.

2. The character of the pain (in particular is it sharp or colicky?). A distinction can usually be made between a colicky pain and other types of pain and this will immediately narrow the diagnostic possibilities, since a colicky pain can arise only from distension of a hollow viscus (including the biliary tree, small and large intestine, the renal pelvis and ureters and the fallopian tubes). A colic is typically intermittent, building up to a climax in which the patient may curl up on his side and roll around with the pain. Even in children the character of the pain is usually obvious following a short period of observation. This contrasts, for example, with the patient who has a generalised peritonitis and who will lie still and flat — avoiding the least movement which accentuates the pain. However, the pain of a perforated ulcer may be so severe that the patient finds it impossible to lie still.

3. What makes it worse or better? (movement, coughing, breathing, micturition).

4. The severity and duration of the pain. Assessment of severity may be difficult in the brief period of contact with the patient in the A & E department and repeated examination (if necessary in an observation ward) may be required before a decision can be reached as to further management. Some help, however, may be obtained from the patient's reactions to a full examination. It is important to make this assessment because in some conditions the severity of the pain is out of all proportion to the physical signs observed. Examples of this are the pain following mesenteric vascular occlusion; rupture or dissection of an aortic aneurysm; pain due to retroperitoneal or posterior peritoneal pathology (such as pancreatitis or a perforation of duodenal ulcer into the lesser sac), retrocaecal appendicitis and injury to the retroperitoneal duodenum. In such patients the abdominal signs may be minimal, but early diagnosis is essential if treatment is to be successful. An impression of the pain can be made by watching the patient as

he is giving his history, noting whether he breathes freely and easily or with the grunting respiration associated with peritoneal irritation, how the patient behaves while undressing and how he responds to sitting up or turning over on his side during clinical examination.

5. Other relevant symptoms. Questions must always be asked about the gastrointestinal tract (bowel habit, constipation, vomiting, appetite, loss of weight, amongst others) and also about the genitourinary system (frequency, burning, dysuria or haematuria), as well as the menstrual history and other related problems. When the pain is in the upper abdomen, particular attention should be paid to symptoms referrable to the respiratory and cardiovascular systems. Symptoms of fever, sweating, shivering or rigors will be supplemented by taking the temperature as well as the pulse and the blood pressure.

The examination is performed to determine the site or sites of tenderness, abdominal distension and enlarged organs or palpable masses. It is important to establish the presence or absence and character of bowel sounds. Having done this decide whether or not the patient has *peritonism*. As the peritoneum becomes involved tenderness is accompanied by *guarding, rigidity* and 'rebound tenderness'. Pressure on the abdomen must be sufficient to depress the peritoneum and the patient must be allowed time to accommodate to this. If sharp withdrawal of the hand produces obvious pain, rebound tenderness is said to be present. Voluntary contraction of the abdominal muscles during examination is guarding. Involuntary contraction is rigidity. The progressive disappearance of bowel sounds accompanies this pathological process. The pain of peritonitis is usually severe and continuous. It may start locally but spreads to involve the whole of the abdomen.

A frightened patient in severe pain will be unable to give a clear history and examination will be difficult. Adequate analgesia will make diagnosis easier and not more difficult as is sometimes thought.

In the acute stages peritonism may be associated with a rigid tender abdomen in a shocked patient. The transverse colon divides the abdomen into a supra- and infracolic compartment. Therefore, peritonitis may be localised to one of these halves in its early stages. Because of the paracolic gutters, fluid tracks down both sides of the abdomen, and symptoms may also be felt more at the sides. A lesion involving the gall bladder, pancreas or peptic ulcer will drain fluid through the right hepatic space and the right paracolic gutter and the pain is more likely to be on the right. The sigmoid colon lies obliquely and will divert fluid out of the pouch of Douglas and towards the left. A pelvic appendix and a pelvic abscess are therefore more likely to produce symptoms on the left.

A patient with acute generalised peritonitis requires resuscitation and monitoring of the urinary output. Blood gases should be estimated and a chest radiograph taken. Blood should be sent for serum amylase, blood culture, full blood count, urea, electrolytes and blood glucose. A 'shocked' patient will require oxygen, analgesia and a plasma expander as detailed in Ch. 13.

Paralytic ileus is associated with abdominal distension and vomiting. It is usually secondary to peritonitis but also occurs with pancreatitis, hypokalaemia and after anticholinergic drugs have been given. It is most commonly seen postoperatively. It can occur with a retroperitoneal haematoma following abdominal or spinal injury. When peritonism is not a feature then there is often little pain. Bowel sounds are usually absent; occasionally a few normal sounds can be heard but these are not associated with pain.

Rectal or vaginal examination

One or other of these examinations should be performed in every patient at some stage of the patient's care in hospital. They are particularly important in patients who are being sent home. However, if the A & E doctor can make a clear decision that admission to hospital is necessary, then it will often be kinder to leave the rectal or vaginal examination to the admitting doctor who will have to make the definitive decisions about treatment.

An empty rectum in the presence of intestinal obstruction will exclude constipation as a cause. The presence of mucus, blood or a melaena stool on the examining finger may help confirm an otherwise uncertain diagnosis. A pelvic abscess may only be diagnosed by a rectal, vaginal or bidigital examination. Vaginal examination should be carried out once only and by the gynaecologist when there is a suspicion of an ectopic gestation. The patient should empty the bladder before any of these examinations is carried out.

Examination of the urine

Not only should the routine chemical tests be carried out, but also urine should be examined by the doctor for its colour, its clarity, its smell and if necessary its microscopic characteristics. A microscope should be available to every A & E department so that the presence of pyuria can be detected. This may sometimes focus attention on the urinary tract of a patient with otherwise unexplained abdominal pain. The detection also of red cells will distinguish haematuria from haemoglobinuria (or porphyria).

Examination of the faeces

This should be performed whenever possible by the doctor — whether on the gloved finger following rectal examination or through a proctoscope. Occasionally, sigmoidoscopy will be indicated (if ulcerative colitis or other rectal pathology is suspected) but will usually be carried out by the admitting surgeon after the patient has left the department.

Pitfalls

1. Steroid therapy. Physical signs following a perforated viscus may be minimal in patients on prolonged steroid therapy (such as the patient with rheumatoid arthritis who perforates an appendix, or the patient suffering from ulcerative colitis whose colon perforates).

2. The very old, the very young and the very ill may not be able to communicate the site or the severity of their pain.

3. The presence of fever will suggest an infective lesion, but its absence will not exclude infections in the old, the very ill or

those on long-term steroid or immunosuppressive drugs.

4. Patients presenting with abdominal pain and the signs of hypovolaemic shock may be suffering from a perforated viscus (such as a duodenal ulcer), a retroperitoneal haemorrhage (e.g. from a ruptured abdominal aortic aneurysm), or a ruptured ectopic pregnancy, but such a combination of symptoms and signs may also occur in acute cardiogenic shock secondary to myocardial infarction, septic shock (often associated with pyelonephritis) and diabetic coma. Such very ill patients may also be unable to give a coherent history.

5. A number of conditions may present with abdominal pain where the pathology is not primarily intra-abdominal. They are set out in Table 21.1 (for a description and discussion of these conditions, see Howard, 1972).

6. Organs which are abnormal (as a consequence of either congenital anomaly or previous disease) may rupture following trivial injury. Examples of this will include rupture of a spleen affected by glandular fever or malaria, and rupture of a hydronephrotic kidney.

Table 21.1 Abdominal pain caused by extra-abdominal diseases

Intrathoracic
Basal pneumonia, pleurisy and pulmonary infarction
Bornholm disease
Myocardial infarction and pericarditis
Dissecting aneurysm of the aorta

Metabolic
Diabetic ketoacidosis
Acute porphyria
Lead poisoning

Neurological
Pain referred from the spine
Tabetic crisis
Herpes zoster

Systemic disease
Polyarteritis nodosa
Disseminated lupus erythematosus
Henoch-Schonlein purpura
Sickle cell crisis
Familial Mediterranean fever

Drug-induced disease
Anticoagulants causing haemorrhage
Barbiturates precipitating a porphyric crisis (see Ch. 15)

Psychogenic
Anxiety and hysteria
Munchausen syndrome

SYSTEMATIC APPROACH TO THE DIAGNOSIS

A definitive diagnosis cannot be made in about 45% of patients. These are often labelled as 'non-specific abdominal pain'. The pain under these circumstances may be present in any part of the abdomen — although most commonly it is central or involving the whole abdomen. There is no marked tenderness, no guarding and no other signs of peritonism. Some of these patients may have mild intestinal colic following dietary indiscretions, some may have

a urinary tract infection and in some there may be a psychogenic component (see Ch. 28). A decision about management may only be possible after a period in the observation ward, which is particularly useful for such patients. However, many will be thought suitable for discharge if the pain is thought not to be severe and if adequate support from friends is available at home (Fig. 21.1).

Intra-abdominal cancer may present following perforation of the cancer in the stomach or large bowel. However, it can also present as unexplained abdominal pain of short duration and must be considered in all patients, but particularly those over the age of 50 years. The more usual presentation involves a change of bowel habit and weight loss over weeks or months. It is the family doctor who is usually consulted, but patients may seek advice from the A & E department.

In the remaining 55% of cases it should be possible to make a provisional diagnosis with some confidence. The following paragraphs start the diagnostic process with the site of pain in the abdomen — upper, central or lower.

Upper abdominal pain

Pain in this region is quite commonly referred from elsewhere (lungs, heart or spine), but if the source of the pain is within the upper abdomen it usually arises from the foregut, i.e. from the lower oesophagus, stomach, duodenum, biliary tree or pancreas.

Severe colicky pain

This may be felt in the midline, just to the right of the middle or under the right costal margin. It is nearly always related to the biliary tree and will often be very acute in onset. There may be a history of previous similar attacks with or without jaundice. In any given attack, the appearance of jaundice (indicating that a stone has passed into the common bile duct) may take a day or more to develop. Nearly all these patients will have a positive Murphy's sign. (Murphy's sign is said to be positive when an inflamed gall

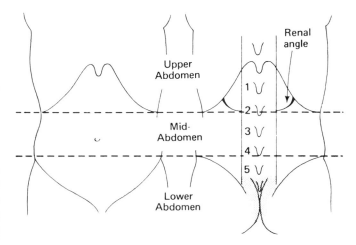

Fig. 21.1 The three abdominal regions described in the text — delineated one from another by costal margins and the top of the iliac crests.

bladder causes a catch in the breath when the patient breathes in with the examiner's fingers in the right hypochondrium.) The urine should be tested for bile. Only about 15% of biliary calculi are opaque to radiographs. It is difficult to distinguish between acute cholecystitis and 'so called' biliary colic. The latter refers to obstruction of the cystic duct without acute inflammation of the gall bladder. It is not a true colic but a gradual pain sustained for several hours and sometimes days. Serum amylase may be slightly raised. Admission will usually be indicated and an analgesic such as pethidine should not be withheld once the admitting doctors have been consulted.

Severe non-colicky pain, developing acutely (without peritonism)

This may indicate an oesophageal perforation, an early pancreatitis or rarely, a dissection of the thoracic aorta. Non-calculous gall bladder disease does not usually present so acutely. However, in all of these conditions the pain may also be felt in the back — pancreatitis, oesophageal perforation and dissecting aneurysm near the midline — whilst gall bladder pain is referred to the angle of the right scapula. Conditions above the diaphragm may be easily confused with the above diagnoses. The patient with a severe myocardial infarction may be sweating and complain of 'gripping' or 'crushing' pain (which is often but not always referred to the shoulder or arm). Pain arising from the lungs will usually be accentuated by respiratory movements and if diaphragmatic, may be referred also to the tip of one or other shoulder.

A *sickle cell crisis* can occur in carriers of haemoglobin S. Some southern Europeans are affected but Negroes are the principal carriers. Homozygous individuals are severely affected but heterozygous carriers can experience symptoms during periods of *hypoxia*. Haemolytic anaemia and multiple infarctions can occur but the commonest presentation is a painful crisis. The pain is severe and often abdominal. It can be difficult to distinguish from appendicitis or cholecystitis. In children the hands and feet are often involved and swelling accompanies the pain. The diagnosis is confirmed by the microscopic demonstration of sickling. A 5 ml specimen of blood in EDTA bottle is required. Treatment is primarily with narcotic analgesia but 100% oxygen and intravenous fluid replacement is also required.

The patient should be referred to the inpatient medical team.

Investigations

Radiographs may show pathology in the lungs, but basal consolidation and a small effusion can be confusing since they may be an indication of pathology beneath the diaphragm. An ECG may not be helpful at this stage, nor may cardiac enzymes. A high serum amylase, however, may distinguish acute pancreatitis from the rest.

All such patients will need admission and should be given intravenous analgesia at the earliest possible moment.

With peritonism. Such pain is usually due to a perforated peptic ulcer or pancreatitis. In either case, pain may be referred to the tip of the right shoulder (or the left if the lesser sac is involved).

Perforation of a peptic ulcer. The mortality and morbidity from this condition is proportional to the duration of the perforation and the age of the patient. As time progresses a chemical peritonitis deteriorates into a bacterial peritonitis. Bowel sounds will be absent from an early stage. Splinting of the diaphragm which occurs in this condition predisposes to complicating chest infection which accounts for the significant mortality in the elderly. These days the patient has often no previous history of peptic ulceration or dyspepsia but the perforation may have been precipitated by the ingestion of alcohol or aspirin. Tobacco is also known to be a predisposing factor. Some perforated duodenal and gastric ulcers produce right-sided signs (but many produce generalised pain starting in the epigastrium). This is because the right hepatic space opens on the right and fluid will track down the right paracolic gutter. An erect chest radiograph may reveal gas over the diaphragm in 50–75% of patients. The serum amylase may be slightly raised but not as high as in acute pancreatitis. Commence intravenous infusion and pass a nasogastric tube. Analgesia with intravenous pethidine should be given immediately and the patient referred to a surgeon.

Pancreatitis. This condition can be associated with gallstones, alcohol abuse, hyperlipidaemia, hypercalcaemia, steroid therapy, pancreatic malignancy and often trauma. The pain is usually sudden and very severe. It is associated with vomiting. The patient may be shocked and occasionally have a fever. The patient requires an intravenous infusion and drainage of gastric contents. Pethidine should be given intravenously. The serum amylase is raised above 1000 i.u. Blood gases should be estimated as hypoxaemia can complicate this condition. Hypocalcaemia is also associated and the serum calcium should be checked at regular intervals. Immediate referral to a surgeon is indicated.

If the condition goes untreated then skin discolouration can occur in the late preterminal stages. This is well described but extremely rare. Discolouration in the loins has been described as 'Grey Turner's sign' and the periumbilical staining as 'Cullen's sign'.

Moderately severe non-colicky pain of fairly rapid onset

This may be due to an exacerbation of a peptic ulcer, acute cholecystitis (in which case the pain is often felt under the right costal margin) or pancreatitis (in which case the pain may often spread towards the left). In all three the pain may be felt also in the back — in the case of the gall bladder at the tip of the right scapula, with duodenal ulcer and pancreatitis towards the midline. Previous episodes of biliary colic or of exacerbations of peptic-ulcer-type pain (typically relieved by alkali or food, and often waking the patient at 2.00 or 3.00 in the morning) will help to distinguish these two. Recurrent pancreatitis is associated with alcohol abuse.

A reflux oesophagitis (associated usually with a hiatus hernia) may also present in this way. However, in this case there will

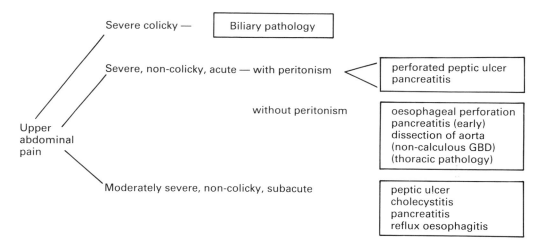

Fig. 21.2 Upper abdominal pain.

usually have been a preceding history of postprandial pain which is worse when lying down or stooping, and relieved (particularly at night) in the sitting posture. Signs of peritonitis (or peritonism) will not be present unless any of these conditions progresses to perforation or acute inflammatory peritonitis. The bowel sounds will therefore usually remain active.

The differential diagnosis from conditions above the diaphragm should be considered as in the preceding section.

Those with suspected cholecystitis or pancreatitis should be admitted but most patients who are thought to have an exacerbation of a duodenal ulcer or of a reflux oesophagitis may be allowed home with an antacid and appropriate advice, together with a letter for their general practitioner. If there is any doubt, a short period in the observation ward and therapeutic trial of antacids may clarify the diagnosis. (Fig. 21.2).

Mid-abdominal pain

Pain in this region may be referred from the spine, but if the source is within the abdomen it may have its origins in the mid or hind gut or in the retroperitoneal organs (aorta, kidneys and ureters).

Severe colicky pain of rapid onset

If this is accompanied by diarrhoea and vomiting, the diagnosis is likely to be gastroenteritis. The absence of abdominal signs (except slight tenderness in the left iliac fossa) and the presence of active bowel sounds will exclude more serious pathology and the patient may be allowed home with symptomatic treatment and a letter for his general practitioner. A Richter's hernia may occasionally present in this way — therefore, the hernial orifices must always be examined. (A Richter's hernia is when the wall of a piece of bowel herniates, but not the whole loop — Fig. 21.3.)

However, if this rapid onset of colicky mid-abdominal pain is accompanied by constipation (as well as vomiting) the diagnosis must be assumed to be intestinal obstruction. Establish whether this is due to an open or closed loop and whether the obstruction is simple or strangulated. The latter is likely to have occurred

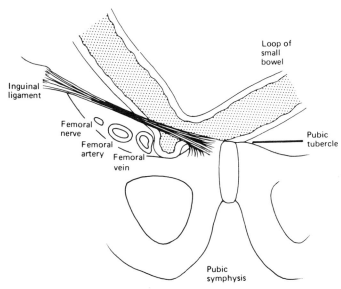

Fig. 21.3 A knuckle of bowel caught in the femoral canal, causing incomplete (partial) intestinal obstruction (Richter's hernia).

suddenly and be associated with shock. Bowel sounds will be increased, rectal examination (after evacuation spontaneously or following a suppository) will indicate the absence of faeces in the rectum. With a high obstruction, vomiting is early and profuse and distension minimal; with a low small bowel obstruction or large bowel obstruction, vomiting may be late but distension early. If the obstruction has been present for some while, or if the abdominal wall is thin, peristalsis may be visible. The bowel sounds are said to be 'tinkling' and come in clusters or rushes, coincident with the pain. In mechanical obstruction the pain comes in waves and the bowel sounds are increased in association with the pain. Strangulated herniae are often missed because it is not realised that local pain is not an essential feature and femoral swellings are too often thought to be inflammatory. The patient may have peritonism particularly if there is an incarceration of a hernia. Gastric aspiration and intravenous infusion of normal saline should be established at once.

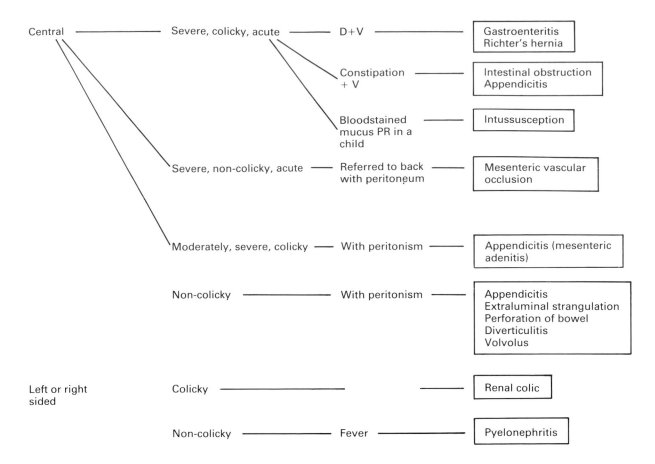

Fig. 21.4 Mid-abdominal pain.

Mechanical obstruction may be:

1. Intraluminal — such as a gall-stone.

2. Intramural — such as intussusception (occuring commonly in babies or young children), or Crohn's disease (commonly in young adults).

3. Extraluminal (pressure on the outside of the gut) — this may be the neck of a femoral or inguinal hernia, or adhesions or congenital bands within the peritoneal cavity causing internal herniae (Figs 21.4 and 21.5).

In the early stages of appendicitis, impacted faecoliths cause typical obstructive gut pain, felt in the centre of the abdomen. As the wall of the appendix becomes inflamed, the pain alters in character and moves to the right iliac fossa.

Intussusception. Occurs in children from the age of two months to two years. It is characterised by sudden intermittent abdominal pain. The spasms may last minutes or sometimes an hour. There may be vomiting. The 'classic' bloodstained mucus p.r. occurs in only 50% of patients. However, detection rate can be improved by inspecting the gloved finger used for rectal examination. An abdominal lump can often be palpated either in the right iliac fossa or somewhere along the course of the large bowel. A diagnosis

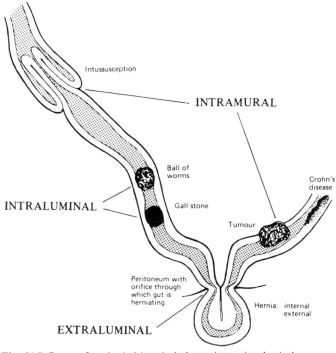

Fig. 21.5 Causes of mechanical intestinal obstruction — intraluminal, intramural and extraluminal.

is confirmed by barium enema. Ths investigation can be used as a therapeutic manoeuvre.

Radiographs may be very helpful under these circumstances (see p. 75). If vomiting has been prolonged or profuse, estimation of electrolytes should be carried out and an intravenous infusion set up. All these patients will need urgent admission and usually operation.

Severe non-colicky pain of sudden onset

When this is referred to the back and accompanied by local or generalised peritonism it is likely to be due to a mesenteric vascular occlusion involving small or large bowel. The pain may be poorly localised and the diagnosis from acute pancreatitis may not be easy. Sometimes tenderness localised above the umbilicus and accompanied by dark blood and mucus in the faeces will indicate that the ischaemic segment is in the transverse colon. Plain radiograph may be helpful (see pp. 65 and 74).

Less severe pain, colicky or non-colicky

Such pain unaccompanied initially by peritonism is most often due to appendicitis, or, in children, to 'non-specific abdominal pain' (mesenteric adenitis). In appendicitis the pain may be felt initially in the right iliac fossa or may subsequently pass to this region and tenderness will usually be maximal at McBurney's point. The diagnosis is more likely when there is tenderness on rectal examination, particularly if this tenderness is referred upwards towards the abdomen. Enquire of all patients about associated urinary symptoms, as a urinary tract infection can often be misdiagnosed for this condition. Pelvic inflammatory disease in the female may be confused but may be differentiated by eliciting cervical excitation on vaginal examination. Mesenteric adenitis occurs in young people, but this is basically a diagnosis of exclusion and is unlikely to be made in the A & E department. Testicular pathology in men may be interpreted as pain in the lower abdomen and external genitalia must always be examined. Computer-aided diagnosis significantly improves performance and should be used wherever possible. A radiograph is unlikely to be helpful and unfortunately the white count is only consistantly raised in those patients in whom the diagnosis is clinically obvious. From a practical point of view, a differentiation between Meckel's diverticulitis and appendicitis is not important at this stage — both require urgent operation. A Meckel's diverticulum occurs in 2% of the human race and males outnumber females 3–1. Twenty per cent of these diverticula have heterotopic mucosa and this is most often gastric. The constant acid secretion leads to peptic ulceration within a Meckel's diverticulum and this may bleed.

The differentiation of appendicitis from 'non-specific abdominal pain' (mesenteric adenitis) may not be easy. The pain of the latter tends to be non-colicky, severe and intermittent, and the fever may be rather higher than in early appendicitis (although a normal temperature is not uncommon). Tenderness is usually close to the umbilicus and, while the pain is felt in the right iliac fossa, tenderness to the left of the umbilicus is common. Pressure on the left of the abdomen does not produce pain on the right side (as is sometimes found in appendicitis) and the 'psoas' sign is never positive. The positive 'psoas' sign occurs when psoas irritation results in flexion of the hip at rest with the patient lying flat. This can be a feature of appendicitis but is not a feature of mesenteric adenitis. Mesenteric adenitis is a virus infection of Peyer's patches which produces subumbilical colic. It can be associated with cervical lymphadenopathy. It is unwise to send a patient home armed only with this diagnosis. It is better to admit the patient and repeat the examination. Mesenteric adenitis is common in childhood, less common in teenagers, and rare after the age of 20.

Non-colicky abdominal pain with peritonism

This may spread to either side of the abdomen. Bowel sounds are usually absent. It may indicate the presence of strangulation (if these signs were proceeded by a period of central colicky obstructive pain), or perforation of small or large bowel or the appendix. As indicated above, the tenderness of acute appendicitis is most commonly in the right iliac fossa but may be under the right costal margin, under the right rectus, over the brim of the pelvis or close to the anterior superior iliac spine. Tenderness in the right iliac fossa may also be due to a solitary ulcer of the caecum or to volvulus of the right colon. The last is uncommon in the UK but is very common in some African countries.

If the tenderness is mainly in the left iliac fossa the likely diagnosis is diverticulitis or volvulus of the left colon. In the latter case, distension is usually very rapid and striking and the radiograph quite characteristic (see pp. 65 and 74).

All of these conditions merit urgent admission and usually operation. An intravenous infusion should be started before the patient is transferred to the ward.

Left or right side pain of the mid abdomen

Colicky pain may start in the loin and spread into the iliac fossae.

Renal colic — the passage of a stone into or down the ureter will usually produce severe pain. This is intermittent and spreads from the loin or abdomen to the groin, testicle or upper thigh. The patient is restless, sweating and may vomit. During the pain the abdomen is rigid but examination may be normal at other times. Urinalysis often reveals haematuria. A plain radiograph of the abdomen is a traditional method of identifying a renal or ureteric stone. It is a very unreliable investigation. An i.v.u. is much more sensitive particularly if repeated follow-up films are done to show stasis within the renal tract. Strong intravenous analgesia (e.g. pethidine) is required to relieve the pain and referral to a surgeon is indicated.

Non-colicky renal pain associated with fever may be due to various pathological entities such as pyelonephritis, carbuncle of the kidney, a perinephric abscess and tumour. The patient often feels alternately hot and cold, with shivering and sweating. In all but the first of these conditions there may be a palpable tumour. A tender palpable kidney in a febrile patient whose urine is macroscopically clear suggests a 'blocked kidney' and urgent admission is required. Any patient who is toxic with a high fever and severe pain will also require admission. Some patients with acute renal colic may be treated initially on an outpatient basis with arrangement being made for an early urological appointment. Sometimes when the pain has been very severe, 24 hours in the observation ward may be appropriate. Investigations including urea and electrolytes and intravenous pyelogram should, however, be initiated at the first visit. The intravenous pyelogram is discussed in the section on radiology at the end of this chapter.

Skillful representation of renal colic (even to the extent of adding a few drops of blood to a sample of urine) may deceive even the most experienced doctor. This problem is discussed further in Chapter 31.

Torsion of the testis.   May produce lower abdominal pain. No age is immune from this condition, but it usually occurs below the age of 18. The majority of lesions occur round about puberty. If the diagnosis is delayed or missed both testes suffer because an autoimmune process reduces fertility on the non-affected side. The other testis is also at risk of torsion. It is characterised by sudden pain in the testis often associated with nausea and vomiting. The skin of the scrotum may be red. It is often confused with epididymo-orchitis, a condition in which the prostate is usually tender and the urine is non-sterile. If the patient is allowed to stand then the opposite testis can be seen to lie horizontally.

Lower abdominal pain

Sudden severe pain, with or without colic and/or peritonism. This combination of symptoms and signs is rarely found in men but may be due to a calculus in the lower end of the ureter. In women such pain, often poorly localised to one or other side, is most likely to be due to an ectopic gestation. At the moment of rupture of the fallopian tube the patient may feel a sharp pain followed a

few minutes later by a feeling of weakness and dizziness. If such a patient gives a history of missing one period, has some vaginal bleeding, is tender in one or other iliac fossa and is hypovolaemic, the diagnosis will not be in doubt. Such a patient should have an intravenous infusion started, blood sent for cross-matching and she should then be referred immediately for surgery. In many patients, however, there may be no signs of peritonism. Occasionally, blood will track up the paracolic gutters to cause pain referred to the right or left shoulder tip. One vaginal examination only should be carried out prior to operation in these patients and this is preferably performed by the surgeon who will be operating on the patient (Fig. 21.6) (see Ch. 24).

Sudden pain with profuse vaginal bleeding

This is most likely to be due to an abortion. The help of the gynaecologists should be sought here also.

Moderate non-colicky pain of gradual onset

In the female, moderate non-colicky pain of gradual onset may originate in one or other fallopian tube or ovary, which will be tender on vaginal examination. Salpingitis is a common cause of this type of pain. Such patients usually (but not always) have urinary symptoms and either a vaginal discharge or pyuria. There is often (but not always) a slight fever. Vaginal examination causes pain when the cervix is moved. No mass is usually felt unless the condition has proceeded to pyosalpinx. Somewhat similar but more severe pain in either the left or the right side may be due to torsion or rupture of an ovarian cyst. For further differential diagnosis a textbook of gynaecology should be consulted.

In either sex the commonest cause of pain in the right iliac fossa is appendicitis, provided the pain is accompanied by local tenderness at McBurney's point (which, as described earlier,

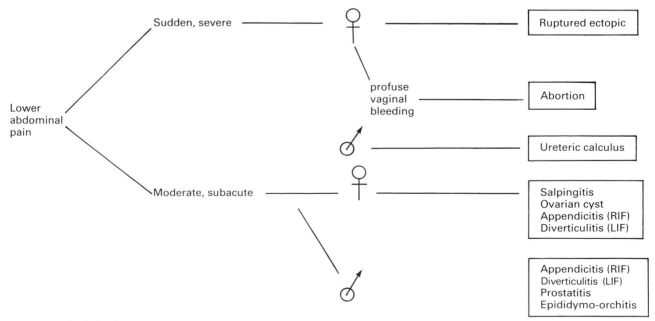

Fig. 21.6 Lower abdominal pain.

differentiates it from mesenteric adenitis). Pain and tenderness on the left side (usually in a middle-aged to elderly subject) is most commonly due to diverticulitis,which may or not be accompanied by peritonism. Either of these conditions may be accompanied by slight fever.

In men, an acute infective prostatitis may cause lower abdominal pain, usually with a high fever, urinary symptoms and a prostate which is acutely tender when palpated through the rectum. Acute epididymo-orchitis may occasionally present with low pain in the right or left side of the abdomen.

Radiograph examination is unlikely to be helpful in these patients and the majority will need admission to a surgical or gynaecological ward.

CONCLUSION

From the above it will be seen that there is considerable overlap between the different regions of the abdomen, but that appendicitis may present with symptoms or signs in any one of them.

Can the patient go home?

Allow the patient home if:
1. They are symptom-free.
2. They are not a child.
3. They are going home to a responsible adult to whom you have spoken.
4. They are on the telephone.
5. Examination of the abdomen was normal and all investigations were negative.

The indications for radiographic investigation have been mentioned and, because of the difficulty in interpreting these radiographs, it is hoped that the following section will be helpful to A & E doctors who have to make a decision at times when the help of a radiologist is not available.

When considering these points it is wise to remember that the taking of such radiographs may be uncomfortable or even harmful for certain categories of patients — besides being costly. Usually the radiographer (or radiologist) is better placed to decide which views are indicated than the referring doctor — provided that clinical details and suspected diagnosis are recorded on the request card. The radiographer, however, will need to know whether the patient is fit enough to have radiographs taken in the erect position; if not, lateral decubitus films should be substituted.

If there is any doubt about interpretation of the radiographs, or if a special investigation is contemplated, a radiologist should be consulted.

Some of the abnormalities which may be detected in the A & E department will now be discussed.

RADIOGRAPHY

Chest radiographs

Whenever possible, posteroanterior films should be taken in the erect posture in inspiration supplemented when necessary by lateral or oblique views. If the patient is too ill to sit up, lateral decubitus views may be of value.

The interpretation of radiographs of the chest should be familiar to the reader, but the following points should be noted.

1. The presence of basal inflammatory disease in the lungs may explain upper abdominal pain.

2. Basal effusions may indicate subphrenic pathology.

3. A gas/fluid level behind the cardiac shadow may suggest the presence of a hiatus hernia.

4. The presence of mediastinal emphysema or a pneumothorax may suggest (in the appropriate clinical context) the presence of a rupture of the oesophagus. Radiographic studies can confirm the presence of an oesophageal rupture,but any contrast medium may of course find its way into the lungs. Barium is contraindicated and both gastrograffin and urograffin are hyperosmolar and can lead to pulmonary oedema. Low osmolar media must be used for this investigation in these circumstances.

5. The appearance of a high left diaphragm may indicate rupture following closed injury (even in the absence of evidence of damage externally to the chest). Inspiration and expiration radiographs are useful to differentiate a simple eventration in which the normal swing remains. A high diaphragm may also indicate paralysis due to the presence of subphrenic blood or pus.

6. Air close under the diaphragm muscle indicates a perforated viscus and may be distinguished by the gas bubble in the stomach from the fact that the latter deviates away from the diaphragm towards its left side. A lesser sac perforation may be more difficult to differentiate (Figs 21.7 and 21.8).

7. Displacement of the gas bubble in the stomach towards the

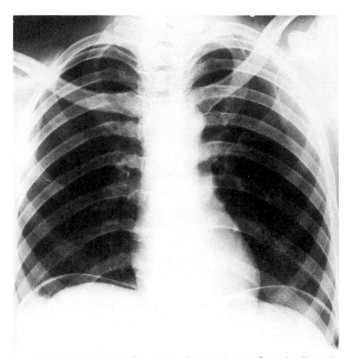

Fig. 21.7 Erect radiograph of the chest of this patient confirms the diagnosis of a perforated viscus (duodenum).

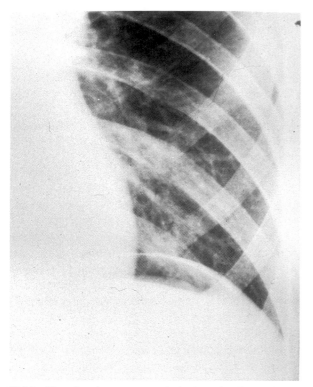

Fig. 21.8 In this patient there was some doubt about the dignosis following clinical examination. In the erect chest radiograph the gas shadow (which was present under the left diaphragm only) was misinterpreted as a normal 'stomach bubble', and the patient was sent home. In fact, the gas shadow followed the line of the diaphragm right across, indicating a perforation of a peptic ulcer in the lesser sac. This patient died.

right may indicate an enlarged spleen or bleeding around the spleen or kidney.

8. Gas under the right diaphragm indicates a perforated viscus. However, this should not be confused with the occasional normal interposition of a loop of colon between the liver and the diaphragm.

9. The interpretation of chest radiographs following injury is discussed in Ch. 8.

Plain radiographs of the abdomen

Plain films in the erect posture will add little to what can be seen on the supine study, provided the latter is combined with scrutiny of an erect chest film. However, the presence of minimally distended loops may be more obvious to the unexperienced observer when identified as air fluid levels on erect views. If the patient is too ill to assume the upright position, a lateral decubitus study with the right side raised will suffice.

Plain films should also be examined for abnormalities of the bony structures, and the soft tissue outlines of the liver, spleen and retroperitoneum. It should also be used to detect the following:

Gall stones and renal calculi:

Differentiation between calcified lymph nodes is usually possible.

Phleboliths can cause confusion, particularly in the pelvis, but usually demonstrate a small central lucency. Approximately 80% of renal calculi are opaque, but they may be exceedingly small and difficult to detect due to overlying bowel shadows, and also when sited over the bony structures of the transverse processes or sacrum. It is important to scrutinize these areas when renal colic is suspected. 10–20% of gall stones are opaque. They may be difficult to identify, especially on overpenetrated films or impacted in the distal ileum. Ultrasound is the examination of choice where gall bladder disease is suspected and plain film studies are unhelpful.

Calcification

Calcification may be identified in the aorta, with or without aneurysmal dilatation. It is also commonly seen in the splenic and ileofemoral vessels.

Punctate calcification may occasionally be seen in chronic relapsing pancreatitis.

Rarely the gall bladder wall is calcified — 'porcelain gall bladder'. Its contents may also show homogeneous calcification — 'limey gall bladder'.

Cysts in the liver and spleen may also be a well defined rim of marginal calcification. Faint speckled areas of calcification may draw attention to gut, liver and renal tract tumours.

Foreign bodies

Pins, buttons and other radio-opaque foreign bodies are commonly swallowed by children, but seldom need to be followed by serial films, as most pass spontaneously. Glass fragments may be difficult to identify.

Bezoars may form in patients who have undergone gastric surgery, particularly vagotomy with reduction in gastric motility. These usually consist of organic vegetable matter and may be recognised as mottled soft tissue masses. Trichobezoars (hair balls) present a similar appearance and are usually present in patients with a psychiatric disturbance. Very rarely in the UK a bolus of roundworms may be seen obstructing the distal ileum.

Gas bubbles

Mottled bubbly gas shadows may be seen outside the GI tract due to retroperitoneal perforation and/or abscess formation. They are easily mistaken for faeces. Streaks of gas can occur in the wall of gut and indicate necrosis. This is usually due to mesenteric infarction. An exception to this are blebs or streaks of gas seen in the gut wall in pneumatosis intestinalis.

Distribution of gas and fluid

The distribution of bowel gas and fluid will now be considered.

Gas is normally present in the stomach and colon. It is rarely present in the small gut in any quantity, but does tend to increase when the patient is confined to bed. This gas is widely scattered in small collections and there is no increase in the diameter of the gut.

In obstruction fluid as well as gas collects in the lumen of the gut and the relative amounts can vary enormously.

Air fluid levels indicate stasis, but do not help distinguish between mechanical obstruction and paralytic ileus. They may also be due to non-specific diarrhoea, administration of enemata or ingestion of large amounts of fluid. Marked gaseous distension may be seen in chronic constipation, particularly in elderly or long-term psychiatric patients. This is usually distinguished by large quantities of faecal residue throughout the colon and extending into the rectum.

Distinction between the small and large gut is usually possible. The valvulae conniventes completely traverse the lumen of the small gut, whereas the haustral markings incompletely divide the colonic lumen.

Paralytic ileus commonly occurs in the immediate post operative period. Other causes include peritonitis, gut ischaemia, severe inflammatory bowel disease, thoracic and abdominal trauma, prolonged immobilisation and electrolyte disturbance, especially hypokalaemia. It is characterised by distension, absence of colic and auscultatory silence. The whole gut may be affected, or it may be limited to a single segment.

The differing positions within the abdomen of small and large bowel also help distinguish between the two. However, notable exceptions are small bowel loops in external inguinal and femoral herniae and caecal and sigmoid volvulus, where significant displacement from the norm occurs.

Difficulties can arise when oedema and distension obliterate the valvulae or haustral markings. Furthermore, the mucosal patterns of the ileum and sigmoid may be scant, causing problems in differentiation.

Aerophagy (meteorism). This is normally seen at the extremes of life. It is due to excessive air swallowing associated with painful conditions such as trauma or renal colic. Gross gaseous distension of the gut may be present. The gut walls are sharply defined and fluid levels are usually absent.

Small bowel

Mechanical obstruction. 1. Distended loops with air fluid levels, or fluid-filled loops proximal to the site of obstruction. Little or no gas may be evident in high obstruction. Such fluid-filled loops are difficult to identify — they are seen as homogeneous sausage-shaped densities.

2. Evacuation of bowel contents distal to the obstruction.

3. Increasing gas and/or fluid distension over several hours.

4. Multiple small air fluid levels resembling a 'string of beads' across the abdomen.

Paralytic ileus. 1. Most often seen for two or three days following surgery.

2. Multiple fluid filled loops in both small and large gut. May be identical to most types of large gut mechanical obstruction.

3. Little change in distension or position of loops over several hours.

4. Contiguous loops may be separated by thickened bowel wall when peritonitis is present.

5. Where ischaemia is present, the thickened bowel wall may present a scalloped or thumb print margin. The valvulae become flattened, indistinct and may disappear.

6. Localised ileus — sentinel loops may be seen adjacent to inflamed organs, e.g. gall bladder, pancreas, appendix. Indistinguishable from the very early stages of small gut mechanical obstruction.

Large bowel

Mechanical obstruction. 1. If the ileocaecal valve is competent, increasing gas and fluid distension of the colon occurs proximal to the obstruction. This is maximal in the caecum. Caecal perforation can occur.

2. Usually evacuation of bowel content occurs distally.

3. If the ileocaecal valve is incompetent (commonest type), the degree of colonic distension is less. Air fluid levels will be seen in both small and large gut, identical to those seen in paralytic ileus.

4. In obstruction to carcinoma, the gas column may taper distally at the site of tumour. The carcinoma may occasionally be outlined with air.

5. Volvulus: sigmoid — a huge distended ahaustral loop arising out of the pelvis, with an inverted U configuration. Gas and fluid distended gut is seen proximally. Caecal — a distended haustrated comma-shaped loop, which usually lies centrally or in the left upper quadrant. Usually contains a single fluid level. The caecum is noted to be absent from the right iliac fossa, which contains distended loops of ileum.

6. In suspected large gut obstruction, without perforation, it is safe to administer a single contrast instant barium enema, terminating the examination when the point of obstruction is reached.

Special investigations

Intravenous urography (i.v.u.)

This is of use chiefly for the investigation of cases of renal colic. There are many advantages in performing an i.v.u. immediately in the A & E department for all patients presenting for the first time with renal colic. It is rare for there not to be some clear radiographic signs to confirm the diagnosis at this time. It may not be necessary to repeat the i.v.u. for every attack in a patient who suffers from repeated attacks of renal colic. However, on the first occasion if the i.v.u. is postponed until a visit to an outpatient clinic, the radiographic signs may have disappeared, and it may no longer be possible to confirm or exclude a renal calculus.

In cases where there is no excretion of dye from the painful side, the possibility of a renal embolus should be remembered and angiography may be indicated.

In some cases the calculus can be clearly seen lying in the line of the ureter. However, some calculi are non-opaque and sometimes the patient has already passed the calculus. The size of the two kidneys should be measured and compared — obstruction causes swelling. Excretion of dye may be delayed on the affected side and there may be dilatation of the renal tract above the point of obstruction. Where excretion is delayed late pictures may show the dye even 12 hours after injection.

Angiography.   This is a comparitively rare investigation for acute abdominal pain. Its use is referred to in Ch. 8.

Ultrasound.   The advantages of this examination presenting in the A & E department have been referred to in Ch. 8. In diagnosing abdominal pain its value is especially in the diagnosis of cholecystitis and pancreatitis.

CT scanning.   The use of CT scanning in the diagnosis of acute abdominal pain is comparatively rare. One condition where it may be of use is in a suspected leak from abdominal aneurysm (see Ch. 8).

REFERENCES

Howard W H 1972 Medical states simulating the acute abdomen. British Journal of Hospital Medicine 7: 443

FURTHER READING

Diagnosis of acute abdominal pain F T de Dombal 1980 Churchill Livingstone, Edinburgh

Plain X-ray diagnosis of the acute abdomen M H Gough, M W L Gear, A S Darr 1986 Blackwell Scientific, Oxford

Abdominal pain in children B O'Donnell 1985 Blackwell Scientific, Oxford

Anorectal problems

Only some of the many conditions which produce symptoms in this area will present as emergencies. It is the duty of the A & E department to establish whether the condition needs any acute intervention or whether the local problem is really a symptom of a more general condition. The extent to which the A & E department is involved in treatment and follow-up will depend upon local custom and practice.

PAIN AROUND THE ANUS

Acute episodes of anal pain are common and patients usually, and often erroneously, attribute these to 'piles'. Internal haemorrhoids may prolapse alarmingly, but it is the *perianal haematoma* (thrombosed external pile) that is usually painful. This tender, dark blue swelling may appear at the anal margin following straining. It is not a haemorrhoid but a haematoma, caused by the rupture of a tributary of the inferior haemorrhoidal plexus. Incision and drainage under general anaesthetic will relieve symptoms, but needs to be carried out within 24 hours of their onset. When haemorrhoids prolapse they may be strangulated by spasm of the anal sphincter. This is painful and reduction under general anaesthesia is indicated. The patient is usually referred to the surgical team.

A *fissure in ano* or tear of the anal margin is a common complaint in adults. Multiple fissures are uncommon and may be associated with Crohn's disease. Examination will show a tight anal sphincter and occasionally a tag of torn epithelium. The fissure itself is seen immediately within the anal opening. Treatment does not usually fall within the remit of an emergency department and referral to a general practitioner is appropriate. If pain is very severe then an urgent surgical appointment can be arranged.

However, the presence of tears around the anal margin in infants and children must alert the doctor to the possibility of sexual abuse. Innocent or spontaneous anal tears are rare in children. Reddening around the anal margin occurs in abuse, but more commonly with diarrhoea and threadworms. Haematoma and other clear signs of

trauma must be assumed to be abuse. Reflex dilatation of the anal canal, venous swelling and loss of tone are also extremely suspicious and such children must be investigated for sexual abuse. Detailed examination and investigations may be more appropriately carried out once the patient has been admitted. Investigation of the anus and rectum, if only with a finger, constitutes a further violation of the child and is to be avoided in the A & E department (see Ch. 5).

Abscesses around the anus are painful and require immediate treatment. This topic is dealt with in Ch. 31.

Prolapse of the rectum may be a presenting symptom, but it is more likely to be an incidental finding. A *partial prolapse* involving only the rectal mucosa can occur at any age. A *complete prolapse* involving all the rectal wall is more common in the elderly, and elderly women in particular. Appropriate referral is indicated.

Pruritus ani or itching around the anus is an uncomfortable symptom, but not an emergency. It is primarily a localised skin condition. However, particularly in children, *threadworms* can cause intense nocturnal itching around the anus. The child may scream with frustration and be brought to the emergency department by their anxious parents. It is not necessary to employ the traditional 'Sellotape' trap to visualise the tiny thread-like worms. Minimal patience and a keen eye will soon be rewarded by the sight of worms looking like small strands of cotton. If doubt exists the worm will move when prodded! An adult with pruritus ani should be referred to his family doctor unless there is evidence of an underlying condition associated with generalised pruritus, e.g. obstructive jaundice, lymphoma or severe iron deficiency anaemia. The patient should be advised to keep the area clean and dry, and avoid ointments, creams and talcum powder.

Patients may present to an emergency department for anonymous advice about perianal warts and condylomata (acuminata or lata). Referral to an appropriate outpatient clinic is indicated.

BOWEL PROBLEMS

Constipation

A change in bowel habit in a middle-aged or elderly patient should always alert the doctor to the possibility of bowel neoplasia. However, constipation affects many people in the western world and is largely the result of a low fibre diet. Immobility and poor fluid intake are also factors and all of these may combine in the elderly patient. However, constipation can be associated with abdominal or more generalised pathology, e.g. hypothyroidism, and is a feature of depression. Patients do not often present to the emergency department solely because of constipation, but sometimes they do. Always examine your patient, even when you feel their attendance is perhaps unwarranted. Exclude intestinal obstruction (see p. 254), and examine the rectum. You may identify the impacted faeces or be surprised by the carcinoma. If the diagnosis remains in doubt, an X-ray of the abdomen may be taken. The presence of large amounts of faeces extending from the proximal colon into the rectum will exclude a large bowel obstruction. Conversely, the absence of faeces in the rectum raises the suspicion of a large bowel obstruction.

Diarrhoea can complicate constipation as a 'retention with overflow' phenomenon. However it is usually the result of an acute infection.

Diarrhoea

Acute gastroenteritis of infancy is a major problem, particularly in the developing world, but all children are at risk if rehydration is inadequate or delayed. An infant requires 120–150 ml/kg each day when healthy and a large fluid deficit is easily accumulated in the presence of diarrhoea. This is usually secondary to gastroenteritis, but can accompany urinary and respiratory infections as well as otitis media and meningitis. Non-infective causes must also be considered, such as intussusception and appendicitis.

The rotavirus is the commonest organism responsible for gastroenteritis in infants. A cough, running nose and sometimes fever may precede the diarrhoea and vomiting. Other organisms responsible include *Shigella, E. coli, Salmonella* and *Campylobacter.* Occasionally amoebic dysentery will be encountered.

Moderate dehydration (5% body wt) might produce few physical signs other than dry mucous membranes. Once the 'classical' signs of sunken eyes, a depressed fontanelle and loss of skin turgor have appeared the child is certainly 5% dehydrated and probably more. When more than 10% of the body weight has been lost there will be circulatory collapse, tachypnoea, oliguria and loss of conscious level. The infant will die if more than 15% is lost.

A child with diarrhoea who looks well and is physically normal could be treated at home. Normal feeds are substituted with a glucose/electrolyte mixture (Dioralyte). Glucose facilitates the transport of electrolytes across the intestinal mucosa. At least 150–200 ml/kg in 24 hours will be required and should be given in frequent small amounts to avoid vomiting. However, regardless of the child's physical status, the parents have brought the child to the emergency department because they aren't coping. Admission is usually required but is mandatory if there are any physical signs.

The child must be weighed. Admission because of dehydration will mean estimation of full blood count, serum urea, sodium, potassium and glucose. Further investigations including arterial blood gases will depend upon the clinical picture. If the child is shocked then an intravenous infusion of 0.9% saline should be established in the A & E department; 10–20 ml/kg should be given rapidly. Further fluid requirements will be based on the overall clinical picture and will be determined by the inpatient paediatric team to whom you have referred the patient.

The signs of dehydration are essentially those of extracellular (sodium and water) fluid loss. Estimation of serum electrolytes may, however, reveal an elevated level of sodium ($\geq$150 mmol/l). Hypernatraemic dehydration can occur when rehydration has been attempted with a high solute milk. The physical signs of dehydration are often absent but cerebral signs such as a decreased conscious level and seizures occur more frequently. The resuscitation of these children is difficult and complex. The A & E doctor should establish venous access and refer the child at once to an experienced paediatrician.

The treatment of diarrhoea is rehydration. Antiemetic and antidiarrhoeal drugs are usually ineffective and some have dangerous side effects (e.g. Lomotil).

Scrombrotoxic fish poisoning can produce diarrhoea, often associated with flushing, sweating and a bright red skin rash. Smoked mackerel is the principle culprit in the UK. The toxic element is histamine, which is produced by bacterial contamination after the fish has been caught. This can be avoided if fish are immediately stored in ice after being caught. The illness is usually mild and no specific treatment other than rehydration is required. Non-infective causes of diarrhoea include:

1. *Chronic inflammatory* — includes diverticulitis, ulcerative colitis and Crohn's disease.

2. *Incomplete obstruction* — fibrous bands, abdominal adhesions and external herniae of the Richter type can lead to a partial obstruction. Rectal polyps and malignant neoplasms of the large bowel should also be considered.

3. *Malabsorption* — many conditions produce this syndrome and the patient will require detailed investigation by the inpatient team.

Enquiries should be made about recent eating habits and trips abroad. Traveller's diarrhoea is often thought to be infective, but is just as likely to be the result of the journey, a change in food and overindulgence in alcohol.

Rectal bleeding

Rectal bleeding may occur with anal fissures, but is usually scanty. More extensive bleeding may occur from internal haemorrhoids. Examination of the rectum, first with a finger and then a proctoscope, will confirm the site of blood loss and may reveal an associated carcinoma of the rectum. Any further investigation, such as sigmoidoscopy is carried out by the surgical team.

Profuse, bright red bleeding from the rectum in adults may be due to a rectal neoplasm, ulcerative colitis, Crohn's disease and, occasionally diverticulitis. Profuse rectal bleeding in children is unusual but may be associated with peptic ulceration in a Meckel's diverticulum. Blood from a peptic ulcer in the duodenum may present in the rectum if bleeding is brisk and transit time short.

A dark red or black melaena stool in an adult is likely to be from a duodenal ulcer, gastric erosions or sometimes oesophageal varices. In infants (usually 9–18 months), the passage of a small amount of blood and mucus, accompanied by abdominal pain and, usually, the presence of a palpable tumour somewhere along the course of the colon, is indicative of intussusception. It is sometimes seen in older children and rarely in adults. In the elderly, this combination of abdominal pain accompanied by the passage of mucus and blood may indicate mesenteric vascular occlusion. The small bowel is usually involved, although a segment of large bowel may be affected.

Chronic, small bleeds will lead to iron deficiency anaemia. A full blood count may indicate whether this should be treated as an in- or outpatient.

Finally, foreign bodies of all shapes and sizes can be inserted into the rectum, usually deliberately and often for pleasure. The patient attends the emergency department because they are unable to remove it themselves having tried usually for some considerable time. It is not the doctor's place to judge, but merely to advise. General anaesthesia is often required to relax the sphincter. The dangers of such practices must be clearly explained to the patient.

When the patient is a child a tactful but comprehensive account of the event must be obtained from all involved. Sexual abuse is not uncommon and must always be considered. The child will usually require inpatient admission for the medical condition and this period of time will allow discreet enquiries to be made.

Male urogenital problems

HAEMATURIA

Beetroot, blackcurrants and blackberries cause red discoloration of the urine in some people. True haematuria always requires investigation.

Renal trauma causes haematuria, except in rare cases of severe injury in which the ureter is avulsed. The haematuria may be immediate or may be delayed by a few hours or even one or two days. A kidney may be injured by a direct blow in the loin or indirectly by compression between the 12th rib and the spine during sudden lateral flexion of the trunk. There may be other injuries, especially fractures of the lower ribs or the transverse processess of the lumbar vertebrae, or rupture of the spleen or liver. Haematuria following trauma is an indication for admission for rest and observation. An intravenous pyelogram is needed to check that both kidneys are working and to look for renal damage. Urine must be kept in clear containers labelled with the time of voiding, so that changes in the amount of bleeding can be assessed. Most cases of renal injury settle without operation.

If there is no history of trauma the likely causes of painless haematuria are tumours of the kidney or bladder, hydronephrosis and acute nephritis. Schistosomiasis and renal tuberculosis are common causes in many tropical countries. Leukaemia, haemophilia and sickle cell disease may cause haematuria. Some patients with cystitis have marked haematuria with relatively little pain. Most patients with painless haematuria can be referred to an early outpatient clinic, but admission may be needed if there is severe haemorrhage, fever, hypertension or oedema. Haematuria associated with pain is usually caused by calculi or blood clot in

the ureter or urethra. Urinary infection may be present. Admission will usually be necessary. Renal colic is discussed in Ch. 21.

ACUTE RETENTION

Acute urinary retention is usually caused by prostatic hypertrophy but may result from faecal impaction, drugs (especially tricyclic antidepressants), or neurological conditions such as multiple sclerosis, poliomyelitis or the Guillain–Barré syndrome.

Elderly men with retention due to prostatic hypertrophy often have a history of urinary frequency and deteriorating stream. Retention may be precipitated by alcohol, diuretic tablets or a long coach journey. Admission for prostatectomy will be required, but the immediate needs are relieving pain and emptying the bladder. Every A & E department should have a plan for such patients agreed with the local surgeons or urologists. Some patients with acute retention will pass urine after an injection of morphine and a warm bath, but most will require catheterisation. Catheterisation must be done gently and carefully with full sterile precautions. The urethra must be anaesthetised and lubricated with sterile gel, containing lignocaine and chlorhexidine, which is left for at least 3 minutes before catheterisation. A Foley balloon catheter of 12 or 14 Charrière gauge is generally satisfactory. Latex catheters are commonly used but the more expensive silicone catheters cause less tissue reaction and are preferred by some urologists. The catheter balloon is inflated with 5–10 ml of sterile water or saline. If unable to pass a catheter do not use force and do not use a catheter introducer without special training. Suprapubic catheterisation is preferable to damaging the urethra.

Acute on chronic retention

Some patients with long-standing outflow obstruction and chronic distention of the bladder and upper urinary tract present as an emergency when complete retention occurs. Such patients may be uraemic, dehydrated and anaemic. Bladder catheterisation will be needed but sudden decompression may cause bleeding from the mucosa: one may try to prevent this by putting a gate-clip on the tubing and letting the urine out slowly.

PAIN ON MICTURITION

Pain on micturition can be caused by urinary infection but this is rare in men with a normal renal tract: obstruction, tumour and renal stone all predispose to infection and so referral for investigation will be needed.

Acute prostatitis causes urinary frequency with pain in the perineum and penis, especially on micturition. The prostate is very tender. Urine cultures and prolonged antibiotic treatment are needed, under the care of a urologist.

Acute urethritis causes pain and frequency of micturition and often a urethral discharge. Gonorrhoea and chlamydia are the common causes. Referral to a venereologist is needed for proper investigation and treatment of the patient and contacts.

INFLAMMATION OF THE PENIS

Acute balanitis, inflammation of the glans penis, is caused by secondary infection in diabetics or by allergic dermatitis or genital herpes. The urine must be tested for glucose. Referral to a venereologist may be needed. Sometimes there is a phimosis requiring referral for circumcision.

Painful ulcers of the penis may be caused by venereal diseases or Behçet's syndrome. The chancre of primary syphilis is usually painless.

PARAPHIMOSIS

In early cases paraphimosis may respond to one of the following methods:

1. A rubber glove is loosely filled with ice chips and the penis inserted into it. After 15 minutes the glans may have shrunk sufficiently to allow reduction of the tight ring by gentle forward traction of the foreskin and pressure on the glans penis.

2. Lignocaine (without adrenaline) and hyaluronidase (Hyalase, 1500 i.u.) are injected into the constricting ring. After a few minutes manipulation may be possible.

If these measures fail, emergency circumcision is needed. If they succeed the patient should be referred for later circumcision to prevent a recurrence of the paraphimosis.

PRIAPISM

Priapism may be associated with leukaemia, sickle cell anaemia, pelvic vein thrombosis or haemodialysis, but in many cases no cause is apparent. The corpora cavernosa remain stiff but the glans and corpus spongiosum become flaccid. The condition is painful and distressing. It may be relieved by making an aperture between the cavernous system and the spongiosum or by anastomosis of the saphenous vein to the corpus cavernosum on one or both sides. Delay makes success less likely and so immediate referral to a surgeon is needed.

TRAUMA OF THE PENIS

The foreskin or penile skin may become trapped in the slider of a zip. Local anaesthesia (with plain lignocaine) may allow removal of the trousers intact, but sometimes it is necessary to cut through the zip slider with bone-cutting forceps.

Lacerations of the glans bleed profusely and need careful repair with fine Dexon under general anaesthesia. Urological referral is needed if the urethra is involved.

Rings placed around the penis cause venous engorgement and strangulation (Fig. 23.1). General anaesthesia is needed for removal by ring-cutters or a hacksaw. Aspiration of the corpora cavernosa with a syringe and needle may be helpful.

Trauma of the erect penis may cause 'fracture' of the penis with severe pain and swelling due to rupture of the corpora cavernosa. The patient should be admitted for repair of the injury.

RUPTURE OF THE URETHRA

Rupture of the urethra may be caused by a kick or by falling astride an object. The perineal urethra is compressed against the underside

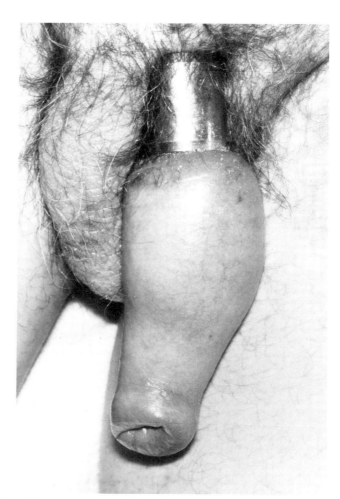

Fig. 23.1 A constricting metal ring which was removed with a hacksaw under general anaesthesia.

of the pubic symphysis and torn. This causes pain, urethral haemorrhage, a perineal haematoma and retention of urine. Pelvic fractures may be associated with injury to the membranous urethra and other internal injuries (see Ch. 14). If urethral injury is suspected, or there is a pelvic fracture, the presence or absence of blood at the external meatus must be recorded. Urological advice is needed if there is urethral bleeding. Suprapubic catheterisation is often required.

PAIN AND SWELLING OF THE TESTIS

Pain and swelling of the testis may be caused by torsion, infection, trauma or tumour. A man with a painful testis must be assumed to have a torsion until proved otherwise and so immediate referral to a surgeon is usually needed.

Torsion of the testis may occur at any age, but it is most common at around puberty. There is usually a sudden onset of pain in the scrotum or groin, but sometimes pain occurs only in the lower abdomen. Nausea and vomiting are common. The testis is swollen and tender and the scrotal skin may be inflamed. Immediate referral to a surgeon is essential: the torsion must be reduced as soon as possible and both testes fixed to prevent a recurrence. In early cases it may be possible to untwist the testis and relieve the pain without operation, but fixation of the testes is still required.

Acute orchitis is usually caused by mumps and is a common complication of mumps after puberty. The testis is swollen and painful. Early surgical decompression may reduce the risk of testicular atrophy, which is common after orchitis, and exploration may also be needed to exclude a torsion. Discussion with a surgeon is therefore advisable.

Acute epididymitis sometimes follows urinary infection with *E. coli,* or occasionally gonorrhoea, but in many cases no organism is found. The epididymis is swollen and tender and the testis may also be involved. Urine culture is necessary and treatment with cotrimoxazole or ampicillin. In patients aged less than 30 years exploration to exclude a torsion is essential before a diagnosis of epididymitis is made.

Trauma may cause rupture of the testis followed by a secondary hydrocoele. Surgical referral is needed if a testis is swollen after injury, since early repair will relieve pain and reduce the risk of later atrophy. Testicular swelling after trauma may also be caused by a testicular tumour and so exploration and careful assessment are essential.

FURTHER READING

Lecture notes on urology, 3rd edn. Blandy J, 1982 Blackwell Scientific, Oxford

Hamilton Bailey's emergency surgery, 11th edn. Dudley H A F (ed) 1986 Wright, Bristol

Gynaecological problems

VAGINAL BLEEDING

When a woman (or girl) presents to the A & E department because of vaginal bleeding, it is likely to be for one of the following reasons:
1. Excessive menstrual loss (menorrhagia)
2. Frequent menstrual loss
3. Frequent, heavy loss
4. Bleeding associated with other factors.

An adequate assessment of the problem will require the following basic information about the patient.

Menstrual status

In concert with the age, it is important to establish the 'normal' pattern of blood loss. Patients will be prepubertal, menstrual, or menopausal.

Age

Abnormal vaginal bleeding in elderly women is indicative, though not conclusive of, malignancy. Regardless of any other finding, the patient should be discussed with the duty gynaecologist. Young girls may occasionally present with their first period. This is unusual, but the girl may not have been prepared for this event, particularly if she is very young. Precocious puberty is not an emergency, but the child should be referred to the next paediatric clinic.

Duration

Establish for how long there has been a problem and is it getting worse (or better). Ask the patient why she thinks this is not a normal period.

Nature of the bleeding

The amount lost can be estimated by the number of sanitary towels used and the passage of clots. Find out if she is concerned because she loses too much each period, bleeds between periods, or does not stop bleeding.

Associated symptoms

The bleeding may be accompanied by pain or other symptoms.

If blood loss has been severe she may have symptoms of anaemia. Breathlessness on exertion and general fatigue are particularly common in elderly women, but also occur in the young. Angina may be precipitated in those with pre-existing ischaemic heart disease and itching can be a feature of iron deficiency.

Precipitating factors

Trauma, both accidental and deliberate, will clearly cause vaginal bleeding. In young girls and children it is essential to exclude sexual abuse. The type of injury and its relevance to the given account of the accident will indicate the need for further investigation. For example, a fall on a bicycle can result in small tears to the labia minora. These can bleed fairly briskly. If haemostasis cannot be achieved with direct pressure, referral to a gynaecologist is indicated.

A thorough examination is always indicated and if any doubt persists the child should be referred to a paediatrician. In any event these children should be followed up by either a gynaecologist, family doctor and, in some circumstances, the A & E doctor. The health visitor should be informed and a visit to the child's home arranged.

Victims of rape will require special attention. It is only men who ever question the need for women in these circumstances to be examined by women whenever possible. Before special attention is given to any perineal injuries, it is essential to ensure that other potentially life-threatening injuries have been identified and the patient is fully resuscitated. The patient can then be referred to the gynaecologist and/or police surgeon for further therapeutic and forensic procedures (see also Ch. 4, Legal aspects)

Normal sexual intercourse may precipitate abnormal vaginal bleeding. It is imperative that gynaecological referral is expedited to ensure that an early carcinoma of the cervix is not missed.

The normal bleeding pattern, if one has been established, and the date of the last normal period should be recorded. Enquire as to the number of previous pregnancies and their outcome. Does the patient think she might be pregnant now? Ask specifically about the signs of early pregnancy — amenorrhoea, breast tenderness, nausea — and enquire about the result of any pregnancy tests.

Examination

Most patients who need to be referred to the gynaecologist will be identified by the history they give. Where such a decision can be made and a gynaecologist is available, the patient may be spared the embarassment of two examinations. However, there will be a number of patients for whom a correct decision about the urgency of referral can only be assessed correctly after examination, and under these circumstances the A & E doctor should proceed.

Record the patient's blood pressure and pulse and make a decision about fluid replacement. Most will not require it, but young people can look remarkably healthy, in spite of significant blood loss. Palpate the abdomen and identify any abnormal masses or areas of tenderness. Inspect the external genitalia and look for signs of trauma.

Internal vaginal examination

If you have received training, are experienced in vaginal examination and have the relevant equipment to hand, it may be reasonable to perform such examinations in the A & E department. You will need an adequate light source, a Cuscoe's or Sim's speculum, and an assistant. If you are male, you will need a chaperon. Absence of any one of these will preclude the examination and the patient must be referred. Furthermore, whenever an experienced gynaecological opinion is clearly required, the patient must not be subjected to an unnecessary intimate examination. The patient's full co-operation must be reserved for the examination which really counts. When products of conception are distending the os cervix a profound vasovagal response may be induced. Digital removal will reduce cervical distension and is probably the only exception to the guidelines outlined above.

Vaginal examination from mid-pregnancy onwards may precipitate an abortion in patients who present with vaginal bleeding. It must not be done in the A & E department.

Diagnoses to consider

In *prepubertal* girls the commonest cause is trauma and bicycles are usually to blame. Self-inflicted injury and insertion of foreign bodies occurs and may be part of early sexual experimentation. Enquires require great tact and sensitivity and a female nurse may more easily broach the subject.

At least part of the interview should be conducted in the absence of the parents and always in the presence of a senior female nurse. If sexual abuse cannot be excluded (but not necessarily proved) the patient must be referred to the duty *consultant* paediatrician. Expert help is essential from an early stage.

In *women of menstrual age* trauma may still be a factor. Rape must be considered, although it might not be declared. Foreign bodies and sexual experimentation must also be considered.

External examination may reveal vulval varicosities. A simple cervical polyp may bleed, but this is only likely to be diagnosed following examination by a gynaecologist.

Vaginal bleeding in a woman who believes herself to be pregnant must be assumed to be an abortion. Slight bleeding can occur at the time of trophoblastic implantation. The diagnosis of implantation haemorrhage should not be made by the A & E doctor alone, but by the gynaecologist to whom he has referred the patient.

A *threatened abortion* is bleeding within the first 28 weeks of pregnancy.

An *inevitable abortion* has the additional features of strong, painful contractions and dilatation of the cervix.

An *incomplete abortion* has the further features of significant blood loss, cramp-like uterine contractions and the passage of the products of conception.

A *complete abortion* implies that *all* the products of conception have been passed.

All patients with bleeding in early pregnancy should be referred to the duty gynaecologist. Local practice may mean that patients with a pregnancy of 20 or more weeks are treated on an obstetric unit.

Incomplete abortion, particularly when it has been criminally induced, can be associated with infection. *Septic abortion* may be limited to the uterus but can lead to generalised sepsis with shock. The patient must be adequately resuscitated prior to antibiotic therapy.

Blood specimens for culture and sensitivity should be taken and plasma expansion with colloid commenced in the A & E department.

In non-pregnant women the bleeding may represent a menstrual problem. Discussion with the duty gynaecologist will help formulate a plan of action for the patient. Great care must be taken to ensure that the patient is not pregnant and this is a menstrual loss and not a threatened abortion.

Ectopic pregnancy

Of greater importance still is the diagnosis of ruptured ectopic pregnancy. Any women of child bearing years who is collapsed and hypotensive must be considered to have a ruptured ectopic pregnancy until proven otherwise. The average delay in diagnosis is still measured in days and is due invariably to the diagnosis having never been considered.

There are certain points to always bear in mind.

1. Many patients with ectopic pregnancy do not realise they are pregnant.

2. There may not have been a missed or late period, or any clues to be gained from the menstrual history.

3. The moment of rupture may be accompanied by pain and a feeling of faintness. This is by no means constant.

4. The possibility of ectopic pregnancy is much more likely in patients who have had pelvic inflammatory disease, fallopian tube surgery or have an intrauterine contraceptive device in situ.

The commonest symptoms are irregular vaginal bleeding, lower abdominal or pelvic pain, shoulder tip pain and fainting. The bleeding follows the pain, may be thought to be menstrual or a threatened abortion, and is usually slight.

Pelvic examination by the gynaecologist may reveal cervical excitation and tenderness. The latter is not always unilateral.

Ultrasound examination of the abdomen may be helpful, but laparoscopy is usually diagnostic.

The emergency managment of these patients rests upon consideration of the diagnosis in *all* women of appropriate age who have abdominal pain and/or vaginal bleeding. Blood loss can be profound and vigorous fluid replacement required.

If the patient is clearly shocked and ruptured ectopic pregnancy is being considered, then the patient must be transferred to the operating theatre while resuscitation is in progress.

Postmenopausal bleeding

Bleeding from the genital tract occurring a year or more after the menopause should be considered due to malignancy until proven otherwise. Immediate consultation with a gynaecologist is indicated.

PELVIC PAIN

The commonest 'gynaecological' cause of pelvic pain is *salpingitis*. There is moderate to severe lower abdominal/pelvic pain, usually bilateral and of sudden onset. There is often a previous history of similar episodes. A vaginal discharge may accompany the symptoms and the patient may be pyrexial. The condition must be differentiated from *appendicitis, ruptured ectopic pregnancy and torsion/rupture of an ovarian cyst*. The patient should be referred to the duty gynaecologist. The infecting organism is often the gonococcus and the patient must be asked (tactfully) about sexual contacts. Mild cases may require only a course of antibiotics, but the gynaecologist will need to take urethral, vaginal and endocervical swabs before treatment is commenced. The antibiotics chosen should be effective against anaerobes and chlamydia as well as gonococcus. A combination of metronidazole (400 mg tds for 1 week) and tetracycline (500 mg qds)/erythromycin (500 mg qds)/augmentin (375 mg tds) is adequate. The more severe cases will require inpatient rest and observation with intravenous antibiotics. The differentation between salpingitis and appendicitis is often unclear and admission in these circumstances will always be required.

Pelvic pain from rupture or torsion of an ovarian cyst is often associated with nausea. There may be a unilateral tender pelvic mass on internal examination and ultrasound is often diagnostic.

Bartholin's abscess

Bartholin's glands are situated in the posterior wall of the vaginal introitus. Their function is to lubricate the vagina during sexual intercourse. If the duct of the gland becomes blocked following infection, the gland below will be infected, enlarge and form an abscess.

A painful swelling will develop over a few days. Occasionally the condition is self-limiting and patients have repeated minor episodes. However, the swelling is usually severe and painful and the patient seeks urgent medical help.

Examination will reveal a tender, fluctuant swelling on one or either side of the posterior introitus. The only conditions likely to cause diagnostic confusion are infected sebaceous cysts and perianal abscesses.

Treatment usually involves excision of an ellipse of skin and abscess wall immediately inside the introitus. The margins of the wound are sutured, and this 'marsupialisation' will allow the gland to continue functioning once the acute crisis is over — an important point in maintaining normal sexual function. The procedure can only be carried out under general anaesthetic and wound swabs are always required. The gonococcus is often involved and partners will need to be traced and councilled. Treatment is usually the province of the gynaecologist, but local arrangements may mean that the A & E doctor is involved.

Vaginal discharge

A slight discharge is normal and any change in this is normally discussed with the family doctor. However, a woman may present with this problem to the A & E department when she prefers the anonymity or has difficulty arranging an appointment with her own doctor.

The oral contraceptive pill will increase the normal discharge and the incidence of the 'creamy' discharge of vaginal candidiasis. The latter is also more common in pregnancy, diabetes and patients taking antibiotics or steroids. Referral of both the patient and her partner to the family doctor is appropriate.

Trichomoniasis may have the additional symptoms of pruritis and urethritis, and the discharge is sometimes said to be green. The advice is as for candidiasis.

If a woman is thought to have a urinary tract infection and it is decided to start antibiotic therapy in the emergency department it is important that a mid-stream specimen of urine is obtained first. The results of microscopy, culture and sensitivity can then be forwarded to the family doctor.

It may be that fear of venereal disease has prompted the consultation. Gonococcal vaginitis may produce only a mild discharge and a minor irritation. The penalty for a delay in diagnosis may, however, be later infertility, if gonococcal salpingitis ensues. Referral to a venereologist in a department of genitourinary medicine is essential in these circumstances. This will also ensure that other diseases, such as syphilis and HIV infection (where appropriate) are also excluded. Contact tracing is also important and the department of genitourinary medicine will organise this.

Emergency delivery

Very occasionally a woman may present to the A & E department already in the final stages of labour, and clearly unlikely to manage even a short transfer to maternity unit. Young girls who conceal their pregnancy and multiparous women who progress rapidly through labour are the commonest such patients. The emergency doctor must summon the paediatrician and the obstetrician on call and prepare for an emergency delivery. Now is not the time to discover that the department does not possess a delivery pack. A paediatric laryngoscope and neonatal endotracheal tubes should be brought to hand and the suction turned on.

It is usually easier for the inexperienced to allow the woman to deliver in a semi-sitting position. Support her back and instruct her to pant to avoid a rapid expulsion of the head. Manually guide the baby's head beneath the symphisis and allow it to rotate. Gently direct the head downwards to deliver the anterior shoulder. The next contraction will expel the other shoulder and trunk which can be directed upwards in an arc to allow the baby to rest on the mother's abdomen.

When the baby is fully delivered, it should be wrapped in a warm towel and the liquor aspirated from its nose and mouth. If the cord is around the neck it must be freed at once or cut between haemostats. If the baby fails to breathe inspite of suction and intubation, ventilation will be required. The umbilical cord will need to be cut between clamps in these circumstances. If the baby is clearly breathing and crying it is not necessary to cut the cord and the baby should be given to its mother. An Apgar score should be estimated immediately (see Table 24.1).

Allow the placenta to deliver without traction. Suckling the breast is a strong stimulus for uterine contraction and should be encouraged.

Pregnancy

All women of child-bearing years are potentially pregnant. This is particularly important to remember when prescribing drugs and ordering radiographs. It must also be excluded when investigationg the symptoms of amenorrhoea, nausea, vomiting, frequency of micturition and breast tenderness. Young girls may vehemently deny the possibility of pregnancy and great tact is required when broaching the subject. Laboratory analysis of urine can confirm the pregnancy as early as two weeks after the first missed period. It is extremely important that pregnant girls under 16 years of age are referred immediately to a gynaecologist. Social services need to be informed and parental consent will be required for any further treatment.

Women of child-bearing age should be asked if they are, or may be pregnant. If the answer is 'no' then it is safe to proceed with radiological examination. If the answer is 'yes' then all requests for radiological investigations should be carefully reconsidered and discussed with the senior doctor on call for the A & E department and preferably with a radiologist.

There are no associated risks in giving a local anaesthetic in pregnancy. A general anaesthetic, however, must only be administered by an experienced senior anaesthetist.

All prescribing in pregnancy and lactation must be questioned. If, however the need is obvious then identify the safest drug to use by reference to prescribing and consultation with senior colleagues.

Table 24.1 The Apgar score

Skin colour	good	= 2
	peripheral cyanosis	= 1
	generalised cyanosis/pallor	= 0
Muscle tone	good	= 2
	flexion movements of the limbs or trunk	= 1
	complete flaccidity	= 0
Respiratory effort	rhythmic breathing or crying gasping	= 2
	gasping	= 1
	apnoea	= 0
Heart rate	> 100 b.p.m.	= 2
	< 100 b.p.m.	= 1
	absent	= 0
Response to stimulation (by suction to nostrils or by flicking the soles of the feet)	brisk	= 2
	poor	= 1
	absent	= 0

Infectious diseases and fever

Fever is usually caused by infection but may result from many other conditions, including tissue infarction, embolism, neoplasia, autoimmune diseases and drug reactions. A febrile adult may have general symptoms such as malaise, sweating and shivering but often has specific complaints, such as cough or dysuria, which help to identify the site of infection. However, in a small child the first evidence of infection may be anorexia, vomiting or a convulsion and no specific symptoms may be obtainable. Many infectious diseases are self-limiting virus infections requiring only symptomatic treatment, but it is important to diagnose the more serious infections which need specific therapy, especially life-threatening conditions such as meningitis and malaria.

DIAGNOSIS OF INFECTIOUS DISEASE

History

The history may be very important in making a diagnosis of an infectious disease. The patient's symptoms and details of drug therapy and allergies must be recorded. One must know about foreign travel, especially to the tropics and subtropics, and about contacts with other ill patients. Knowledge of the incubation periods of diseases (Table 25.1) and periods of infectivity (Table 25.2) may be helpful.

Examination

Careful examination is necessary for signs of infection and to assess the severity of illness, especially complications such as dehydration. The skin and mouth, ears, chest and abdomen must be examined. Lymph nodes should be palpated. In small children the bones should be palpated for tenderness (suggesting osteomyelitis) and the fontanelle examined for evidence of dehydration. Signs of meningitis, such as photophobia and neck stiffness, must be assessed and recorded, although in early meningitis there may be no specific signs, especially in small children.

Table 25.1 Incubation periods of infectious diseases

Incubation period less than 1 week	
Bacillary dysentery	1–7 days
Cholera	Hours–5 days
Diphtheria	2–5 days
Gonorrhoea	2–5 days
Meningococcaemia	1–7 days (usually 3 days)
Scarlet fever	1–4 days
Incubation period usually 1–3 weeks	
Brucellosis	7–21 days
Chickenpox	14–21 days
Lassa fever	7–21 days
Leptospirosis	4–21 days (usually about 10 days)
Malaria	10–14 days (sometimes much longer)
Measles	7–14 days (usually 10 days)
Mumps	12–21 days (usually 16–18 days)
Poliomyelitis	3–21 days (usually 7–10 days)
Rubella	14–21 days
Typhoid fever	7–21 days
Typhus	7–14 days
Whooping cough	7–10 days
Incubation period usually more than 3 weeks	
Amoebiasis	2 weeks – many months
Hepatitis A	2–6 weeks (usually about 4 weeks)
Hepatitis B	6 weeks – 6 months
Rabies	1 week – 2 years (usually 2–10 weeks)
Syphilis	10 days – 10 weeks

Table 25.2 Duration of infectivity of infectious diseases

Chickenpox	5 days before rash until 6 days after last crop of spots
Hepatitis A	1 or 2 weeks before until two weeks after the onset of jaundice
Measles	From onset of prodromal symptoms until 4 days after onset of rash
Mumps	3 days before to 1 week after salivary swelling
Rubella	1 week before to 4 days after onset of rash
Scarlet fever	10–21 days after onset of rash (1 day if treated with penicillin)
Whooping cough	1 week after exposure until 3 weeks after onset of symptoms (1 week if on antibiotics)

Investigations

The investigations needed depend on the history and clinical findings. In many common diseases such as otitis media and measles no investigation is necessary. If no diagnosis is apparent on examination the urine should be examined microscopically and cultured, a chest radiograph performed and blood taken for a full blood count and examination of the blood film. Special precautions are needed if taking blood from patients who may have hepatitis B, AIDS, or Lassa fever (p. 275).

GENERAL MANAGEMENT OF INFECTIOUS DISEASES

Many patients with infectious diseases can be treated at home with follow-up by the general practitioner. However admission may be needed, depending on the type and severity of illness and the home circumstances. Febrile babies aged less than two months should usually be admitted to hospital since they may deteriorate rapidly and serious illnesses such as meningitis and septicaemia must be excluded.

Fluids should be given orally or intravenously as necessary. Paracetamol helps to relieve pain and pyrexia. If the temperature is 40°C or higher the patient should be cooled by sponging with tepid water (see section on heat stroke, Ch. 28).

Notifiable infectious diseases

A doctor who knows or suspects that a patient is suffering from any of the diseases listed in Table 25.3 is required by law to notify the local authority's medical officer for environmental health. Notification forms are provided by the local authority. Initial notification should be made by telephone if control of an outbreak of disease may be needed.

MANAGEMENT OF SPECIFIC CONDITIONS

Diseases discussed in other chapters include:

Epiglottitis and croup	Chapters 10 and 44
Tonsillitis	Chapter 44
Otitis media	Chapter 44
Pneumonia	Chapters 11 and 19
Whooping cough	Chapter 19
Gastroenteritis	Chapter 21
Osteomyelitis and septic arthritis	Chapter 35
Tetanus	Chapter 15

Febrile convulsions

Febrile convulsions are common in children aged between 6 months and 5 years, especially at about 18 months. The fit is caused by a rapid rise in temperature, often due to infection of

Table 25.3 Notifiable infectious diseases in Britain

Anthrax
Cholera
Diphtheria
Dysentery (amoebic or bacillary)
Acute encephalitis
Food poisoning
Infective jaundice
Lassa fever
Leprosy
Leptospirosis
Malaria
Marburg disease
Measles
Acute meningitis
Ophthalmia neonatorum
Paratyphoid fever
Plague
Acute poliomyelitis
Rabies
Relapsing fever
Scarlet fever
Smallpox
Tetanus
Tuberculosis
Typhoid fever
Typhus
Viral haemorrhagic fever
Whooping cough
Yellow fever

A local authority may make additional diseases such as rubella and glandular fever notifiable in its district.

the ears or throat. Febrile fits are generalised rather than focal and last less than 10 minutes, with no residual limb weakness.

The fit has usually stopped before the child reaches hospital, but if not the airway must be cleared and an anticonvulsant given (Ch. 12). The clothes should be removed and paracetamol given as soon as possible to reduce the temperature. The blood glucose should be checked. The child must be admitted to hospital. A lumbar puncture is often necessary to exclude meningitis.

All children with simple febrile convulsions recover completely. If there was no previous neurological problem and no family history of epilepsy the risk of a child having epilepsy at age 7 is only about 1%. The parents may be reassured about this but should discuss the matter with the paediatrician.

Meningitis

Some patients with meningitis present with the characteristic features of pyrexia, headache, neck stiffness, photophobia and drowsiness. However in early cases, and especially in children aged under 2 years, the clinical diagnosis of meningitis may be very difficult. If there is any reasonable suspicion of meningitis the patient must be admitted to hospital immediately and a lumbar puncture performed.

Meningococcal meningitis is associated with a septicaemia and there is often a purpuric rash. Deterioration may be rapid, with septicaemic shock, disseminated intravascular coagulation and adrenal haemorrhage (the Waterhouse-Friderichsen syndrome). If meningococcal meningitis is suspected blood should be taken for culture and treatment started immediately with intravenous penicillin (initial adult dose 2 g of benzylpenicillin). Chloramphenicol should be used in patients allergic to penicillin. Meningococcal infection is spread by droplets from the nose of an infected carrier, who may be asymptomatic. Cases must be notified immediately to the medical officer for environmental health (p. 274). Prophylactic treatment with rifampicin should be arranged for the patient's family and close contacts. Hospital and ambulance staff usually need prophylaxis only if they have given mouth-to-mouth resuscitation. The dose of rifampicin, given twice daily for 2 days, is 5 mg/kg for children aged 3–12 months, 10 mg/kg for ages 1–12 years and 600 mg for older children and adults. Rifampicin makes the urine orange or brown, stains soft contact lenses and reduces the effectiveness of the contraceptive pill and other drugs: appropriate warnings should be given.

Tuberculosis

Tuberculosis may present in many different ways in an A & E department. It is relatively common in alcoholics and vagrants and in Asian immigrants. Pulmonary tuberculosis may cause fever, malaise, weight loss and haemoptysis. Mycobacteria are usually apparent in the sputum on Ziehl-Neelsen staining. In *primary pulmonary tuberculosis* there is a patch of consolidation which may be anywhere in the lung and rarely cavitates. The ipsilateral mediastinal lymph nodes are often enlarged and a small pleural effusion is common. In adults the presenting feature may be a large solitary effusion. *Miliary tuberculosis* produces fine slightly indistinct mottling throughout the lung fields. These lesions may later coalesce. Choroidal tubercules may be visible in the retinae. Chronic pulmonary infection is characterised by fibrosis and distinct mottled areas containing calcified foci, usually in the upper lobes. There may be thin-walled cavities, especially at the apices, and sometimes emphysema and elevation of the hila. In reactivation disease there are ill-defined areas of consolidation, which may cavitate.

Tuberculous meningitis, which may be associated with miliary tuberculosis, causes a gradual onset of headaches, fever and malaise and sometimes confusion or cranial nerve signs (Ch. 17). Other presentations of tuberculosis include cervical lymphadenopathy, skin sinuses and symptoms of osteomyelitis, pericarditis, erythema nodosum and chronic abdominal infection. Admission to hospital for investigation and treatment will be necessary.

Viral hepatitis

Hepatitis A is transmitted by contaminated food or water and has an incubation period of 2–6 weeks. There is often a sudden onset of fever, aching limbs, upper abdominal discomfort, anorexia, nausea and vomiting. After 3–6 days the urine becomes dark, the stools pale and jaundice appears. The jaundice fades after 1 or 2 weeks and full recovery is usual. Treatment is symptomatic and many patients can be treated at home with follow-up by the general practitioner. Infectivity is greatest before jaundice appears and so isolation is of limited value. Undiagnosed asymptomatic cases are common. Immunoglobulin is sometimes needed for short-term protection against hepatitis A. Falciparum malaria may present with jaundice and fever and be misdiagnosed as viral hepatitis: blood films must be examined for malaria if this infection is possible.

Hepatitis B is transmitted by contaminated blood or needles, or by sexual intercourse. It is common in drug addicts. The clinical features are similar to those of hepatitis A although the onset is more gradual. Arthralgia and an urticarial rash may occur. The liver is often swollen and tender and the spleen may be palpable. Treatment is symptomatic, but referral to an infectious diseases unit is advisable.

Particular care is needed to avoid infection from the blood of patients suspected of having hepatitis B. Disposable gloves and aprons should be worn when taking blood. Needles should be placed in 'burn bins' without being resheathed. Blood sample tubes should be separate from the request forms in polythene bags marked with warning stickers. Any spilt blood should be cleaned up with hypochlorite solution (Geddes 1986).

In Britain about 1 in 1000 people are asymptomatic carriers of the hepatitis B virus. Medical and nursing staff in A & E departments are sometimes exposed to patients' blood and so immunisation against hepatitis B is a sensible precaution. Hepatitis B immunoglobulin (available from the Public Health Laboratory Service) reduces the risk of infection in staff accidently pricked by needles from carriers of the virus. After needlestick accidents bleeding should be encouraged by venous occlusion and the wound cleaned with antiseptic solution. The accident should be carefully recorded and a serum sample sent for storage in the laboratory in case later analysis is needed.

Non-A non-B hepatitis is transmitted by infected blood and has similar clinical features to hepatitis B.

HIV infection and AIDS

AIDS (acquired immune deficiency syndrome) is caused by the human immunodeficiency virus HIV (previously known as HTLV–III, LAV or ARV). The virus is transmitted by infected blood or blood products or by sexual intercourse. Infection with the HIV virus is common in homosexual and bisexual men, haemophiliacs and intravenous drug abusers. Heterosexual transmission can also occur and may become more common. Transplacental infection can occur in the babies of infected women. Needlestick accidents rarely result in infection and the risk is much less than for hepatitis B.

Antibodies to HIV develop about 4–7 weeks after exposure to the virus. One or two weeks after infection some patients develop an illness similar to glandular fever with fever, a macular rash and lymphadenopathy. In most cases this is transient, but sometimes a persistent generalised lymphadenopathy occurs. HIV infection may also present with neurological features such as encephalitis, meningitis, neuropathy or myelopathy. About 30% of people infected by HIV virus develop clinical evidence of AIDS, after a latent period of 1–5 years. However most people infected by HIV remain asymptomatic.

Patients with AIDS may present with non-specific symptoms such as malaise, weight loss, fever and night sweats. They may have joint pains, rash, diarrhoea, lymphadenopathy or infection with candidiasis, herpes simplex or herpes zoster. Central nervous system involvement may occur with confusion, fits or focal signs due to encephalitis or meningitis. However, the commonest presentations are with *Pneumocystis carinii* pneumonia or Kaposi's sarcoma. Pneumocystis pneumonia causes a persistent dry cough with dyspnoea on exertion and marked hypoxia. The chest radiograph may be normal but usually shows a perihilar 'ground glass' appearance followed by bilateral patchy shadowing. Kaposi's sarcoma may initially be a localised red or purple lesion on the skin, similar to a bruise or angioma (Adler 1987, Farthing et al 1986).

Contamination with blood or other secretions from known or suspected carriers of HIV must be avoided. This includes all haemophiliacs and drug addicts. The necessary precautions are the same as for hepatitis B (Adler 1987, DHSS 1985, 1986, Geddes 1986). Patients suspected of having AIDS should be admitted to hospital (preferably to an infectious diseases unit) for investigation and treatment. If such a patient refuses admission and is likely to infect other people the problem should be discussed with the medical officer for environmental health. AIDS is not a notifiable disease, but a justice of the peace may order a patient with AIDS to be detained in hospital if there is a risk to other people.

Malaria

Malaria is common in most tropical and subtropical countries and is a parasitic infection transmitted by mosquitoes. There are four varieties of malaria caused by *Plasmodium falciparum, P. vivax, P. ovale and P. malariae.* Of these falciparum malaria ('malignant tertian malaria') is the most important since it may be rapidly fatal and drug-resistant strains are common, especially in South-East Asia, East Africa and South America. Serious complications are uncommon with the other varieties of malaria but febrile convulsions may occur in children.

Each year more than 2000 cases of malaria are recorded in Britain in travellers from malarious areas. Most of these patients have vivax malaria from the Indian subcontinent or falciparum malaria from Africa. Occasionally malaria is found in people who have not been in a malarious area but have been infected by a blood transfusion or by a mosquito brought in an aeroplane from the tropics. Some people die of falciparum malaria because of delays in diagnosis and treatment. Antimalarial tablets reduce the risk of malaria but do not always prevent it and are often taken incorrectly.

Clinical features

The incubation period of malaria is usually about 10–14 days but may be much longer, sometimes over 1 year, in *P. malariae* and *P. vivax* infections. The incubation period of *P. falciparum* is rarely more than four weeks.

Fever is the most common presenting feature of all forms of malaria. The fever is often irregular, but in vivax and ovale infections it sometimes occurs on alternate days with rigors and shivering, followed by a high fever and then profuse sweating as the temperature falls. Haemolytic anaemia, splenomegaly and jaundice may occur with all varieties of malaria.

Falciparum malaria can present in many different ways and may cause diagnostic difficulty. The fever, headache, malaise, nausea, vomiting and limb pains may be misdiagnosed as influenza or gastroenteritis. Abdominal pain may occur. Deterioration may be sudden with cerebral malaria, hyperpyrexia, renal failure and severe anaemia, sometimes with haemoglobinuria. Cerebral malaria may be manifest as confusion, coma and focal neurological signs. Cardiac failure, pulmonary oedema, diarrhoea, hypoglycaemia, septicaemia and shock may occur.

Diagnosis and management (Gilles 1984, Weatherall et al 1987)

If anyone is ill after travelling in a malarious area blood films must be examined for malaria, even if antimalarial prophylaxis has been taken. If falciparum malaria is possible antimalarial treatment should be started at once without waiting for the results of blood films. The full blood count, urea and electrolytes and blood glucose should be checked.

Patients with severe malaria, especially those with cerebral malaria, should be treated in an intensive care unit. Other patients with falciparum malaria should be admitted to a medical ward or an infectious diseases unit without delay. Patients with vivax malaria can often be treated as outpatients if suitable follow-up is arranged: treatment with primaquine will be needed to prevent relapses.

The initial treatment of malaria involves either quinine or chloroquine, given orally or by intravenous infusion, depending on the severity of illness. Chloroquine is used for vivax, ovale and malariae malaria and for falciparum malaria from West Africa (adult oral dose 4 tablets, i.e. 600 mg of chloroquine base, then 2 tablets after 8 hours and 2 tablets daily for 3 days; intravenous dose 200 mg of chloroquine base in dextrose/saline over 8 hours). Quinine is used for falciparum malaria from South East Asia, East Africa and South America (adult oral dose quinine sulphate 600 mg 8 hourly for 7 days; intravenous dose quinine dihydrochloride 10 mg of base/kg in 500 ml of dextrose/saline over 4 hours, repeated every 8 hours). Quinidine may be used if quinine is not available. Patients from Thailand and nearby parts of Asia may have drug-resistant falciparum malaria requiring higher doses of quinine and also tetracycline, 'Fansidar' or other drugs. Expert advice should be obtained from a tropical diseases hospital (Table 25.4) in such cases and in other patients with severe malaria.

Table 25.4 Tropical diseases units in Britain

	Telephone
Hospital for Tropical Diseases, London	01-387-4411
East Birmingham Hospital, Birmingham	021-772-4311
Liverpool School of Tropical Medicine	051-708-9393
Ruchill Hospital, Glasgow	041-946-7120

Typhoid fever

Typhoid fever occurs throughout the world and is common wherever hygiene is inadequate. Typhoid and malaria are the first diagnoses to consider if a patient develops a fever within two weeks of returning from the tropics. Typhoid is spread by contamination of food or water with urine or faeces from a patient or an asymptomatic carrier. The incubation period is usually 7–14 days, but may be up to 21 days. The onset is often gradual with headache, malaise, fever, anorexia and a dry cough. Constipation is common but diarrhoea may occur, especially in children. The patient may become confused. Physical examination may be normal or there may be a fever with a relative bradycardia, abdominal tenderness and splenomegaly. Rose coloured spots appear transiently on the upper abdomen in about 50% of cases. There may be signs of pneumonia and dehydration. Intestinal perforation or haemorrhage occur occasionally. The white cell count is usually low with a neutropenia. Paratyphoid causes similar clinical features but is usually less severe.

Patients with suspected typhoid require barrier nursing and admission to an infectious diseases unit. The medical officer for environmental health should be informed so that further cases can be prevented.

Viral haemorrhagic fevers

Lassa fever

Lassa fever is endemic in many rural parts of West Africa. The viral infection is transmitted by accidental inoculation or by contamination of broken skin or mucous membranes by infected blood or secretions. The incubation period is up to three weeks. The early symptoms are often non-specific with fever, malaise and headache. Lassa fever must be considered in any pyrexial patient who has been in rural West Africa in the previous three weeks. However, malaria and typhoid are much more common than Lassa fever and need urgent diagnosis and treatment. If Lassa fever is possible the patient should be barrier nursed in a cubicle by the minimum number of staff, who should wear gloves, gowns and masks. The case should be discussed at once with a tropical diseases unit (Table 25.4). Blood films should be examined for malaria but the laboratory must first be warned of the possibility of Lassa fever. Treatment with chloroquine should be started immediately in case the patient has falciparum malaria. The patient will be admitted to an isolation bed in an infectious diseases unit or, if there is strong suspicion of Lassa fever, to a special high security unit (Banatvala 1986, DHSS 1986).

Marburg disease and *Ebola disease* are viral haemorrhagic fevers which occur in Central Africa. *Congo/Crimean haemorrhagic fevers* occur in Africa and western Asia, where they are transmitted by tick-bites or by contact with infected blood. The initial clinical features of these diseases are similar to those of Lassa fever. Later features are rashes, haemorrhage, jaundice and shock. The initial management is similar to that for Lassa fever.

REFERENCES

Adler M W (ed) 1986 ABC of AIDS. British Medical Journal, London

Banatvala J E 1986 Lassa fever. British Medical Journal, London

DHSS 1985–1986 Acquired immune deficiency syndrome (3 booklets covering different aspects of AIDS). DHSS, London

DHSS 1986 Memorandum on the control of viral haemorrhagic fevers. HMSO, London

Farthing C F et al 1986 A colour atlas of AIDS, acquired immune deficiency syndrome. Wolfe, London

Geddes A M 1986 Hepatitis B and HTLV 3 — infection in injured patients. Injury 17: 293–294

Gilles H M 1984 Malaria. Medicine International 2: 141–145

Weatherall D J, Ledingham J G G, Warrell D R (eds) 1987 Oxford textbook of medicine, 2nd edn. Oxford University Press, Oxford

FURTHER READING

A colour atlas of infectious diseases, 2nd edn. Edmond R T D, Rowland H A K, 1987 Wolfe Medical Publications, London

The natural history of human T lymphotropic virus-III infection: the cause of AIDS Melbye M 1986 British Medical Journal, 292: 5-12

Neurological problems

Over the years an A & E doctor will see examples of many different diseases affecting the patient's nervous system and many different manifestations of common neurological diseases, such as multiple sclerosis. The recognition and management of conditions commonly seen in the department are discussed. They are listed in Table 26.1.

Table 26.1. Common neurological problems

Strokes	Transient cerebral ischaemic attacks, the completed stroke and the evolving stroke
Fits	See also Ch. 12.
Syncope	Vasovagal faints, postural hypotension, forced Valsalva manoeuvres, exercise syncope, Stokes-Adams attacks, other cardiac dysrhythmias, carotid sinus syncope, hyperventilation syndrome (see Ch. 31) and other miscellaneous causes
'Weakness'	See Table 26.2
Dyskinesias	Tremor, chorea, myoclonus, tic and torsion dystonia (or athetosis) — also myokymia, fasciculation and tetany
Incoordination	
Miscellaneous	*AIDS and hysteria*
Vertigo	See Ch. 44

STROKES

Transient cerebral ischaemic attacks (TCIAs)

TCIAs are caused principally by emboli arising either from the heart or from atheroma in the great vessels, especially in the neck. Cerebral blood flow may also be temporarily compromised by atheromatous arterial stenoses, osteophytes associated with cervical spondylosis, transient cardiac dysrhythmias and hypotensive episodes (e.g. postural hypotension associated with various drugs). Occasionally short-lived symptoms, mimicking ischaemia, are caused by brain tumours or subdural haematomas.

By definition the symptoms and signs disappear within 24 hours. Most attacks last less than 30 minutes (in the case of amaurosis fugax, less than 5 minutes) but they tend to be recurrent. The onset is abrupt and there is no tendency for the neurological deficit to spread as occurs in the vasospastic aura of migraine or at the onset of focal epilepsy. Rarely chest pain or palpitations herald an attack, which is precipitated by a cardiac dysrhythmia. Either the *carotid* or *vertebrobasilar* arterial territory may be involved. Common manifestations of *carotid* ischaemia are transient uniocular blindness (amaurosis fugax), hemiparesis or monoparesis, clumsiness, dysphasia, hemianopia and unilateral paraesthesiae. The commonest symptom produced by *vertebrobasilar* ischaemia is vertigo. Other manifestations include ataxia, dysarthria, diplopia, cortical blindness, hemianopia, deafness, tinnitus, vomiting, dysphagia, facial paraesthesiae (especially around the mouth), occipital headaches and weakness or sensory disturbances affecting one or both sides of the body. *'Drop attacks'* are probably also caused by vertebrobasilar ischaemia in many instances. The patient, usually a middle-aged or elderly woman, suddenly falls to the ground while standing or walking. Consciousness may be lost fleetingly, but, unless injured, the person is often able to get up immediately. *Transient global amnesia* is another much rarer manifestation of brain stem ischaemia. The typical patient is a man aged between 50 and 70 and the attack may be provoked by taking a shower or by physical exertion. The patient suddenly becomes confused, agitated and restless and repeatedly asks where he is and what he is doing. He retains no memory of recent events but is able to continue normal daily activities such as dressing, eating or even driving a car. Recovery is normally complete in a few hours but memory for the time during the attack itself is not regained. The attacks are usually solitary but up to three or four episodes may occur.

Apart from the various neurological features which may still be present when the patient arrives in hospital any of the following relevant abnormalities may be found: anaemia, polycythaemia, postural hypotension, hypertension, cardiac dysrhythmias, evidence of ischaemic or valvular heart disease, unequal arterial pulses, arterial bruits in the head and neck, or limitation of neck movements suggestive of cervical spondylosis. Neurological symptoms related to arm exercise should lead to the measurement of the blood pressure in both arms. Inequality suggests subclavian artery stenosis leading to the 'subclavian steal' syndrome. Sometimes turning the patient's head will precipitate an attack or produce nystagmus or an extensor plantar response. Occasionally emboli may be seen passing through the retinal arterioles.

Management

Investigations in the A & E department can usually be limited to an ECG, red cell count and haematocrit. Radiographs of the skull and cervical spine are rarely helpful.

The importance of TCIAs is that they may herald an impending completed stroke, especially if they occur in the territory supplied by the carotid artery. Patients who have a demonstrable neurological deficit, even though it may be improving, and those who have recently had frequent TCIAs ('the stuttering stroke') should all be admitted. Immediate hospital admission should also be arranged for patients with electrocardiographic changes suggesting myocardial infarction, any cardiac disorder which might provide a further source of emboli, polycythaemia (haematocrit above 46%) or a significant degree of hypertension (diastolic blood pressure greater than 110 mmHg). Transient focal neurological signs can be the first manifestation of hypertensive encephalopathy, in which case the diastolic blood pressure is usually greater than 130 mmHg and there are retinal haemorrhages, papilloedema and proteinuria. The emergency treatment of severe hypertension is described in Chapter 11.

Individuals whose neurological signs have resolved by the time they arrive in hospital and who have no evidence of the other conditions mentioned above can often be allowed home, perhaps after a period of observation. The prognosis is unpredicatable and the risk of a later stroke and/or death has been calculated at about 10% per annum. The commonest cause of death is myocardial infarction and control of risk factors such as smoking, obesity and hypertension are therefore important. Daily low dose aspirin probably confers some benefit particularly in men. Patients with symptoms arising in the carotid territory, especially if a bruit is heard, have a high risk of the development of a completed stroke and should be referred for urgent outpatient investigation. Local investigative facilities, available surgical expertise and the age of the patient will determine the referral procedure. It would be unusual for surgery to be contemplated in someone over the age of 70. Vertebrobasilar ischaemia does not impose the same degree of urgency unless it has caused transient hemiplegia or hemianaesthesia. A soft collar to prevent sudden neck movements may abolish the attacks. A routine neurological outpatient consultation can be arranged for patients under the age of 60, patients with incapacitating attacks or those with bruits near the junction of the vertebral and subclavian arteries.

Completed strokes

The criteria of the World Health Organization for the diagnosis of a stroke are:

'rapidly developing clinical signs of focal and at times global loss of cerebral function, with symptoms lasting more than 24 hours or leading to death, with no apparent cause other than that of vascular origin'.

Recognition is not usually difficult. Although commoner in later life, the condition is not exclusive to old age. An increasing number of young men with widespread atherosclerosis and young women taking the 'pill' are being affected. Hypertension is a major risk factor. A stroke may also be the presenting feature of polycythaemia, leukaemia, bacterial endocarditis or a vasculitis. It may also occasionally follow an alcoholic binge, but in that situation an associated head injury is a much more likely cause.

All possible information should be obtained regarding the time and mode of onset, the subsequent progression and any premonitory symptoms. The description will help the doctor to decide if the stroke is in fact completed (i.e. the neurological defect is maximal) or still in the process of evolution. The patient's management may depend to some extent on this information. It is therefore important to question relatives or any other witnesses to the illness, especially when the patient is confused or dysphasic.

It may be possible from the history and physical signs to distinguish a cerebral haemorrhage from a cerebral infarct. The sudden onset of paralysis accompanied by severe headache, vomiting, impairment of consciousness, neck rigidity and signs of long-standing hypertension point to a haemorrhage. A few patients may have had a previous subarachnoid bleed or history of headaches caused by an aneurysm or angioma. The onset of cerebral infarction tends to be slower and headache not so severe. The patient is more often conscious and there may be a history of TCIAs. Infarction may be caused by a thrombosis-in-situ, in many cases in the extracranial rather than the intracranial arteries, an embolus or a sudden hypotensive episode (e.g. following myocardial infarction or a gastrointestinal haemorrhage).

The following points should receive particular attention during the examination.

1. Elicit the neurological signs carefully — they help to pinpoint the anatomical site of the lesion. Also the signs may change over the next few hours indicating that the stroke is in evolution. Before a patient is sent home it is important to assess in detail the deficits which the stroke has caused. How severe is the paralysis? Is there a hemianopia? Can he swallow and can he understand?

2. The blood pressure should be measured but should not be taken as representative of the 'prestroke' level. A reflex rise is common; occasionally a fall occurs. Examination of the heart and fundi may reveal signs of sustained hypertension.

3. Look for sources of emboli. Is the patient in atrial fibrillation or are there signs of valvular disease?

4. Listen for bruits over the neck vessels and orbits.

Infarction of the ventral pons or medulla may cause the 'locked in syndrome'. Such patients are rendered tetraplegic and mute but have preserved sentient consciousness. They are thus immobile, but can communicate by blinking and vertical eye movements. Patients thought to be in a coma should be asked to raise their eyes and to blink otherwise the rare alert but helpless patient may be overlooked.

Conditions which may simulate a stroke include a subdural haematoma, a brain tumour, postictal paralysis (Todd's paralysis), hypoglycaemia and hemiplegic migraine. When the patient has a head injury it can be difficult to ascertain whether the stroke caused a fall or the hemiparesis followed the injury. In general, however, the patient with a subdural haematoma has had a well defined injury to the head followed by headaches and a fluctuating neurological deficit which has become slowly progressive. Dysphasia and ocular field defects are rare. The patient with a brain tumour usually has a longer history of headache plus, perhaps, epileptic fits. Papilloedema is more likely. When haemorrhage occurs into a cerebral tumour the clinical presentation is indistinguishable from an ordinary cerebrovascular accident. Hypoglycaemia occasionally produces focal neurological signs which resolve when the blood sugar is corrected. Hemiplegic migraine should rarely be diagnosed in the absence of a family history of this problem.

Management

A chest radiograph should be obtained and an electrocardiogram recorded on all stroke victims. If consciousness is impaired the blood sugar should also be estimated. The ECG may indicate a 'silent coronary' or paroxysmal dysrhythmia. The chest film will display the overall size of the heart and may reveal an unsuspected malignancy. If the patient's head has been injured or an injury cannot be excluded, skull films should also be obtained. Significant midline shift (greater than 3 mm) suggests intracerebral haemorrhage or a subdural haematoma rather than infarction. Shift may be seen on a plain skull film if the pineal gland is calcified. It may also be demonstrated by echoencephalography.

The patient's condition on arrival at hospital may range from the mildly affected to the deeply unconscious (see Ch. 12). In the UK about 50% of stroke victims are admitted to hospital. A severe stroke or living alone are major determinants in this decision. Other reasons for admission to hospital include:

1. The need to make or confirm the diagnosis; in this regard one should be particularly wary of patients under the age of 55.
2. The presence of complications or associated conditions which require intensive medical treatment, e.g. myocardial infarction, pneumonia or heart failure.
3. Inadequate nursing and rehabilitative care in the community.

There is no dramatic treatment for a patient who has suffered a stroke. No particular medical treatment has been shown unequivocally to improve the functional outcome. Comatose patients have a very bad prognosis and require appropriate positioning, the placement of a nasogastric tube and intravenous fluids. Convulsions may also need to be controlled (see Ch. 12). All 'stroke patients' should be given oxygen. A low blood pressure should be raised and all but severe hypertension (systolic pressure greater than 180 mmHg) can be temporarily ignored. If blood pressure adjustments are indicated they should be made by tilting the patient appropriately. The use of agents to reduce cerebral oedema, such as dexamethasone or intravenous mannitol, has been disappointing. There is some evidence that the early administration of slow channel calcium-blocking agents such as nimodipine may decrease morbidity and mortality. A stroke is a particularly catastrophic event for the relatives of the patient, especially the spouse, and discussions with them require particular sensitivity and tact.

Treatment at home may be decided in the following circumstances:

1. Onset of symptoms 24–48 hours previously.
2. No evidence of progressive weakness.
3. Disability slight.
4. No acute cardiorespiratory disease.
5. Adequate social circumstances.
6. Agreement of the general practitioner.

The expressed wishes of the patient and the relatives should be taken into account. After an explanation of the management plan the patient may prefer home to hospital. Also relatives may prefer a moribund patient to be allowed to die at home. Proper home care requires a good community nursing and rehabilitation service. The patient must be actively encouraged and retrained to use paralysed limbs. Depression after a stroke is greatly underestimated*.

In summary, the decision to admit the patient to hospital or not is influenced by the severity of the stroke, the age of the patient, his previous mental status and the likelihood or benefit from anticoagulation or remedial surgery. Two instances when anticoagulation may be beneficial are: 1. when the stroke has been caused by a cerebral embolus and 2. when the thrombotic process is still considered to be in evolution. Often social factors are the main reasons for admission as many of those patients are elderly and living alone.

FITS (see also Ch. 12)

Repetitive attacks with similar features are essential for the diagnosis of epilepsy. The attacks may cause alteration of consciousness or mood or produce abnormal sensory, motor or visceral symptoms or signs. An eye witness account of the attack is essential for a clinical diagnosis. Helpful diagnostic characteristics are the description of an aura, tonic-clonic movements, incontinence,

*A useful leaflet for the patient and family is published by the Chest, Heart and Stroke Association, Tavistock House, London WC1H 9JE.

tongue biting and the nature of recovery after the episode. Postictal confusion, headache and drowsiness are common. The description may indicate a focal origin and enable differentiation of partial from generalised seizures. Prolonged syncope may result in a few clonic movements in the limbs but full-blown seizures are rare. Most fits occurring in children aged between 1 and 5 are simple febrile convulsions.

Management

Many patients brought to the A & E department after fits have a known epileptic tendency and have already been fully investigated. Common trigger factors are intercurrent illness, over- or undertreatment, alcohol abuse or alteration of the seizure threshold by other drugs (e.g. chlorpromazine or tricyclic antidepressants). It may be necessary to telephone the general practitioner for relevant information. Patients who have a known epileptic tendency, who rapidly recover clear consciousness, have not been injured and have not had any recent increase in the frequency of their seizures do not usually require admission to hospital. A short period of rest under observation is more appropriate. An early neurological outpatient appointment may be arranged.

The following categories of patients require hospital admission either for observation or specific inpatient treatment.

1. First fit.
2. Two or more fits within a short time.
3. Fit following a head injury.
4. Significant injury as a result of a fit.
5. All fits in early childhood.
6. Fits symptomatic of tumours, meningoencephalitis, cerebrovascular disease, alcoholism, hypoglycaemia, drug withdrawal or overdose, electrolyte disturbances, or other systemic disease.
7. Probable over- or undertreatment.
8. Prolonged postictal confusion.

A local cerebral lesion is suggested by a fit of focal onset, a history of personality change or the recent onset of headaches. Idiopathic epilepsy rarely presents after the age of 25.

Epileptic fits in the neonate are often either tonic or clonic in type and rarely show the characteristic progression seen in adults. They may be simulated by apnoeic attacks. Hospital admission is mandatory for all infants who have had either a convulsion or an apnoeic period.

The initial part of the examination is directed towards looking for evidence of a head injury and checking the vital signs. A careful neurological examination including the fundi is particularly indicated in patients who have sustained their first fit. Remember that transient neurological signs may persist for up to 24 hours after a fit (Todd's paralysis). Neck stiffness should be sought. Evidence of tongue or cheek biting helps confirm the diagnosis. Some confusion is common. Although not commonly a herald

of an intracranial haematoma this diagnosis must be excluded when fits occur shortly after an injury (see Ch 14).

Skull and chest radiographs should be obtained in patients who have had a first seizure. The skull film should be examined for:

1. Signs of increased intracranial pressure — in children diastasis of the suture lines (Fig. 26.1) and in adults thinning and erosion of the dorsum and floor of the sella (see Fig. 17.5, p. 222).
2. Significant pineal shift (see Fig. 17.2, p. 222).
3. Abnormal intracranial calcification which may be focal (Fig. 26.2) or diffuse (Fig. 26.3).
4. Unsuspected skull fractures, especially in old people.

The chest film is taken mainly to exclude a primary tumour.

The EEG is not a useful acute investigation as it is often abnormal for several days after the ictus whatever the cause. It is better carried out one to two weeks after the episode. Occasionally a normal 'postictal' tracing is put forward as evidence of syncope or hysteria. However, the usefulness of the EEG recording in differentiating epilepsy from other conditions associated with real or apparent loss of consciousness is limited. Many hysterics have 'unstable' records and in up to 30% of epileptics the tracing is normal. Furthermore, an EEG abnormality does not necessarily confirm a diagnosis of epilepsy which is essentially a clinical decision.

If the patient is still twitching on arrival in the A & E department or has experienced two or more fits in rapid succession, a single intravenous dose of diazepam (10 mg in adults or 0.1 mg/kg in

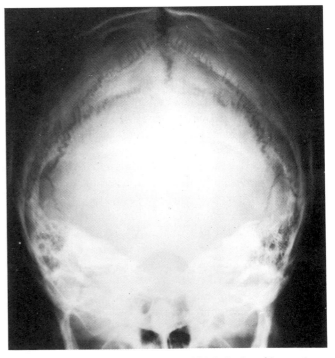

Fig. 26.1 Diastasis of the suture lines in a child, indicative of increased intracranial pressure.

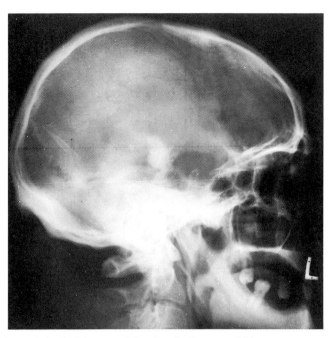

Fig. 26.2 A calcified tumour lying deep in the temporal lobe.

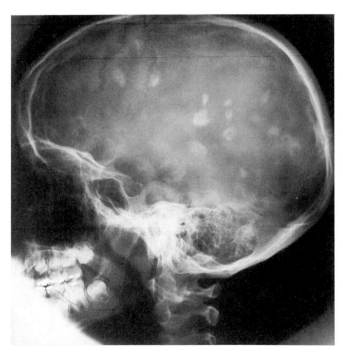

Fig. 26.3 Diffuse intracerebral calcification in a child (tuberous sclerosis).

children) should be given before arranging transfer to the admitting ward. A preparation of diazepam for rectal administration ('Stesolid') is very effective and easy to give to young children. Normally patients who have experienced a first fit will be admitted directly to a neurological or medical ward. However, some individuals in whom the diagnosis is unclear may be sent to the observation ward.

They should be carefully re-examined the next day — a minor neurological abnormality may have been overlooked during the initial examination. If this examination and the radiographs are normal the patient can be referred for outpatient investigation. It is most important that every detail of the history and examination recorded in both the A & E department and the observation ward is forwarded to the specialist clinic. Especially useful is a description of any attack witnessed. The patient should be told not to drive, work near dangerous machinery or at a height, or indulge in potentially dangerous sports (e.g. swimming) until seen by the specialist. A person should never be labelled epileptic and started on anticonvulsant drugs after an isolated fit.

In patients with confirmed epilepsy the margin between overtreatment and undertreatment is often narrow. Omission of anticonvulsants is more common than toxicity from overdosage. Signs of the latter include confusion, drowsiness, nystagmus and ataxia. Serum drug levels can be used as a guide to dosage. A random blood sample taken in the A & E department can also be helpful in assessing the patient's compliance with treatment. Unless there is obvious evidence of toxicity it is better to leave the dosage unaltered and await specialist advice.

SYNCOPE

Syncope is sudden, brief loss of consciousness due to transient impairment of cerebral circulation. Confusion after recovery is very unusual. The onset typically develops over a few seconds and is heralded by blurred vision and dizziness. The patient may get enough warning to sit down or else may go limp and sink to the ground. The loss of consciousness can be prolonged if the person is propped up.

The patient with syncope may also describe previous funny spells or dizzy turns in which consciousness was altered but not lost. Many forms are instantly recognisable from the context in which they occur. The duration of attacks, trigger factors and presyncopal activity should help differentiate syncope from epilepsy, hypoglycaemia, asphyxia, poisoning, hysteria, the hyperventilation syndrome and narcolepsy. Adverse reactions to drugs may mimic virtually every form of syncopal attack. As with epilepsy a witness's description of an attack can be invaluable. Unless the episode was an obvious simple faint all these patients should have an ECG recorded and many will require a full blood count. Some common causes of syncope are described below.

Vasovagal faints

Simple faints occur after prolonged standing, especially in warm surroundings, or in mentally distressing situations, e.g. with venepuncture. Transient loss of consciousness while sitting or lying is rarely due to a simple faint. The diagnosis should be made with great caution in middle-aged and elderly patients in whom cardiac dysrhythmias or drugs are more frequently to blame.

The patient often feels nauseated and dizzy beforehand and has enough warning to sit or lie down. A history of previous attacks is common. During the attack the patient is pale, sweaty, hypotensive, bradycardiac, has dilated pupils and sighing respirations. Recovery is rapid if the person is placed recumbent with legs elevated. No further action is needed.

Postural hypotension

Postural hypotension is a common side effect of many drugs, most usually antihypertensive agents and sedatives (e.g. chlorpromazine), but also levodopa, some diuretics, nitrates and alcohol. It may also be a symptom of diabetes, hypoadrenalism, renal disease, Parkinsonism, tabes dorsalis, polyneuropathy or occur after surgical sympathectomy. There may be associated autonomic disturbances such as impotence and lack of sweating. It can also be an early sign of occult bleeding. A typical history is that the patient experiences dizziness or momentarily loses consciousness in the act of getting up from the sitting or lying position. Symptoms tend to be worse on rising in the morning and after eating. The elderly are particularly susceptible. A difference of more than 30 mmHg between the supine and standing systolic blood pressures confirms the diagnosis. Commonsense advice about avoidance of sudden postural changes is usually all that is necessary. Sometimes a reduction in the dosage of a particular drug or a change to another preparation may be required. For instance β-adrenergic blocking drugs are effective antihypertensive agents but produce little postural hypotension compared with many of the older drugs. The patient should be referred back to his general practitioner for any alteration of medication. The more complicated case should be referred to a specialist who may recommend that the patient sleeps with his head and trunk raised 20% to reduce nocturnal diuresis and, in addition, may prescribe fludrocortisone or a non-steroidal anti-inflammatory agent.

Atrial myxoma or thrombus are rare causes of posture-related syncope.

Forced Valsalva manoeuvres

Forced expiration against a closed glottis is the cause of micturition and cough syncope, weightlifter's blackout in adults, and syncope following breath-holding attacks in children. Micturition syncope typically occurs at night, in men who have some degree of prostatic obstruction and have to strain to pass urine. A prolonged bout of coughing may cause fainting by the same physiological mechanism (i.e. reduced venous return to the heart).

Breath-holding attacks may occur as early as 3 months and up to 4 years of age. They more usually begin between 9 and 18 months. The child cries vigorously once or twice and then suddenly holds his breath, becomes cyanosed and, in the most severe cases, loses consciousness. The limbs may become rigid and there may be a few clonic movements but no real convulsions. The attack is ended by the child taking a deep breath and immediately regaining consciousness. There may be transient confusion afterwards. The most significant feature is that the attacks always occur when the child has been physically hurt or psychologically thwarted. The often frightened parents should be reassured that the attacks are benign, that the child will not die and that they will diminish with age. The child should be placed in the coma position during an attack. The general practitioner should be requested to refer the child to a paediatrician.

Exercise syncope

Effort syncope is classically associated with tight aortic stenosis in which the cardiac output is virtually fixed. It is occasionally due to pulmonary stenosis, hypertrophic obstructive cardiomyopathy, severe left ventricular disease or constrictive pericarditis. Syncope specifically associated with the use of an arm suggests the subclavian steal syndrome.

Stokes-Adams attacks

Stokes-Adams attacks are caused by self-limiting episodes of complete heart block resulting in ventricular standstill. The patient is often elderly and the history is characteristic. The person falls to the ground, deathly pale and pulseless. About half to one minute later his face suffuses and consciousness returns with no residual confusion or neurological deficit. Recovery may be hastened by a precordial thump or a few thrusts of external cardiac massage.

The ECG may show various degrees of heart block between attacks. On the other hand the tracing may be entirely normal, in which case *gentle* massage of the carotid sinus may expose an underlying atrioventricular conduction defect. This manoeuvre must be done on one side only at a time, under continuous ECG monitoring and with full resuscitation facilities at hand. The ECG will, of course, be diagnostic if recorded during an attack.

These patients require admission for cardiological evaluation with a view to pacemaker implantation.

Other cardiac dysrhythmias (see also Ch. 18)

Intermittent disturbances of rhythm are common causes of syncope in older patients, e.g. paroxysmal ventricular tachycardia or sinoatrial block. Again the latter may only be brought to light by carotid sinus massage. Patients with paroxysmal supraventricular tachycardia may faint if they stand up during an attack. Many such patients will have experienced previous bouts of palpitations. A short PR interval and abnormal QRS complex is diagnostic of the pre-excitation syndromes (e.g. Wolff-Parkinson-White syndrome). A prolonged QT interval should warn of the possibility that life-threatening tachydysrhythmias are a danger. The presence of a paroxysmal dysrhythmia per se should not automatically be assumed to be the cause of syncope unless symptoms occur simultaneously. Suspicion of such events should lead to referral to a cardiologist for 24-hour ambulatory electrocardiographic monitoring.

Carotid sinus syncope

Carotid sinus syncope is very rare. The patient may notice dizziness or faintness when wearing tight collars or turning his head quickly.

Careful massage of the hypersensitive carotid sinus may produce bradycardia and/or hypotension.

Miscellaneous conditions

Syncope may be the presenting feature of myocardial infarction, pulmonary embolism, a dissecting aneurysm of the aorta, a subarachnoid or intestinal haemorrhage, a ruptured ectopic pregnancy or basilar migraine. (For a discussion of syncope complicated by concussion, see Ch. 40.)

Note: Any syncopal attack may be followed by a true epileptic seizure and any transient loss of consciousness may result in injury to the patient.

WEAKNESS

This symptom may be confined to one or more limbs or it may be generalised. It should not be confused with stiffness as occurs in Parkinsonism and polymyalgia rheumatica. Generalised weakness is often due to underlying systemic disease or neurosis. When weakness is not generalised the mode of presentation and the pattern of disability are of great diagnostic importance. Often there are associated symptoms which suggest the diagnosis, e.g. pain or paraesthesiae. Some of the more important conditions are listed in Table 26.2.

If weakness is generalised and rapidly progressive consider the Guillain-Barré syndrome. Chronic progressive weakness is typical of muscular dystrophies and motor neurone disease. Exercise-related fatiguability suggests myasthenia gravis, a metabolic myopathy or the postviral fatigue syndrome (see Ch. 31). In multiple sclerosis weakness is widespread in anatomical distribution and in time and associated ocular and sensory problems are common.

Apart from a detailed description of the site of the weakness and its rate of progression, it is most important to elicit a family and drug history from these patients. Is there anything similar

Table 26.2 Causes of weakness

Neurological	Hemiplegia (see before), acute paraplegia, spastic mono- and paraparesis, poly- and mononeuropathies, myasthenia gravis, poliomyelitis and motor neurone disease
Muscular	Hereditary muscular dystrophies, myopathies (drugs, electrolyte disturbances), polymyositis, rhabdomyolysis (see Ch. 15), postviral fatigue syndrome, muscle wasting secondary to joint disease and diabetic amyotrophy
General diseases	Malnutrition, carcinomatosis, cardiorespiratory insufficiency, anaemia, drugs, infections (tuberculosis, brucellosis, AIDS), autoimmune disease, electrolyte disorders (hypokalaemia, hypomagnesaemia and hypophosphataemia), diabetes, thyrotoxicosis and adrenal dysfunction
Psychogenic	Depression and hysteria

Table 26.3 MRC grading of muscle power

0	No contraction
1	Flicker of contraction
2	Active movement with gravity eliminated
3	Active movement against gravity
4	Active movement against gravity and resistance
5	Normal power

in other members of the family? Corticosteroids can damage muscles directly but other drugs such as diuretics, purgatives and liquorice derivatives, may cause weakness secondary to hypokalaemia. The patients' jobs may be relevant especially if they work with chemicals or metals, e.g. lead, arsenic or thallium. If weakness of the legs is the problem, specific questions should be asked about spinal pain, sensory disturbances, bladder function and impotence. Peripheral paraesthesiae in a 'glove and stocking' distribution are typical of polyneuropathies, commonly caused by diabetes or alcoholism.

After a complete general and neurological examination particular features should be sought. The strength of each muscle group should be tested and recorded using the Medical Research Council (MRC) grading (see Table 26.3).

The muscles themselves should be examined for wasting, tenderness, fasciculation and myotonia. At the end of the examination the patient should be asked to stand and walk, and abnormalities of posture and gait noted.

Acute paraplegia

Acute paraplegia is most commonly caused by trauma (see Ch. 14). The injury is usually all too obvious unless the patient is unconscious. Quite minor neck injuries may cause paraplegia in the presence of cervical spondylosis, rheumatoid arthritis or ankylosing spondylitis. Paraplegia advancing over a few hours or days is usually due to spinal cord compression from a tumour or abscess, sometimes tuberculous (Pott's paraplegia). It may also be caused by spinal arterial or venous thrombosis, acute transverse myelitis (postinfective or caused by multiple sclerosis), epidural haemorrhage (anticoagulants), or an acutely prolapsed intervertebral disc. Many of these conditions produce pain at the site of the lesion and associated girdle pains in the appropriate dermatomes. Transient weakness after exercise suggests lumbar spinal stenosis.

The main physical sign is a flaccid paraplegia of the lower limbs. Variable sensory loss will be present, depending on the extent of the cord damage, and there may be a sensory 'cut-off' level indicating the site of the spinal pathology. Local spinal tenderness may indicate vertebral body collapse due to osteoporosis or metastases.

All these patients must be admitted to hospital immediately as spinal decompression may be necessary.

Impairment of bladder function constitutes an urgent neurological emergency.

Poliomyelitis should always be considered in any patient with asymmetrical flaccid paralysis of the limbs especially if there has been a febrile illness.

Chronic spastic paraparesis

Chronic spastic paraparesis is usually due to lesions which compress the spinal cord or to intrinsic diseases of the cord itself. Roughly in the order of their frequency, the causes are tumours, multiple sclerosis, spondylotic myelopathy (commonly cervical), prolapsed intervertebral discs, tuberculosis, motor neurone disease, syringomyelia and subacute combined degeneration of the cord.

Multiple sclerosis most commonly presents with a weakness in one or more limbs. There may be associated nystagmus, pallor of the optic discs, incoordination of the limbs, exaggerated tendon reflexes, urinary retention and extensor plantar responses.

In any case an urgent neurological opinion should be sought and often hospital admission will be necessary in order to establish the diagnosis.

Polyneuropathies

In the polyneuropathies the neurological symptoms and signs are usually symmetrical and start peripherally in the limbs. Postinfective polyneuropathy (Guillain-Barré syndrome) has an onset over a few days but most of the other types are insidious in their evolution. They are caused by processes which act diffusely on the peripheral nervous system, such as: metabolic disturbances (diabetes, porphyria, uraemia and amyloidosis), toxic agents and drugs (alcohol, acrylamide, lead, arsenic, isoniazid and nitrofurantoin), vitamin deficiencies, neoplasia and rare inherited disorders.

Muscle weakness and wasting usually starts in the legs causing bilateral foot drop and a high stepping gait. The ankle jerks are the first reflexes to be lost. Paraesthesiae are frequent and consist of numbness, tingling and unpleasant burning sensations. Neuropathies caused by alcohol and diabetes are notorious for the unremitting pain they can produce in the soles of the feet.

Weakness and sensory changes in the legs caused by compression of the cauda equina can be difficult to distinguish from the onset of a polyneuropathy. Important features of cauda equina lesions are a history of bladder and erectile difficulties and demonstrable loss of sensation in the perineum.

Mononeuropathies

Bell's palsy is one of the commonest mononeuropathies seen in the A & E department (for a description see Ch. 44). Nevertheless, diabetes and severe hypertension should be excluded in any person presenting with a lower motor neurone facial weakness. Sudden *oculomotor* palsies, especially of the 6th cranial nerve, are quite common in the elderly and are usually due to atheroma, sometimes associated with diabetes.

The other mononeuropathies which the A & E doctor is likely to see are examples of entrapment or pressure neuropathies. In the *carpal tunnel syndrome* the median nerve is compressed as it passes deep to the flexor retinaculum. The patient complains of numbness, tingling and burning sensations in the hand and fingers, worse at night. The hand feels clumsy and useless on waking but recovers quickly with use. The pain sometimes radiates up the whole arm which may erroneously lead to suspicion of cervical spondylosis or a cervical rib. Tapping over the median nerve at the wrist may reproduce the pain (Tinel's sign).

The classical story in *Saturday night paralysis* is that the individual has fallen asleep when drunk with his upper arm over the back of a chair. Paralysis of the radial nerve produces wrist drop and sensory impairment on the back of the hand. Recovery is usual over several weeks and a cock-up wrist splint is helpful while it is awaited.

Entrapment of the *anterior interosseous nerve* should be considered in any patient with an inability to pinch.

Sciatica is described in Ch. 20.

Meralgia paraesthetica is caused by compression of the lateral cutaneous nerve of the thigh as it passes under the inguinal ligament. The patient is often a man who has gained weight recently. It may be unilateral or bilateral. The person experiences numbness on the outer aspect of the thigh and burning paraesthesiae during prolonged standing or walking. The symptoms usually subside spontaneously.

Because of its superficial position at the neck of the fibula, the *common peroneal nerve* is another nerve which is exposed to compression, e.g. by sitting with the legs crossed for long periods or by a tight short leg plaster cast. Damage leads to foot drop and sensory impairment over the lateral aspect of the lower leg and dorsum of the foot.

While not strictly a mononeuropathy, this seems an appropriate place to mention idiopathic brachial plexus neuropathy (otherwise known as neuralgic amyotrophy or brachial neuritis). This condition presents with severe pain in the shoulder, soon followed by paralysis of various muscles of the shoulder girdle. There may be associated sensory loss. It sometimes follows an immunising injection, an operation, or an intercurrent illness, but often there is no recognisable antecedent event. Spontaneous recovery is the rule although it is occasionally recurrent. Steroids have no therapeutic part to play.

When the diagnosis is in doubt, or active treatment is planned (e.g. surgery for carpal tunnel syndrome) the patient should be referred to the appropriate outpatient department, which may be neurological, surgical or in physical medicine. Some may turn out to have lesions of the central nervous system or primary muscle disorders which are only uncovered by electromyography and nerve conduction studies. These electrodiagnostic techniques also enable an estimate to be given of the likely duration until recovery.

Limb girdle weakness

Weakness of the shoulder and pelvic girdle musculature is a feature of many generalised muscle disorders. Patients may complain of difficulty holding their arms above their heads for any length of time (e.g. brushing their hair or hanging up the washing). If the pelvic muscles are involved, it is climbing steps or getting out of a low chair which presents the difficulty. Various metabolic (vitamin D deficiency), endocrine (thyrotoxicosis) and drug-induced myopathies can present in this way as can polymyositis, carcinomatous neuropathy and limb girdle muscular dystrophy. Unilateral quadriceps wasting may be due to hip or knee disease, lumbar disc protrusion or diabetic amyotrophy. Therefore the joints and spine should be examined clinically and where appropriate, radiographically, and the urine tested for sugar.

Drugs which may cause complaints of muscle weakness, with or without pain, include corticosteroids (especially the fluorinated compounds), chloroquine, clofibrate, ϵ-aminocaproic acid (EACA), vincristine, diuretics, purgatives, liquorice derivatives, β-adrenergic blocking agents, lithium, methyldopa and chronic alcohol or opiate abuse.

Most patients with muscle disorders can be referred to the appropriate outpatient clinic.

DYSKINESIAS

Unless the disorder is so violent that the patient may injure himself (e.g. hemiballismus), or there is a possibility of Sydenham's chorea, most patients suffering from involuntary movements can be referred to a neurological outpatient clinic.

In taking a history the perinatal circumstances should be noted and a detailed family history obtained. Anoxia or jaundice at birth may be significant and many of the causative diseases are inherited. The patient's occupation may be relevant ('hatters' shakes'), as may a history of 'sleeping sickness' (encephalitis lethargica) or rheumatic fever. A list of current medications may also help to solve a seemingly bizarre clinical problem. Neuroleptic agents such as chlorpromazine and haloperidol can produce a spectrum of involuntary movements which range from acute dystonias, akathisia (restlessness), Parkinsonism and akinetic mutism to so called tardive dyskinesia.

In the course of the clinical examination it should be possible to define the movement disorder (see below) and to decide if any other parts of the nervous system are involved.

Tremor

Tremor is an unwanted movement caused by rhythmic muscle contractions. A diagnosis can usually be made by observation of the tremor at rest, on sustained posture and on active use of the limb.

A fine tremor of the outstretched fingers is physiological. The common causes of exaggerated postural tremor are anxiety, alcohol, drugs (e.g. lithium and tricyclic antidepressants) and benign essential or familial tremor which may be of the late onset (senile tremor) type. The essential type tends to increase in severity with time and a helpful diagnostic feature is that it may be strikingly improved by modest quantities of alcohol. Less common causes of postural tremor are thyrotoxicosis, mercury poisoning, cerebellar diseases and Wilson's disease. An intention tremor is characteristic of diseases of the cerebellum and its pathways, e.g. multiple sclerosis, tumours or vascular lesions. Classically it is most clearly seen towards the end of the movement in the finger to nose test.

Parkinson's disease produces a coarse 'pill-rolling' tremor occurring at rest in a middle aged person. It begins in one limb and spreads initially to the unaffected limb on the same side. Within months bradykinesia, rigidity and other features of Parkinsonism usually become apparent.

A 'flapping' tremor (asterixis) seen when the hands are outstretched and dorsiflexed may occur in hepatic, renal or respiratory failure.

Chorea

Chorea consists of continual jerky movements which pass unpredictably from one part of the body to another. The movement appears to be a fragment of a normal movement.

Sydenham's chorea occurs between the ages of 5 and 20 years. About one-third of patients have a prior history of rheumatic fever 2–3 months previously. Often there are associated personality changes. The patient should be admitted to hospital for assessment, rest and sedation. A similar disorder occasionally occurs in pregnant women or women taking contraceptives.

Choreiform movements in the 30–50 age group may signify the onset of Huntington's disease. Increasingly more grotesque movements are accompanied by behavioural changes and progressive mental deterioration. The disease is inherited as an autosomal dominant trait.

Myoclonus

The term myoclonus is applied to rapid shock-like twitches. It is physiological when it occurs upon falling asleep or awakening. Intermittent generalised benign myoclonus is found in a large number of patients with idiopathic epilepsy. In children, however, it may signify the onset of one of a number of dementing illnesses.

Tic

Tics are repetitive and stereotyped muscular twitches. They are usually innocent motor phenomena but may, rarely, be symptomatic of organic brain disorder (e.g. the syndrome of Gilles de la Tourette). In a minority of people simple tics may become so marked that they seek medical help. The tics are then sometimes an expression of underlying psychological distress.

Torsion dystonia (athetosis)

Sustained muscular spasms causing characteristic contortions of the head, trunk and limbs is known as torsion dystonia. The condition may be either idiopathic, or symptomatic of serious underlying brain disease (e.g. cerebral palsy or Wilson's disease), or, more commonly, an idiosyncratic reaction to a drug. The best known offenders are phenothiazines, haloperidol, metoclopramide and domperidone. In the characteristic posture the head is twisted to one side (torticollis), the trunk forced into lordosis and scoliosis, the arm extended and hyperpronated and the leg is also extended, the foot being plantar flexed and inverted.

When athetosis is symptomatic of a neurological disease, evidence of damage to other parts of the nervous system will be found. In the idiopathic variety, apart from the movement disorder, the rest of the neurological examination will be normal.

Orofacial dyskinesias secondary to drug therapy can be treated by the A & E physician. The bizarre facial contortions may appear after the first dose of the drug and are significantly more common in young women. These patients are easily misdiagnosed as hysterical unless a careful history is taken. The condition will clear spontaneously within 24 hours of stopping the drug. Resolution can be hastened by the intravenous injection of benztropine (2 mg) or procyclidine (10 mg) followed, if necessary by two or three oral doses.

Spasmodic torticollis, writer's cramp and blepharospasm are all examples of segmental torsion dystonia and some patients may need neuropsychiatric advice.

Miscellaneous

Twitching of the lower eyelid (*myokymia*) is a normal accompaniment of fatigue in some people and of no significance.

Fasciculations are spontaneous contractions of individual muscle fasciculi. A few coarse twitchings of the muscles of the face, thenar eminence or calves are often seen in normal individuals and are physiological. However, widespread, persistent fasciculations usually indicate disease of the anterior horn cells.

Tetany is characterised by carpopedal spasm and general neuromuscular irritability. It may develop in the presence of alkalosis, potassium and magnesium deficiency as well as in hypocalcaemia. The hyperventilation syndrome (see Ch. 31) is the most common cause seen in the A & E department. Treatment is that of the underlying disorder.

INCOORDINATION

The problem may range from unsteadiness of gait, through minor clumsiness, to a complete inability to perform fine motor tasks. Disability due to weakness, tremor, dystonia and sensory neuropathy should first be excluded. If the presentation is in childhood, hydrocephalus should be considered. The hereditary ataxias tend to present in adolescence and early adulthood. Alcohol and drugs (benzodiazepines, anticonvulsants) are the commonest causes in adults. Cerebellar signs suggest multiple sclerosis or a tumour while Rombergism may point to a diagnosis of vitamin B_{12} deficiency or tabes dorsalis. Rarely, ataxia may be a non-metastatic manifestation of neoplasia or a feature of myxoedema.

MISCELLANEOUS

AIDS (see also Ch. 25)

More and more neurological manifestations of human immunodeficiency virus (HIV) infection are being recognised. At the time of seroconversion an acute reversible encephalopathy may develop. The illness is characterised by fever, general malaise, disorientation, loss of memory, personality change and sometimes fits. Atypical meningitis, neuropathy and myelopathy have also been described as part of the acute seroconversion illness. The atypical features of meningitis include recurrence, chronicity, cranial nerve involvement and long tract signs. The neuropathy may be of the mononeuritis multiplex type or a bilateral sensorimotor disturbance with weakness, paraesthesiae, ataxia and incontinence.

In full blown AIDS the most common neurological syndrome is a subacute encephalitis. In the early stages there are subtle cognitive changes which may progress to serious dementia over several weeks or months. The general lethargy and loss of interest at the outset can easily be mistaken for depression arising as a reaction to the illness. Patients with AIDS may also develop a chronic symmetrical sensorimotor neuropathy with painful dysaesthesiae.

All these neurological disorders are caused by direct infection of nerve cells by the HIV. AIDS sufferers' misery may be further compounded by opportunistic infections of the central nervous system and an increased liability to develop tumours therein.

The neurotropic propensities of HIV may eventually allow it to inherit the title of 'the great mimic' previously ascribed to neurosyphilis.

Hysteria

Patients with hysteria may imitate many neurological disabilities. The most common presentations are weakness of the limbs, unconsciousness, blindness and fits. The inconsistent history, the patient's inappropriate indifference to their disability and the odd clinical features should alert the doctor to the correct diagnosis. For instance, the patient may use a 'paralysed' limb when apparently unobserved. Motor and sensory loss is often anatomically incompatible with an organic neurological lesion. Obvious lack of genuine effort in complying with tests of power may be accompanied by tensing of muscles other than those under scrutiny. In feigned unconsciousness there is often a tell-tale tremor of the eyelids and active resistance to forcible eye opening. Hysterical fits may be provoked by suggestion. For a more detailed consideration of non-organic symptoms see Ch. 31.

FURTHER READING

Peripheral nerve disorders: a practical approach Asbury A K, Gilliatt R W 1984 Butterworths International Medical Reviews; Neurology 4 Butterworths, London

Brain's clinical neurology, 6th edn. Bannister R 1985 Oxford University Press, Oxford

Paediatric neurology Brett E M 1983 Churchill Livingstone, Edinburgh

A clinician's view of neuromuscular diseases, 2nd edn. Brooke M H 1986 Williams & Wilkins, Baltimore

Movement disorders Marsden C D, Fahn S 1987 Butterworths International Medical Reviews; Neurology 6 Butterworths, London

McAlpine's multiple sclerosis Matthews W B, Acheson E D, Batchelor J R, Weller R O 1985 Churchill Livingstone, Edinburgh

Neurological differential diagnosis: an illustrated approach Patten J P 1983 (Reprint of 1977 edn.) Harold Starke, London

The epilepsies Porter R J, Morselli P L 1985 Butterworths International Medical Reviews; Neurology 5 Butterworths, London

Stroke: a critical approach to diagnosis, treatment and management Wade D T, Hewer R L, David R M, Skillbeck C E 1985 Chapman & Hall, London

Brain's diseases of the nervous system, 9th edn. Walton J N 1985 Oxford University Press, Oxford

Limb pain

Spontaneous limb pain severe enough to bring a patient to the A & E department most commonly has a neurological or vascular origin. It may also be due to localised or generalised disease of the skin, muscles, bones, tendons, joints or periarticular structures. Muscle disorders which cause pain range from simple conditions such as 'strains' from overuse and viral myalgia, through fascial compression syndromes, to much rarer diseases such as polymyositis, trichinosis and paroxysmal myoglobinuria. Common musculoskeletal disorders are described in Ch. 35. This chapter is confined to a description of the vascular and neurological causes of limb pain.

History

A diagnosis can often be made from a detailed description of the characteristics of the pain alone. The points to note are as follows:

1. *The date and mode of onset.* Was it sudden (suggesting an arterial blockage or lumbar disc herniation), or gradual as occurs with many neuropathies? What was the patient doing before or at the onset of the pain? Had he been indulging in unusual exercise, heavy lifting, or been involved in a car accident?

2. *The subsequent progression of the pain.* Is it easing or getting worse?

3. *The nature, site and severity of the discomfort.* Neurological pain often has a very unpleasant character, although the possibility of serious disease should not be dismissed if the discomfort is not very severe. Referred pain may mislead the unwary. For example, pain in the arm (whether or not this is associated also with pain in the neck) should lead to a search for pathology in the spinal cord, the nerve roots or the cervical spine. Similarly, pain in the region of the knee may indicate disease in the hip joint. Pain of vascular origin is not confined to any nerve or root distribution and, apart from intermittent claudication in the calf, sole of the foot or the buttock, is usually peripheral (in the tips of the fingers and toes or in the foot) and will be accompanied by signs of arterial or venous obstruction. The pain produced by sudden arterial blockage may be very severe initially but tends to diminish with

time. The pain of deep venous thrombosis is often unimpressive; but the pain of superficial thrombophlebitis in the veins of the leg may be quite severe and located in the veins themselves.

4. *Aggravating or relieving factors.* Exercise-induced pain is typical of intermittent claudication. Elevating the affected limb tends to relieve the pain of venous obstruction while 'rest pain' due to arterial insufficiency may be lessened by hanging the limb in a dependent position. Stooping, coughing or straining may aggravate 'root' pains due to intervertebral disc protrusions.

5. *The presence of associated symptoms.* Angina pectoris suggests widespread arterial disease when it occurs in patients complaining of intermittent claudication.

Painful neurological disorders may be associated with paraesthesiae, muscle weakness or bladder complaints.

The possibility of diabetes or alcoholism, both common causes of a painful peripheral neuropathy, should be considered. Diabetes is also a potent accelerator of peripheral vascular disease.

Any tablets the patient is taking should be noted, as there is a long list of substances which may cause peripheral neuropathy or painful muscle cramps. For the same reason an occupational history may be relevant. Enquiry into the family history may reveal an inherited predisposition to occlusive vascular disease or to a genetically determined neurological disorder.

Examination

The colour, temperature and size of the affected limb should be noted and compared with the normal side. The skin should also be examined carefully for ulcers and other trophic changes. Points of tenderness should be precisely located. Examination should include palpation of arterial pulses and listening for bruits over major arteries. Where the pain is not obviously vascular or musculoskeletal in origin, a careful neurological examination must be carried out. The mobility of joints should be tested, especially the hip joint if pain in the knee or thigh is the problem. The spine should be examined for local tenderness or deformity, and the circulatory system assessed, especially if the symptoms are thought to have a vascular origin.

Finally, the urine should be tested for sugar, particularly in the older age group when diabetes is often asymptomatic.

VASCULAR LIMB PAIN

Arterial

Generalised *atherosclerosis* is the commonest cause of peripheral arterial insufficiency, and the incidence is increasing at an alarming rate. Not only is the age of onset falling, but more people are surviving to ages at which the degenerative diseases are common.

The pain of *intermittent claudication* is characteristically related to exercise in a way that is constant for each individual. It commonly occurs in the calf muscles, although it may also affect gluteal, foot and arm muscles. Gradual progression of the atherosclerotic process or an intercurrent thrombosis may result in pain at rest, from which the patient may attempt to get some relief by warming the affected part or keeping the legs dependent. However, sudden *embolic or thrombotic obstruction* of a main line artery gives rise to very acute pain, for which the patient may seek urgent relief in an A & E department. Such pain usually reaches a maximum within minutes, although occasionally it may build up over several hours. Sensations of numbness, coldness, tingling or weakness are frequently associated features and are due to progressive ischaemia of nerve tissue as well as of muscle and connective tissues. The limb becomes pale initially, but later turns a mottled, cyanotic colour. Later still, blisters appear and gangrene supervenes.

The pain of early peripheral arterial insufficiency may be confused with that of an associated paronychia or infected ingrowing toe nail. If these conditions are then treated surgically, using a tourniquet and a digital nerve block, gangrene may be precipitated and amputation will become necessary. The leg pulses should therefore be palpated in all such patients irrespective of age, and are usually absent or reduced in amplitude below an arterial blockage. Sometimes the pulses are palpable at rest but disappear after a short period of exercise. The Doppler ultrasound flow velocimeter is very useful for the detection of flow differences which may not be discernible clinically. Auscultation over the larger arteries may reveal a bruit. The colour of the skin and the appearance of the superficial veins should be examined in the erect and the supine posture. These signs will usually serve to distinguish venous from ischaemic ulcers. The latter are very painful and, unless the patient is hypertensive, are usually situated below the ankle. Since atherosclerosis is a generalised disease, accessible arteries elsewhere should also be palpated, the heart examined carefully and the common sites for xanthomata scrutinised. The patients should be weighed and their urine tested for sugar. Anaemia, polycythaemia and hyperlipidaemia should be excluded and an ECG recording made. Any such patients who require surgery, however minor, should be admitted to hospital or referred to a vascular surgeon for careful preoperative evaluation, which may include arteriography. One form in which the ischaemic foot may present is slightly swollen, bright red, shiny and tender to the touch. The appearances are very similar to cellulitis, for which it can be easily mistaken. However, if the patient lies down and the leg is elevated to 45°, the redness fades and is replaced by a striking pallor.

When symptoms suggest either acute or chronic arterial occlusion, the family history, past medical history and drug history may provide corroborative evidence. Whilst the ingestion of oral contraceptives may be associated with an increased risk of arterial thrombosis, the presence of an aneurysm and a history of previous arterial surgery suggest significant sources of emboli.

Limb ischaemia due to aortic dissection is frequently transient. The patient is invariably hypertensive and there is usually a history of sudden severe retrosternal or interscapular pain.

Treatment

The same general principles apply to the initial management of the ischaemic limb whether it be due to thrombosis or to embolism. Immediately the diagnosis is made, a vascular surgeon should be contacted and 10 000 units of heparin given intravenously. This prevents distal propagation of the thrombus and should be given even if emergency arterial surgery is necessary, since the surgeon can reverse its effect with intravenous protamine sulphate. The contraindications to heparin therapy include active peptic ulceration, severe hypertension, hepatocellular disease and a bleeding diathesis. Pain should be relieved with appropriate analgesics and the ischaemic limb maintained at room temperature in a slightly dependent position. Heart failure, cardiac dysrhythmias, uncontrolled diabetes or hypertension may also need treatment. Low molecular weight dextrans should not be administered until a surgeon has examined the patient and has made a decision regarding the need for surgery. Likewise, the indications for the use of thrombolytic agents are not yet generally agreed, and their use is therefore best left to the specialist who will be undertaking the surgery.

Arm pain of vascular origin

Although much less common than in the legs, acute and chronic arterial occlusion may occur in the vessels supplying the arms; for example, axillary artery thrombosis may follow trauma or unusual exercise, especially if the artery is atherosclerotic. Claudication mainly affects the forearm muscles.

Two other conditions which may cause pain in the arms are the *aortic arch syndrome* (Takayasu's disease, pulseless disease) and the *thoracic outlet compression syndrome*. In the latter the subclavian artery is narrowed at the point of compression and this results in a bruit and reduction of the distal pulses, especially when the shoulders are retracted and the arms hyperabducted. A poststenotic aneurysm may result, developing mural thrombi which release emboli. These lodge in the digital arteries, often causing severe pain and tenderness in the fingers. However, embolism may be asymptomatic until trophic changes appear in the finger tips. Such a patient may present in the A & E department with a finger infection which will be exceptionally painful, and may result in spreading gangrene if the diagnosis of the underlying condition is not made and appropriate treatment begun without delay. Depending on the severity of the symptoms and the extent of the trophic changes, these patients may require admission to hospital or an early outpatient appointment may be satisfactory.

Raynaud's syndrome is a useful eponym for the collection of symptoms and signs caused by arterial insufficiency of the fingers, whatever the cause. Whilst Raynaud's disease mainly afflicts young women, identical symptoms may herald the onset of an autoimmune disorder, or indicate neurovascular compression from a cervical rib. Therefore all patients with Raynaud's syndrome should be investigated to exclude these disorders. Cold hypersensitivity may also occur among the users of rapidly vibrating tools (e.g. stone cutters, grinding tools and chain saws).

A painful finger with an area of terminal necrosis indicates *digital artery thrombosis or embolism*. The patient is usually a middle-aged man and the symptoms may be quite gradual in onset. Cold sensitivity may be an early feature, but the fingers are more often cyanosed than white during the ischaemic stage. Absent digital artery pulsation may be felt alongside the proximal phalanges, and confirmed using an ultrasound probe. The thrombosis is usually secondary to atherosclerosis, polycythaemia, cold agglutination, cryoglobulinaemia, leukaemias, other malignant diseases or generalised autoimmune disorders. The patient should be admitted or referred urgently for investigation. Ischaemic fingers have a great capacity for spontaneous recovery and early surgical interference should, therefore, be avoided.

Foot pain

Swollen, painful, blue toes or feet, with a history of cold water immersion, may progress to extensive tissue loss. This is called *trench foot* (Fig. 27.1). White (or eventually dusky) numb extremities (fingers, toes, nose or ears) following exposure to dry cold is called *frost bite*. The management of these conditions is described in Ch. 28 — Environmental emergencies.

Venous

Venous disease may also cause pain in the legs or, much more

rarely, in the arms. Ache and tiredness in the calves are common symptoms of varicose veins. The discomfort increases in severity in proportion to the time the patient spends standing, and is gradually relieved by elevation of the feet. It may be more pronounced during the premenstrual period. If there is deep venous insufficiency, a severe, bursting pain may be brought on by exercise. It is quite unlike the pain of intermittent claudication.

An inflamed *venous ulcer* should be covered with a non-adhesive tulle dressing. A non-adherent, dry, absorbent dressing will suffice for an uninflamed ulcer. In either case the leg should be bandaged from toe to kee and the patient instructed to keep the leg elevated as much as possible. Further dressings may be applied by the community nurse, but arrangements should be made to review the patient's progress from time to time at an appropriate hospital outpatient clinic. Patients with intractable ulceration may need to be admitted under the care of a dermatologist or vascular surgeon. Carcinomatous change can occur in a chronic venous ulcer (Marjolin's ulcer, Fig. 27.2). A biopsy of the edge, taken under a local anaesthetic, will confirm or refute this diagnosis.

Pain localised to an inflamed vein (usually the long saphenous vein) and accompanied by a tender reaction along the line of the vein indicates a *superficial thrombophlebitis*. It is common near

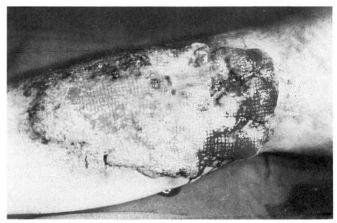

A

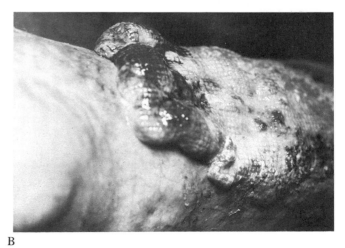

B

Fig. 27.2 A and **B** A Marjolin's ulcer — note the raised, rolled margin.

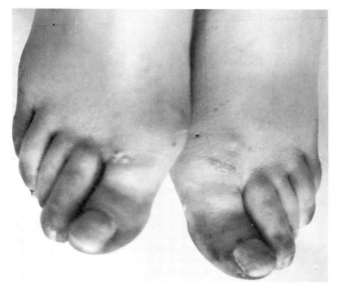

Fig. 27.1 Trench foot in a vagrant.

venous ulcers and after intravenous injections and infusions. The tender vein is felt as a thick cord underlying reddened skin. Simple analgesics, bandaging and rest of the affected limb are all that is necessary. The risk of embolisation is very small and anticoagulants are not indicated.

Migratory thrombophlebitis may be associated with occult intestinal neoplasia or Buerger's disease.

Deep vein thrombosis

Pain in the leg, which is sudden in onset, becomes maximal within a few hours and is quickly followed by swelling, starting behind the malleoli, may indicate deep venous thrombosis. The skin may be warm, the superficial veins prominent, and there may be local tenderness on deep palpation in the centre of the calf. Homans' sign and the tibial tap sign are notoriously unreliable. A slight pyrexia and tachycardia may be present. However, nearly three-quarters of the patients with a deep venous thrombosis have minimal or no symptoms and few clinical signs at the onset. Nevertheless, the condition ranks with acute arterial insufficiency as the most important vascular cause of limb pain, as early treatment gives the best chance of complete recovery. The veins of the soleal plexus and the ileofemoral vein are those most frequently involved.

Occasionally *thrombosis of the axillary vein* occurs after unaccustomed use of the arm, direct trauma or as a complication of chronic congestive heart failure.

Whilst all patients thought to have a deep venous thrombosis should be admitted to a medical ward for investigation and appropriate treatment, the following conditions, although easily recognised, are often mistaken for a deep venous thrombosis; they must not be treated with anticoagulants. Furthermore, patients with these conditions often *do not* require admission to hospital.

> 1. A tear at the musculotendinous junction of the calf muscles (often in middle-aged men and women who begin to play football with their grandchildren).
> 2. Stress fractures of the tibia or fibula.
> 3. Aneurysm of the popliteal artery.
> 4. Rupture of a Baker's cyst.
> 5. Superficial thrombophlebitis, which does not carry any of the serious implications of a deep venous thrombosis.

An occasional patient in whom a deep vein thrombosis cannot be excluded clinically, may be investigated in the observation ward if facilities for emergency venography are available.

Burning pain and redness of the skin of the forefoot is associated with a rare disease called *erythromelalgia*. It may sometimes also affect the hands, and the pain is initiated when the extremity is warmed (e.g. by walking or being under the covers of the bed).

Chronic lymphoedema may also cause an ache similar to that found in patients with chronic venous insufficiency.

NEUROLOGICAL PAIN

Pain in the limbs which has its origin in the nervous system is most commonly caused by diseases affecting the lower motor neurons, but may also be a manifestation of a wide variety of pathology involving the cerebral cortex, the thalamus or the spinal cord (see Ch. 26, Neurological problems). In Table 27.1 are listed the neurological conditions which are either commonly encountered in the A & E department or, although uncommon, must be instantly recognised because they constitute neurological emergencies.

A neurological origin for spontaneous pain in a limb is suggested by one or more of the following features.

Its character is often of an unpleasant burning, tearing or deep boring nature.

Other paraesthesiae may have preceded or may accompany the pain. Thus patients may complain of numb, heavy, burning, itching or tingling sensations. They may also have noticed skin hypersensitivity in the areas affected.

The pain is limited to the cutaneous areas supplied by the affected spinal or peripheral nerves or, in the case of polyneuropathies, is glove and stocking in distribution.

Motor weakness and other neurological abnormalities may also be present.

Apart from defining the exact site and duration of the pain, its radiation and any aggravating factors should be determined. For example, spinal root pains may be accentuated by coughing, sneezing or changes in posture. If there is any suspicion of spinal

Table 27.1 Neurological causes of limb pain

Peripheral nerves
1. Post-traumatic — painful neuroma, causalgia and 'phantom limb'

2. Pressure (entrapment) neuropathies — compression of the median nerve (carpal tunnel syndrome), ulnar nerve (at the elbow or Guyon's canal at the wrist), the radial nerve ('Saturday night palsy'), the lateral cutaneous nerve of the thigh (meralgia paraesthetica), the lateral popliteal nerve, Morton's metatarsalgia and others

3. Shoulder girdle neuritis — following viral infection and immunisation procedures

4. Polyneuropathies — alcoholism, diabetes, vitamin deficiency, infections, autoimmune diseases and poisoning with heavy metals, organic substances and various drugs

5. Referred pain — from the heart, oesophagus and gall bladder

Spinal nerve roots
1. Compression — associated with congenital anomalies (spondylolisthesis), trauma, herniated intervertebral disc and narrowed intervertebral foramina (often associated with spondylosis)

2. Inflammation — herpes zoster and syphilis

3. Diseases of the vertebral column — tuberculosis, Paget's disease, and primary and secondary tumours

4. Subarachnoid haemorrhage

Spinal cord
1. Compression — by abscesses and tumours
2. Infection — poliomyelitis
3. Ischaemia — spinal artery thrombosis

cord compression, specific questions should be asked concerning bladder function.

The nervous system as a whole should be examined carefully, as limb pain may be just one manifestation of a generalised neurological disease. Examination of the painful area should seek to answer the following questions. Is it anaesthetic or hyperalgesic? Are the reflexes intact? Are there trophic changes in the skin due to impaired sensation and loss of autonomic nerve function? Do the muscles fasciculate?

An episode which follows trauma, such as heavy lifting or a whiplish injury, may be due to an *acute muscle strain or to intervertebral disc disease*, or may be associated with *vertebral osteophytosis*. Disc disease may be distinguished from the others if there is tenderness localised to one or two spinous processes, if there is scoliosis or if there are symptoms or signs of sciatic or lumbar nerve involvement, including altered sensation, diminished or absent reflexes or limited straight leg raising. If the tenderness is localised to a point in the paravertebral muscles, an acute muscle strain is more likely.

Similar symptoms, however, can be caused by less common lesions, such as primary or secondary *tumours* within either the spinal canal or the vertebral bodies, by *ankylosing spondylitis*, *spondylolisthesis* and *arthritis of the hip*. Tumours usually produce slowly progressive symptoms with more marked sensory and motor changes than seen with spondylopathies. Arthritis of the hip will

be accompanied by limitation of movement and pain on rotation and abduction, movements which do not stretch the sciatic nerve. All patients with chronic lumbosacral pain should be examined rectally and/or vaginally.

Anteroposterior, lateral and oblique X-rays of the appropriate part of the spine should be obtained in all these patients whether the presentation is acute or chronic. In general, neoplastic processes tend to affect the central part of the vertebral bodies (Fig. 27.3), and their appendages (Fig. 27.4), while inflammatory processes occur adjacent to the end-plates (Fig. 27.5). Thus the only evidence of a secondary deposit may be an absent pedicle (Fig. 27.6). Intraspinal masses should be suspected when there is widening of the interpedicular distance with erosion of the medial aspects of the pedicles (Fig. 27.7). Diffuse myeloma may be dismissed as osteoporosis (Fig. 27.8) unless the erythrocyte sedimentation rate is measured. If there are clinical pointers to hip disease, the suspect joint(s) should also be X-rayed.

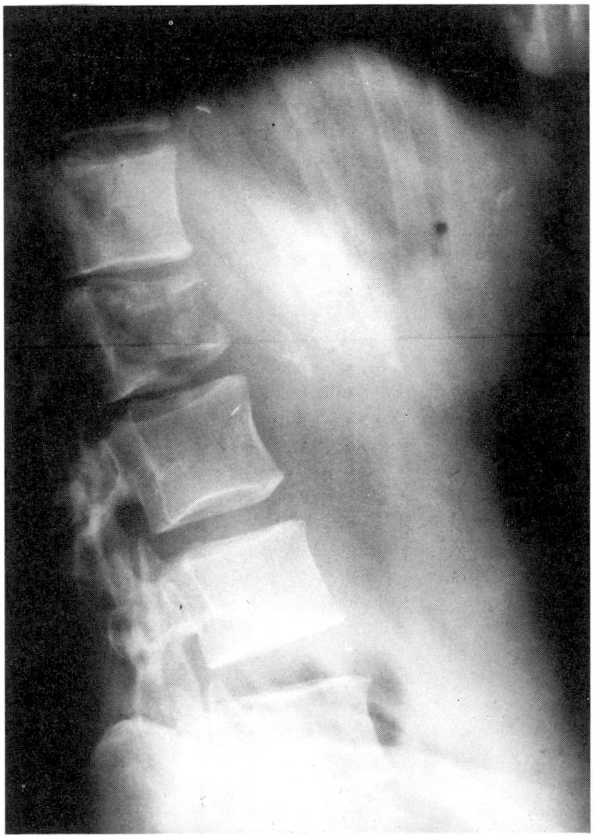

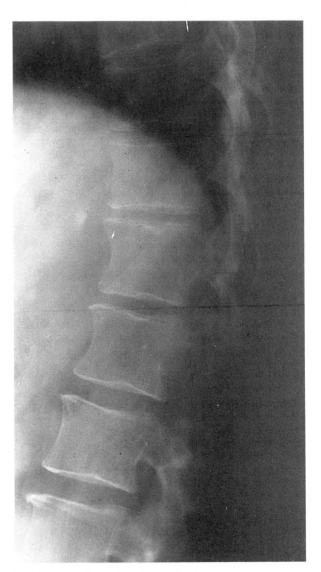

Fig. 27.3 An osteolytic secondary deposit in the lumbar spine.

Fig. 27.4 Malignant destruction of a neural arch.

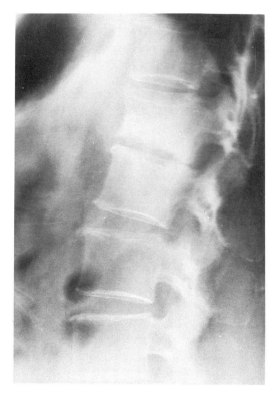

Fig. 27.5 Osteomyelitis of the spine — not the bony sclerosis beside the end-plates.

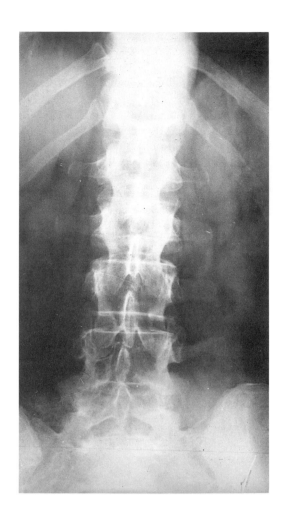

A

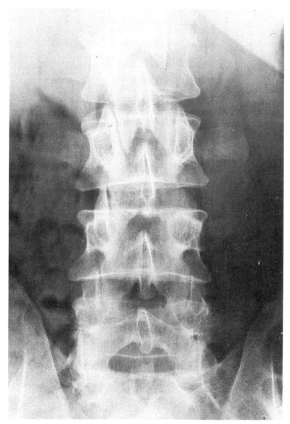

Fig. 27.6 Absence of a pedicle in the second lumbar vertebra, due to a secondary deposit.

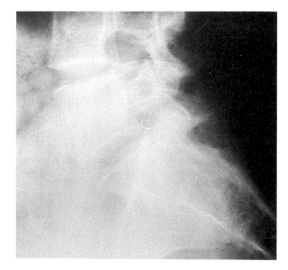

B

Fig. 27.7 A Widening of the interpedicular distance and erosion of the medial aspects of the pedicles of the third and fourth lumbar vertebrae, caused by a large intraspinal tumour. **B** A lateral view of the same patient, showing scalloping of the posterior aspects of the bodies of the third and fourth lumbar vertebrae.

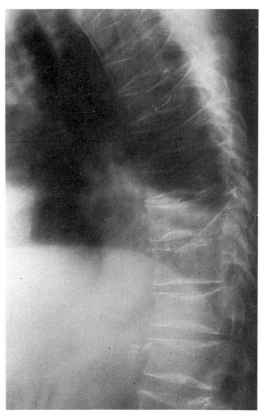

Fig. 27.8 Diffuse osteoporosis due to multiple myeloma.

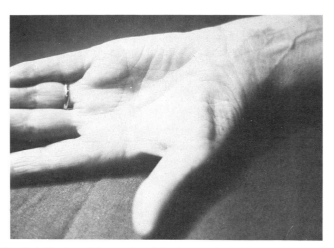

Fig. 27.9 Wasting of the muscles of the thenar eminence, due to compression of the median nerve in the carpal tunnel. Note the preservation of adductor pollicis which is supplied by the ulnar nerve.

Patients should be admitted to hospital if they have:
1. Very severe symptoms unrelieved by analgesics.
2. Neurological symptoms or signs of bladder dysfunction.
3. Suspected malignant or generalised neurological disease.
4. Not responded to conservative measures.

A more detailed description of the causes and management of back pain is given in Ch. 20.

Pain in the arm accompanied by wasting of the small muscles of the hand, or by a Horner's syndrome, which is gradual in onset, referred to the ulnar side of the forearm and hand and occasionally relieved by raising the hand above the head, may be associated with a cervical rib (thoracic outlet syndrome). The differential diagnosis includes an apical lung tumour (Pancoast's syndrome), syringomyelia, motor neurone disease, compression of the ulnar or median nerves and a cervical disc lesion.

Patients with *compression of the median nerve* in the carpal tunnel may occasionally present in the A & E department complaining of pain in the thumb, index and middle fingers and occasionally radiating up the arm as high as the shoulder. They are usually middle-aged women. The pain is often at its worst during the night, and patients frequently complain that their fingers feel like sausages on first awakening. Wasting and weakness of the muscles of the thenar eminence are late signs (Fig. 27.9). A light blow with a patella hammer to the area overlying the

median nerve on the anterior surface of the wrist may reproduce the pain or paraesthesia (Tinel's sign). If no primary cause can be identified and treated, and pain is persistent, local steroid injections should be tried. If there is no relief, the patient may require surgical division of the transverse carpal ligament and should be referred to the appropriate outpatient clinic.

The *ulnar nerve* is vulnerable to damage where it passes behind the medial epicondyle of the humerus and, less commonly, at the wrist (Fig. 27.10). Repeated blows on the thenar or hypothenar eminences, as when striking the end of a chisel or hammer, may cause acute median or ulnar paraesthesiae. In both median and ulnar nerve entrapment syndromes, measurement of nerve conduction velocities may assist in making the diagnosis.

Pain and numbness on the lateral side of the thigh may be due to a high lumbar disc lesion or to constriction of the *lateral cutaneous nerve of the thigh*, either in the pelvis or where it passes through the fascia lata. This condition (meralgia paraesthetica) is often associated with recent weight gain.

The patient who displays a symmetrical, flaccid muscle weakness, accompanied by sensory disturbances, suggests the diagnosis of a *polyneuropathy*. The paraesthesiae affect the distal more than the proximal parts of the limb, and the reflexes tend to be diminished or lost, and the patient ataxic. Sometimes the cranial nerves are involved and there may also be disturbance of the higher cerebral functions. Alcoholism and diabetes mellitus

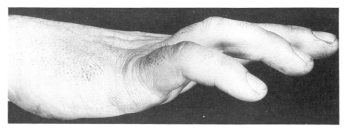

Fig. 27.10 Typical attitude of the hand after interruption of the ulnar nerve.

are two common causes of painful polyneuropathies. Most of these can be investigated at an outpatient clinic, but the patient who is suspected of having acute infective polyneuritis (the syndrome of Guillain and Barré) must be admitted urgently to hospital. The history in such patients is usually of an initial febrile illness, followed by a latent period of days or weeks. The patient then develops headache, vomiting, mild pyrexia, generalised myalgia and meningism. Paralytic symptoms usually come on suddenly, both proximal and distal limb muscles being affected. All sensory modalities are impaired. The reason for urgent hospital admission is that the process can spread rapidly to involve bulbar and respiratory muscles. Acute infective polyneuritis is distinguished from paralytic enterovirus infections by the relative absence of muscular wasting, and by the presence of sensory loss.

Pain in the back which is referred to the distribution of one or more spinal nerve roots, either unilaterally or bilaterally, may be due to *acute compression of the spinal cord*. The pain is often made so much worse by movements of the spine or by coughing or sneezing that the patient tries to avoid any movement. Localised pain at the site of spinal lesions is common. Pain in the legs may be a feature of cervical disease as well as of lumbosacral disease. Weakness usually develops later than sensory symptoms. Sphincter disturbances may occur early and are of great prognostic

significance. The patient should be asked specifically about difficulties with micturition.

Hypersensitivity or analgesia may occur at the level of the lesion, while compression of the spinothalamic tract causes dissociated thermoanaesthesia below the level of the lesion. Variable loss of posterior column sensibility may also be evident.

The spine itself should be examined carefully for deformity, local tenderness and pain on movement.

The underlying causes include trauma, an acute disc lesion, spondylolisthesis, rheumatoid arthritis (affecting the upper two cervical vertebrae), tuberculosis or a neoplasm, a primary tumour arising within the spinal cord, involvement of the spinal column by metastases, or haematological disorders such as leukaemia.

Patients who exhibit features of spinal cord compression must be admitted to hospital urgently. The advice of a neurosurgeon should also be sought because emergency myelography, followed by a decompression operation, may be necessary within hours.

Finally, a pain which does not appear to fit any obvious disease pattern may not have an organic cause. Such patients often complain that the skin feels cold when its temperature is normal. Conversely, if the patient complains of the skin feeling hot when in fact it is cool, a peripheral nerve lesion should be suspected. Non-organic symptoms are discussed further in Chapter 31.

FURTHER READING

Peripheral nerve disorders: a practical approach Asbury A K, Gilliatt R W 1984 Butterworths International Medicine Reviews: Neurology 4, Butterworths, London

Vascular surgery Bell P R F, Tinley N L 1984 Butterworths, London

A clinician's view of neuromuscular diseases, 2nd edn. Brooke M H 1986 Williams and Wilkins, Baltimore

Vascular emergencies Haimovici H 1982 Appleton-Century-Crofts, New York

Environmental emergencies

The topics to be discussed in this chapter include accidental hypothermia and cold injuries, drowning and scuba diving emergencies, illnesses and injuries due to heat, lightning, radiation and toxic gases and venomous bites and stings.

Conditions due to ultraviolet light are discussed in Chapter 37 (sunburn) and Chapter 43 (snow-blindness/arc eye).

ACCIDENTAL HYPOTHERMIA

Hypothermia is defined as a core temperature below 35°C. There are many possible causes of accidental hypothermia (Table 28.1) and in many patients there is more than one cause.

Table 28.1 Causes of accidental hypothermia

(The commoner causes in A & E departments are in italic type)
Poverty and social isolation in old people
Poor thermoregulation in old age
Falls, immobility (e.g. fractured neck of femur)
Alcohol intoxication
Drug overdosage
Hypoglycaemia
Immersion hypothermia
Exposure to cold, wet and wind (e.g. mountain hypothermia)
Prematurity in babies
Heat loss during operations
Endocrine disorders: hypothyroidism, hypopituitarism, hypoadrenalism, diabetes
Malnutrition
Neglect of children
Skin conditions: widespread burns, psoriasis, erythroderma.
Cerebral disorders: stroke, tumour, encephalopathy
Spinal cord injury
Septicaemia

The effects of hypothermia vary depending on the patient's previous fitness, associated diseases and the duration and severity of cold exposure. Thus the problems and the necessary management may differ between a young fit person rescued from cold water and an old ill person gradually developing hypothermia in a cold house.

Diagnosis of hypothermia

Hypothermia may be missed if it is not suspected or if a patient's temperature is measured incorrectly. The rectal temperature should be measured in every patient who is unconscious or whose oral or axillary temperature is less than 35°C. A low reading thermometer must be used. A mercury thermometer must be shaken down to below 25°C before use or it may give a falsely high reading. The rectal temperature is usually the same as the temperature of the body 'core' but may differ by as much as 1°C from the core temperature during rapid heating or cooling. The temperature measured in the oesophagus (using a thermister probe) or in the ear (using a special zero-gradient thermometer) may be closer to the core temperature but these methods are usually impracticable in an A & E department.

Effects of hypothermia

Hypothermia affects most organs of the body, but the effects on the heart and brain are usually the most important. In mild hypothermia (32–35°C) confusion and apathy are common and most patients are pale and shivering. Shivering stops at about 32°C and muscle rigidity occurs. Consciousness is usually lost at 28–30°C.

Cardiac effects are common at core temperatures below 33°C. Bradycardia and hypotension often occur. The electrocardiogram may show a sinus bradycardia or slow atrial fibrillation with prolongation of the PR, QRS and QT intervals and a characteristic deflection (the 'J wave') of the down-stroke of the R wave (Figure 28.1). Ventricular ectopic beats are common and ventricular fibrillation may occur, sometimes precipitated by sudden movements or by endotracheal intubation. At temperatures below 28°C electrical defibrillation is often unsuccessful.

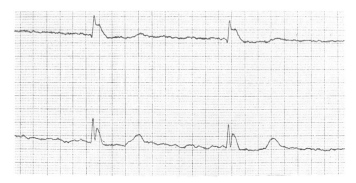

Fig. 28.1 Electrocardiogram in hypothermia (rectal temperature 25°C).

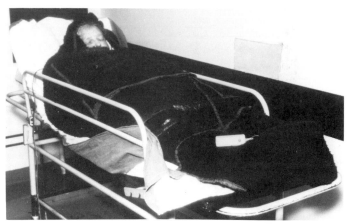

Fig. 28.2 Hypothermic patient in fibre-pile rewarming blanket with monitoring of rectal temperature by thermister probe.

Respiration may be rapid in mild hypothermia, due to the effects of shivering, but as the core temperature falls respiration slows until it is imperceptible. Exposure to cold causes a diuresis which contributes to hypovolaemia. Haemoconcentration and thrombosis may occur. Metabolism in the liver slows and pancreatitis may occur in severe hypothermia.

At core temperatures below 25°C the patient may appear dead, with no movement or response, no palpable pulse or audible heart beat and complete muscle flaccidity. However, survival may still be possible even if the electrocardiogram shows asystole. Death should only be diagnosed if the patient fails to revive after rewarming.

Treatment of hypothermia

The initial treatment depends on the situation and the facilities available. The first essential is insulation from the cold and protection from wind and rain. In some mild cases of hypothermia it may be best to rewarm the patient on the mountainside or at home by proper insulation and hot drinks. Patients should be carried in the recovery position and flat or head down: reduction in cerebral blood flow may cause fits and brain damage if the patient is tilted feet downwards.

Treatment in the A & E department

The main problem in the A & E department is usually keeping the patient adequately insulated despite the necessary medical and nursing attention. The room must be warm and the doors kept shut. The patient must be wrapped in blankets, or preferably in a thick fibre-pile rewarming blanket (Fig. 28.2) which covers the whole body, including the head, but allows access via flaps for examination and treatment. Metallised 'space' blankets are no more effective at conserving heat than sheets of polythene.

An electric thermometer allows continuous recording of the rectal temperature without disturbing the patient's insulation. The patient should be moved as little as possible, since sudden movements may precipitate ventricular fibrillation. A quick general examination for signs of illness or injury is needed and later a full examination after rewarming. The cardiac rhythm should be monitored. An intravenous infusion should be started. Arterial blood gases should be measured and the results corrected for temperature: hypoxia and a metabolic acidosis are common and oxygen may be needed. Blood should be taken for measurement of full blood count, glucose, urea and electrolytes. Radiographs of the chest and for injuries such as fractured neck of femur can usually wait until the patient is warm.

Hypotension may be caused by hypovolaemia but more often by cardiac depression. Large amounts of fluid are rarely needed and may cause pulmonary oedema. Artificial ventilation is needed if respiration is inadequate, but endotracheal intubation should otherwise be avoided since it may precipitate ventricular fibrillation. Cardiac massage is necessary if cardiac arrest occurs.

Most hypothermic patients will rewarm spontaneously if kept adequately insulated. This passive rewarming may be used in patients of any age and is the treatment of choice in old people suffering from mild or moderate hypothermia. However, young adults who have fallen into cold water, but are still conscious, may be treated by immersion of the trunk (but not head or limbs) in a hot bath at 42°C.

The real problems occur in patients with severe hypothermia (especially below 25°C) or patients in cardiac arrest. Active rewarming is needed in such patients and, if possible, the body core should be warmed before the periphery. Ventilation with humidified oxygen at a maximum temperature of 45°C helps by providing a small amount of heat via the respiratory tract and may reduce the risk of cardiac arrhythmias. The many other rewarming techniques which have been tried include heat cradles, warm gastric lavage, peritoneal dialysis, cardiopulmonary bypass and opening the chest and pouring warm saline over the heart. Expert help is needed in the management of severely hypothermic patients.

PERIPHERAL COLD INJURY

Immersion foot

Immersion foot ('trench foot') is caused by immersion of the feet for many hours in cold, but not freezing, water or in wet boots. Vasoconstriction induced by the cold and venous stasis due to tight boots and prolonged standing result in tissue ischaemia. Although the tissues do not freeze, there may be severe damage and disability.

The feet are initially cold and numb and walking is difficult due to loss of sensation. The skin is pale or mottled and the arterial pulses may be impalpable. After rewarming the feet become painful, hyperaemic, swollen and blistered. Secondary infection may occur. The hyperaemic phase often lasts for two months but the pain gradually resolves and sensation usually recovers. However, there may be muscle wasting and permanent sensitivity of the feet to cold.

If the feet are cold and pulseless they should be rewarmed in a warm room or a warm bath. They should be kept clean and dry and elevated to reduce oedema. The patient must not walk. Analgesics are often needed. The prevention of further damage from cold should be emphasised.

Frostbite

Frostbite is caused by temperatures below freezing and involves the extremities and exposed parts of the body. Mountaineers may suffer from frostbite, especially at high altitude, but many cases in cities result from intoxication with alcohol or drugs. Wind increases the risk of frostbite of exposed areas. Contact with cold metal or liquids such as petrol may cause frostbite due to rapid heat loss. Frostbite and hypothermia may occur in neglected children.

In 'frostnip', the first stage of frostbite, the skin becomes numb and white but recovers rapidly when protected from the cold. In superficial frostbite the skin is white, numb and frozen but still pliable. On rewarming the area becomes swollen, mottled and purple and blisters develop within one or two days. The blisters resorb leaving a hard black eschar which eventually separates. Deep frostbite involves muscle, nerves and other structures as well as skin and superficial tissue. The area remains blue, mottled and swollen and may not blister. Non-viable tissue separates after several months, but the tissue loss is much less than the area initially involved by frostbite.

The frozen area should be thawed rapidly by immersion in warm water (40–42°C) for about 20 minutes. Parenteral analgesia may be required. No active warming should be done if the area has already thawed when the patient is seen. The patient is admitted for elevation and exposure of the part. Frequent cleaning in a whirlpool bath is helpful. Division of eschars may be needed but no tissue should be removed surgically for many months. Smoking and anticoagulants are contraindicated. Sympathectomy, vasodilators and dextran are of no proven value in reducing tissue loss, but aspirin may be helpful.

DROWNING AND NEAR-DROWNING

Drowning is a common cause of death in children and young adults, but some of these deaths could be avoided by better treatment at the scene and in hospital. 'Near drowning' is the term used when there is at least temporary survival from suffocation

Table 28.2 Conditions associated with drowning and near-drowning

Hypothermia
Cervical spine and cord injury (especially in diving accidents)
Head or other injuries (due to falls or boating accidents)
Alcohol or drug intoxication
Hypoglycaemia (e.g. diabetics, alcohol intoxication)
Epilepsy
Cerebral air embolism (in scuba divers)
Non-accidental drowning (suicide, homicide, child abuse)

by submersion. Most patients inhale water, but in about 10–20% asphyxiation occurs without water entering the lungs ('dry drowning'). In many cases of near drowning there are additional factors (Table 28.2.) which alter the necessary management and the outcome. Immersion in water often causes hypothermia, which allows longer survival from hypoxia. Indeed survival is possible after as long as 40 minutes of submersion in cold water. Sudden immersion in very cold water may cause immediate cardiac arrest.

Initial resuscitation

Treatment of a near-drowned patient begins with rescue from the water and cardiopulmonary resuscitation (see Ch. 10). The airway must be cleared but attempts to empty water from the lungs waste time and are ineffective. Mouth-to-mouth ventilation must start immediately. Water in the lungs reduces the lung compliance and so greater inflation pressure than usual may be needed. If the chest does not rise despite attempts at ventilation, an abdominal thrust (Heimlich manoeuvre) should be performed and ventilation restarted. External cardiac compression is necessary if no pulse is palpable.

Resuscitation should continue for at least 1 hour if there is no response, or longer if the patient is very cold. Most patients who survive start to breathe within 5 minutes of rescue, but much longer resuscitation may still be successful. Profuse vomiting is common when breathing starts. An unconscious but breathing patient must be transported to hospital in the recovery position.

Hospital management

On arrival in hospital cardiopulmonary resuscitation is continued if necessary. Oxygen must be given. Intubation of a cold and hypoxic patient may cause bradycardia or asystole but this parasympathetic reflex can be blocked by atropine and oxygen. The level of consciousness must be assessed and recorded and the rectal temperature measured with a low-reading thermometer. Crackles in the lungs are good evidence of aspiration of water. Details of the history must be obtained and trauma and the other conditions associated with near-drowning considered.

Investigations

A chest radiograph and an electrocardiogram should be obtained and blood taken for measurement of arterial gases, glucose, urea and electrolytes. Near-drowning causes severe shunting of blood in the lungs and marked hypoxia is common. Changes in plasma electrolytes large enough to be clinically important are rare after either fresh or salt water immersion.

The chest radiograph may show pulmonary oedema, especially in the perihilar and mid zones. If a large amount of water is inhaled there may be complete opacification. These changes may be delayed for one or two days. Inhalation of vomit or other material may cause patchy secondary pneumonia with atelectasis.

Treatment

Even if the patient appears well, admission for observation is essential because of the risk of pulmonary complications. If there is any evidence of aspiration of water the patient should be in an intensive care unit. 'Secondary drowning' is pulmonary oedema caused by loss of surfactant and damage to alveolar cells. This may develop up to 48 hours after rescue and requires treatment with oxygen, diuretics and sometimes ventilation. Pneumonia may also occur. Prophylactic antibiotics and steroids are often given but are of doubtful benefit.

Mechanical ventilation is needed if respiration is inadequate (e.g. PaO_2 less than 8.0 kPa on 50% oxygen). Positive and expiratory pressure (PEEP) is helpful but may cause hypotension.

Intravenous fluids may be started with dextrose or saline but plasma expansion is often needed if PEEP is used. The treatment of near-drowned patients who remain unconscious after admission to hospital is controversial. Hyperventilation and infusion of barbiturates (controlled by intracranial pressure monitoring) may aid survival by reducing cerebral oedema. Deliberate induction of hypothermia has also been recommended but its effectiveness is unknown.

If the patient is in asystole, but hypothermic, on arrival at hospital resuscitation must be continued while a history is obtained and the rectal temperature measured. The decision to stop resuscitation is difficult, especially in children. The patient should be rewarmed to 35°C before being pronounced dead.

SCUBA DIVING EMERGENCIES

Patients suffering from diving emergencies are uncommon in most A & E departments but may be seen at any time. Most divers breathe compressed air from scuba (self-contained underwater breathing apparatus) equipment which allows descent to 50 metres. In commercial diving below this depth mixtures of oxygen and helium are used. The water pressure increases by 1 atmosphere absolute every 10 metres and so at a depth of 30 metres the pressure is four times atmospheric pressure. The pressure changes during diving and surfacing and the corresponding changes in gas volumes may cause barotrauma, air embolism and decompression sickness.

Pulmonary barotrauma

The lungs are compressible and give no trouble during descent but may be injured during ascent as the compressed air expands within them. A diver must exhale during ascent but sometimes fails to do so if in a panic, or if suffering from laryngospasm after inhaling water. The expanding air may rupture the lung causing a pneumothorax or leakage of air into the mediastinum resulting in subcutaneous emphysema of the neck. If pulmonary veins are torn when the lungs rupture air reaches the systemic circulation via the left side of the heart. The diver is usually upright at the time of ascent and so the air often enters the carotid arteries causing cerebral air embolism.

Cerebral air embolism

Cerebral air embolism causes symptoms as soon as the diver surfaces: the diver collapses with chest pain and develops confusion, coma or convulsions and sometimes a hemiparesis. Ventilation is needed if the patient stops breathing. Urgent recompression in a recompression chamber is needed.

Decompression sickness

During a dive nitrogen from the compressed air dissolves in solution in the body tissues. The amount of nitrogen varies with the depth and length of the dive. The nitrogen is released as the diver ascends but if he surfaces too quickly bubbles of nitrogen form in the tissues and blood causing decompression sickness. This may present with a very wide range of symptoms. The time of onset is variable and symptoms may appear immediately or be delayed for up to 24 hours. Decompression sickness may develop if one flies in a plane within 24 hours of a dive.

The symptoms and signs of decompression sickness may be divided into minor and severe. Minor decompression sickness is 'the bends' with pain in joints at the shoulder, elbow, hip or knee. The pain may be mild or severe and may persist for days or weeks if untreated. Severe decompression sickness often involves the central nervous system. Involvement of the brain may cause hemiplegia, convulsions, vertigo, diplopia or other manifestations. Spinal cord involvement may present as backache, paraesthesiae and weakness in the legs, urinary retention or abdominal pain. If untreated, permanent paraplegia or tetraplegia may develop. Pulmonary decompression sickness ('the chokes') causes chest pain, dyspnoea, cyanosis and haemoptysis. Any symptom arising within 24 hours of a dive may be due to decompression sickness and must not be ignored. Specialist advice must be obtained immediately and the need for recompression considered. Sources of advice in the United Kingdom are listed in Table 28.3. When asking for advice it is helpful to know about all dives in the previous 24 hours, the maximum depth and duration of each dive, the volume of air used, the time of surfacing and the time of onset of symptoms.

Table 28.3 Information on diving emergencies and recompression chambers

Portsmouth	0705-818888
Aberdeen	0224-871848
Northern Ireland	0762-336711

The treatment of cerebral air embolism or decompression sickness is immediate recompression in a pressure chamber. 100% oxygen should be given during transport to the chamber. Entonox and analgesics are contraindicated. If cerebral air embolism is suspected the patient should be carried head down and on the left side.

Barotrauma of ears and sinuses

The pressure changes during diving may damage the ears and sinuses. Ear damage occurs if the Eustachian tube is blocked or the diver does not do a Valsalva manoeuvre to clear his ears during descent. The ear drum is stretched and becomes erythematous after the dive, or it may rupture, causing transient vertigo. Sometimes blood vessels rupture filling the middle ear with blood. These conditions resolve within three weeks if no diving is done. Prophylactic antibiotics may help avoid secondary infection.

Vertigo and tinnitus after a dive may result from rupture of the round window between the middle ear and the labyrinth. Pressure on the tragus will exacerbate the symptoms, which must be distinguished from vertigo due to decompression sickness. Surgical repair of the round window should be considered.

ILLNESSES DUE TO HEAT

Illnesses due to heat are common in the tropics but may also occur in temperate climates during a hot summer.

Heat stroke is particularly likely if unacclimatised people perform heavy physical work or take part in endurance sporting events in hot weather. Small children are also at risk if wrapped too warmly during febrile illnesses or left in closed cars in direct sunlight. Malaria and other infections predispose to heat stroke, as do anticholinergic drugs such as the tricyclic antidepressants. Malignant hyperpyrexia during anaesthesia is discussed in Ch. 9.

Heat cramps are common in people who exert themselves in the heat. The painful muscle cramps are due to salt deficiency and the patient recovers rapidly when extra salt is given.

Heat exhaustion is more serious and results from water and salt deficiency. It develops gradually over a few hours or days with vague malaise, headaches and fatigue. There may be sudden collapse with confusion and often vomiting. Oral treatment with salt and water is often adequate but in severe cases intravenous saline is needed.

Heat stroke is the most severe form of heat illness and may be rapidly fatal. The body temperature rises rapidly to 40°C or higher and sweating may stop. Coma, convulsions, vomiting and diarrhoea are common. Hypotension and kidney and liver damage occur. Rapid cooling of the patient is essential. The best method is to expose the maximum amount of skin and wet it repeatedly with tepid water while fanning strongly with air at room temperature. Ice should not be used since it causes vasoconstriction and shivering. Active cooling should be continued until the rectal temperature falls to 39°C. Oxygen should be given and a patent airway maintained. Injections of chlorpromazine are helpful to prevent shivering, reduce the temperature and sedate the patient. Diazepam may be needed if fits occur. Intravenous fluids are started with 1 litre of 4% dextrose and 0.18% saline in the first half hour. Hartmann's solution or dextrose/saline with added potassium is then given, adjusted according to the blood pressure and electrolytes. The urine output should be monitored and frusemide or mannitol given to promote a diuresis. Haemorrhage may occur and fresh plasma and blood may be needed. Haemodialysis is necessary if renal failure occurs.

LIGHTNING INJURIES

A person struck by lightning receives a direct current electric shock of very high voltage (up to 100 million volts), but short duration (0.1 to 1 ms). This causes different effects from electric shocks from high voltage power lines, which usually involve much longer contact with an alternating current and severe tissue destruction.

Mechanism of injury

Lightning may strike a person directly or a 'splash injury' may occur when the current jumps from the primary conductor, such as a tree, on to the victim. 'Ground current' injury occurs when lightning strikes the ground close to a person, setting up a current between his legs. Many people in a group may be affected in this way at the same time. Lightning often flashes over the outside of a person vapourising sweat and rain-water and blasting off the clothes or shoes. Blunt trauma may result from the explosive heating of the air or from falls caused by the strike.

Lightning injuries

Lightning may cause cardiac arrest with asystole. The heart often restarts spontaneously but respiratory arrest may then cause hypoxia and secondary cardiac arrest, which is fatal without immediate resuscitation. Coma may result from direct brain injury, closed head injury from a fall or from cardiac arrest. Fits and transient paralysis may occur. Survivors may be confused and amnesic for several days. The limbs are often cold and mottled due to arterial spasm, which usually resolves in a few hours. Burns are very superficial and may have a characteristic feathered appearance. Deep muscle damage is rare and so myoglobinuria seldom occurs. Many victims are deaf and suffer ruptured ear drums. Ocular injuries are common and cataracts often develop.

Treatment of lightning injuries

Most deaths occur at the scene of injury due to cardiac arrest. Patients reaching the A & E department alive are likely to recover with supportive care. Examination is needed for trauma and for eye and ear injuries. An electrocardiogram should be performed and the patient admitted for observation and cardiac monitoring.

RADIATION ACCIDENTS

Radiation accidents involving nuclear power stations and nuclear research establishments cause much publicity and concern but are actually much rarer than accidents from radiation sources used in industry, universities and hospitals.

It is important to distinguish between external irradiation of a person and contamination with radioactive material. A person exposed to X-rays or to gamma rays used in a radiation sterilising unit receives no further radiation after removal from the source and there is no risk of 'spreading radioactivity' to anyone. However, a person contaminated with radioactive material is still exposed to radiation and requires urgent but careful decontamination to minimise the risks to himself and to other people. Certain hospitals in Britain have been designated for the care of casualties contaminated with radioactive substances (DHSS 1976). If, however, a patient needs life-saving treatment for any injury or illness he may be taken to the nearest A & E department, even if it is not in the designated list. All departments must therefore have plans for dealing with radiation emergencies.

On receipt of a message that a patient from a radiation accident is being brought to hospital the consultant in charge of the A & E department should be informed. Advice and help from a radiation physicist (usually from a medical physics department) should be obtained. Organisation of the department is needed and arrangements made to deal with enquiries from journalists.

Treatment of contaminated casualties

Any necessary life-saving treatment has priority over all other actions. Patients must be assumed to be contaminated until cleared by the radiation physicist, who should monitor for radioactivity as soon as possible. Contaminated patients may occasionally need to be treated in the resuscitation room, but if possible treatment should be given in a decontamination room near to the ambulance entrance (see Ch. 2). Care is needed to avoid spreading contamination and the patient should be treated as if he was suffering from a contagious disease requiring barrier nursing. Movement of people in and out of the room must be restricted and recorded. The minimum number of staff should be involved. They should wear gloves, plastic aprons and overshoes or rubber boots. Operating theatre clothing is preferable to ordinary clothes, if time allows. The patient should be brought from the ambulance on a stretcher covered by a large plastic sheet. The ambulance crew must wait for monitoring of themselves and their vehicle. Everything that may have come into contact with radioactive material should be kept for radiation testing. The patient's clothes, dressings, swabs and other items used should be collected in plastic bags and fluid used for washing retained in buckets or other containers.

Decontamination of the patient

The aim is to remove contaminating material and minimise absorption into the body, especially via the mouth, nose and wounds. The radiation physicist should determine the sites of contamination and monitor the effectiveness of treatment. Radioactive material can usually be removed from intact skin by simple washing with soap and water or cetrimide solution. Gentle scrubbing may be needed but it is important to avoid damaging the skin. The mouth, nose, eyes and ears should be cleaned carefully and swabs kept for measurement of radioactivity. The mouth is cleaned using a mouthwash and if necessary a soft toothbrush, with care to avoid swallowing of any fluid. The patient should blow his nose into paper handkerchiefs. If the nose is still contaminated it should be irrigated with small amounts of water. The eyes should be irrigated from the medial side outwards to avoid draining of contaminated water into the nasolacrimal duct. The hair is cleaned by washing with shampoo and by clipping if contamination persists, but the scalp should not be shaved. Wounds are carefully cleaned and irrigated with water or saline.

If monitoring shows that all contamination has been removed, the patient should then be treated as for an irradiated but uncontaminated patient. However, if contamination of skin or wounds persists or if any radioactive material has been ingested or inhaled, further treatment will be needed after discussion with a radiation specialist. Potassium permanganate solution is occasionally needed to decontaminate the skin but should only be used with specialist advice. All staff involved in treating the patient must be checked for radioactive contamination before leaving the treatment area.

The irradiated patient

A patient who has suffered external irradiation or radioactive contamination may be at risk of radiation sickness or other ill effects of radiation. He must be admitted for assessment and follow-up by a radiotherapist or other specialist. The initial symptoms of radiation sickness are often malaise, nausea, vomiting and diarrhoea, starting a few hours after exposure. There is then a latent period before the main effects of radiation sickness appear. Any symptoms and the time of onset should be carefully recorded. It may be difficult to distinguish symptoms due to anxiety and stress from the prodromal symptoms of radiation sickness and so the effects of irradiation on the blood must be determined as soon as possible. Measurement of the lymphocyte count and analysis of chromosomes at known times after exposure are helpful in assessing the amount of radiation received and determining the prognosis. A low (less than $1.0 \times 10^{9}/l$) or falling lymphocyte count indicates serious radiation exposure.

EXPOSURE TO TOXIC GASES

Carbon monoxide

The incidence of carbon monoxide poisoning in Britain fell considerably when the domestic gas supply was changed from coal gas to natural gas. However, carbon monoxide poisoning is still seen from exposure to car exhaust fumes and from incomplete combustion of gas or coal due to faulty appliances or blocked vents.

Poisoning may also occur from the use in a confined space of paint strippers containing methylene chloride, which is metabolised to carbon monoxide. Carbon monoxide is strongly bound to haemoglobin in place of oxygen and also inhibits cytochrome oxidase systems, causing tissue hypoxia.

The early symptoms of carbon monoxide poisoning are headache, dizziness, nausea and vomiting, which may be wrongly diagnosed as gastroenteritis. Coma occurs with hyperventilation, hypotension and increased muscle tone and reflexes. Cherry-red colouring of the skin due to carboxyhaemoglobin may be seen after death, but is rare in live patients, most of whom are cyanosed or pale. Pressure blisters and muscle necrosis may occur if the patient has been unconscious for some hours. Cerebral oedema may be present. The electrocardiogram may show myocardial ischaemia. There is usually a metabolic acidosis with a normal oxygen tension but reduced oxygen saturation in the arterial blood. Carboxyhaemoglobin can be measured on venous blood taken in an arterial gas syringe.

The patient must be removed from the toxic atmosphere and given oxygen in as high a concentration as possible in order to displace carbon monoxide and relieve tissue hypoxia. An unconscious patient should be intubated and ventilated on 100% oxygen and given mannitol and dexamethasone to relieve cerebral oedema. Hyperbaric oxygen therapy is usually impracticable but in severe cases it should be discussed with a poisons specialist (Ch. 16). Patients who reach hospital alive are likely to survive but some have permanent brain damage.

Smoke inhalation

People involved in fires often suffer from inhalation of smoke. The respiratory tract may be damaged by heat and by smoke particles. Hypoxia and carbon monoxide poisoning are common. Combustion of plastics and foam produces toxic chemicals such as hydrogen chloride and hydrogen cyanide. Many patients have pre-existing chronic bronchitis due to smoking cigarettes.

Coughing, breathlessness and chest tightness are common. There may be central cyanosis and widespread rhonchi and crepitations in the lungs. Hypoxia is often severe and myocardial ischaemia may occur. The chest radiograph is often normal but may show multiple pulmonary opacities, which may become confluent, caused by acute pulmonary oedema. Patchy pulmonary vascular congestion may also occur.

Maintenance of the airway and breathing is essential, especially if there are burns of the face or mouth (Ch. 14). High concentrations of oxygen should be given and the arterial blood gases and carboxyhaemoglobin concentration should be measured. Admission for observation and physiotherapy is necessary. Bronchodilators and mechanical ventilation may be needed. Corticosteroids are unhelpful and increase the risk of pulmonary infection. The cyanide antidote dicobalt edetate (Kelocyanor) should be considered in patients who arrive moribund after inhalation of smoke in house fires. However, this antidote is itself toxic in the absence of cyanide ions and should only be used in patients with severe poisoning, i.e. those who are unconscious.

Chlorine

Exposure to chlorine causes choking, burning of the eyes and skin, coughing, breathlessness and chest pain. Acute laryngeal and pulmonary oedema may occur within a few hours of exposure. There is often cyanosis with tachypnoea and widespread pulmonary rhonchi and crepitations. Treatment consists of removal from exposure and administration of oxygen and bronchodilators as necessary. Admission for 12 hours for observation may be needed.

Tear gas

CS (chlorobenzylidene malononitrile) is an harassing agent which is used for riot control. It is an aerosol or smoke rather than a gas. Exposure to CS causes immediate lacrimation, uncontrollable sneezing and coughing, a burning sensation in the skin and throat and tightness of the chest. Vomiting may occur. These symptoms usually disappear within 10 minutes in fresh air but conjunctivitis may persist for 30 minutes. Exposure in a confined space may cause symptoms for some hours. Treatment after removal from exposure consists of washing the skin and irrigating the eyes. The attendants should wear gloves. By the time patients reach the A & E department the physical effects of tear gas are usually over but the emotional reaction may be intense, resulting in overbreathing and tetany.

CN (chloroacetophenone) is used in some countries for riot control and in personal defence devices. CN has similar effects to CS but is more toxic.

VENOMOUS BITES AND STINGS

Bee stings

Bee stings are painful and can occasionally be fatal. In most cases of bee sting all that is needed is to scrape out the sting (without squeezing it) and clean the wound. Asphyxia may occur if a sting in the throat causes oedema and obstructs the airway: cricothyrotomy (Ch. 10) is then needed. However, most deaths from bee stings result from anaphylaxis in people who are allergic to the venom. The clinical features and treatment of anaphylaxis are discussed in Chapter 13. Allergic reactions to stings are more common in patients taking non-steroidal anti-inflammatory drugs. A patient who has had an anaphylactic reaction should carry an adrenaline inhaler (Medihaler-epi, Riker Laboratories) for use if he sustains a sting.

Stings by marine animals

Sea urchins, sting-rays and venomous fish such as weaver fish may cause painful stings. In most cases the pain may be relieved by immersing the affected part in uncomfortably hot water, which deactivates the venom. The stung part should be removed from the water to prevent scalding and then reimmersed when pain recurs. This treatment is usually needed for about 30 minutes. Alternatively, local anaesthesia may be used. Spines should be removed from the wound as soon as possible. Systemic poisoning is rare and treatment is symptomatic.

The tentacles of jelly fish and related species such as the Portuguese man-of-war contain thousands of nematocysts which discharge on contact causing lines of painful wheals. Intact nematocysts may be inactivated with vinegar and any remaining tentacles removed with forceps. Systemic symptoms are uncommon but may include fever, colic, vomiting, diarrhoea, collapse and muscle weakness. Symptomatic treatment is required. Fatal poisoning may be caused by the box jellyfish or sea-wasp (*Chironex fleckeri* and other species), which occur in Australian and Pacific waters and for which an antivenom is available.

Adder bite

The only native venomous snake in Britain is the European adder, *Vipera berus,* which occurs throughout the mainland. More than 100 people a year are bitten by adders but serious poisoning is rare and there have been only 14 deaths in the last 100 years. Many bites occur in men who try to pick up snakes. Venom is injected in less than 50% of bites.

The bite comprises two puncture marks about 1 cm apart. When venom is injected there is usually immediate pain and swelling is often apparent within 1 hour. Occasionally serious poisoning occurs without a local reaction. Vomiting, abdominal pain, diarrhoea, hypotension and coma may occur within a few minutes or many hours. Oedema of the bitten limb may increase for two or three days and in severe cases the face and tongue may swell. Shock, coma, abnormal bleeding, oliguria, ECG changes and a neutrophil leucocytosis (over 20×10^9 per litre) indicate severe poisoning. Deaths have occurred 6–60 hours after the bite (mean 34 hours).

The symptoms of envenomation may be difficult to distinguish from those of anxiety. Reassurance of the victim is important. The snake should not be handled even if dead since reflex biting may occur for up to an hour. The bite should be cleaned and dressed but must not be incised or sucked. The bitten limb should be immobilised and the patient taken to hospital. If the journey will take more than 30 minutes a firm bandage should be applied above the bite to restrict venous return without obstructing arterial pulses. An antiemetic may be needed and an antihistamine if facial oedema occurs.

On arrival at hospital any constricting bandage should be released. Every patient should be admitted for at least 24 hours observation with hourly recording of pulse, blood pressure and fluid balance and frequent measurement for limb swelling. The white cell count and plasma urea and electrolytes should be measured, an ECG performed and the rhythm monitored if hypotension occurs. Zagreb antivenom is needed if there is evidence of severe envenomation. Antivenom should also be considered if an adult is seen within four hours and has swelling extending up the limb, since it may reduce the disability from the local effects of the bite. A history of asthma or other allergy is a relative contraindication to antivenom. Sensitivity test doses are unhelpful and may be misleading. Antivenom must be given by intravenous infusion in a dose of 2 x 5.4 ml ampoules (for adult or child) diluted in 100 ml of saline at a rate of 15 drops per minute. Immediate reactions to the antivenom can be controlled by temporarily stopping the infusion and immediate intramuscular injection of 0.5 ml of 0.1% adrenaline, which must be drawn up in the syringe before antivenom is given. Zagreb antivenom is stocked at many hospitals in Britain. Advice is available via the Poisons Information Service (Ch. 16).

Bites by other poisonous snakes

The principles of treatment are the same as for adder bites. Antivenom is indicated if there is a risk of local skin necrosis or evidence of severe poisoning (as shown by hypotension or changes in the electrocardiogram, abnormal bleeding after viper bites or muscle weakness after elapid bites). Specialist advice should be obtained via the Poisons Information Service. Stocks of antivenom against foreign snakes are kept at Walton Hospital, Liverpool (telephone 051–525 3611), The Poisons Unit, New Cross Hospital, London (telephone 01-407 7600 or 01-635 9191), and at the University Hospital of Wales, Cardiff (telephone 0222-755944).

FURTHER READING

General references

Management of wilderness and environmental emergencies Auerbac P S, Geehr E C (eds) 1983 Macmillan, New York

Environmental emergencies Kizer K W (ed) 1984 Emergency Medicine Clinics of North America 2 (3)

Environmental emergencies Nelson R N, Rund D A, Keller M D 1985 Saunders, Philadelphia

Oxford textbook of medicine, 2nd edn. Weatherall D J, Ledingham J G G, Warrell D A (eds) 1987 Oxford University Press, Oxford

Hypothermia, frostbite and other cold injuries Wilkerson J A, Bangs C C, Hayward J S 1986 The Mountaineers, Seattle, Washington

Hypothermia
Accidental hypothermia Maclean D, Emslie-Smith D 1977 Blackwell, Oxford

Frostbite
Frostbite Ward M 1974 British Medical Journal i: 67–70

Drowning
Drowning and near drowning Harries M 1986 British Medical Journal 293: 122–124

The management of near drowning Pearn N 1985 British Medical Journal 291: 1447–1452

Diving emergencies
The physiology and medicine of diving, 3rd edn. Bennett P B, Elliot D H 1982 Baillière Tindall, London

Medical problems of sport diving Douglas J D M 1985 British Medical Journal 291: 1224–1226

Heat stroke
Management of heat stroke Anonymous 1982 Lancet ii: 910–911

Heat stroke: a review Shibolet S, Lancaster M C, Danon Y 1976
Aviation, Space and Environmental Medicine 47: 280–301

Radiation accidents

**National arrangements for dealing with incidents involving radioactive
substances** Department of Health and Social Security 1976 HMSO,
London

Emergency medicine Evans R 1981 The irradiated patient (Schofield GB),
pp 405–429. Butterworths, London

The management of radiation accidents Stott A N B 1979 Practitioner
223: 54–58

Toxic gases

Inhalation of products of combustion Cohen M A, Guzzardi L J 1983
Annals of Emergency Medicine 12: 628–632

Medical aspects of riot control (harassing) agents Sanford J P 1976
Annual Review of Medicine 27: 421–429

Bites and stings

Adder bites in Britain Reid H A 1976 British Medical Journal ii: 153–156

Bites and stings by venomous animals in Britain Warrell D A 1979
Prescribers' Journal 19 (6): 190–199

The elderly patient

'Die young as late as possible'

Sir Richard Doll

INTRODUCTION

More and more people are surviving into their 70s and the proportion of elderly people in the population is likely to increase for at least another two decades. The consequence of this for A & E medicine is an ever increasing amount of time spent in the management of the problems of elderly patients. There are many reasons why apparently similar disease processes may have entirely different medical and social implications in elderly compared with younger patients. It is important that these differences are understood and considered by all A & E staff.

Physiological ageing occurs in all bodily organs and systems but they do not all deteriorate at the same rate. There is also an increasing prevalence of disease in old age, the result being a summation of pathological and age-induced disabilities. The disabilities are often multiple and affect most commonly locomotion, the brain, the special senses and cardiorespiratory function. Muscular weakness, arthritis and loss of neuromuscular coordination leads to increasing difficulty with walking, an increasing risk of falling and, in some, a progressive decline to a 'housebound' state with its attendant social isolation. Diminishing cerebral function causes forgetfulness, poor concentration, in some cases depression and, in an ever larger number, overt dementia. Poor eyesight, deafness, failing cardiorespiratory fitness, malnutrition, dehydration and alcohol abuse may compound these difficulties. Due to the diminished functional reserve of all the bodily systems, infections and minor trauma, which might have been shrugged off in earlier years, tend to have a cumulative effect. The reduction in physiological reserves often remains concealed until the stress of an illness, an accident or some toxic condition tips the precarious balance into failure and precipitates a crisis. Elderly patients are often prescribed drugs and are particularly likely to suffer from toxicity and adverse drug reactions. The possibility of iatrogenic disease either as the primary or a compounding problem must therefore always be considered in the sick old person.

While it is important to inquire into the background of all patients, it is of especial importance in the elderly. Social circumstances have a much greater influence on physical and mental well-being and may be the major determinants prompting the patient to seek help at a hospital. Increasing frailty or illness in the patient's chief 'carer' is a common last straw. Those living alone in poor conditions with low incomes are particularly vulnerable. Many old people become increasingly isolated by poor mobility, deteriorating special senses, rehousing projects and the deaths of close relatives and friends. Many cannot afford to eat properly and also keep warm. A 'tea and toast' diet often leads to vitamin deficiency. A few progress to an extreme of gross senile neglect (Diogenes syndrome) where they become apathetic, reclusive, never wash, hoard rubbish and live in total squalor behind locked doors, resenting any outside interference. Most of these senile recluses are psychiatrically ill.

The foregoing has been a broad outline of some personal and social backgrounds against which illness arises in old age and they should be in the forefront of the doctor's mind when he sees an old person being brought into the A & E department. More problems can occur at this juncture. An accurate history is often difficult to obtain, especially if the patient arrives in hospital unaccompanied, ill, confused or deaf. Information from relatives, neighbours, community workers, ambulance men and witnesses of any sort can be invaluable and anyone arriving with the patient should not be allowed to leave before being cross-questioned. The elderly often do not react to illness with clear-cut physical signs. Thus they may merely go off their feet and become too weak to get out of bed or become a bit confused and perhaps incontinent. Pain tends to be poorly localised. The physical examination must therefore be carried out with great care and patience — this requires considerable skill, especially when dealing with the confused and uncooperative. The elderly, like the newborn, can quickly become hypothermic (see Ch. 28). If there is any question that the person has been lying in unheated surroundings for any length of time or the skin feels cold, the rectal temperature must be measured with a low reading thermometer.

Phrases such as 'social problem' should be banished from the doctor's mind. Most old people referred to hospital as 'social problems' in fact have medical problems. It cannot be emphasised often enough that relatively minor conditions frequently lead to loss of independence in elderly people who have hitherto been struggling to maintain themselves in the community.

The following four conditions pose special problems in the elderly and each will be discussed in turn: *trauma (falls), mental impairment, infections* and *terminal illness*.

TRAUMA (FALLS)

Many attendances are the results of accidents, mostly falls. About three-quarters occur in the patient's own home. Old people's bones are brittle and break easily. Upper limb fractures are of much more significance as a threat to independence in the old as opposed to the young. A relatively minor blow to the head can cause subdural bleeding. Therefore extra vigilance is required in the management of relatively minor head injuries in the elderly. Virtually all should have a skull radiograph taken and if there is a fracture any neurological deficit (e.g. a hemiparesis) should be assumed to be caused by a traumatic intracranial haematoma and not a stroke. Confusion is common after head injuries in the elderly due to their reduced cerebral reserve. However, if the confusion persists for more than 12 hours or the patient's neurological status deteriorates, again an intracranial haematoma must be suspected and CT scanning considered.

Having carefully assessed the physical damage incurred in an accident the next problem to consider is the cause of the fall. Some are clear-cut tripping accidents due to loose carpets, trailing wires, steep or poorly lit stairs and outside, pavement irregularities or ice on the ground. Most at risk are people with locomotor instability related to osteoarthritis of the hips and knees, dementia, previous 'strokes', Parkinson's disease, alcohol abuse or visual impairment. In many other cases, however, the fall is due to a transient episode of dizziness or syncope.
Common causes are:

1. Transient cardiac dysrhythmias
2. Postural hypotension
3. Vertebrobasilar arterial insufficiency
4. Side effects of drugs
5. Straining to pass urine (micturition syncope)
6. Aortic valve disease
7. Epilepsy

The autonomic nervous system degenerates with age, leading to postural hypotension. The elderly diabetic is especially prone to this disorder, as are individuals taking phenothiazines, antihypertensive agents, hypnotics, L-dopa and antidepressants.

Often the patient's history will give the clue that the fall was not a simple trip or slip. 'I blacked out' is easy to interpret but more subtle is, 'I must have tripped' which usually means that the patient did not in fact trip. One of the most useful questions to ask is, 'What were you doing at the time you fell?' If the answer is 'Nothing', again this often implies underlying disease. A record of several previous falls has the same implication.

The most important part of the examination consists of getting the patient to stand and walk a few steps. A tendency to clutch on to objects and/or to walk with short irregular steps means the person is at risk of further falls. As already mentioned, people who have been lying on a floor for more than an hour need their body temperatures carefully measured. Multiple bruises and previous admissions with poorly explained trauma should alert the examining doctor to the possibility of 'granny or grandad bashing'.

If the patient is being discharged from hospital after treatment two major aspects need to be considered. Firstly, will there be adequate care at home? This is of particular importance in those living alone. Trivial injuries may seriously threaten independence. Secondly, is there an opportunity to prevent further falls? This may be a relatively simple matter of organising the provision of a walking aid or requesting a health visitor to go to the patient's home.

Falls among old people are often indicative of impaired general health and have serious prognostic significance. Such patients have a greatly increased mortality in the months after the fall when compared with a control group. Even when they do not break bones, after a heavy fall old people often need several days in hospital to recover from the pain, stiffness and lack of confidence that is engendered. While it is important to inform the general practitioner immediately when any old person is being discharged from hospital, it is particularly so in the above group of patients. The general practitioner, as leader of the primary health care team, can then organise early visits to the patients' homes in order to assess their ability to care for themselves.

MENTAL IMPAIRMENT

There are three major causes of mental impairment in the elderly: an acute or subacute toxic confusional state (delirium), dementia and depression. Toxic confusional states have a relatively sudden onset usually over hours or days. Consciousness is clouded and the mental state fluctuates. The patient is often restless, rambling and irrational. Hallucinations and delusions are common. Virtually any illness and many drugs can render an elderly person delirious, e.g. infections, heart failure, head injuries, metabolic disturbances, poisoning, dehydration and 'strokes'. A dysphasic 'stroke' victim can easily be misdiagnosed as confused. Many drugs, including self-prescribed medications and alcohol, are potent causes of confusion. The common offenders are sedatives, tranquillisers, antidepressants, antiparkinsonian agents and digoxin. A mild, early dementia may be unmasked by a relatively trivial illness. Poor sight and hearing and sudden changes of environment all exacerbate confusional states. Virtually all delirious old people require admission to hospital. The development of confusion after admission to hospital is commonly due to withdrawal of alcohol or drugs (e.g. benzodiazepines).

Dementia, in contrast, is a chronic disorder developing over many months or years. About 5% of those over 65 and 20% of those over 80 suffer from this disorder. The intellectual decline comes on insidiously and gradually worsens. Recent memory is impaired first, more remote memory being preserved. General alertness wanes and the person's range of activities narrows. Insight into the waning cerebral powers can cause profound depression during this early phase. Eventually personality changes, behavioural disturbances and frank disorientation occur. The sufferer may become irritable, suspicious, humourless, aggressive, and self-centred and display inappropriate social behaviour. Care for personal cleanliness is lost. Appetite diminishes. Sleep reversal with night-time wandering and frequent cat-naps is common. The end result is an almost vegetative existence which is very distressing to relatives. About one-third will have evidence of previous 'strokes' but the majority do not have lateralising neurological signs. A stooped posture, poverty of movement and a liability to fall are common.

Demented patients present many problems to the A & E doctor. Getting accurate information about the individual is often the first one. Telephone calls may have to be made to relatives, the general practitioner, community social workers and other social agencies. Acute illnesses arise in the demented as in any other patient group. However, in many cases old people are brought to the A & E department because of a breakdown of their care in the community. In some there has been a slight increase in disturbed behaviour which can be attributed to a 'cold' or constipation. In many the decline has been the gradual, natural history of the condition which puts increasing demand on inadequate community resources until they are finally exhausted. The death of a caring spouse or other relative is a common precipitant. Each A & E department should have a policy for the management of these patients who are not actually ill but cannot look after themselves at home. Ideally they should be brought into hospital for a two- to three-day assessment period. This 'breathing space' admission gives time for information about living conditions and social support to be gathered. The patient can be thoroughly examined physically. Mobility, dressing, feeding and toileting capabilities can be assessed and possible reversible causes of dementia considered (e.g. drugs, nutritional deficiencies, alcoholism, hypothyroidism, a subdural haematoma or depression). The geriatric medical unit is the best place for such an admission but in some hospitals observation beds are used for this purpose. Confusion often worsens in the unfamilar hospital environment and thioridazine is a useful sedative in these circumstances. If hospital admission is not possible and someone is willing to care for the patient for a few days, the next best arrangment is an early domiciliary visit from a geriatrician. The management plan must be carefully discussed with and communicated to the patient's relatives, the general practitioner, the geriatrician and the district social services.

Depression is a common accompaniment of declining physical and intellectual powers with age and can be mistaken for dementia. The prevalence of both increases with age. It is important to recognise this pseudodementia caused by depression as it is eminently treatable. The depressed patient may complain of memory loss, which is a rare complaint in true dementia, yet does surprisingly well on memory tests. He/she will often say, 'I can't remember' when asked a direct question. The demented patient, on the other hand, is more likely to hazard a guess or make an excuse for not knowing the answer. The diagnosis will frequently be obvious in the patient's general demeanour, in which a sense of distress is communicated to the doctor. There may also be a past personal or family history of depression and the state may occasionally be due to drugs.

Depressed old people are at great risk of suicide and this aspect of their thinking should always be probed with the patient and relatives. At special risk are the recently bereaved, those living alone in poor circumstances, alcohol abusers and people with chronic painful, debilitating or terminal diseases.

In all apparently mentally confused patients it is useful to carry out a short mental test score (Table 29.1) which can be recorded in the notes and provides a base-line for future comparisons (see also Ch. 30).

Table 29.1 Abbreviated mental test score (each question scores 1 mark)

1. Age
2. Time (to nearest hour)
3. Address for recall at end of test — this should be repeated by the patient to ensure it has been heard correctly.
4. Year
5. Name of hospital
6. Recognition of two persons (doctor, nurse)
7. Date of birth
8. Year of First World War
9. Name of present monarch
10. Count backwards, 20–1.

A score between 0–3 indicates severe mental impairment and 7–10 is regarded as normal. It is important that mental impairment is recognised when planning all aspects of a patient's management, but especially when it comes to making decisions about discharge from hospital care. Unless community support commensurate with the patient's intellectual and social capabilities is available he/she will soon be back in hospital or worse.

Occasional inability to recall names or trivial past events is common in the over 60 age group, especially among men and alone carries no significance.

INFECTIONS

The elderly as a group are particularly prone to infections, especially chest infections. The symptoms and signs may be poorly localised and they are more likely to suffer complications, e.g. perforated viscera in diverticulitis and appendicitis. It is a popular fallacy that many old people remain afebrile, even when the infection is severe. In fact the majority will be found to be pyrexial if the temperature is measured properly, i.e. the thermometer is left in place for at least five minutes.

A common clinical presentation of many types of infections is the development of mild confusion, incontinence and general physical decline often in a person with a pre-existing disability such as Parkinson's diesease, chronic bronchitis or heart failure. Electrolyte imbalance occurs quickly if the patient loses interest in eating and drinking.

Old people with chest infections should be admitted to hospital, especially if:

> 1. They are confused, dehydrated or have recently become incontinent
> 2. They have a background of chronic bronchitis
> 3. They have failed to respond to a course of antibiotics
> 4. They have developed signs of heart failure
> 5. They have a serious associated disease such as diabetes or renal failure which is likely to get worse during an acute illness
> 6. If they cannot cough effectively.

An often neglected physical sign in the diagnosis of a lower respiratory tract infection in the elderly is an increased respiratory rate (commonly above 30 breaths/minute).

Pulmonary tuberculosis should not be forgotten. In Western society it is now primarily a disease of the older age group occurring either as a primary infection or as a reactivation of previous disease.

So called 'significant bacteriuria' ($>10^5$ bacteria in 1 ml urine) is found in about 20% of elderly women and 10% of elderly men. If the patient is asymptomatic the condition is essentially benign and requires no treatment. A course of antibiotics is only needed if there are pus cells in the urine and symptoms of dysuria, frequency, urgency or incontinence. The antibiotics of choice are amoxycillin or trimethoprim given either as a 3-day course or, in the case of amoxycillin, as a 3 g stat dose. The possibility of an acute urinary tract infection should also be considered in any confused elderly person who is vomiting and complaining of abdominal pain. Rigors, loin discomfort and 'collapse' due to septicaemia may also be present. These patients require immediate admission to hospital.

The following types of patients are at increased risk of urinary tract infections:

> 1. Those with anatomical abnormalities of the urinary tract, especially obstructive lesions
> 2. Those with faecal or urinary incontinence
> 3. Women with vaginal prolapse
> 4. Those with organic brain disease
> 5. Following cystoscopy or catheterisation
> 6. Those living in institutions.

A diagnosis of pruritis vulvae in the female or balanitis in the male should immediately lead to testing the urine for glucose.

TERMINAL ILLNESS

Elderly people moribund as a consequence of a massive 'stroke' or severe pneumonia will often be brought to the A & E department. In many cases death is inevitable and attempted resuscitation unkind. Essential treatment should be given which is specifically aimed at the relief of distress, while background information is rapidly gathered from relatives, the general practitioner and from previous hospital notes. Cardiopulmonary resuscitation should rarely be carried out in the very elderly, patients with advanced cancer or those with severe chronic cardiorespiratory disease. The nursing staff should always be informed of such decisions and the reasons for making them. A useful guide for the junior medical staff is to ask them to imagine what they would like done if the patient was their beloved elderly relative. The relatives require the utmost sensitivity in this type of situation (see Ch. 5).

Patients with advanced cancer whose survival may be measured in weeks or even months may also arrive in the A & E department. The most common reasons are the development of distressing symptoms and/or the inability of the relatives to cope with the patient at home. Sometimes the visit is due to poor communication or misunderstanding concerning the patient's true state of health. However, the A & E department is not the place to attempt to explain to a patient and relatives that a cure for the condition is unlikely and the best that can be offered is comfort through symptom relief. Few people are able to assimilate information about a life-threatening condition if given the bad news at one point in time. These patients need admission to hospital for at least a few days, preferably to a specialised cancer unit, so that all the medical facts can be marshalled, a therapeutic strategy for symptom control devised and a scheme for further care organised. During the admission the understanding which the patient and his relatives have of the illness can be explored. The general practitioner and district social services will need to be contacted if home care is planned. Some simple aids, such as incontinence pads or a commode, may be required. The local hospice can often provide support and help, either in the form of highly trained nurses visiting the patient at home or by admitting the patient in the final stages of the illness. In evolving the management plan it should be remembered that the family may need more time spent with them, more information given and more confidence inspired than the patient. Three useful publications in the care of the terminally ill are listed at the end of the chapter.

SUMMARY

Elderly patients require great care in their assessment and management in the A & E department. Many have multiple diseases and disabilities and it is particularly important to recognise the inter-relationship of medical, social and psychiatric factors in their problems. They often present as the result of a medicosocial crisis precipitated by an apparently trivial accident or illness which overstretches inadequate community resources. The fact that they do not appear to be acutely ill should not be written off as 'dumping' by uncaring relatives.

Some departments use their observation beds for assessment of the elderly, especially those who have sustained minor injuries in falls. However, admission to hospital is not always the most appropriate method of dealing with the problems of the elderly as it is linked with increasing morbidity and dependence.

A medical social worker and a liaison nurse specifically attached to the A & E department are invaluable in the gathering of background information about the patient, giving advice about financial and other entitlements and coordinating community help when the patient is being discharged from hospital. The decision to allow an infirm elderly person to go home should not be taken lightly by the A & E doctor. It should certainly not be based solely on the patients' own assessment of their ability to look after themselves. They take longer than young people to recover from illnesses and injuries and, due to residual disability, their level of dependency is often increased after a hospital admission. It is important for the A & E department to develop close cooperation with the community social services and the district geriatric service in order that back-up arrangements are routinely made before the patients' discharge from hospital. Each patient's family doctor must be forewarned of the imminent discharge so that a member of the primary health care team (e.g. health visitor, district nurse or trained volunteer) can immediately visit the person at home and discuss support arrangements. While there must be direct communication between the hospital and the family doctor, a liaison nurse can bring much detailed information from the department to the general practitioner and provide feedback in the opposite direction. In some cases it may be appropriate to suggest a domiciliary visit from a geriatrician. The staff of the A & E department should be aware of the full range of services for the elderly available in its locality and the clinical managment principles recommended by the department of geriatric medicine. A good rapport with the local geriatricians is essential when seeking help with difficult problems. The British Geriatrics Society has recently issued the following 'broad guidelines of good practice for the discharge of elderly patients from an A & E department':

1. Elderly patients seen between 10.00 p.m. and 8.00 a.m. should not be discharged during the night, unless they are accompanied by family or friend. Preferably, such patients should remain in an overnight or observation ward.

2. Medical staff should ascertain whether or not all elderly patients living alone are able to cope independently prior to their discharge from the department.

3. If an injury has occurred necessitating a plaster cast or a collar-and-cuff, the medical staff should ascertain that the elderly patient can walk and perform safely tasks vital for daily living. If not, and the discharge is still considered appropriate, the general practitioner, district nurse and social services should be informed to provide extra support.

4. If a minor injury has occurred necessitating sutures or a simple dressing, the district nurse and general practitioner should be alerted, in order that they can supervise further treatment in order to prevent the elderly person having to return to the hospital for removal of dressing or sutures.

5. The general practitioner, social services department, and district nursing service should be informed and contacted for further information when an elderly confused person presents with a minor injury, or has been found wandering in the street. Responsibility rests with medical staff.

6. All elderly patients, presenting with a drug overdose or other method of attempted suicide, e.g. cut wrists or placing polythene bag over head, should be seen by the duty psychiatrist prior to discharge. The patient's general practitioner should also be informed.

7. Repeated attendances to an A & E department by an elderly person over a short period of time should be taken seriously. The case should be reviewed in the light of information from the general practitioner, district nurse, family and social services. A further plan of action should then be made prior to the next discharge from the A & E department.

8. If a case of non-accidental injury is suspected, the patient's general practitioner and health visitor should be informed, and possibly the social services department.

9. If an elderly person is taken to the A & E department for social reasons and is not found to have an acute physical or mental illness after full medical assessments, the on-call social worker should be contacted prior to discharge.

10. The staff of an A & E department should give full consideration to the manner and the mode of transport by which the elderly people are returned to their home. Preferably such patients should be accompanied by family or a friend.

11. The on-call geriatric and psychogeriatric teams should be available for liaison duties in the A & E department.

The A & E doctor should regard himself as part of a surveillance team aiming to provide anticipatory and preventive care for the elderly. The inappropriate attendance of an elderly person to an A & E department should be regarded as a 'warning light' and suggest the need for referral to the appropriate community service. The doctor should be aware that certain old people are particularly vulnerable and take special care with their management. Such 'high-risk' old people are:

Over 70 years of age
Housebound
Demented
Living alone
Recently bereaved
Recently discharged from hospital.

The elderly are particularly prone to the side effects of drugs, including anaesthetic agents. They should therefore be taking a minimum of tablets and have clear directions how to take them. Whenever possible, treatment should not be changed in the A & E department as dangerous confusion can result. If a change is thought necessary the general practitioner should be contacted and asked to review the patient's medication.

In the best possible world of adequate community and hospital resources and vigilant surveillance in general practice many old peoples' visits to the A & E department would be unnecessary.

FURTHER READING

Health care of the elderly: essays in old age medicine, psychiatry and services Arie T 1981 Croom Helm, London

Terminal care: drug control of common symptoms Baines M St Christopher's Hospice, London

Meeting the needs of older people — some practice guidelines Cloke C 1986 Age Concern, England

Practical geriatric medicine Exton-Smith A N, Weksler M E 1985 Churchill Livingstone, Edinburgh

Birmingham care of the dying National Association of Health Authorities

Living with dying: the management of terminal disease Saunders Dame C, Baines M, 1983 Oxford University Press, Oxford

Psychiatric emergencies

The management of mental illness in the emergency department, like many other conditions, is often described by experts in the inpatient management of disease. Their authority stems from detailed knowledge of individual conditions and their advice revolves around the establishment of a diagnosis. Emergency work, however, often involves the management of a particular crisis before a definitive diagnosis can be made. In psychiatric emergencies the management of the condition may in fact prevent a definitive diagnosis being made, at least for a time. With this in mind, this chapter draws on psychiatric experience but is intended only to give advice about particular crises.

THE DISTURBED PATIENT

The 'casualty department' or emergency room is often the receptacle for any person found wandering the streets. The police, social services and the general public will relieve themselves of such a burden at the only open-access, 24-hour a day medical agency. To be effective, the staff of the emergency department must have a clear idea of what they can and cannot do. This usually means being able to distinguish *medical* from *non-medical problems*. We all share a human responsibility for each other's welfare but we must equally recognise what special responsibilities society has invested in us. The two are not mutually exclusive but clearly the latter must always take priority. The special responsibilities of staff in the accident and emergency department are to exclude or treat any immediately reversible physical condition and recognise the need for psychiatric referral. The degree of urgency for a psychiatric referral can often be discussed with the duty psychiatrist.

When faced with a disturbed patient your immediate priority is the safety of yourself and others. After all, if you or your staff are injured nobody gets any treatment. A patient who is damaging property but not people should be isolated by removing others from the vicinity. Verbal reassurance must always be attempted first and as much information as possible gained from friends, relatives, etc. You must attempt to establish if this is a civil or medical matter. Talk to the patient and listen for evidence of disordered thought or confusion. If in doubt, err on the side of illness. If, however, this is clearly a civil matter and is not medical, contact the police. Attempts at physical restraint must be premeditated and part of a management plan. Simply restraining a patient will only provoke a struggle and reinforce and confirm any paranoid ideas. However, physical restraint may be employed in order to facilitate the administration of a tranquilliser or dextrose to a hypoglycaemic patient, for example. Ensure you have enough personnel to overpower the patient and preferably ensure that they have had some training. Seek assistance from the police if there is time. Four adults and two mattresses is one way of controlling a violent individual. The use of straps is an extremely effective method of securing a patient to a trolley. It is, however, extremely distressing and must be accompanied by the administration of tranquillising drugs. The administration of tranquillising drugs will prohibit a diagnosis until recovery is complete. Chlorpromazine intramuscularly can be given in 100 mg aliquots every 20 minutes until sedation is achieved. Nevertheless they are indicated when:

> A disturbed patient is thought to be suffering from an acute psychiatric/medical condition, although the precise nature may not yet be known, and:
> 1. The patient's actions are such that it is thought they will harm themselves or others if not restrained
> 2. Investigation and treatment of a potentially life-threatening physical condition is prohibited by the patient's behaviour.

Many doctors are unsure about treatment in these circumstances and attempt to delay intervention until the patient can be 'sectioned' under the Mental Health Act. Unfortunately this often takes too long and the patient can cause or incur serious harm in the meantime. However, it is rarely, if ever, the responsibility of the emergency department to 'section' a patient. This falls upon the department of psychiatry which services the A & E department. An emergency unit unserviced by a department of psychiatry cannot be considered adequate for the reception of disturbed patients. It is important to note that personality disorders and alcoholism are not in themselves sufficient reasons for compulsory admission to a psychiatric hospital.

The administration of treatment without the prior consent of the patient is *battery* . To give a clear indication to the patient that this is about to happen is an *assault* . However, treatment may be administered without consent under 'common law', when there is 'urgent necessity'. This is not clearly defined in law but is usually meant to describe circumstances when '*life-saving* ' treatment is given but also involves any '*emergency*'! An emergency in these circumstances is when immediate action is necessary to preserve life or to prevent a serious and immediate danger to the patient or other people. Any treatment or physical restraint employed in these circumstances must be '*reasonable* ' and sufficient only for the purpose of bringing the emergency (not necessarily the underlying condition) to an end.

Consent itself is not always clearly understood. Even when not expressed it can be implied. For example, presenting oneself to an emergency department implies at least some degree of consent to treatment. Expressed consent may be oral or more commonly written. The document itself, however, is not absolute proof of consent. Certain other criteria must also be fulfilled.

1. The patient must be *informed* of the true nature of the procedure and any inherent risks.

2. The patient must be *competent* to understand the nature of the procedure. An adult is technically anyone of 18 years or above. However, a 16-year-old is usually accepted as capable of giving or withdrawing their consent. Below the age of 16 the situation is unclear. However, the preferred view is that the consent is valid as long as the child is competent to understand the nature and purpose of the treatment. Let common sense prevail. Clearly if there is doubt and the treatment can wait — then wait. If the treatment is urgent then common law and indeed common sense prevails. Administer treatment sufficiently to resolve the emergency but no more until consent can be obtained.

3. The consent must clearly be *voluntary* . Any degree of duress, fraud or deceit will invalidate the consent — implied or expressed.

In summary. Common law powers of detention (i.e. those powers not embodied in statute) entitle any individual to apprehend and restrain a person who is mentally disordered and who presents an imminent danger to himself or others. The degree of medical or physical intervention used should be sufficient to bring the emergency to an end but no greater. The degree and duration of the force involved must be proportional to the risk which is presented.

Compulsory admission

The emergency admission to hospital, under the Mental Health Act of 1983, of a patient from the A & E department will usually, if not always, involve the duty psychiatrist. The act can be invoked when a patient 'requires detention for his own health and safety, or for the protection of others'.

An *emergency order* (section 4 of the Act), can be signed by any member of the medical profession, but a psychiatrist is clearly preferable. The signature of the nearest relative *or* a social worker is also required. There are no conditions as to the patient's whereabouts, and so it is commonly used to secure the admission of a patient to hospital from the community. It can only be enforced for a maximum of 72 hours.

If assessment alone is not enough then *urgent treatment* can be given under section 62 of the Act. This must be immediately necessary to save life, prevent serious deterioration or suffering, and represent the minimum interference necessary to prevent the patient from behaving violently or being a danger to him/herself or others.

Further assessment, up to 28 days, can be secured by invoking section 2 of the Act. This *assessment order* requires the signatures of two medical practitioners, *plus* that of the nearest relative or approved social worker. One of the doctors involved must have been approved for this purpose under section 12 of the Act. As for section 4, there are no restrictions as to the patient's location prior to admission. The same conditions must be fulfilled to complete a *treatment order* (section 3 of the act) which will allow detention for up to 6 months.

The 'doctor in charge' of a patient already in hospital can detain him or her under section 5(2) of the Mental Health Act 1983 with an *admission order* for up to 72 hours. Similarly a qualified nurse has a *holding power* and can detain hospital inpatients under section 5(4), but only up to 6 hours.

Finally a police officer may take a person to hospital against their will for *admission by police* under section 136 of the Act. This can be enforced for up to 72 hours.

Differential diagnosis

Having assumed that the disturbed patient is 'ill' and that restraint is unnecessary at the moment, consider what illness he or she may have and what if anything need be done in an emergency. A patient aged more than 40 years must initially be assumed to have a physical cause for their first episode of confusion or abnormal behaviour, particularly if there are any physical signs.

1. Ask yourself —
   a. Is this a civil matter?
   b. Is this mental illness?
   c. Is this physical illness masquerading as mental illness?
   d. Is this mental illness exacerbated by physical illness?
2. Ask the patient
   a. His or her name, address, telephone number and age.
   b. Who does he or she live with? Whom should we contact.
   c. The day, date, time and place.

Disorientation, loss of recent memory and clouding of consicousness are features of a toxic confusional state (see 318).

3. Perform a simple mental state examination. An example for adults with no mental handicap is as follows:
   a. Ask the patient to remember three numbers; count from 1

to 10, then repeat the original three numbers.

   b. Repeat the days of the week backwards.

   c. Give a simple sum.

   d. Ask them to remember three simple words.

   e. Record the time interval each time.

   f. Ask for simple opposites and groups, e.g. the opposite of up .... Pounds and pennies are both ....

   g. Give the meaning of common proverbs.

   h. Take 7 from 100 and 7 from that, etc.

4. Ask a friend or relative:

   a. Is this the first episode?

   b. Has it come on gradually or suddenly?

   c. What do they think precipitated it?

5. If the decision is that this is not a civil matter, complete a physical examination and take blood for:

   a. FBC

   b. U & E

   c. Glucose

   d. Toxicology

6. Obtain a skull and chest radiograph. Consider estimation of arterial blood gases.

The common physical conditions that must be excluded include:

Hypoglycaemia

Confusion and often aggression accompanies a fall in blood sugar. If this condition is suspected then administer 50 ml of 50% glucose intravenously *immediately*. In children there are more dangers in the administration of hyperosmolar solutions and 2 ml/kg of 25% dextrose should be given after reagent strip estimation of the blood glucose.

A very disturbed patient will require restraint. Intramuscular glucagon may be safer in these circumstances (see p. 141), since extravasated dextrose is extremely damaging to tissue.

If i.v. dextrose is to be given it is essential to give 'parentrovite' first if chronic alcohol abuse is a possibility. The two 5 ml ampoules of the intravenous high potency preparation must be mixed in the syringe prior to administration. Vitamin B_1 deficiency often accompanies chronic alcohol abuse. The vitamin is required in the Kreb's cycle. If a glucose load is given to a severely depleted patient then the last remaining B_1 will be consumed and a Korsakov's psychosis will be precipitated.

Finally, patients who are taking β-blockers may not exhibit any of the sympathetically mediated compensatory responses, e.g. tachycardia and sweating. The diagnosis of hypoglycaemia may be extremely difficult clinically in these circumstances. It is therefore essential that you know the blood sugar of all disturbed patients.

Dementia

Dementia does not often of itself present as an acute behavioural disturbance. Rather an acute infection or other illness precipitates decompensation.

Drug toxicity

Either by accident or intent, this is probably the most common and important reversible cause of behavioural disturbance. The most common drug involved is alcohol.

Thyroid disease

Thyroid disease may present as an acute anxiety when thyrotoxicosis is severe. Myxoedema is usually associated with reduced activity, but 'myxoedema madness' with increased and disturbed activity is an unusual but well-recognised occurrence.

Cerebral hypoxia

Either as an acute event or an exacerbation of a chronic condition, cerebral hypoxia is an important cause of disturbed behaviour. Cyanosis is usually not a feature and so the diagnosis must actively be looked for. Often it is a summation of several acute and chronic conditions rather than a single event. Chronic obstructive airways disease is usually present and a superimposed infection can often be found. The patient may be anaemic and this will exacerbate other causes of hypoxia.

One should exclude cardiac failure and consider pulmonary embolus. Carbon monoxide poisoning may have occurred accidentally or deliberately. The 'classic' pink discoloration of the skin, like most 'classic' signs is in fact rare. The percentage of carboxyhaemaglobin must be greater than 60% for this to occur and so it is usually a postmortem finding. Indeed, cyanosis is probably more common.

If hypoxia is suspected, then clearly you must measure arterial blood gases and administer oxygen.

Many *intracerebral catastrophies* precipitate disturbed behaviour. A *cerebrovascular accident* with hemiplegia will be obvious, but *subarachnoid haemorrhage* when not accompanied by collapse can progress insidiously and the diagnosis may be delayed. If an epileptic fit was unwitnessed, the confusion of the *postictal* state may be unrecognised. Similarly, a *head injury* may have been unwitnessed and if external signs of injury are unusual or missed a serious error in diagnosis may be made.

Subdural haematoma

Subdural haematoma, with or without fracture, may develop several days after a head injury. The most common misdiagnosis is CVA, but behavioural changes alone can occur early. Other *space-occupying lesions* may present in this way although they are uncommon.

CNS infections

CNS infections involving brain and/or meninges clearly involve behavioural change. However, pyrexia is usually present and the patient is obviously 'ill'. Occasionally syphilis will present in this way but the diagnosis is only likely to be made later.

The conditions described above are specific causes of a 'toxic confusional state'. This syndrome may be the result of a more generalised condition or, as said earlier, a combination of conditions. *Dehydration* and *pyrexia* either by themselves or in combination, are important and probably the commonest general causes. Rare conditions such as *systemic lupus erythematosis* can cause severe acute mental changes but are likely to be diagnosed by the inpatient team. *Acute intermittent porphyria* is an inherited disorder of porphyrin metabolism. There is *no* photosensitivity in this type. The acute clinical picture can be extremely confusing but involves abdominal pain, peripheral neuropathy and 'psychosis'. A family history may be available, or more likely the patient is already known to the hospital. An acute episode is usually precipitated by drugs and in particular:

1. Alcohol
2. Barbiturates
3. Sulphonamides.

Fortunately, chlorpromazine (and morphine) are safe in this condition and so the general guidelines for sedation of the disturbed patient can be applied without prejudice even if this diagnosis is missed.

In summary, the commonest process that leads to a toxic confusional state is:

Acute/chronic brain syndrome + decompensation = confusion.

The commonest cause of 'decompensation' is an intercurrent infection but changes in environment or domestic circumstances are potent factors in many elderly people.

THE VIOLENT PATIENT

Violent behaviour in patients attending emergency departments appears to be an increasing hazard of emergency practice throughout the world. Some of this is related to underlying mental illness, but most is not. The majority is related to drug intoxication, most commonly with alcohol. The emergency physician must bear several things in mind:

1. Alcohol and drug intoxication 'is no excuse'! A patient is still responsible in law for any action taken whilst under the influence of such substances.
2. Alcohol and drug ingestion may:
   a. be a symptom of underlying medical or psychiatric disease
   b. mask such conditions.
   c. predispose to such conditions.
3. Don't judge — just help.
4. Take all threats seriously. Many episodes of physical violence are preceded by verbal violence. It is easier to respond appropriately and effectively to the latter. If this is done early the situation may be more easily defused. It is unlikely to precipitate an event that would not have occurred anyway.
5. Violent aggressive or abusive behaviour is inappropriate to the hospital setting. It should be explained carefully and neutrally to the patient that his/her behaviour is upsetting others. Many outbursts of violence are an exaggerated response to a legitimate grievance. Explain repeatedly to patients the reason for any delays and do not hesitate to apologise for any short-comings in your system.
6. Finally recognise what is a civil matter and call the police. When a violent person has left the emergency department the police should still be informed. The common 'medical' conditions to consider in a patient who is violent are:
   a. alcohol intoxication
   b. other drug intoxication
   c. hypoglycaemia — often in association with a.
   d. post-ictal
   e. head injury
   f. the causes of a toxic confusional state outlined earlier
   g. A distended bladder, especially in a drunk who is being restrained, but also sometimes in a head injured patient

It must be stressed that, most commonly, violence is a civil matter and is not the direct result of physical illness. Similarly, mental illness, although a cause of disturbed behaviour, is not often the sole cause of a patient's violent behaviour.

In dealing with any disturbed or violent behaviour it is important to be able to recognise the essential features of the common psychiatric conditions.

The brief mental state examination should be followed by specific enquires about symptoms characteristic of specific diseases. Throughout the examination attempt to determine if the patient has any degree of insight into their conditions and so differentiate *neurosis* from *psychosis*.

Schizophrenia

'Dementia praecox' is primarily a disease of young people. Disordered thought with thought block, ideas of reference, passivity and delusions are distressing, but in fact an unusual reason for disturbed or violent behaviour. Affect is flattened and may be inappropriate to the idea being expressed. Behaviour can be extremely unusual. Delusions and hallucinations (almost invariably auditory) can contribute to a profound paranoia. The 'voices' continuously comment on their behaviour. If the patient's behaviour is met with hostility or attempts at physical restraint then violent outbursts may ensue and the paranoia becomes justified. If sedation is required then 100 mg aliquots of chlorpromazine intramuscularly every 20–30 minutes until behaviour is controlled may be used.

Violence is an unusual feature of schizophrenia. The disease is characterised by passiveness, withdrawal and loss of self. These features are unlikely to permit the self-assertiveness of aggression. Violence may occur as a response to threats — real or imagined.

It is unusal for 'new' cases of schizophrenia to present 'ab initio' to the emergency department. Most patients will already be under treatment.

Mania

The term 'hypomania' is used more frequently when often there is no clear distinction between hypomania and mania. The mood is elevated and inappropriate to the patient's condition. 'Pressure of thought' and 'flight of ideas' may be easily identified in speech. The patient is restless and perhaps excessively good humoured. Such patients are not usually violent but may strongly resist any attempts to persuade them to accept treatment.

DEPRESSION

Occasionally an acute depressive illness may be seen in the emergency department because of the condition itself. More frequently, however, it is because of the consequences of the pathological mood change. We all feel sad, but a depressive illness involves profound feelings of worthlessness, auditory hallucinations, physical retardation and sleep disturbance. Early morning wakening is characteristic and adds to the patient's misery. The physical retardation produces symptoms which can only add to the depression. The patient often feels he/she has an underlying illness — usually cancer — both as a delusion and as an explanation for his/her condition. Weight loss and constipation may trigger a whole series of medical investigations.

Perhaps of more importance to the emergency department is the fact that many of these patients will attempt to take their own lives. Consider anyone you have diagnosed to be depressed as 'at risk' for suicide and discuss their care with a psychiatrist.

Puerperal psychosis

The puerperium may precipitate or be associated with a variety of psychiatric conditions. 'The blues' is a commonly recognised phenomenon after delivery, but it may be severe and it may persist. The baby and/or other children may be neglected and it can lead to suicide. Any psychiatric presentation in this period is serious and must be referred to a specialist.

ANXIETY REACTIONS

Palpitations, overbreathing, atypical chest pain and sometimes fear of sexually transmitted disease (particularly AIDS) are all features of anxiety. The fear is usually based on some relevant symptom, but the reaction to it is often extreme. The patient usually has insight into the problem and so may be described as having a 'neurosis'. The term 'neurotic', however, has gained a social and derogatory meaning and is best not used. The danger for the emergency physician is that a truly life-threatening condition may be misdiagnosed as anxiety. One should exclude physical illness as far as is appropriate and then refer the patient to their own doctor.

DELIBERATE SELF-HARM

People poison or injure themselves for a variety of reasons, including frustration, a cry for help, in response to hallucinations

and as a deliberate attempt to take their own lives. The response of the public to this action, and the medical profession in particular, can often be uncaring and sometimes frankly hostile. Yet other acts of deliberate self-harm are greeted only with sympathy. Heart and lung disease in smokers and injuries to motor cyclists, for example, are avoidable conditions yet little blame is attached to their victims. It is possibly the delay in onset of symptoms from the time of exposure to risk and the degree of risk itself that influences our response. Nevertheless all these people are clearly suffering and the relief of their suffering is our duty. The emergency physician must decide on the following:

1. What is the degree of physical harm?
What is the degree of physical risk?
Does the patient require admission because of the physical injury?
2. What is the mental state of the patient?
What is the risk of suicide?
Does the patient require admission to hospital because of his/her mental state?
Does the patient require admission to hospital because of the risk of suicide?
3. Can the patient go home?

The degree of physical harm incurred and risk of future harm is usually the simplest parameter to assess. Poisons are discussed in Ch. 16. Wrist cutting, immolation and other acts of violence directed towards the self can result in a variety of injuries and should be treated as outlined in the relevant section of this book.

The decision to admit the patient for the physical injury of course depends on the injury.

The mental state of the patient can briefly be assessed as outlined above. The risk of suicide should be assessed first by the emergency physician and, if appropriate, later by a psychiatrist. When assessing the 'degree of intent' it is essential to acknowledge that a patient's perception of what might be harmful is different to that of a doctor. The details of the act per se are far less significant than what the patient expected the act might achieve. Furthermore, the possibility of rescue in the circumstances of the event is a further indication of intent and this risk/rescue ratio is important to establish.

Factors which indicate the risk of a completed suicide were high are:

1. The *risk/rescue ratio* — as perceived by the patient (vide supra). Establish whether any overt or covert attempts at summoning help were made.

2. The *degree of isolation* at the time of the event and in the future.

3. Any *history of previous attempts*.

4. *Final acts in anticipation of death* — for example, did the patient make a will or leave a suicide note?

5. *Expected outcome* — did the patient believe he would die.

6. *Relief/remorse* — how does the patient feel now that the 'suicide' has been unsuccessful. Is he glad to be alive?

7. *Impulsive or planned*? — how much preparation went into the act? Clearly the risk of suicide is highest in those who made meticulous preparations perhaps over several days

8. *Alcohol* (or other drugs). Many acts of deliberate self-harm

occur in a setting of alcohol intoxication. More significantly the overall risk of suicide is enormously increased in patients with chronic alcohol problems.

9. *Mental illness* — people who already suffer from mental illness attempt and complete suicide more frequently than the general population. When deliberate self-harm occurs in the setting of overt mental illness and, in particular, psychosis, the risk of completion is extremely high. Such patients must be closely monitored.

10. *Age/sex* — men over 40 years of age, living alone, have a higher incidence of suicide than the rest of the population. However, the incidence is now increasing in younger men, especially those who are socially isolated. The unemployed are particularly at risk.

Women aged less than 35 years are more likely to harm themselves deliberately. Difficult domestic circumstances (poor housing, errant husband) are involved and the act can be intended to precipitate a change in these circumstances. The first such attempt often proves to be a successful catalyst for a change, although the effect is less for any subsequent attempts. Women who have children before they are 20 years old and live in poor social circumstances have been shown to be particularly at risk.

Finally, don't accept too readily that an adult's poisoning has been accidental or inadvertant. Treat 'wrist cutters' in exactly the same way as 'overdoses'. If any of the 'risk factors' are present — discuss the case with a psychiatrist.

The decision to allow a patient who has deliberately harmed himself/herself to go home must be based on positive criteria:

1. The patient does not require immediate inpatient treatment for the self-inflicted injury/illness.

2. The absence of suicide risk factors (vide supra).

3. The patient is over 16 years of age.

4. You have spoken to a responsible friend/relative who will escort the patient home and will look after him/her there.

5. The patient is on the phone.

6. You can ensure appropriate follow-up within the next few days.

ALCOHOL AND OTHER DRUGS

As mentioned above, alcohol and other drugs are often underlying factors in the violent or disturbed behaviour of patients who attend A & E departments. It is germain to the practice of emergency medicine to expand a little about these substances.

Alcohol

This is the most widely used drug of abuse in the western world. If you define a narcotic as a drug that has anaesthetic, analgesic and addictive properties, then alcohol is also the most widely abused *narcotic* in the western world. What is more, it is legal, over the age of 5 at home, 18 in public, although there are restrictions on its sale. It is primarily consumed for its psychotropic properties and almost exclusively in the form of alcoholic beverages. One standard glass of wine, one measure of spirit or half a pint of beer is usually taken to be one unit of alcohol or approximately

9 g of pure ethanol. It is rapidly absorbed from the stomach and small intestine. The liver possesses the enzyme alcohol dehydrogenase (ADH) in sufficient quantity to detoxify the minute but regular amounts of ethanol produced by bacterial breakdown of food. It is easily swamped by a single unit of alcohol and free ethanol is released into the bloodstream. Eventually the ADH enzyme system will convert all the free ethanol to acetaldehyde and then to acetate. The blood alcohol concentration will fall about 15 mg/dl per hour. There is an alternative enzymatic pathway — MEOS (microsomal ethanol oxidising system). If large amounts of ethanol are regularly presented to the liver then the amount of MEOS in the liver is increased (along with the size of the liver) and the rate of detoxification may be increased. It is extremely difficult therefore to back-calculate accurately what the blood alcohol level was at any given time in a particular individual.

As soon as alcohol becomes measurable in the blood its effect on the CNS becomes demonstrable. Tolerance does occur, but this is primarily behavioural and objective psychomotor testing will reveal changes of which the subject is unaware, even in the most practised drinker. The effects of ethanol on the CNS are all depressive. The reduction in activity of the frontal cortex results in early loss of inhibitions which is often misinterpreted as stimulation. Cerebrovestibular impairment follows with ataxia, nystagmus and dysarthria. Eventually consciousness may be lost if the blood alcohol level continues to rise. The irritant effects of ethanol upon the gastric mucosa induce vomiting and if this occurs when the conscious level is depressed, inhalation may ensue. It is this, rather than alcohol-induced apnoea, that accounts for most deaths from 'alcohol poisoning'.

Extreme caution must be exercised in the interpretation of blood alcohol levels. The relationship between conscious level and blood alcohol concentration (BAC) varies widely between individuals. Apnoea may ensue at 400–500 mg/dl in most of the adult population but practised drinkers will walk and talk at levels well above this. Conversely inexperienced drinkers will die at levels less than 400 mg/dl. Never attribute a change in conscious level to alcohol alone. Assume another cause and look for it. After all if alcohol is the only cause, they will simply sober up.

Acute alcohol intoxication is probably the commonest cause of disturbed behaviour in the A & E department. Drunkenness itself is not necessarily a crime but can be if associated with other behaviour and in public, e.g. drunk and disorderly; drunk and incapable, etc. It is essentially a civil matter. The drunk in law is assumed to be responsible for the consequences of his/her actions. Drunkenness is not a mental illness and in itself is not a permissable reason for compulsory admission to hospital. However, the drunk is physically at risk from the following:

1. *Inhalation* of vomitus and other airway difficulties.

2. *Head injury* — ataxia plus reduction in protective reflexes means drunks fall and bang their heads. Movement of the head is often uncontrolled and superficial cerebral veins are more easily torn. Skull fracture and extradural haematoma occur but subdural haematoma, perhaps without fracture must be considered.

3. *Hypoglycaemia* — alcohol inhibits the release of glucose from the liver and thereby potentiates some of the effects of insulin.

If food is not taken with alcohol then hypoglycaemia without adequate compensation occurs. The circulating catecholamines rise in an attempt to release glucose from the liver but this is blocked by the alcohol. Tachycardia, sweating, confusion and aggression may owe more to low glucose and high adrenaline levels than alcohol itself. Occasionally a transient hypoglycaemia may occur when alcohol is taken with a concentrated glucose mixture, e.g. gin and tonic. The glucose stimulates hyperinsulinaemia and a rebound fall in blood glucose. The alcohol may inhibit compensatory release of glucose from the liver. The hypoglycaemia is not usually severe in these circumstances but it may be accompanied by aggression and mild confusion. Severe hypoglycaemia is common in children, however, even with small amounts of alcohol and is seen not infrequently in teenagers who take excess alcohol. If alcohol and parenteral insulin are combined then severe refractory and sometimes fatal hypoglycaemia may ensue.

4. *Other injury* — drunks fall down. Rib fractures may be incurred without complaint. Moreover serious intra-abdominal injuries can occur with minimal apparent discomfort and physical signs. Drunks are particularly vulnerable to assault.

5. *Self poisoning,* with other substances — either deliberately or by accident. (Particularly common in teenagers.)

6. *Brainstem apnoea.* Drunks may drink enough to paralyse the respiratory centre.

It is clear therefore that a 'simple drunk' may have other serious pathology masked by his intoxication. Skull radiographs and blood glucose are mandatory. If glucose is required it should be preceded by thiamine.

If the patient appears to be drunk and totally refuses to co-operate with treatment, it is, in the first instance, a civil matter. Call the police if the patient refuses to leave. If the police are to arrest the patient then advise them to contact a police surgeon.

If you are uncertain that the disturbed behaviour is due to drunkenness then restrain the patient for the purpose of examination and withdraw a blood sample for glucose estimation. In children it is useful to analyse the sample for ethanol, although this need not be done immediately.

The alcohol withdrawal syndrome

This is a common condition and its features include — tremulousness, sweating, tachycardia, agitation and nausea. Clouding of consciousness, disorientation and memory disturbances are not features of the alcohol withdrawal syndrome but suggest *delirium tremens*. This is an organic brain syndrome associated with alcohol abuse and epileptic seizures. Mortality can be high and is usually the result of uncontrolled fitting. It is extremely important that the term 'DTs' is not used by medical staff. This implies a more benign condition and is usually a misnomer for the alcohol withdrawal syndrome. This condition is also associated with fits as alcohol lowers the threshold for epilepsy in all of us. Chlormethiazole and chlordiazepoxide can be used in reducing doses over 5 days to alleviate the symptoms of the alcohol withdrawal syndrome. They must then be discontinued. There is no indication for long-term maintenance of patients on these medications in the mistaken belief that they prevent 'alcoholism'. Chlormethiazole in particular has cross tolerance with alcohol and will add to, rather than relieve, the patient's burden of dependence. In overdose the combination can be rapidly fatal. A chlormethiazole infusion can be associated with cardiorespiratory depression and must be used with extreme caution, if at all.

Delirium tremens requires inpatient therapy in an intensive care environment.

The term *rum fits* merely describes the association between alcohol abuse and epilepsy. Fits more commonly occur in the withdrawal phase but can occur during intoxication.

Dependence

Dependence implies *tolerance* — you drink more for less effect, *craving* — you want more, *withdrawal* — you suffer if you can't get more. To become dependent on a substance you have to take a certain amount on a regular basis. The safe level of alcohol ingestion is not known but liver disease and alcohol dependence are very unlikely if the intake is less than 2–3 pints of beer (4–6 units) 2–3 times a week for men (half this for women).

Alcoholism

This simply implies that someone is drinking more than they can cope with and are suffering as a result.

Many such people will be dependent — but not all. A feature of alcohol dependence is the withdrawal syndrome and is managed as above. The more serious the dependence the greater the risk of delirium tremens.

Patients with alcohol withdrawal syndrome and particularly those with delirium tremens may become extremely disturbed. Sedation in the first instance can be achieved with chlorpromazine. Give 100 mg i.m. then repeat with 50–100 mg aliquots every 20–30 minutes until the patient's behaviour is controlled. This regime is suitable for any acutely disturbed patient.

Wernicke's encephalopathy is a neurological condition involving ophthalmoplegia, ataxia and peripheral neuropathy. It is related to thiamine deficiency as is *Korsakov's syndrome*. This 'dysmnesic' syndrome usually occurs with some of the features of Wernicke's and the term Wernicke-Korsakov syndrome is now widely used. The dysmnesia takes the form of a complete loss of short-term memory. Attempts by the patient to restore some order results in confabulation. This symptom has probably been somewhat overplayed by diagnosticians and in practice is not a very dramatic feature.

Other drugs

Heroin

Heroin and other narcotics are extremely addictive — more so than alcohol. The withdrawal syndrome, particularly from heroin, is not as severe and often requires no medication. The difficulty for the heroin addict is usually not 'coming off' but staying off.

Cocaine

Cocaine and particularly its base 'crack' is extremely addictive and marked behavioural changes may occur. These are usually manic in form and very disturbed patients may require sedation.

Amphetamines

Amphetamines cause hyperactivity, but it is usually in withdrawal that the most serious behavioural changes are experienced. A psychosis involving paranoid delusions may occur, which in the short-term is indistinguishable from schizophrenia.

LSD

Lysergic acid diethylamide (LSD) can provoke vivid, visual hallucinations. These can sometimes be associated with bizarre behaviour when the images are particularly frightening. 'Flashback' experiences have been described where hallucinations occur long after the drug has been taken.

Solvent inhalation

This causes rapid mood change and, particularly in the very young, bizarre behaviour. Fortunately the volatile substances are quickly expired once the solvent is removed and the patient is allowed to breathe freely. In the western world, any child or young adult found to have acute neurological changes particularly involving behaviour and gait must first be assumed to be a solvent or drug abuser.

It is not only deliberate drug abuse that produces disturbed behaviour. The side effects of drugs taken for legitimate medical purposes may induce quite bizarre changes. *Extrapyramidal* side effects in the form of *dystonic reactions* are important and often not initially appreciated. 'Maxolon' (metoclopramide) and the phenothiazines are the commonest drugs to cause such reactions in practice, although many others have been described. Facial grimacing, torticollis and writhing movements of the arms are frightening for the patient and alarming for the doctor. Furthermore, the patient may appear to have a certain degree of 'control' and a diagnosis of 'hysteria' is often made in error. Consider the diagnosis in all patients with abnormal movements or posturings and seek a history of drug ingestion. Even if a confirmatory history is not forthcoming, it is worth giving benztropine 1 mg i.v. If it is a dystonic reaction then fairly rapid improvement should ensue.

Lithium toxicity primarily depresses the central nervous system, but giddiness and ataxia can occur. Clearly, such symptoms can be precipitated by a decreased renal clearance, or giving a diuretic to a patient already taking lithium.

Physical symptoms for which no organic cause can be found

In the A & E department, as in every other place where patients are interviewed, some individuals will have symptoms which are caused by mental stress or conflict alone. Some may suffer from definitive psychiatric illnesses, e.g. depression, anxiety states, hysterical conversion disorders, phobias or other psychoses. Others are responding to transient life situations. Patients also feign symptoms and fake physical signs for innumerable reasons (the 'deceivers'), e.g. malingerers, chronic artifactualists and examples of the Munchausen syndrome. Many do not fit any of these categories yet spend a lifetime visiting different doctors and hospitals with various complaints. Whether one calls this last condition hypochondriasis, a 'somatising' disorder, a personality problem or hospital dependency syndrome, illness for such people is a way of life, due in many cases to a learned pattern of aberrant behaviour beginning in childhood. The guises in which all these types of 'patients' present are endless. The symptoms can appear mild or severe and can affect a single or several bodily systems. The following points are important when dealing with this difficult area of medicine.

1. Psychologically determined illness can present with symptoms highly suggestive of physical illness. In western cultures a doctor's training is heavily biased towards the recognition of organic disease ('the scientific technician'), and a diagnosis of psychogenic disease tends to be arrived at, if at all, by exclusion. The training system is understandably designed to minimise the chances of overlooking physical pathology and to forestall the consequences of such a mistake — the potential adverse effect on the patient's health, loss of personal esteem and possible litigation. The upshot of the doctor's enslavement to the disease model tends to be multiple consultations and investigations which merely serve to reinforce the patient's illness behaviour.

2. A wide variety of medical illnesses can present with mental symptoms. For example, organic brain disease must always be excluded when hysterical conversion symptoms develop de novo in middle age. Likewise, occult malignancies may cause depressive symptoms many months before physical signs appear.

3. The borderline between psychoneurotic and physical illness is often vague. Some illnesses which were formerly considered 'functional' in origin have since been shown to have an organic basis (e.g. torsion dystonias, globus hystericus and postviral fatigue syndrome).

4 The symptoms of some organic illnesses can be exacerbated by psychological stress (e.g. bronchial asthma, angina and peptic ulceration).

5. Every physical illness is associated with some sort of emotional reaction. The patient's personality type may determine the type of reaction. For example, the immature, labile, hysterical personality often enjoys being the centre of attention despite the discomfort of illness, whereas the rigid obsessional individual is more likely to become anxious or depressed.

6. Within the presently accepted diagnostic framework, whether a patient is described as hysterical or malingering depends on the doctor's ability to attribute consciousness to the act, frequently an impossible task. In fact the borderline between hysteria (illness as a comfort), hypochondriasis (illness as a hobby), Munchausen syndrome (illness as a profession) and malingering (illness as a purpose) (Asher 1972) is very indistinct and, in many cases, largely semantic.

GENERAL POINTERS TO NON-ORGANIC ILLNESS

Although non-organic illness arises across the whole spectrum of humanity there are certain clues which may be given in the history and the physical examination which should alert the physician. Bizarre and exaggerated descriptions of symptoms (e.g. pain that is 'blinding', 'sickening' or 'like a red hot poker being pushed through me') accompanied by facial grimacing and abnormal postures is common. Alternatively there may be a marked disparity between the description of the severity of the symptoms and the patient's equable demeanour. Often the symptoms do not fit a readily identifiable disease pattern and they may be multiple and trivial, each systematic question from the doctor being answered in the affirmative. Such patients tend to have a heavy file of hospital notes, sometimes in several volumes, containing records of consultations with many different doctors, numerous investigations with mostly negative results, several small operations (e.g. otolaryngological or gynaecological) and, if anything, only minor ailments discovered. A history of psychiatric disease in the patient or his family, of previous neurotic personality traits and episodes of deliberate self-harm are also highly significant. Obvious secondary gain from the illness role may also become apparent during the history taking. Other situations which should bring on warning lights include:

1. Gross social deprivation, especially when the person is living alone in very straitened circumstances
2. Drug and alcohol abuse
3. Severe illness in a close relative or friend
4. Sexual problems
5. Recent bereavement, divorce or loss of job
6. Impending examinations or legal actions.

Doctors should especially beware of men who come from another hospital area complaining of severe pain. A number may be drug addicts and others may be examples of the Munchausen syndrome. Some attempt at corroboration of such patients' names and addresses and the identities of their family doctors should always be made.

Characteristic symptoms, ascribable to a bodily system, are common in functional states and are described under the appropriate disease heading. *Pain* is a unique symptom as it crosses all system barriers. It is very much a subjective experience and its intensity and the behaviour associated with it, vary from person to person. Also an individual's perception of pain at any one time depends on an interplay of emotional and environmental factors. Abnormal learned pain behaviour often begins in childhood, the most common site being the abdomen. Expressions of pain elicit sympathetic attention from oversolicitous parents and enable unpleasant activities to be avoided. With repetition, a pattern of behaviour is laid down which persists into adult life. Psychogenic pain tends to have some of the following characteristics:

1. Improbable descriptions
2. An onset which is vague with no obvious precipitant
3. Ill-localised and not corresponding to nerve distributions
4. Progression in severity and extent with time
5. Mood dependent variability
6. Relief by alcohol or tranquillisers
7. Multiple previous treatments.

Examination may reveal any of the following:

1. Exaggerated facial expressions
2. Abnormal postures
3. Frequent grunting, sighing and rubbing of the sore parts
4. Over-reaction to examination with apparent skin hypersensitivity and excessive guarding responses which can be partially or wholly eliminated by distracting the patient
5. Sensory disturbances which cross conventional dermatomes.

Using such clues, positive evidence can be built up, strongly suggestive of a psychogenic origin for a patient's pain. Simulated renal colic and low back pain are favourite complaints of drug addicts and other 'deceivers' wishing admission to hospital. However, it must never be assumed that inability to find a physical cause for a person's pain necessarily implies abnormal psychology or deception. In the A & E department, initially at least, all pain must be assumed to have a physical origin.

The non-organic disorders most likely to be encountered by the A & E physician are listed below and the recognition and management of each condition are described in turn:

Hypochondriasis
Depression
Anxiety (hyperventilation syndrome, panic attacks)
Conversion hysteria
Malingering (factitious illness)
Munchausen syndrome
Borderline disorders — compensation neurosis, irritable bowel syndrome, and postviral fatigue syndrome.

The A & E doctor should try to understand that most of these patients are 'dis-eased' and asking for help.

HYPOCHONDRIASIS

These patients manifest a distinctive triad. They become convinced that they have a disease, fear the consequences and are preoccupied with their bodies. In some cases the hypochondriacal complaints are secondary to a general psychiatric disturbance such as:

1. A depressive illness — in this case hypochondriacal preoccupations and delusions carry a high risk of suicide. Psychiatric advice should be sought immediately for such patients.
2. An anxiety state — hypochondriacal ideas are misinterpretations of normal physiological changes experienced at some time or another by nearly everyone.
3. A delusional illness such as schizophrenia, dementia or toxic confusional state.
4. Conversion hysteria or some other general neurotic disorder.

However, many patients with hypochondriacal beliefs have only mild, if any, disturbance of affect. They are convinced that they are physically ill, seek repeated medical consultations and steadfastly deny psychological complaints. Most have experienced maladaptive patterns of learnt behaviour as outlined in the description of non-organic pain, i.e. they find the sick role more rewarding than a healthy one. Many come from unhappy families with an unusual prevalence of alchohol abuse, sociopathic behaviour, illness and early death of a parent. A history of truancy is common, as is an inability to form lasting personal relationships. Such patients have little self-esteem, are often lonely and meeting and being touched by the doctor is very important to them. Women become particularly vulnerable around the menopause when they are likely to present at gynaecological clinics with pelvic pain, vaginal discharge or menstrual irregularities. After a careful physical examination these patients should be reassured that no evidence of serious disease has been found. They should then be referred back to their general practitioners for appropriate follow-up, as many will require reinforcement of the reassurance and, in some cases, family counselling.

DEPRESSION

Depression is a particular hazard of the convalescent period, especially after a life-threatening illness such as myocardial infarction, and is associated with delayed return to work and chronic invalidism. Common complaints are general lethargy, insomnia, loss of appetite and weight, constipation and reduced libido. Features of the mental state include:

1. Depression of mood
2. Feelings of guilt, unworthiness, self-blame and self-depreciation
3. Loss of hope in the future
4. Suicidal ideas or intentions
5. Depressive delusions
6. Hypochondriasis.

The clinical picture may be one of withdrawal or agitation. Often the diagnosis is obvious in the patient's mien.

The identification of the severely depressed patient who may also be actively suicidal is more fully described in Ch. 30. Such patients must be admitted to hospital and assessed urgently by a psychiatrist.

ANXIETY

Acute anxiety can lead to a variety of somatic symptoms such as tremulousness, dryness of the mouth, air swallowing, retching, stomach pains, diarrhoea, polyuria, chest pain and shortness of breath. Consequently, the patient may be suspected of having thyrotoxicosis, a cardiac dysrhythmia, peptic ulceration, diabetes

mellitus or ischaemic heart disease. The real basis of the symptoms is often given away by the tenseness of the individual — the flexing and unflexing of the fingers, the rhythmic contraction of the facial muscles and the staccato nature of speech. Having begun by asking questions relevant to the most likely organic disease suggested by the symptoms, some tactful probes into the patient's family life and job may uncover a major source of stress. Hypochondriacal ideas often appear following serious illness in a near relative and are caused by misinterpretation of normal physiological sensations amplified by anxiety.

Common physical findings are a fine tremor of the outstretched fingers, excessive perspiration, a sinus tachycardia and generalised hyper-reflexia. A diagnosis of thyrotoxicosis is unlikely in a young individual with the above symptoms in the absence of a goitre and 'eye signs' (see also factitious thyrotoxicosis). Also, feelings of depersonalisation are unusual in thyroid disease but are common in anxiety states.

A careful explanation of the mechanism of production of these unpleasant symptoms is essential. Some patients may deny that they have any worries. The illness has replaced the anxiety. The symptoms are unpleasant but not as unpleasant as the anxiety. One reason that patients resist treatment and doctors sometimes evade giving it is that, in order to restore health, the patient must first be given back his anxiety. Reassurance and some practical suggestions given in an atmosphere of confidence will often show the patient a solution to his problems. Many individuals find the mere situation of being a patient in an A & E department anxiety-provoking. The symptoms and signs produced by this anxiety can then override those due to organic disease. This possibility should always be kept in mind.

Panic attacks and hyperventilation syndrome

These are two particularly severe, interrelated forms of acute anxiety. Panic disorder is characterised by the sudden onset of an overwhelming sensation of terror, impending doom and imminent collapse, usually without any external understandable cause. The most common symptoms experienced during an attack are dyspnoea, palpitations, chest pain and faintness. Others include choking or smothering sensations, dizziness, trembling, tingling in the extremities, feelings of unreality and loss of control. The individual episodes do not usually last long but if they are not recognised and treated they lead to secondary avoidance responses with the development of agoraphobia. Depending on the severity and chronicity of the attacks, these patients should either be referred back to their general practitioners or to a psychiatrist.

Hyperventilation may be a prominent symptom during an attack. If it is followed by a Valsalva manoeuvre a faint, sometimes progressing to an epileptic fit, may ensue. Prolonged overbreathing can also result in tetany. These patients should be sedated and persuaded to rebreathe out of a paper bag. During mild attacks or when the hyperventilation is chronic the patient is often unaware of overbreathing and the symptoms may be so non-specific that making the diagnosis can be extremely difficult. Many sufferers are young women and simple instructions in relaxation and breathing control can help considerably. If there is any doubt about the diagnosis the arterial blood gases and pH should be measured. In psychogenic hyperventilation the PaO_2 will be normal, the $PaCO_2$ reduced and the patient alkalotic. Occasionally the clinical presentation of diabetic ketoacidosis superficially resembles that of the hyperventilation syndrome. Measurement of the arterial pH will prevent a potentially tragic misdiagnosis as diabetics will be acidotic.

CONVERSION HYSTERIA

At the outset it should be understood that 'hysterical conversion symptoms' and 'hysterical personalities' are two quite separate entities. Conversion hysteria is a condition in which physical symptoms are produced as a result of severe psychological stresses by a mechanism of which the subject is not fully aware. A hysterical personality, on the other hand, is the rather manipulative, theatrical person who likes the centre of the stage. The majority of patients developing hysterical conversion symptoms have never shown evidence of a hysterical personality.

Medicine has limitations in the detection of physical illness and psychiatrists have generally become very wary of diagnosing conversion hysteria. There are many recorded cases of 'hysterical' symptomatology being the first manifestation of serious physical illness. For this reason the label should be restricted to patients in whom the psychopathology has been clearly established. Two important points in this regard are: first, that the symptoms should be related to emotional conflict; and, second, that possible primary or secondary gain to the patient through the illness should be identified.

Keeping the above remarks in mind, the following points should lead to a suspicion of conversion hysteria. In few other types of patients are the symptoms likely to be described in more colourful language, heavily loaded with superlatives and exaggerated similes. Such descriptions may be emphasised by the use of contorted facial expressions and dramatic gestures or, alternatively, the most severe pain may be described with complete serenity (la belle indifference). Great detail is often used in recounting hysterical symptoms and they commonly involve more than one bodily system. However, it should be remembered that some patients exaggerate real symptoms because they think doctors will not otherwise take them seriously.

The most common hysterical symptom seen in the A & E department is pain. The pain may be very real to the patient but, unless he has some specialised knowledge, it is not usually typical of a particular disease. The general characteristics of non-organic pain have already been outlined. Other hysterical symptoms commonly involve the central nervous system — they include paralyses and pareses, sensory abnormalities, fits, coma, vertigo, aphonia, visual disturbances, urinary retention and dysphagia. A hysterical paralysis may appear to be flaccid yet, during handling of the limb, resistance to movement may develop. Sometimes contraction in the 'paralysed' limb can be felt while examining the opposite limb (Hoover's sign: downward movement of the 'paralysed' leg when the patient is asked to raise the normal leg). Sensory loss is often inconsistent and does not follow anatomical rules. Normal limb reflexes are usually present. In psychogenic paraplegia the sphincters remain unaffected. The classic visual field defect is a tubular constriction. Often the patient is very hesitant about his answers to testing of the visual fields and seems to be weighing up the pros and cons of his replies. In feigned unconsciousness there is often a tell-tale tremor of the eyelids and resistance to forcible eye opening. Hysterical seizures are one feature of Briquet's syndrome. These patients are young women with numerous somatic complaints, sexual problems being prominent and multiple hospital admissions. The fits may be provoked by suggestion. The patient may talk, scream or burst into tears during or immediately after the attack and tongue biting is uncommon. A particularly confusing association is that between true epilepsy and various hysterical manifestations. Bona fide grand mal fits may be interspersed with hysterical fits, and gross non-organic ataxias may mimic anticonvulsant drug intoxication.

Hysterical conversion symptoms are occasionally accompanied by fugue-like states, amnesia and pseudodementia (see Ch.30). The amnesia tends to be patchy and typically concerns details of personal life, especially personal identity. Amongst school-children, epidemics of imitative behaviour (e.g. fainting) have been described and hysterical amblyopia sometimes occurs in children stressed by imminent examinations.

Patients with hysterical complaints may present in the opening episode but, as is the case with hypochondriacs, many have a long medical history strewn with normal investigative results and notes of operations at which no pathology was found. It is often obvious from the medical records that several people have considered the symptoms to be psychoneurotic in origin.

Management

On first meeting a patient in the A & E department it is often extremely difficult and potentially dangerous to make an immediate diagnosis of a non-organic disorder. In most instances a physical cause for the symptoms has to be assumed and the examination and investigations directed towards identifying possible organic disease. Many patients will require referral to appropriate specialists either directly or via their general practitioners.

However, when the A & E doctor seriously suspects that the problem is non-organic the possibility should be openly discussed with the patient. If the patient knows that an open mind is being kept on the possibility that the true cause is organic, and that this is just a tentative examination of another possibility, then he/she will usually agree to co-operate. Sometimes the background psychological stresses and strains will be openly expressed, but more often it will be of the nature of an exploratory conversation. Great tact and patience needs to be exercised during the interview and at first the presenting symptom(s) should not be focused upon. Friends and relatives should not be present at the initial interview, as they may have helped precipitate or perpetuate the symptomatology. If the patient appears very anxious, a small amount of oral diazepam (5–10 mg) should be administered.

In the process of unravelling the stresses in the patient's life and demonstrating a temporal relationship with episodes of disease, the patient may become convinced of the truth. As the symptoms have arisen at an unconscious level to help the person cope with a stressful life situation, a simple explanation that there is nothing physically amiss is not enough — the underlying problem will remain but the coping mechanism will have been removed.

It is therefore important to spend some time explaining the nature of the illness to these patients and never to let them feel rejected. For instance, in dealing with the symptom of psychogenic pain, an explanation along the following lines might be attempted. To begin with, it should be realised that since the patient will have difficulty understanding that such pain could exist without an organic lesion, some mental picture of the mechanism of pain is necessary. It may be suggested to the patient that the upper part of the brain is more concerned with thinking and the lower part with the control of bodily functions such as the heart rate, respiration rate, peristalsis in the gut, secretions of different juices and co-ordinated movements of muscles. For health a careful integration of the functions of different organs and opposing muscle groups is necessary. If the thinking part of the mind is faced with very painful thoughts and feelings, these may be got rid of by pouring out one's grief to friends, crying, shouting and making scenes. It is also possible to get rid of them by repressing them, burying them deep in the mind and/or deciding not to think of them. It is these buried thoughts and feelings which, when pushed downwards, interfere with the co-ordinating function of the brain. The different organs or muscle groups then act out of harmony and symptoms are produced.

This type of explanation has the advantage of depicting the cause of pain as a genuine bodily dysfunction — a localised conflict. One is therefore not implying that the patient is dishonestly pretending to have pain. It also connects the relief of symptoms and understanding of the strains and worries which are its true cause. Naturally, any explanation of psychogenic symptoms has to be tailored to the intellectual capabilities, mood and personality of each patient.

Once the individual has insight into the root cause of his complaint, he can be assisted to face up to and deal with the underlying problem. Doctors who fail to diagnose psychogenic illness or fail to talk to their patients about it, co-operate with the neurotic factors in the situation and thereby help to make the illness more deep seated and difficult to reverse. Too much sympathy can have the same effect. A straightforward practical approach is best.

Patients who develop hysterical symptoms of sudden acute onset related to recognisable personal or social stresses have a good prognosis. Formal psychiatric help is rarely necessary. By contrast, patients with chronic personality disorders may be very difficult to treat and should be referred to a psychiatrist. Hysterical symptoms appearing for the first time in middle life should be treated with great suspicion. An underlying organic illness or depressive psychosis must be excluded.

DECEPTION

Malingering

Malingerers are individuals who deliberately feign or exaggerate illness or disability for a particular purpose. Depending upon the person's intelligence and knowledge of medicine, the clinical presentation may be a very obvious fake or may closely resemble a real illness. Thus children may want a rest from school or adults from an uninteresting job. Complaints of vague pains in the abdomen or chest may achieve this objective. Doctors and nurses, on the other hand, may present with sophisticated facsimiles of actual diseases (see below, 'factitious illness'). The clever malingerer picks one symptom and sticks to it. He knows that evasivenesss is a sure give-away. He may even try to put the unwary doctor off the scent by pretended dislike of illness.

Low back pain is clearly related to physical strain and therefore commonly experienced by people in occupations involving heavy manual labour. The malingerer is usually well versed in the straight leg raising test and cannot elevate one or both legs above 30° without apparent excruciating pain. However, when asked to sit up on the examination couch, he may not realise that this movement also tests hip flexion and give himself away.

The malingerer will be identified if it becomes clear that the act has been performed for a clear objective. Examples of typical situations are avoidance of a police summons, or of conscription, escape from intolerable life situations (e.g. family, job, prison or battlefield), a desire for free board and lodging, and drug addiction. Most A & E departments keep a list of people, with their physical descriptions and aliases, who repeatedly feign severe pain, usually either abdominal or pectoral, in order to obtain an injection of a narcotic analgesic. Because it may be difficult to attribute 'consciousness' to the act, there is considerable overlap between malingering and hysteria, especially when monetary gain is involved (see 'compensation neurosis' below). Indeed, the diagnosis may say more about the doctor than the patient. For many patients an episode of malingering is a once only phenomenon and, when recognised, should be dealt with in a perfectly straightforward fashion. Unfortunately doctors often display great unwillingness to consider malingering and confront the 'patient'. There are some other individuals who repeatedly mimic signs of disease. The Munchausen syndrome is rare and is described below. The larger group is much more ill-defined and comprises people who fabricate illness, often in very subtle and elaborate ways, with appropriate physical signs and abnormal laboratory findings (factitious illness). Any secondary gain from the illness, apart from puzzling the hospital staff, is hard to discern. Many are intelligent young women employed in medically related work. The range of abnormalities they may produce is extensive, e.g. hypoglycaemia produced by self-injection of insulin or ingestion of sulphonylureas; pyrexial illnesses either related to manipulation of thermometers or due to self-injection with contaminated materials; factitious thyrotoxicosis caused by taking thyroxine tablets; diarrhoea due to abuse of purgatives; bizarre skin lesions (dermatitis artefacta) induced by corrosives, needles or scalpels and apparent bleeding problems where patients have secretly put blood in their urine or sputum. A more recently recognised group are mothers who either spuriously complain of, or actually cause, illnesses in their children (Meadow's syndrome, see also under Child abuse, Ch. 5). All these patients lie in the vague hinterland between malingering and the Munchausen syndrome. They tend to have immature personalities and crave caring attention. Their relations with the ward staff are usually polite but aloof. Investigation and management can be very difficult as attempts are made to uncover the deception. In the end exposing the fraud is often thankless as it leads to criticism from relatives, a feeling of rejection in the patient and a prompt change of doctor. Direct confrontation should therefore be avoided if possible and, instead, some sort of roundabout approach employed.

Munchausen syndrome

This eponymous title was coined by Richard Asher in 1951 to describe patients who repeatedly feign a wide variety of illnesses in order to gain hospital admission. They appear to be addicted to medical or surgical care. They usually have thick files of notes in several hospitals (hence the alternative term 'hospital hoppers'), have undergone numerous uncomfortable investigations, and even operations, most of which have failed to uncover any abnormality, and have rapidly discharged themselves from hospital when challenged. Some carry diaries recording their hospital peregrinations. False names and addresses are often given to further the deception. Typically they are young to middle-aged males from the lower socioeconomic groups, who 'collapse' in the street far from home. The corollary is that patients who take ill in their own homes and are sent to hospital by their family doctors are rarely examples of Munchausen's syndrome. The presenting symptomatology ranges from acute abdominal emergencies, through bleeding from various orifices, to epileptic fits. The most unlikely diseases have been simulated (e.g. decompression sickness). If closely questioned these individuals tend to become increasingly truculent and leave hospital precipitously. The psychopathology of this condition is probably as varied as its physical presentation. A gross personality disorder underlies many cases and psychiatric treatment appears to do little to alter the aberrant behaviour pattern.

In considering all the foregoing conditions it cannot be emphasised often enough that organic disease must be carefully excluded. The coroner will not be impressed by a diagnosis of malingering or hysteria.

BORDERLINE DISORDERS

Compensation or post-traumatic neurosis

Recovery from illness, or in sociological terms 'relinquishing the sick role', is determined by many factors. These may be cultural or psychological. In a modern society, a very powerful influence is the prospect of monetary gain following litigation. The advantages of illness may then far outweigh the advantages of health.

Patients may prolong and elaborate their symptoms in relation to a claim for injury compensation. This is more likely to happen after an industrial or road traffic accident than after a sporting injury, and the incident may be quite trivial. Many cases are examples of more or less sophisticated fraud, but among others, especially unskilled workers of limited education, a compensation motive does not appear to have been consciously formulated. A major problem for the doctor is to decide how, in the absence of objective physical abnormalities, he should assess the severity and significance of complaints such as headaches, dizziness, fatigue, inability to concentrate, insomnia and alleged personality change (for a more detailed discussion see Ch.40). However difficult it may be, it is the responsibility of the senior A & E doctor to take a detailed history from and carefully examine these patients, and then give his honest opinion, both to the patient and the solicitor. Suspicion of simulation must not be evaded (see also Ch. 4).

Usually symptoms remit with settlement of the claim, although this is not always the case. They may persist if a disability pension is involved or if there is an underlying neurotic personality disorder, or if the claim is not settled for several years. Medicine would appear to have little to offer these latter patients. The answer probably lies in a simpler and more efficient medicolegal system.

Irritable bowel syndrome

Common abdominal symptoms of this disorder are a sensation of distension, rumbling, crampy or 'dragging' pains and constipation or diarrhoea, or both. The pain is sometimes relieved by defaecation or the passage of flatus and a change in stool frequency and consistency may occur at the onset of the abdominal discomfort. Defaecation may be accompanied by the passage of mucus and a sensation of incomplete evacuation. A major diagnostic criterion is the exclusion of organic disease. There is a strong association between psychosocial stress and this condition and, apart from alcohol abuse, a much weaker association with dietary change. Problems of coping with difficult life situations tend to precipitate exacerbations of symptoms. In order to exclude organic disease many of these patients have barium enema examinations. Occasionally a significant degree of spasm may be seen during fluoroscopy, usually in the descending colon. More commonly no abnormality is identified.

In most cases careful reassurance is all that is needed. The patient should be told that it is accepted that they have a 'real' condition but that it is not dangerous. An explanation of the effect of stress on the bowel can be followed by some simple advice on how to relax mentally. If abdominal symptoms are particularly troublesome, depending on their nature, an intestinal relaxant, antidiarrhoeal or laxative may help.

Postviral fatigue syndrome (also known as myalgic encephalomyelitis or Royal Free disease)

Some patients, following acute viral illnesses, continue to feel ill for many weeks or months. Typical symptoms include excessive tiredness and muscular fatiguability, unsteadiness and episodic amnesia and inability to concentrate. Such patients were originally thought to be hysterical, but within the past five years many have been demonstrated to have an abnormality of their immune response mechanism. Appropriate advice for sufferers is to take plenty of rest and not push themselves to their physical and mental limits.

SUMMARY

A discrepancy between symptoms and physical signs should raise the suspicion of a psychogenic disorder. Organic disease must always be carefully excluded. Drugs, carbon monoxide poisoning and many systemic diseases can produce a bewildering variety of symptoms and signs.

The diagnostic label attached to a patient is very important because it can erroneously influence subsequent medical decisions.

As it is often impossible to make a definitive diagnosis of non-organic disease in the A & E department the diagnostic labels mentioned in this chapter should be used sparingly. Many of these patients need to be observed over several weeks or months while background information is gathered and specialist investigations performed, before a clear picture emerges. Appropriate referral of the patient from the A & E department is therefore most important. When the A & E doctor uncovers underlying psychological problems he should give the patient support. Sometimes a clue to an impending episode of deliberate self-harm is half-hidden in the consultation.

REFERENCES

Asher R 1972 In: Jones Sir F A (ed) Richard Asher talking sense. Pitman Medical, Tunbridge Wells, p 149

Minor Conditions

INTRODUCTION

Most of the patients with minor conditions are ambulant. A designated area of the department is often set aside for their care. There are many more patients with minor than major conditions attending the department. Although the conditions from which they suffer are usually referred to as minor, and most of the patients are not very ill, nonetheless, improperly treated wounds, musculoskeletal disorders and septic conditions can lead to weeks of incapacity, and even permanent disability. It has been said that there are no such things as minor illnesses — only minor doctors. A well-trained doctor in A & E medicine should take pride in the correct diagnosis and treatment of these patients.

Most patients who should be called back for a review visit will have been seen initially in this area. It should be possible to review a few patients every day of the week. It should also be possible to perform minor surgery every day. At weekends, operating can be curtailed to a minimum, but the treatment of conditions such as acute abscesses or amputation of a finger-tip should not be postponed.

The number of specialist clinics held will vary from one department to another. The practice will depend largely on the special interests of the doctors in a particular department. There is much in favour of special clinics for head injuries and for hand injuries.

Patients who arrive at the walking area of an A & E department come to have a particular complaint or injury dealt with. This is not the place to elicit a detailed medical history and carry out extensive investigations. A patient presenting with a cut finger should be questioned about the circumstances of the injury, and then the finger should be thoroughly examined. Similarly, a patient who goes over on his ankle should have the main attention focused on the injured ankle. However, a good doctor will always be on the look-out for disease and will take pride in spotting the hypothyroid patient with a hoarse voice or the alcoholic with his shaking hand, even though the patients make no reference to these complaints.

It is very important to undress the patient sufficiently widely to allow a really adequate examination of the injured part. For knee injuries, trousers must be removed; for back injuries, everything but the underpants. On occasion patients lie about their accident and the doctor should always be prepared to suspect more widespread injury and to undress the patient completely. This is particularly true of non-accidental injury to children and 'battered wives'.

32

David H. Wilson

Wounds

INTRODUCTION

The excision and suture of wounds is a field of especial responsibility in the accident and emergency department. Many of the wounds are quite small in size, but none is too small to become infected. Some wounds, especially on the face, can have serious cosmetic implications; others, for instance on the hands, can result in serious disability, and wounds of the shin in an elderly patient require considerable expertise to obtain primary healing.

Every A & E department must have a departmental policy for the management of wounds. This should be reviewed frequently so that modifications and improvements can be introduced when necessary. The reputation of the department can be made or marred by the consideration given to the wounded patient and the skill with which the injury is treated.

The logical sequence to be followed for every patient is as follows:

1. Assessment of the wound, including the consideration of possible complications, such as damage to nerves (Fig. 32.1), tendons, major vessels or the underlying bone and the risk of infection.
2. The operation:
   a. preparation of the patient and the wound
   b. anaesthesia
   c. cleansing and excision of the wound
   d. repair of the wound
   e. dressing of the wound
   f. recording the treatment.
3. Follow-up treatment:
   a. removal of sutures
   b. rehabilitation.

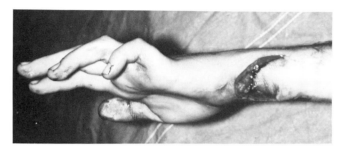

Fig. 32.1 A clean incised wound which has divided the ulnar nerve, causing clawning of the ring and little fingers. The nerve, the tendon of flexor carpi ulnaris and the skin were all repaired as a primary procedure.

ASSESSMENT OF THE WOUND

During assessment of the wound the patient should be screened from the view of others and a couch should be available. A relative or friend should accompany a child or an adult with communication problems (such as deafness, mental deficiency or language barrier).

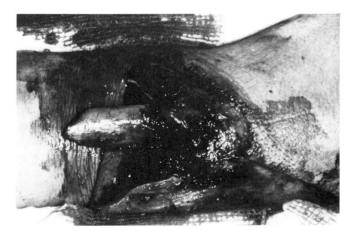

Fig. 32.2 This contaminated, open fracture of the forearm had occurred 3 hours earlier when the patient, a miner, was injured by machinery at the coalface.

The history of the accident must be recorded, including the time, circumstances and mechanism of the injury (Fig. 32.2). In a road traffic accident it is necessary to note the speed of impact to appreciate the possibility of internal shearing stresses. The possibility of oil, grease or foreign body penetration into the wound must be considered (Fig. 32.3). The patient must also be questioned about previous tetanus immunisation, any sensitivity reactions or other significant illnesses.

Patients with major wounds or wounds in special sites (stab wounds or gunshot wounds of the trunk) should be admitted to hospital after the application of a sterile dressing. If analgesia, antitetanus or antibiotic injections are given in the A & E department before admission to hospital, the dosage, time and route of injection must be clearly indicated on the patient's record.

Wounds in special sites, such as the eye or the hand are discussed in the appropriate chapters. Burns and the problem of foreign bodies, gun shot wounds and bomb injuries are also all dealt with in their respective chapters.

The description of the wound must include the anatomical site (a diagram or drawing is often helpful) and also the type of wound. An appreciation of the different types of wound is essential for planning the appropriate treatment and anticipating any complications.

Incised wound

A clean incised wound is unlikely to pose problems for repair of the skin, but haemorrhage and damage to tendons or nerves may be a problem. A dirty incised wound will require thorough surgical toilet and possible prophylactic antibiotic therapy.

Contused wound

In this condition the skin has split due to blunt trauma. Tendons and nerves are less likely to be damaged but the skin will heal less readily. Dead or devitalized tissue must be resected or the wound will become infected. Ragged skin edges must be trimmed to give as neat a scar as possible (Fig. 32.4).

Penetrating wound

When a knife, nail, wire or needle has penetrated deeply into the tissues, it is usually impractical to explore and excise the whole track (Fig. 32.5). In such circumstances more reliance must be placed on prophylactic antibiotics.

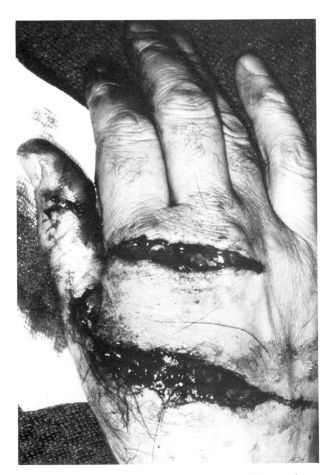

Fig. 32.3 This injury occurred in a brush-making factory. The wounds were contaminated by bristles and oil. Primary healing was obtained after thorough cleaning and removal of all foreign material.

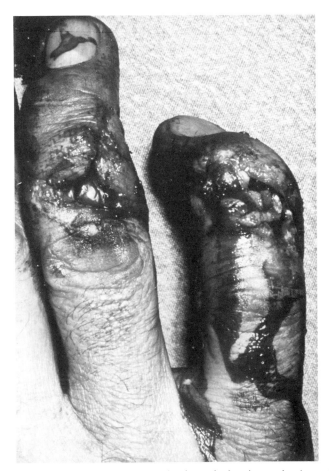

Fig. 32.4 These contused wounds require thorough cleansing, exploration and resection of devitalised tissue. Temporary splinting will aid wound healing.

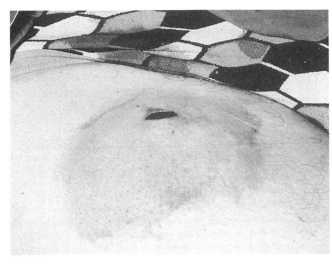

A

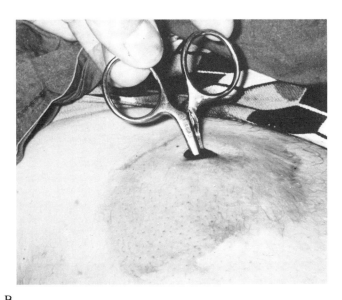

B

Fig. 32.5 A This small wound occurred when a butcher's knife slipped in the course of his work and penetrated his groin. **B** Artery forceps give an indication of the depth of the penetrating wound shown in **A**.

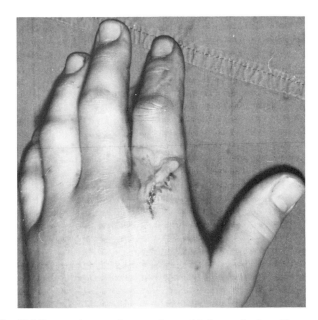

Fig. 32.6 Pus running out of a wound caused 3 days earlier by a blow against human teeth.

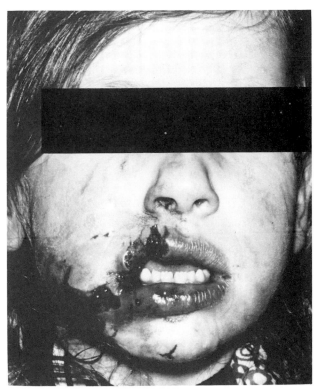

Fig. 32.7 Dog bites of the face of a young girl. Prompt reconstruction by a plastic surgeon is required to give a good cosmetic result.

Bites

Animal or human bites are always contaminated by a variety of oral bacteria (Fig. 32.6). The wounds should be treated with an antiseptic dressing and not sutured. If necessary, secondary suture can be considered after three days if the wounds are then clean. An exception to this policy is the problem of facial wounds, as for instance when a dog savages a child (Fig. 32.7). The excellent blood supply to the facial skin and importance of obtaining minimal scarring justify the risk of primary suture under an antibiotic cover. It is advisable to refer such a patient to a plastic surgeon for initial treatment. This problem is discussed more fully in Ch. 33.

Degloving wounds

When skin has been torn or sheared off from the underlying subcutaneous tissue, whether or not it will survive if repositioned depends on several factors: the width of the base compared with the length of the degloved flap, the degree of trauma and contamination of the loose skin and underlying tissue, the natural blood supply to the area, and the skill with which the wound is treated (Fig. 32.8). Contrasting examples are the scalp, which has a rich blood supply and usually heals well, and the skin on the front of the shin which has a poor blood supply and is slow to heal. The problem of the shin wound is discussed later in this chapter. Degloving of the ring finger usually necessitates amputation.

Friction wounds

These are of two varieties. One is when the patient skids over an immovable surface, as when a cyclist slides along a road (Fig. 32.9). The other is when part of a patient, usually the forearm, is trapped between moving rollers. The first wound will heal well because only the epidermis has been removed, but it is essential (under an anaesthetic) to scrub out any embedded gravel or dirt using a sterile nail brush. Otherwise the wound will become infected and there will be permanent tattooing of the skin. The second type of wound may not look so serious on the surface but, because the skin has often been sheared off the underlying subcutaneous tissue, the blood supply has been interrupted and the skin will die (Fig. 32.10). This latter type of wound should

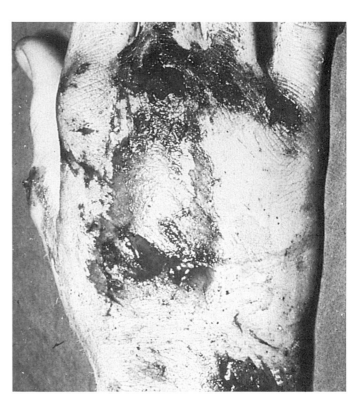

Fig. 32.9 This patient's hand slid along the road. Under a general anaesthetic dirt and gravel were removed by a scrubbing brush and the point of a scalpel.

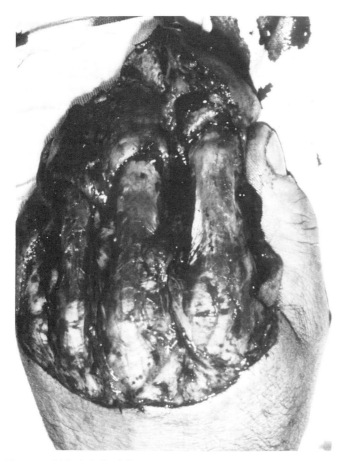

Fig. 32. 8 This degloving injury occurred at work. Most of the skin was still viable; only a small portion had to be resected and replaced by a skin graft.

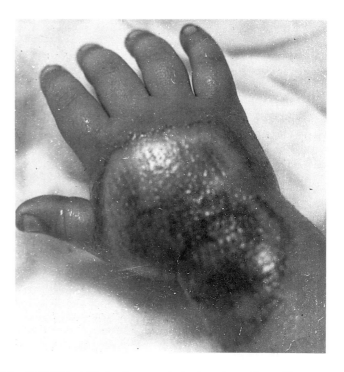

Fig. 32.10 This child's hand was caught in the wringer of a washing machine. The skin was anaesthetised and was later removed and replaced by a skin graft.

be referred to a plastic surgeon, who will consider the necessity of excision and skin grafting.

Wounds contaminated by foreign bodies

Metal or glass embedded in a wound will be demonstrated on a soft tissue radiograph (Fig. 32.11). If this type of foreign body is only 1–2 mm in size and deeply embedded, searching for it may cause more harm than is justified. The procedure should only be undertaken with the help of radiographic fluoroscopy in the operating theatre (see Ch. 39).

Larger pieces of metal or glass and all embedded pieces of wood or radiotranslucent plastic or crayon should be removed when exploring the wound. Oil or grease in the wound is particularly troublesome. If not completely removed, it will subsequently create a painful oil granuloma.

The optimum result of the treatment of the wound depends largely on a full and correct assessment. It is at this early stage that mistakes are so easily made, when the full implication of the injury and the possible complications are not appreciated. An extra minute or two spent on making a comprehensive assessment can save the patient from unnecessary suffering, can save the hospital and the staff the expense and time involved in treating complications, and can save the doctor from possible litigation.

THE OPERATION

Preparation of the patient and the wound

It is essential to explain to the patient the proposed programme

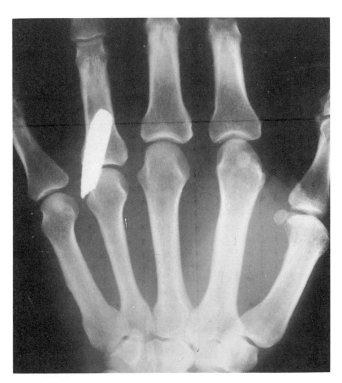

Fig. 32.11 This metallic foreign body, lying alongside the flexor sheath, was not detected at the initial clinical examination.

of treatment and how long it will take. If general anaesthesia is to be used, the patient must sign a consent form and questions must be asked about the last time he took food or drink. Ideally four hours should elapse between the last ingestion and the anaesthetic. Any problems with previous anaesthetics should be noted. Negro patients should be screened for sickle abnormality.

Dirty wounds can undergo preliminary cleansing before reaching the operating theatre — by soaking in a bowl of 0.5% cetrimide and 0.05% chlorhexidine and the use, if necessary, of an industrial hand cleanser to remove grease or oil. With minor industrial hand injuries, the patient can slowly and gently do this preparatory work himself.

Anaesthesia

This is described in Ch. 9.

Cleansing and excision of the wound

Although cleaning the skin around the wound with a sterile, antiseptic solution is an essential part of wound treatment, it is not adequate to prevent infection. The depths of the wound must also be cleansed with a non-irritant solution such as 0.5% aqueous cetrimide and 0.05% chlorhexidine. Then all foreign matter, solid objects, dirt, grease or oil must be removed.

Next, using scapel and dissecting forceps, all devitalized tissue is excised. It requires surgical judgement to decide between inadequate excision of the dead tissue and unnecessary mutilation of the patient. Dead tissue will not spring back to life; it will only form a focus for infection. Too wide an excision may result in a cosmetically unacceptable scar which will subsequently require reconstructive surgery.

In a wound already more than 6 hours old (even though it was originally a clean incised wound), bacteria will have penetrated into the exposed tissue, making it necessary to excise the edges of the wound. In areas of rich blood supply, such as the face, only 1–2 mm of tissue should be removed, but in less vascular areas the excision should extend to 4–5 mm. Even in fresh clean wounds, jagged edges of skin should be removed to give a near linear scar.

Before starting to repair the wound, the degree of haemostasis must be such that healing will not be disrupted by haematoma formation. Stagnant, clotted blood in the depths of a wound will retard healing and invite infection. It is also important to check again for severed tendons or nerves and to probe for any fracture in the proximity of the wound or any retained foreign body.

Repair of the wound

Wounds may be repaired by (1) primary closure, (2) delayed primary closure, or (3) skin grafting.

Primary closure

In a wound which involves skin and subcutaneous tissues only, one layer of sutures is usually sufficient. However, if the wound is deep enough to breach the deep fascia or (in a scalp wound) the galea, these structures should be repaired using an absorbable suture.

Skin closure should be achieved using the smallest size of suture which is strong enough for the purpose. Either catgut or synthetic monofilament sutures, swedged onto an atraumatic cutting needle, in the 0.5–3.0 metric gauge (6/0 to 3/0) range are recommended (Table 32.1).

Catgut sutures are recommended for wounds in children (except on the face) and for hand wounds in adults, because they dissolve in 10–14 days and do not need to be removed.

If the wound is linear, place the first suture in the middle to divide it into two equal halves, then introduce the second and third sutures at the quarter and three-quarter points along the wound. This technique, as opposed to starting from one end, avoids distortion of the wound as it is closed. If the wound is jagged, the first few sutures should be used to appose angles and corners which serve as anatomical markers. The needle should take an equal 'bite' of tissue at each side of the wound and the knot should be tied so as to appose the wound edges precisely, without either leaving gaps of exposed subcutaneous tissue or, conversely, inverting the wound edge. Healing is a biological process and the wound is not to be 'tied up like a parcel'. A knot tied too tight strangles the tissue within it so that it dies and becomes infected.

An alternative to sutures is the use of sterile strips of reinforced microporous tape. These can be applied without causing any pain, and are therefore suitable for clean superficial wounds in children. The main objection to their use is that they are so quick, simple and convenient that doctors and nurses are tempted to use them for wounds which require proper cleansing and exploration under anaesthetic, either local or general. However, provided that high standards of exploration and excision are maintained, there is no valid objection to their use.

The technique of application is to stretch the skin smooth on one side of the wound and apply the tape there. The free end of tape is then used to pull this edge towards the opposing side of the wound, the skin of which is also held slightly stretched during application. If a little blood emerges from the wound, it can be mopped up with gauze — the blood has no difficulty in passing through the pores of the tape. It should not be applied in overlaping layers: this destroyes its porous quality, and leaves a pabulum of blood for the growth of bacteria close to the wound. A space of 3–6 mm should be left between one strip and the next. Strips of tape are particularly valuable for the thin skin of patients on long-term steroid treatment.

Table 32.1 Recommended suture sizes

Suture size	Adult	Child
2.0 (3/0)	Scalp, trunk arm, leg	—
1.5 (4/0)	Hand	Scalp, trunk, arm, leg
1.0 (5/0)	Face	Hand
0.5 (6.0)	—	Face

Delayed primary closure

This technique should be used for most wounds caused by animal or human bites or where there has been obvious contamination by anaerobic organisms as in farmyard injuries. If, after excision of any wound, there is still doubt about the viability of some of the surrounding tissue, or if the wound is more than 12 hours old when first seen, primary closure is inadvisable. After thorough toilet these wounds should be covered by a tulle gauze supported by an absorbent dressing and firm bandage.

The need for systemic antibiotic therapy should be considered. After three to five days, when the dressing is removed, a clean bright red granulating wound should present. If this cannot be sutured without tension, partial-thickness skin graft should be used.

Skin grafting

Free partial-thickness skin grafts are occasionally necessary for primary or delayed primary closure in the A & E department. They are used to replace small areas of skin loss where primary suture is impossible or would create tension in the wound. Their disadvantages are that they shrink as they heal, they never achieve normal sensory innervation and they cannot be used over exposed tendons, bone or joints. When such tissues are exposed and primary suture is not practicable (or when there is extensive tissue loss), full-thickness grafts are less likely to take than partial-thickness grafts and should seldom by used in an A & E department.

Wounds in special sites

These are dealt with in the appropriate chapters: wounds in the hand in Ch. 34, in the eye and eyelids in Ch. 43 and in the ear, nose and throat in Ch. 44.

Scalp wounds

Hair around scalp wounds should be shaved to a distance of at least 2 cm but, if possible, the hair margin of the scalp should be preserved. Hair will grow again or, if not, there will not have been much there in the first place to be missed! However, *do not shave the eyebrows;* they will only regrow slowly and imperfectly. Careful cleansing and excision of scalp wounds is followed by palpation of the skull under the wound, using a gloved finger or a sterile proble, to detect or exclude a fracture. Bleeding occurs from vessels which are superficial to the galea and they cannot easily be grasped by artery forceps. Digital pressure around the wound edges will diminish the bleeding, which will be controlled as the galea and skin are sutured.

The shin

The circulation of the skin on the front of the leg is poor and wounds in this site heal slowly — particularly in the elderly and in patients who have been on steroids for long periods. Wounds

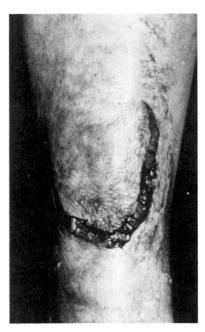

Fig. 32.12 This proximally based flap on the shin of an elderly patient can be sutured — but tension must be avoided.

in such patients are usually produced by blunt injury and are often triangular in shape. If the subcutaneous fat is still intact in the flap and if the flap is based proximally, it is reasonable to replace it and suture the wound wholly or partially, provided that this can be done without tension (Fig. 32.12).

Alternatively the wound edges can be brought together with sterile adhesive strip dressings which peel off if the tension is too great (Fig. 32.13). Any unclosed portion may require a delayed skin graft. If, however, the flap is distally based and if the skin has been stripped off the underlying fat, it will be anaesthetic and avascular and is better removed (together with any underlying loose fat) at the initial visit (this requires no anaesthesia). Some 3–5 days later, the exposed fat (or deep fascia) is covered with a spilt skin graft taken from the thigh, using a lateral femoral cutaneous block. The graft is carefully laid (without anaesthesia) onto the defect and covered with carefully tailored non-adherent gauze and polyurethane sponge. These are kept in place with strips of microporous tape, and should then be covered with gauze, wool bandage and an elastic stocking. The limb should be kept elevated at home, and reviewed again in a week. This method of delayed primary closure need not involve general anaesthesia or hospitalisation, and if primary healing follows (as it usually does) the patient is saved repeated journeys to the hospital for dressings, which are necessary if one waits for the slough to separate before secondary skin grafting can be carried out.

Dressing the wound

This is discussed in Ch. 38.

Recording the treatment

This is the essential concluding part of the opertaion. It must be done immediately while the details are fresh in the mind, and should include the following items.

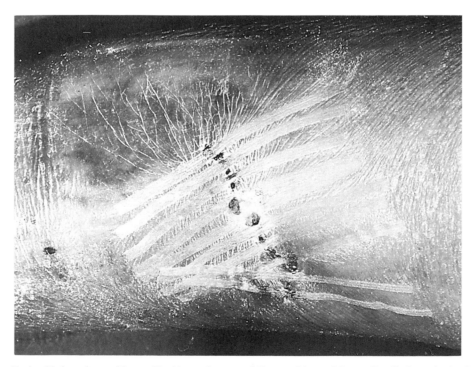

Fig. 32.13 Wounds of the skin in elderly patients with atrophic skin can be successfully treated by applying sterile adhesive strip dressings. This must only be done after thorough cleansing of the wound.

1. The type, dosage and route of anaesthesia used.

2. The anatomical site and extent of the wound (drawings are useful).

3. The operative findings, including a note on the presence or absence of associated injuries to tendons, nerves or vessels.

4. The nature, size and number of sutures used.

5. The type of dressing applied (if any).

6. Details of injections (especially antitetanus) and any analgesics prescribed for the postoperative period.

7. An indication of the instructions given to the patient about follow-up treatment.

8. The operator's signature.

FOLLOW-UP TREATMENT

Removal of sutures

The use of catgut sutures which drop off in 10–14 days obviates much of the tedious and painful work of removing sutures. This is particularly valuable in children and in patients with finger injuries. When patients leave the department, they should be told to return at once if they are worried; otherwise they should attend for the removal of non-absorbable sutures at times for which a guide is set out below. Changing the dressing or inspecting the wound before then is meddlesome and painful and should be avoided if possible.

Time for removal of sutures
Face, head and neck — 3 or 4 days
Arm and hand — 7 days
Trunk, lower limb and the extensor surface of joints 10–14 days.

Rehabilitation

After removal of the sutures the majority of patients can be discharged and return to their normal activities. However, some patients with more serious wounds may require a period of rehabilitation. This is particularly relevant in hand injuries (see Ch. 34). Patients who engaged in contact sports should be given precise advice about training and as to how soon they can play again (see Ch. 36). Elderly patients with wounds on the shin may be well advised to wear a protective dressing for some weeks until the skin becomes sufficiently strong to withstand further minor trauma.

PREVENTION OF INFECTION IN WOUNDS

General principles

Attention to personal hygiene is the first contribution to avoiding wound infection. Farmers, gardeners, people working with animals and employees exposed to oil, dust or chemicals in industry, must all maintain an adequate level of personal cleanliness. People who tend to suffer from recurrent sepsis can use a chlorhexidine soap, but the repeated use of antibiotics must be avoided.

The prompt and efficient treatment of minor wounds is also important; be it a mother caring for her children at home or a school teacher attending to a pupil's injury. Health and safety at work legislation has improved and regularised first aid care in industry.

When a patient seeks professional medical care for an injury the level of responsibility is greatly increased. Doctors in emergency departments must be expert in the assessment and appropriate treatment of open wounds. Wound toilet, exploration, excision and closure, by either primary suture or skin graft, should preclude the development of infection. As described above, delayed primary closure is indicated if the wound is seriously contaminated as with animal bites or farmyard injuries or if the viability of the skin is in doubt. After toilet and excision the wound can be dressed and reassessed in 3 or 4 days time. Leaving debris or dead tissue in a wound, neglecting to remove a foreign body, allowing a haematoma to develop in the wound or suturing the skin under tension, all predispose to wound infection.

Tetanus prophylaxis

Prevention of the catastrophe of developing tetanus depends mainly in good surgical toilet and excision of a wound, secondly on tetanus immunisation and least of all on the use of prophylactic antibiotics. The occasion of the injury should be used to start or renew tetanus immunisation, whether or not the particular wound carries a serious risk of tetanus. The following programme is now widely agreed.

The patient's state of immunity is first classified as follows.

Category A   The patient has had a complete course of tetanus toxoid or a booster injection within the past five years. (A complete course is three injections given at day 1, 6 weeks and 6 months. Each injection is 0.5 ml.)

Category B   The patient has had a complete course of tetanus toxoid or a booster injection between 5 and 10 years ago.

Category C   The patient has had a complete course of tetanus toxoid or a booster injection more than 10 years ago.

Category D   The patient has not had a complete course of tetanus toxoid or his state of immunity is unknown.

The wound is then classified as clean or tetanus prone, and treatment given as follows.

Clean wounds: less than 6 hours old, non-penetrating, tidy and not contaminated, negligible tissue damage

Category A	Nothing more required
Category B	Toxoid booster
Category C	Toxoid booster
Category D	Toxoid — full course

Tetanus prone wounds: those which do not fulfil all the criteria of a clean wound.

Category A	Nothing more required
Category B	Toxoid booster
Category C	Toxoid booster + 1 ml human antitetanus serum
Category D	Toxoid — full course + 1 ml of human antitetanus serum.

Note. When giving both toxoid and human antitetanus serum, they should be injected at different sites. If the wound is already old and infected when first seen, antibiotic therapy will be indicated to treat the infection but it should not be relied upon to prevent tetanus on its own.

Rabies prophylaxis

Patients also present at A & E departments because of real or suspected contact with rabid animals while abroad. The following recommended procedure is taken from the DHSS 1984 publication *Immunisation against infectious disease.*

Should an outbreak in animals occur, and a rabies-infected area be declared, vaccination would need to be offered, as appropriate, to those persons directly involved in control measures and to veterinary surgeons within the infected area and their ancillary staff.

Human rabies is a notifiable disease. In the event of a case of human rabies, the medical officer for environmental health or, in Scotland, the chief administrative medical officer, should be informed. Detailed advice on the management of an outbreak appears in the *Memorandum on Rabies* issued by the DHSS in 1977, and this should be referred to. Scottish arrangements are detailed in the SHHD *Memorandum on Rabies* of 1977.

The treatment of persons with a history of exposure, i.e. a bite, a scratch or an abrasion by an animal suspected or known to be suffering from rabies should be started as soon as possible after exposure and should consist of both local and systemic approaches using active and passive immunisation.

Human diploid cell vaccine (HDCV) is the vaccine of choice. 1 ml of vaccine should be given by deep subcutaneous or intramuscular injection on days 0, 3, 7, 14, 30 and 90. (Day 0 is the day the patient receives the first dose.)

Passive immunisation with human rabies immunoglobulin (HRIG) provides rapid immune protection for a short period and can be used in combination with HDCV in postexposure treatment to cover the delay associated with active immunisation. Human rabies immunoglobulin is obtained from the plasma of vaccinated human donors. Its content is standardised to 150 i.u. per ml and dosage is dependent on body weight. Up to half the dose should be thoroughly infiltrated in the area of the wound, and the rest administered intramuscularly. No more than the recommended dose should be given. A total dose of 20 i.u. per kg body weight should be administered. Local pain and low grade fever may follow receipt of rabies immunoglobulin, but no serious adverse reactions have been reported.

Soft-tissue infections

This chapter deals with soft-tissue infections, which arise spontaneously or follow an injury. Systemic infections are only discussed when they may complicate the local infection. The chapter is divided into three main sections:

> 1. Factors which may precipitate or aggravate infections
> 2. Diagnosis
>   a. general principles
>   b. specific infections
> 3. Treatment
>   a. general principles
>   b. treatment of abscesses and soft-tissue infection in specific anatomical sites

FACTORS WHICH MAY PRECIPITATE OR AGGRAVATE A SOFT TISSUE INFECTION

Age

Very young children are unable to give a history and may be unable to locate their pain precisely. The elderly often have less resistance to infection and sometimes hesitate to 'trouble the doctor' until infections are well advanced.

Metabolic and systemic diseases

Patients with rheumatoid arthritis are particularly liable to develop suppurative arthritis (and many of such patients are also on steroids). Although the diabetic patient does not develop infections more commonly than other patients, when he does, the infection tends to spread rapidly. The patient's dosage of insulin will usually need to be increased until the infection is overcome. Patients who are in chronic renal failure are particularly liable to infection and must be managed promptly and carefully. Ulcerative colitis and

Crohn's disease may be associated with odd infections (such as pyoderma gangrenosum), as may the collagen vascular diseases and some of the blood dyscrasiae. The acquired immune deficiency syndrome (AIDS) will become an increasingly frequent underlying cause of skin and soft tissue infections.

Drugs

Many of the patients with the conditions mentioned above may need treatment which includes the use of steroids, immunosuppressive drugs or cytotoxic drugs. In the presence of infection the dose of these drugs may need to be modified.

Ischaemia

Poor peripheral circulation in a toe or a finger is paricularly liable to be followed by a spreading infection which, because of its demand for an increased blood supply, may progress to peripheral gangrene (Fig. 33.1). This in turn may be complicated by anaerobic

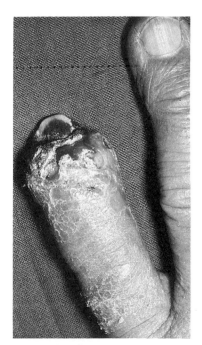

Fig. 33.1 Diabetic gangrene in a finger tip.

infection, followed by further tissue destruction and proximal spread. In the fingers particularly, the presence of a diminished blood supply may not be suspected until an infection brings the patient to hospital. In such patients the severity of the pain may be out of all proportion to the physical signs. In the fingers a poor peripheral circulation may follow injury to the arterial blood supply in the limb, atheromatous changes, collagen vascular disease or Raynaud's phenomenon. In the toes, arteriosclerosis, diabetes and Buerger's disease are common causes of peripheral arterial disease.

Neurogenic dysfunction

The response to infection is modified in such patients due to a lack of pain. In the foot, so-called 'perforating ulcers' may be associated with diabetic neuropathy (Fig. 33.2). Such ulcers occur in association with other diseases of the nervous system, including peripheral nerve injuries, long-standing anterior poliomyelitis, leprosy (Fig. 33.3), syringomyelia (Fig. 33.4), spina bifida and paraplegia.

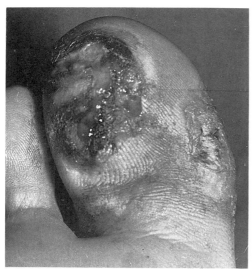

Fig. 33.2 This undiagnosed diabetic patient had a mild diabetic neuropathy which contributed to this poorly localised necrotising infection in the pulp of his right big toe.

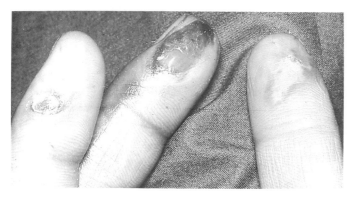

Fig. 33.3 Finger tip burns in a patient with a peripheral neuropathy caused by leprosy.

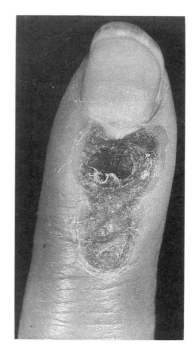

Fig. 33.4 This patient, who suffered from syringomyelia, did not come to hospital with this infection earlier because he did not feel pain.

Lifestyle and mental illness

The chronic alcoholic patient or the person who is addicted to intravenous drugs is prone to develop soft-tissue infections. Patients who are depressed, malnourished or vagrant and who will not, or cannot, care for themselves, frequently present with a variety of such infections. It is always important to consider if the infection is indicative of a more general and more serious malady.

DIAGNOSIS

The diagnosis of soft tissue infection is usually easy. The patient complains of a characteristic throbbing pain, which, in a limb, is made worse by movement. They may also feel ill and have a raised temperature. Inspection and palpation reveal an area of redness, swelling and tenderness.

The infection may be contained within the dermis or may also involve the subcutaneous tissue. Localisation of the infection by the body defences can lead to abscess formation. Conversely, if the infecting organism secretes a fibrinolysin, the inflammation can spread widely, creating a cellulitis.

Further clinical evidence will be seen if the infection is carried proximally by the lymphatics to the regional lymph nodes. The ascending lymphangitis presents as red lines passing up a limb to axilla or groin, where the lymphadenitis produces painful and tender swollen lymph nodes.

The differential diagnosis is important because many conditions masquerade as infection. They include trauma, metabolic diseases such as gout, acute exacerbation of rheumatoid arthritis, and even neoplasms (such as the 'so-called' inflammatory carcinoma of the breast). An acute reaction to a sting or an injection of tetanus toxoid may be misdiagnosed as an abscess, as may some congenital lesions, such as a branchial cyst.

The true diagnosis can usually be made on clinical grounds alone, provided an accurate history is obtained and a thorough physical examination is performed. The history must include details of any previous illness or injury and the time relationship involved. Not infrequently the patient will relate his present painful symptoms to an injury, but careful questioning will reveal that the onset of symptoms were quite unrelated to the injury.

The superficial symptoms may arise from a deep-seated infection through a sinus or fistula or may lead eventually to the discovery of a retained foreign body or osteomyelitis in an underlying bone. Cellulitis overlying a long bone should always raise the possibility of a diagnosis of osteomyelitis.

Aids to diagnosis include the use of a stethoscope to detect crepitus, a sterile probe to explore a sinus or sound a foreign body and a soft-tissue radiograph to demonstrate gas in the tissues or a radio-opaque foreign body.

Specific infections of the skin

Staphylococcal infection occurs in the skin as a furuncle or boil arising in an infected hair follicle; a carbuncle results from infection developing in many adjacent hair follicles. A sebaceous cyst may have been present for months or years before it becomes infected and presents as a painful swelling with a characteristic punctum.

Streptococcal infection of the skin, *erysipelas*, is now an uncommon condition. It produces an acutely red area of thickened skin with a precise border, and typically appears on the skin of the face.

Tuberculosis of the skin, *lupus vulgaris*, is now extremely rare in the developed countries.

Anthrax, usually contracted from handling raw hides or carcasses, is fortunately also now rare in the UK. Inoculation of the skin produces a dark coloured necrotising malignant pustule, which may be accompanied by a fulminating septicaemia. (Inhalation can result in a haemorrhagic bronchopneumonia, wool sorters' disease.) Fortunately the anthrax bacillus remains sensitive to penicillin and either form of the disease can be treated successfully with this antibiotic.

Pseudomonas pyocyanea and *Proteus vulgaris* often colonise and infect burns. Although of low grade pathogenicity these organisms may occasionally cause a dangerous septicaemia. A *Pseudomonas* infection has a characteristic odour and forms green-colour pus.

Infection of the subcutaneous tissues

This sometimes presents as a spreading cellulitis, usually due to streptococcal infection. More frequently the infection is localised, pus forms and an abscess is produced.

Staphylococcus aureus is the most common organism found in subcutaneous abscesses; sometimes it participates in a combined infection with the *β-haemolytic streptococcus* and this may result in a severe necrotising local inflammation with destruction of tissue, proximal spread along the lymphatics, and possibly septicaemia.

Escherichia coli, together with *Bacteroides,* are frequently found in lesions around the anal canal, such as perianal and ischiorectal abscesses. The foul smell of the pus is characteristic. Wounds in the proximal part of the thighs, the buttocks or the perianal region may also be contaminated with other anaerobic organisms such as *Clostridium welchii* which can produce gas gangrene.

Mycobacterial infections. *Tuberculosis* may present as a subacute infection in the skin and soft tissues: this is seen particularly in the Asian population in the UK. Infection in wounds sustained in swimming pools, aquaria and fish tanks may be caused by *Mycobacterium marinum* (formerly *M. balnei*). Acid-fast organisms should be sought in any such wound which is slow to heal.

Other sources of soft tissue and skin infections which may present to an A & E department include *herpes simplex* or *herpes zoster,* especially if it is secondarily infected (Fig. 33.5). Fungal infections around the toes or finger nails and infections due to parasites such as scabies, ticks, lice and bed bugs are not uncommon.

Bites and other infections transmitted by animals

Human saliva contains a mixture of staphylococci, streptococci and

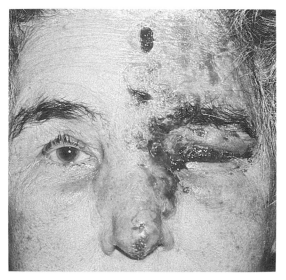

Fig. 33.5 Secondary infection of ophthalmic herpes requires antibiotic therapy.

Proteus vulgaris and other organisms which can produce extensive tissue destruction and spreading infection.

Cats and dogs and some other mammals' bites transmit the organism *Pasteurella multocida* which, whilst producing a virulent local infection, is sensitive to penicillin.

Bite wounds are all potentially infected and it is wise to clean them, remove any dead tissue or broken tooth left in the wound and then, apart from wounds on the face, leave them to heal by secondary intention.

Monkey handlers may be either bitten or scratched. Again, local treatment is important but the possibility of infection by Marburg's disease must not be overlooked.

Cat scratch

This may produce severe local cellulitis, but often presents as an abscess in one of the regional lymph nodes draining the area which has been scratched. When such an abscess is incised, seropurulent fluid only will be found and the bacterial culture will be sterile. The organism responsible is a member of the Chlamydia group but the antibody titre may not show elevation for two weeks. Fortunately the infection is usually self-limiting.

Dogs

The risk of rabies is described in Chapter 32. Many dog bites produce only scratches on the skin, but even these may result in infection, in which the predominant organism is the penicillin-sensitive organism *Pasteurella multocida*.

Sheep

Characteristically, a scratch on the back of the hand or fingers from barbed wire against which sheep have been rubbing will produce a localised vesicle (orf) (Fig. 33.6) which should be distinguished from an abscess or carbuncle and must not be incised because of the risk of introducing a secondary infection. The natural history of orf is of spontaneous healing in the course of three weeks. Only occasionally does the infection spread into lymph nodes or into the blood stream to produce a fever.

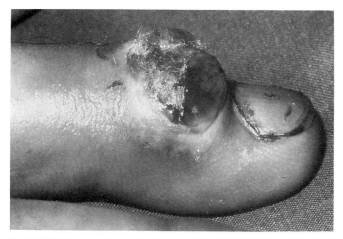

Fig. 33.6 Orf — note the vesicle with surrounding erythema, characteristic of a viral infection.

Cattle

Vaccinia may be transmitted to humans, as may anthrax. Patients who have worked in slaughter houses often have infections caused by β-haemolytic streptococci. Cattle ringworm may be transmitted to children or to those who milk cows in the traditional way with their head against the cow's flank.

Geese and other farmyard fowl

Scratches and bites have been known to cause tetanus and all patients injured by contact with animals must be protected against this possible complication.

Necrotising infections

Fortunately these conditions are rare. Reference has already been made to the 'malignant pustule' caused by the anthrax bacillus.

Meleney's synergistic gangrene usually develops around an abdominal wound. The subcutaneous tissue dies and the skin ulcerates. Underlying muscle may also be destroyed. A wide variety of both aerobic and anaerobic bacteria can be cultured from the wound and this may indicate the choice of antibiotics.

Fournier's gangrene is a similar condition, which develops around the scrotum, perineum and lower abdominal wall or around the vulval area in the female. Once the infection is eradicated by surgery and antibiotic therapy, the skin reveals remarkable powers of regeneration.

Necrotising fasciitis is a generic term used for infection passing along fascial planes, usually in the limbs, but occasionally in the trunk. A well-defined example of this is seen in Central Africa, caused by *Mycobacterium ulcerans*, and known in Uganda as Buruli ulcer.

Vincent's angina is a spreading infection caused by oral flora. It may not be necrotising to local tissue, but as pressure builds up around the pharynx and upper air passages, surgical decompression and antibiotic therapy are necessary to prevent a fatal result.

Gas gangrene. When clostridial gas-forming organisms, e.g. *Cl. welchii*, become established in a wound, the tension within the tissues rises until venous return is impeded. Swelling in the periphery is quickly followed by necrosis as the pressure in the tissues continues to rise and the arterial flow is occluded. Crepitus under the skin on palpation and gas within the muscles on radiographic examination confirm the diagnosis (Fig. 33.7). Absorption of toxins and necrotic products into the remainder of the circulation produces malaise and fever and death ensues unless urgent treatment by decompression or amputation, antibiotic and hyperbaric oxygen therapy are rapidly introduced.

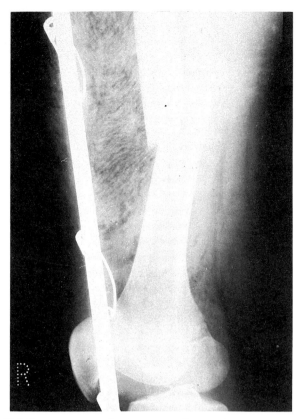

Fig. 33.7 Gas gangrene complicating an open fracture of the femur. After amputation, hyperbaric oxygen and antibiotic therapy, the patient recovered.

TREATMENT

General principles

The aim of treatment is to help the body eradicate the infection. A correct diagnosis is essential; a retained foreign body or an underlying osteomyelitis will perpetuate the infection indefinitely. Similarly, indolent wounds infected by mycobacteria will be helped only by appropriate antibiotics.

Rest and elevation for the infected part reduces the pain and discourages the formation of oedema. A high sling for an infected hand and resting a leg on a stool or the end of a settee have considerable therapeutic value.

Analgesic tablets may be required for additional pain relief, both before and after any surgical treatment.

Antiseptic dressings or a povidone iodine spray will help to eradicate superficial infections in the skin or exposed tissue. Chlorhexidine and sodium hypochlorite (Eusol) are also widely used. Magnesium sulphate paste is useful for drawing out the pus from a furuncle or carbuncle. Slough, debris and dead tissue may be cleaned from the depth of a wound by the use of anodal galvanism. The infected part is immersed in an antiseptic ionic solution and a weak direct current is passed from an anode placed in the solution, through the infected area to the cathode placed proximally on the limb. Because dead tissue carries a negative charge it tends to break away from the wound, traverse the solution

and coat the anode. The dressing of wounds is further discussed in Chapter 38.

> Antibiotics should be used sparingly and selectively.

They may be required in the following circumstances:

1. Early in an infection before pus has formed, in the hope that resolution may occur without abscess formation. Once pus and slough have formed and surgery is to be undertaken, healing will be virtually as quick without antibiotics.

2. If there is evidence of systemic infection, such as a fever or a rigor?

3. In the presence of other factors such as systemic disease (including patients on steroids, cytotoxic or immunosuppressive drugs), malnutrition, ischaemia, or certain specific infections (dog bites, anaerobic infections and chronic specific infections such as tuberculosis).

The choice of antibiotic will depend (pending the results of culture and sensitivities from the pus obtained at operation) on which organism it is thought most likely to be responsible for the infection. For examples a breast abscess, a boil or a carbuncle are likely to be caused by *Staphylococcus aureus* and would be treated with flucloxacillin (and not amoxicillin or ampicillin); a cellulitis associated with lymphangitis will usually be due to a streptococcus, and would best be treated with crystalline penicillin or penicillin V; so also would be *Pasteurella multocida*. If either a staphylococcus or streptococcus might be responsible, a drug such as erythromycin (to which the majority of both these organisms are at present sensitive) might be chosen. It would be wrong to use an antibiotic with the widest possible spectrum in all such patients. Perianal sepsis is best treated with clindamycin or metronidazole because of the frequent association of the anaerobic *Bacteroides fragilis* with the commonly cultured *Escherichia coli* and staphylococci.

Lymphangitis, cellulitis and erysipelas are conditions which do not produce pus, so the choice of antibiotic is made entirely on clinical grounds. They are usually due to streptococcal infection so treatment with penicillin or erythromycin is effective.

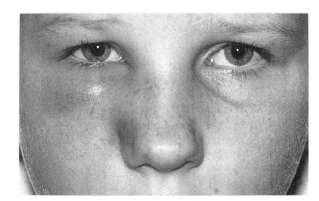

Fig. 33.8 Sepsis at the side of the nose has now caused cellulitis below the eye. Further spread to the cavernous sinus was prevented and the infection resolved on antibiotic therapy.

Localised infection on the face or a spreading cellulitis demand urgent and effective antibiotic therapy to prevent the spread of the infection to within the cranium where a cavernous sinus thrombosis can develop (Fig. 33.8). Because of the ample blood supply to the face, surgical incision, with a consequent scar, is hardly ever indicated.

Surgical treatment

If the infection has developed in a sutured wound, removal of some or all of the sutures will release the pus (from which a swab must be taken) and also ease the pain. The wound should be probed or examined radiologically if there is the remotest possibility of a foreign body being present. Irrigation with an antiseptic solution and application of an antiseptic dressing are indicated, but the introduction of a wick can only delay healing.

Treatment of abscesses

When an abscess is suspected, if the patient's sleep has been disturbed by throbbing pain from an infected area, pus will have formed in the tissues and surgical incision is necessary to release it. Provided the incision is done under an appropriate antibiotic cover given intramuscularly 1 hour before surgery, there is no need to wait for the abscess to become 'ripe' or 'point'. Poulticing to draw the abscess to the surface is an archaic treatment which has no place in the antibiotic era. The incision should be performed under regional or general anaesthesia and due attention paid to Langer's lines and to nearby important anatomical structures. A bacteriological swab is taken from the first pus to emerge. Then all remaining pus and debris are expressed and removed by curetting and gauze toilet of the cavity. By thorough curettage or sharp dissection all dead and infected tissue is removed and the cavity becomes filled with antibiotic-laden blood which effectively sterilizes it.

For large abscesses this, now sterile, area can be closed by deep, encircling, monofilament mattress sutures and it will heal by first intention within 5–7 days. There is no place in modern surgery for introducing a foreign body, in the form of a cotton gauze wick, into the cavity; this merely serves to delay healing and produces an ugly scar. (Small abscesses, 1.5 cm or less, will heal equally well without sutures.)

Postoperative management

Following incision, a sterile dressing is applied and, after recovering from the anaesthetic, the patient can return home and be treated as an outpatient. For relatively small abscesses, such as an axillary abscess, the next attendance at hospital should be after 5 days. By this time the wound will be healed, the sutures can be removed, a small dry dressing applied and the patient discharged. For larger abscesses in, for instance, the breast or anorectal area, the sutures can be removed after 5–6 days and the lesion should be healed within seven to eight days. Provided the preoperative antibiotic

has been effective and the operation was performed correctly, there is no need for postoperative antibiotic therapy.

Abscesses in the hand are treated along the same lines. Sutures are usually not inserted, the cavity being closed by firm bandages. Because of the importance of maintaining or restoring function in the fingers as quickly as possible, it is important to have the hand elevated in a high sling to reduce oedema formation. Splinting of the hand and fingers to rest the healing area is advisable for 5–7 days, but this should be followed quickly by mobilisation, if necessary helped by a physiotherapist. Failure to attend to these details of operative technique, postoperative management and rehabilitation may permanently impair a worker's livelihood.

Infected sebaceous cyst

The patient is often unaware that a cyst was present before it became infected. Treatment is the same as for abscesses, but it is desirable to get rid not only of the infected contents but also the cells which line the cyst — otherwise it will recur. This will be done by very brisk and thorough curettage or by a total excision of the infected cyst. When excising such a cyst if often bursts. Even so, healing by primary intention is usual after suturing.

Infections in the neck and jaw

A child aged 2–3 years may develop a painful red swelling beneath the lower jaw. It is difficult or impossible to examine this alveolar abscess because the patient objects vigorously to palpation. Experience has shown that when the skin over the swelling is red, pus has formed. Under a general anaesthetic an incision under the cover of the lower border of the mandible reveals a mass of granulation. Careful blunt dissection is required to release a few millilitres of pus from the centre of the inflammatory mass. Once the pus has been cleared away with a small curette, no pack or drain is required. The preoperative antibiotic injection is the only necessary therapy to ensure healing within 4 or 5 days.

Suppurative lymphadenitis in a deep cervical lymph node should be viewed with caution since this may arise from an infected branchial cyst or may be tuberculous in origin. An exploratory aspiration under local anaesthetic infiltration may give a lead to the diagnosis.

Axillary abscesses

These are common in patients who shave the axilla or use a deodorant. Treatment by incision, curettage and primary suture under an antibiotic cover will give healing within a week. Should an abscess recur within a short time, a biopsy should be taken. This may reveal hidradenitis suppurativa, which requires either prolonged treatment from a dermatologist or excision of the axillary skin by a plastic surgeon.

Infections in the hand

A precise knowledge of the detailed anatomy of the hand is an essential prerequisite for anyone who operates on an infected hand. Surgical procedures should be done under anaesthesia, either a digital or regional block. Local infiltration into inflamed tissue must not be employed, nor an ethyl chloride spray. General anaesthesia may be required for children or when there is spreading sepsis. A bloodless field is essential for any surgery in the hand. Incisions must be carefully planned so as not to cross flexor creases nor leave a scar on the tactile areas and the surgeon must carefully avoid damage to nerves, vessels, tendons and joints. There is no place for wicks or drains in hand surgery.

Paronychia.   This is the commonest finger infection, usually caused by a staphylococcus, but nail biters and hairdressers may have a variety of other organisms. Pus should be released by making an incision parallel to the edge of the nail and 2 mm away from it (Fig. 33.9). After curetting away all the pus and necrotic tissue there is no need for sutures. The finger dressing will hold the skin edges in apposition. Occasionally a patient presents with a viral paronychia. This occurs particularly in nurses who have been doing tracheal toilet on unconscious patients without wearing gloves. This 'herpetic whitlow' forms a vesicle containing clear fluid. Pus will only develop if the lesion becomes secondarily infected after an inappropriate incision. Aspiration of the vesicle and the application of 100% tincture of povidone iodine will help the lesion to resolve. Paronychia caused by a fungal infection affects many fingers simultaneously and has a much slower onset. It is seen in children and people who work with their hands in cold water. Provided the skin is allowed to dry out, applications of an antifungal ointment will achieve a cure and, as with the viral paronychia, surgery is not indicated.

Pulp space infection.   Infection in the extremely sensitive, terminal pulp of the finger is very painful and patients usually seek medical help very early. If they have been kept awake the previous night, pus is present. Under a digital block, and using a finger tourniquet, an incision is made under the cover of, and following the line of the end of the nail. After curetting out the

pus and debris, no sutures are required. A dressing and a high sling will facilitate a cure within five days.

Web space infection.   Patients with this condition present with a hand that is swollen over the dorsum but, when asked where the pain began and where the tenderness is, they point to the volar side of the web space. Under antibiotic cover, an anaesthetic and with the aid of an arm tourniquet, a superficial incision is made in the line of the flexor crease at the base of the adjacent finger.

Deep palmar space infections.   Pus forming in the thenar, mid palmar or hypothenar spaces is now a very rare occurrence. If it is suspected because of pain, swelling and tenderness over the palm, which is aggravated by finger movements, the patient should be admitted under the care of a hand surgeon.

Suppurative tenosynovitis.   This condition presents as a sausage-shaped, red swelling, extending from the distal flexor crease of a finger, along the volar surface to the distal third of the palm. The finger is held semi-flexed and any movement in either direction is painful (Fig. 33.10). If the patient attends early in the evolution of the infection, antibiotic therapy, preferably with Clindamycin, and elevation of the hand should ease the symptoms within eight hours, otherwise surgical decompression and irrigation of the flexor sheath are required to prevent necrosis of the flexor tendons within the sheath.

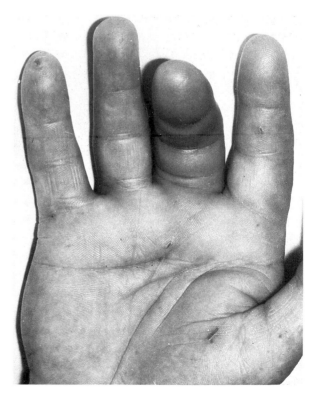

Fig. 33.10 Suppurative tenosynovitis of the middle finger. The finger is held semiflexed; further extension is too painful and only a few degrees of flexion are possible.

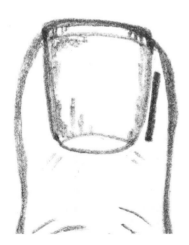

Fig. 33.9 The line of incision in an acute paronychia should be parallel to the edge of the nail and 2 mm away from it.

Septic arthritis. The small joints of the fingers are at risk from thorns and splinters. In septic arthritis the tenderness is located precisely at the joint. As with suppurative tenosynovitis, Clindamycin is the antibiotic of choice because of its penetration into synovial tissue.

After-treatment

Any doctor who undertakes the treatment of an infected hand has not fulfilled his obligation to the patient until everything possible has been done to restore full function in the hand. This may require the help of a physio- or occupational therapist. The doctor must consult with the therapists to ensure a comprehensive and co-ordinated programme of rehabilitation.

Breast abscess

Breast abscesses may be subareolar or more deeply situated in the substance of the gland. In the former case, a small radial incision is suitable. Following excision of dead tissue, such an abscess may be closed by deep obliterating sutures. More deeply situated breast abscesses usually occur in the lactating breast. Breast feeding can be safely continued provided an appropriate antibiotic is administered (this may be flucloxacillin or erythromycin, but not tetracycline). The continuation of lactation will hasten resolution of the congested breast and will lessen the mother's discomfort. Incision should not be delayed beyond two to three days from the onset of throbbing pain and the development of a tense tender swelling. If fluctuation is awaited and antibiotic therapy continued, a slowly spreading granulomatous infection will destroy a large section of the breast. The incision (usually radial) (Fig. 33.11) should, if possible, be placed away from the areola so that breast feeding can continue. The abscess cavity should be curetted so that all dead tissue is removed, and the residual cavity closed by deep obliterating nylon sutures. Packs and drains should not be used. The wound can then be sealed off and need not be disturbed until the sutures are removed on the fifth day. If little or no pus

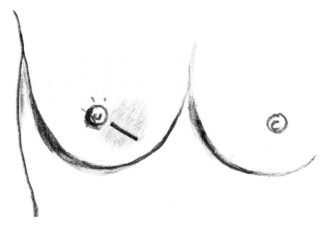

Fig. 33.11 The incision for a breast abscess should extend away from the nipple in a radial direction and should not breach the areolar margin.

is found, a biopsy should be taken to exclude tuberculosis infection or a rapidly growing carcinoma.

Anorectal abscesses

Anorectal abscess is commonest in patients aged 30–50 years. If the painful, throbbing swelling has kept the patient awake the previous night, pus is present and incision will be necessary. Under general anaesthetic, sigmoidoscopy should be performed to search for the presence of a fistula or associated rectal pathology. The abscess is then incised. Dead tissue and pus are carefully removed. If a deeper extension through the ischiorectal fascia is found, this is enlarged and this space also curetted. The cavity is then obliterated using deep 2.5 metric gauge (2/0) nylon sutures guided into place with a finger in the cavity. The sutures are tied together after all have been inserted. The preoperative antibiotic must be active against staphylococci and bacteroides. Metronidazole or Clindamycin are a suitable choice. It is important that the details of surgical technique should be followed carefully. The patient then may return home to rest in bed. The sutures are removed on the fifth day, when healing is well advanced. No further hospital visits are usually necessary.

If the patient develops a recurrent abscess within 3–6 months, the possibility of the presence of a fistula-in-ano must be considered and advice sought from a colorectal surgeon.

Natal cleft — pilonidal abscess

A pilonidal abscess is caused by hair of the buttock growing inwards through the skin; a sinus forms around the hair and becomes infected. As the natal cleft is bound down to the sacral spines, the abscess veers to the left or right. It is treated like any other abscess except that a small area of skin including the sinus should be excised. Large mattress sutures should obliterate the abscess cavity. They are removed after five days.

Infected olecranon and prepatellar bursae

These seldom need incision since the inflammation usually responds to antibiotic treatment (such as a local injection of benzylpenicillin or oral erythromycin or clindamycin) and rest. Aspiration followed by the injection of 0.5 g of benzylpenicillin is usually effective. Occasionally, however, incision is required, and in order to discourage a recurrence of the bursa, a small plastic drain may be sutured in place. A small safety pin in the end of the drain will prevent loss of the drain in the infected bursa. This drain should be left in place for two weeks, by which time the cavity will have largely been obliterated by the healing process. Excision of uninfected bursae is unrewarding since recurrence is usual. Obliteration following infection and prolonged drainage is a tedious but satisfactory method of treatment.

Ingrowing toe nails

Sepsis resulting from ingrowing toe nails causes much discomfort

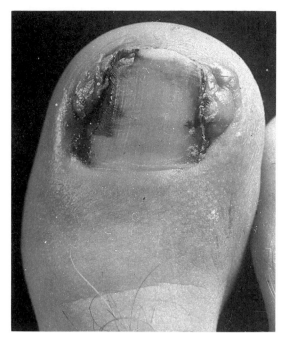

Fig. 33.12 Severe sepsis accompanying ingrowing toe nail.

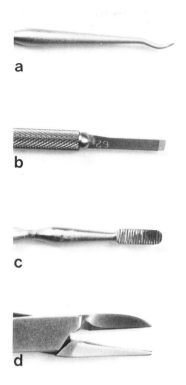

Fig. 33.13 Initial instruments required for resection of ingrowing toe nails: **A** dental probe; **B** Beavor chisel, **C** Black's file, (d) Thwaite's nibblers.

and may be disabling (Fig. 33.12). It has been encountered at all ages (from 10 days to 75 years) but is most commonly seen in young people. The assistance of chiropodists should be sought in dealing with this problem and the patient should preferably be seen jointly with them in the A & E department.

Extensive research in recent years has shown that wedge resection and phenolisation of the nail bed is the treatment which gives the best results.

Technique

A simple suture pack is used to which a few special instruments are added. These instruments are shown in Figure. 33.13 and make the operation both easier and more precise.

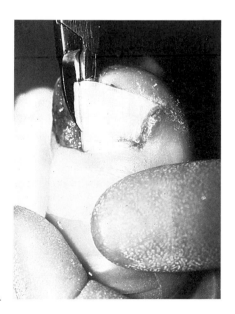

A

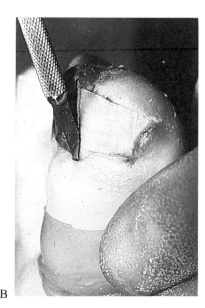

B

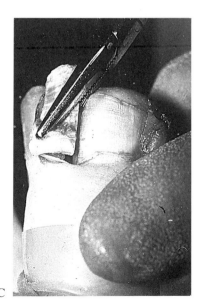

C

Fig. 33.14 **A** The use of Thwaite's nibblers allows the affected portion of the nail to be cut cleanly to the nail fold without disturbing the unaffected portion of the nail, using a digital tourniquet and local analgesia. **B** This cut can then be carried out to the base of the nail under the nail fold using the Beavor chisel. **C** The wedge of nail thus separated is then carefully removed in its entirety.

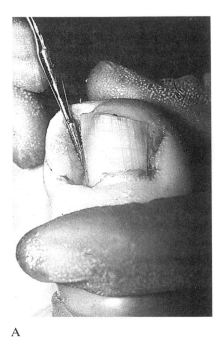
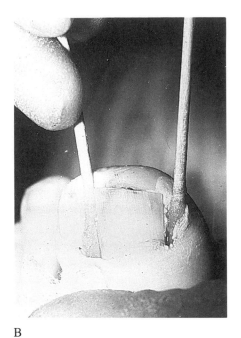
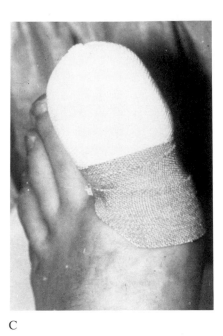

A   B   C

Fig. 33.15 The granulations are removed and the remaining cavity cleansed with the use of a Black's file, which removes any loose tags of epithelium or nail. A small stick wrapped in cotton wool and soaked in 80% phenol is then twisted into the remaining cavity and kept in position for three minutes. At the end of three minutes the excess phenol is washed away with a stream of surgical spirit, the tourniquet removed and a non-adhesive dressing secured in place.

The steps are:

1. The usual aseptic precautions are employed in preparing the field. A digital nerve block is followed by application of a broad latex rubber tourniquet around the base of the toe.

2. Using Thwaite's nibblers, the nail is cut proximally as far as the nail fold. Using the Beavor chisel, this cut is continued under the nail fold to the base of the nail.

3. The whole wedge of nail is then removed (Fig. 33.14).

4. Loose fragments of epithelium are also removed with the assistance of the Black's file.

5. A wisp of cotton wool wound around the end of a 'cocktail stick' is dipped in pure (80%) phenol, rotated into the empty cleft under the nail fold, and kept there for three minutes. Vaseline may be applied to protect the surrounding skin before applying the phenol.

6. The remaining phenol is then washed away using a stream of spirit from a plastic bottle.

7. A non-adhesive dressing is applied and the tourniquet removed (Fig. 33.15).

8. The patient should be asked to rest and elevate the foot for the remainder of the day, but may be able to return to work the following day.

9. The dressing is changed on the second and third day and thereafter at infrequent intervals until healing is complete at 10 days to 3 weeks.

This operation has produced results which are comparable to the best of the more complicated surgical procedures and with none of their complications. The operation can be carried out in the presence of sepsis and the patient is able to walk home and to go back to work the next day. Postoperative pain is minimal, the recurrence rate is small and the operation can be repeated if necessary. If both sides of one nail are affected, then a wedge may be removed from both sides; alternatively, the whole nail may be removed and phenol applied to the whole of the nail matrix (Fig. 33.16).

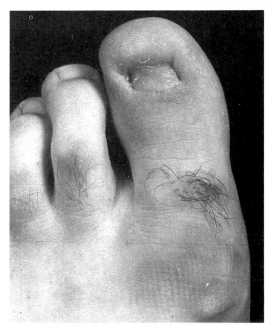

Fig. 33.16 This patient had had the whole nail removed a year previously and the nail bed phenolised. There has been no regrowth of nail.

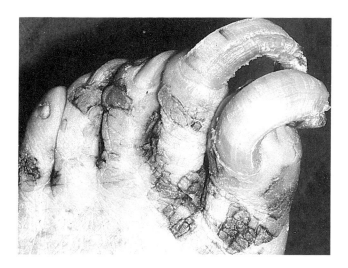

Fig. 33.17 'Onychogryphosis maxima'.

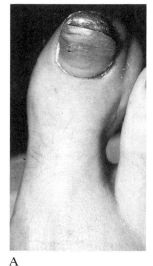
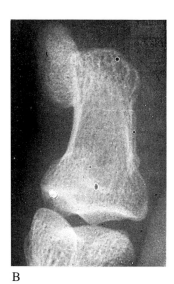

A   B

Fig. 33.18 A This young woman's big toe nail has been lifted forwards by granulations covering an underlying osteoma which shows clearly in **B** the accompanying radiograph.

Onychogryphosis

This is not an infection and strictly speaking is not a condition for A & E departments at all, but many patients will present along with patients with ingrowing toe nails. In onychogryphosis the whole of the nail bed develops germinal properties, so that instead of a thin nail growing forwards as a plate, a horn grows out from the entire nail bed area (Fig. 33.17). This can be treated by removing the whole nail and cauterising the entire area of the nail bed with phenol for three minutes. If this is not successful, the nail bed will have to be excised surgically.

Subungual osteoma

This lesion may present at any age as a 'septic toe nail' which is painful and elevated above the nail fold. Its presence is confirmed by radiography (Fig. 33.18). The nail should be removed and the sepsis treated before the osteoma is excised.

David H. Wilson

Hand injuries

INTRODUCTION

The main purpose of the shoulder, arm and forearm is to give mobility to the hand. This complex systems of levers allows the hand a remarkable range of movement in relation to the rest of the body. The hand itself is a combined sensory and motor organ used for gestures, sensory exploration, holding objects, scratching and creating movement. It is used for feeding, dressing and toilet manoeuvres, and most people depend on their hands for their livelihood, their recreations and their pleasures. However, because of the way we use our hands in work and play and in the exploration of our environment, they are the most exposed and most frequently injured part of the body.

Hand injuries constitute one-tenth of all the cases presenting at an accident and emergency department. In an industrial area, half these injuries occur at work and most of the other half are accidents at home; there is a small but important group which results from sports injuries, mostly at weekends.

Patients injured at work and in sport are usually young men, therefore these injuries may have economic and social repercussions for the next 40–50 years in loss of skill and consequent loss of earnings. This means that these patients should have the optimum surgical care and management to minimise the resulting morbidity.

ASSESSMENT OF THE INJURED HAND

The reader is referred to Ch. 32 for a general account of the examination and assessment of wounds. Because of the complex nature and the importance of the hand, there are certain questions and precise points of examination which are appropriate to hand injuries as distinct from wounds in other parts of the body.

For anything other than the most minor injury, the patient should be screened from public view and examined on a couch in case he feels faint at the sight of his injury. A few minutes taken to enquire about and record the circumstances of the accident enables the doctor to establish rapport with the patient and to assess his reaction to the injury.

Preliminary questions will cover the location, circumstances and cause of the accident and first aid treatment, if any. Then for an injury of any consequence, the work requirements and/or domestic responsibilities and the patient's hobbies and recreational interests should be noted. Enquiry should also be made as to which is the dominant hand. While posing these questions it is helpful to establish rapport by holding the injured hand and so making skin-to-skin contact before the actual physical examination takes place.

The examination of the injured hand should then be undertaken systematically along the classic path of 'look, feel, move and x-ray'.

Look

Inspection begins by looking at the whole patient, assessing his general physique and his physical and emotional reaction to the accident. Inspection of the hand may also give valuable information about disorders of general health, such as clubbing of the fingers or rheumatoid disease. Inspection of the injury itself may show an obvious deformity due to a fracture or dislocation, a finger or fingers hanging in an abnormal position due to a tendon injury (Fig. 34.1) or a part of the hand partially or totally amputated. Inspection of the wound follows the lines described in Ch. 32. In hand injuries there is a high risk of contamination by grease or oil or by anaerobic organisms, and foreign bodies are often embedded in these wounds. It is always necessary to inspect both sides of the hand; there may be more than one wound. As the patient turns the hand over, watch for fingers assuming an abnormal posture due to a tendon or nerve injury. Look for deviation of a flexed finger indicating rotation of the bone in a fracture of a metacarpal or proximal phalanx.

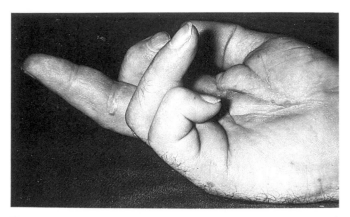

Fig. 34.1 Division of both flexor tendons to the middle finger have produced the characteristic 'hang-out' sign.

Feel

In making physical contact with the injured hand, the approach should be just as gentle as that used for examination of the acute abdomen. Feel for swelling, tenderness, creptus and areas of sensory loss. Confirmation of sensory nerve damage takes time and care. Obscure the patient's view of the hand and instruct him to respond 'yes' if he feels you stroke your finger on the hand. Then lightly touch both uninjured and injured areas alternately at irregular intervals. The validity of the patient's response can be tested by making a gesture of stroking a part of the hand but not actually making contact. Within half an hour of an accident, denervated areas of the hand will have ceased to sweat and the skin will be dry. Drawing the plastic shaft of a ballpoint pen over the area is a valuable way of establishing this change. Over a denervated area it will slide with minimal friction, whereas on normal skin it will drag due to the moisture on the surface (Fig. 34.2).

Move

Begin by examining active movement — those which the patient performs himself. First ask him to make a fist and then to extend the fingers. Then examine flexion and extension of the thumb and opposition of the thumb tip to the fingers. These movements will demonstrate any tendon injury except for an isolated flexor digitorum superficialis (FDS) lesion. To test the integrity of this latter tendon, hold the other three fingers in extension; if the patient can now flex the injured finger at the proximal interphalangeal joint, the FDS tendon is intact (Fig. 34.3).

Passive movements of the fingers are useful to determine whether loss of active movement is due to pain or to a tendon or nerve injury. Fingers paralysed by a tendon or nerve injury usually have a good range of passive movement. If the patient will not move the finger because of the pain of local trauma, then he will resist passive movement as well.

The presence or absence of damage to the radial, median or ulnar nerves is the next point to be decided. If there is a lesion of the radial nerve, at or above the elbow, or of its posterior interosseous branch, then the patient will have a 'drop wrist' and be unable to extend the wrist or fingers (Fig. 34.4). There may also be a variable area of anaesthesia over the dorsum of the first web.

In the presence of a high lesion of the median nerve in the region of the elbow, there will be no active flexion in the index finger (Fig. 34.5), but in the much more common low lesion, at the level of the wrist, the only motor deficit in the hand will be abduction of the thumb. To test for this the hand must be held palm upwards on a flat surface and the patient must make the thumb point to the ceiling. In both high and low lesions of the median nerve the sensory loss in the hand will be the same, usually involving three and a half radial digits.

Occasionally the median nerve supplies two and a half fingers (and the ulnar nerve therefore two and a half fingers); and sometimes the radial nerve may have no sensory distribution extending on the back of the hand — or, alternatively, may have a sensory distribution extending onto the back of the thumb and the index finger. Isolated motor median loss can occur if the motor

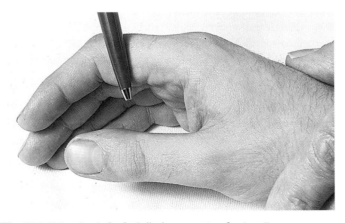

Fig. 34.2 Using the shaft of a ballpoint pen to test for dry, slippery, denervated skin.

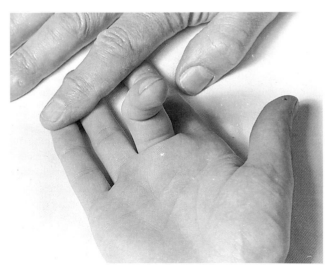

Fig. 34.3 Holding three fingers in extension also immobilises the profundus tendon to the other finger. Any active flexion must now be due to the action of flexor digitorum superficialis.

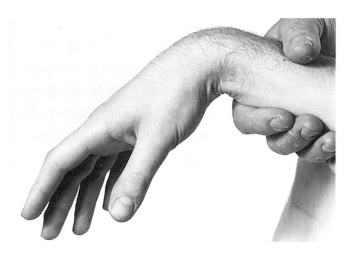

Fig. 34.4 A 'drop wrist' results from an injury to the radial nerve.

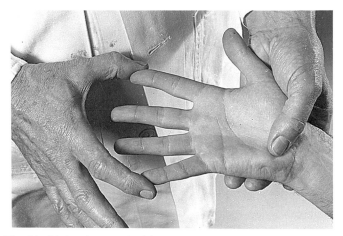

Fig. 34.6 Testing the strength of finger abduction to show the integrity of the motor branch of the ulnar nerve.

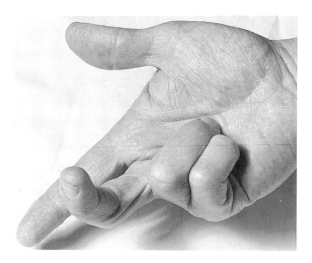

Fig. 34.5 A patient with a high lesion of the median nerve, in the region of the elbow, can still flex the ring and little fingers, and may partially flex the middle finger, but the index finger hangs out in extension.

branch is cut (as, for example, by a piece of glass) — and this is readily missed if the examination is hurried.

A complete ulnar nerve lesion at or above the elbow results in paralysis of the flexor carpi ulnaris as well as of flexor digitorum profundus to the ulnar two fingers and the relevant intrinsic muscles of the hand. This is demonstrated by asking the patient to spread the fingers against resistance (Fig. 34.6). In addition, there will be sensory loss of one and a half (occasionally two and a half) fingers on both the dorsal and the palmar aspect. A complete lesion near the wrist may spare the dorsal branch, leaving intact sensation on the dorsum of the fingers. Sensory loss in the palmar distribution, not accompanied by motor loss, may result from repeated blows with the 'heel' of the hand on a hard object, or from a glass wound affecting the superficial branch just distal to the pisiform bone. Motor ulnar loss (without ulnar sensory loss) may occasionally occur if the deep branch is cut or damaged in (or distal to) Guyon's canal by a glass wound or other pathology.

Finally, there is a rare anomaly in which the motor component of the ulnar nerve crosses from the median to the ulnar nerve in the lower forearm, so that a high median nerve lesion results in total motor paralysis in the hand (plus sensory loss of median distribution); however, a high ulnar lesion will result only in sensory loss of ulnar distribution (and no motor loss).

Thus precise anatomical definition of nerve lesions in the forearm and hand is usually possible if a careful preoperative assessment has been carried out.

X-ray examination

AP and lateral films of the hand will show dislocations or fractures and the presence of most foreign bodies. Nearly all glass is radio-opaque but many plastic substances cast very little shadow on the x-ray film. It will help the radiographer if the doctor indicates whether he suspects bony damage or a foreign body in the soft tissues, and if he specifies the precise site of injury. If the patient has a finger tip injury, it is important to know if the terminal phalanx has been fractured and, if so, whether the joint is involved. In injuries likely to lead to litigation, it is valuable to have a film to document whether or not a radiological abnormality was present. Finally, the radiograph may show evidence of a pre-existing bony abnormality, old trauma or bone disease.

TREATMENT OF UNCOMPLICATED WOUNDS

Uncomplicated wounds are described in Ch. 32 but mention must be made of two common injuries of the finger nail: the subungual haematoma and avulsion of the finger nail.

A subungual haematoma arises from a blunt blow causing bleeding under the nail. It can be very painful. Decompression of the haematoma is achieved by trephining the nail with a red-hot wire. A paper clip opened out and heated in a methylated spirit flame is pushed vertically into the centre of the nail. There is a moment of extra pain as the wire penetrates to the nail bed; then, as the imprisoned blood flows out, the pain is relieved. A simple dressing is applied to absorb the blood. A malignant melanoma of the nail bed should not be mistaken for a subungual haematoma.

Avulsion of the finger nail is often accompanied by a fracture of the terminal phalanx, or a displaced epiphysis. The injury must be cleaned and the nail replaced and secured beneath the nail fold using one absorbable mattress suture. Antibiotics should be administered. Failure to deal with these injuries adequately carries a risk of osteomyelitis (Fig. 34.7).

TREATMENT OF TENDON INJURIES

Extensor tendons

Injuries to the extensor mechanism on the dorsum of the hand and fingers are relatively simple to treat and carry a good prognosis. Division of a flexor tendon is a serious injury which requires expert management.

The extensor tendon mechanism may be injured at one of three levels, as described below.

Division of a tendon or tendons on the dorsum of the hand

Because of the interconnecting bands which pass between the extensor tendons and oblige them to work in a mass action, if one or two tendons are divided the cut ends will not retract up the forearm. These tendons are amenable to a simple end-to-end repair. However, permanent stiffness of the metacarpophalangeal joints may result if there is sepsis following the primary repair, or if the original injury involved a crushing injury to the

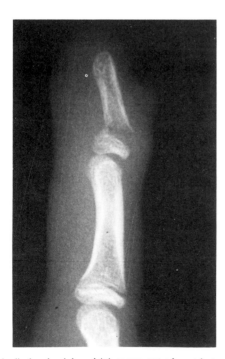

Fig. 34.7 This displaced epiphyseal injury was not adequately treated and has become infected.

metacarpophalangeal joint. Under such circumstances, it may be more appropriate to obtain primary healing of the skin alone, followed by early mobilisation of the metacarpophalangeal joints. Secondary repair of the extensor tendons followed by immobilisation of the joints in extension is then less likely to result in permanent stiffness.

Repair of the tendon is carried out under local or general anaesthesia and using a tourniquet. The wound is excised and extended to allow exposure of the tendon ends, which are then trimmed with a sharp knife or fine scissors. The proximal end is then drawn down into the wound and retained there by passing a sterile needle through the skin-tendon-skin. Dorsiflexion of the affected finger will bring the distal tendon into apposition with the proximal end, thus avoiding tension on the suture line. An interlacing, non-absorbable monofilament suture is inserted, whose precise pattern is less important than accurate apposition of the flat tendon ends. The skin is closed carefully and the metacarpophalangeal joints and the wrist are held in extension using either a plaster of Paris volar slab or Zimmer splint, which must remain in position for 17–21 days. Then a few days supervised exercises in the physiotherapy department should result in a return of full function 4 weeks after the initial injury.

Delayed rupture of the extensor pollicis longus tendon may follow a Colles fracture or, in rheumatoid arthritis, rupture by attrition may occur. In neither case is primary repair appropriate. The patient requires an extensor indicis transference operation and should be referred to a hand surgeon.

Middle slip rupture

Over the dorsum of the proximal phalanx of each finger the extensor mechanism divides into two lateral slips (which, after rejoining, are inserted into the base of the distal phalanx), and a middle slip which terminates in the base of the intermediate phalanx. If a patient detaches or ruptures the middle slip he can no longer fully extend the proximal interphalangeal joint. The lateral slips will still extend the distal interphalangeal joint — indeed they often hyperextend it. This position of flexion at the proximal, and hyperextension at the distal, interphalangeal joints is called a 'boutonniere deformity' (Fig. 34.8). The condition may be secondary to a closed dislocation of the proximal interphalangeal joint (which may have been reduced before the patient reaches hospital), or it may result from an open injury caused by glass or a sharp instrument. The sooner it is corrected surgically, the better will be the result. As soon as the diagnosis is made the finger should be splinted in extension and the patient referred to a hand surgeon.

Mallet finger deformity

This common condition is caused by forced flexion to fingers which are being held taut in the extended position. The insertion of the lateral slips of the extensor mechanism is wrenched off the distal phalanx and may bring a fragment of bone with it. The distal segment of the finger droops like the nose of Concorde. It may

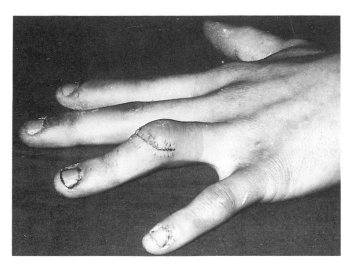

Fig. 34.8 The wound on the ring finger was sutured but the injury to the middle slip of the extensor tendon was missed and a boutonniere deformity has developed.

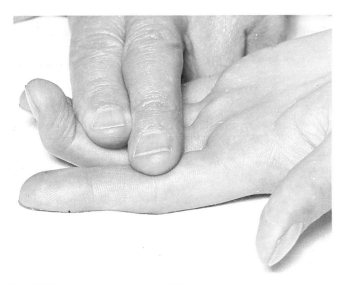

Fig. 34.9 Demonstrating the action of flexor digitorum profundus.

also be caused by a wound on the dorsum of the finger, dividing skin and extensor tendon. Although various surgical procedures are described, it is doubtful if any of them gives a better result than is achieved from immobilising the distal interphalangeal joint. A light plastic splint is used and the patient must be instructed to wear it day and night for 6 weeks to give the tendon time to reattach itself to the bone. If the patient is unable to keep the finger dry (as often happens if he continues to work), the skin may become macerated unless the patient is instructed how to change the splint while maintaining extension at the distal joint. Occasionally resolution of the injury takes longer than 6 weeks, but it will occur if the patient perseveres with the treatment.

Flexor tendon injuries

The A & E doctor must be able to diagnose a flexor tendon injury, but the surgical repair should be performed by an experienced hand surgeon. Lesions of both flexor tendons are usually obvious: there is no active flexion at the interphalangeal joints. A lesion of the superficial flexor tendon is demonstrated by the examiner holding the other three fingers in extension. Then, because the deep tendons must work together or not at all, any flexion in an injured finger will be produced by the action of the superficial tendon alone, thereby establishing its integrity. An isolated division of the flexor digitorum profundus tendon can only be demonstrated by holding the proximal interphalangeal joint so that it cannot move and asking the patient to flex the finger tip (Fig. 34.9). Even 15–20° of movement at the distal interphalangeal joint shows that the deep tendon is intact. The profundus tendon is occasionally ruptured subcutaneously by a sudden strain against the flexed finger tip. This injury is readily missed unless it is carefully sought. Partial division of flexor tendons may be followed up to three weeks later by delayed rupture, or by a trigger finger.

If any of the flexor tendons in the fingers or thumb are divided, surgical repair by a hand surgeon should be arranged as soon as possible. Primary repair of flexor tendons at any level of injury is now generally recommended. The fear of adhesions forming between the tendons, or between the tendons and the flexor sheath, has diminished over the past 10 years because of improved technique and better suture materials. Also, the possibility of replacing an unsatisfactory repair by a Silastic rod and performing a two-stage tendon graft operation has provided an acceptable alternative if primary repair fails.

Trigger finger

Patients with this common complaint may come to the A & E department. There is a congenital variety seen in small children but the usual presentation is in an older person who, following some trivial injury, finds that a finger or thumb tends to lock. On making extra effort to move the digit, there will be a painful click and it will become free again. Palpation in the region of the mouth of the fibrous flexor sheath in the distal half of the palm, or at the base of the thumb, will reveal a tender lump. It is at this point that the swollen tendon is becoming temporarily impacted in the stenosed mouth of the sheath. The condition may respond to a local injection of hydrocortisone into the region of the mouth of the flexor sheath but, if not, it is always cured by surgical incision of the mouth of the sheath.

TREATMENT OF NERVE INJURIES IN THE HAND

The diagnosis of a nerve injury in the hand has already been discussed on page 356. Primary repair of the injured nerve carries the best prognosis for the recovery of sensation. It should be performed by an experienced hand surgeon using an operating microscope (Fig. 34.10).

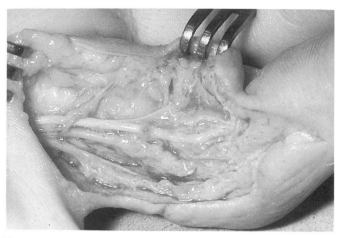

Fig. 34.10 This digital nerve injury was repaired using 0.4 (8/0) monofilament sutures under an operating microscope. Recovery was satisfactory.

INJURIES TO BONE, CAPSULE AND LIGAMENT

Simple sprains and some stable fractures may be treated in the A & E department. Complete ruptures of ligaments and unstable or open fractures are injuries which should be referred for the care of a surgeon skilled in the acute and long-term management of such injuries. The A & E doctor must therefore be able to select, at the first attendance, those patients who have injuries which require more specialised care than he can be expected to provide within the A & E department.

Crushing injuries (or direct blows)

Sprains, dislocation and fractures of the fingers and hand will be considered from the point of view of the mechanism of the injury — which may be 'crushing', 'end-on', or 'angulating' (into extension, or laterally to one or other side) (Fig. 34.11). Critical scrutiny of the mechanism of the injury, the physical signs and correctly positioned radiographs will allow an anatomical diagnosis to be made for most so-called 'sprains' of the fingers. Only if this sort of care is taken will the lesions which require active intervention

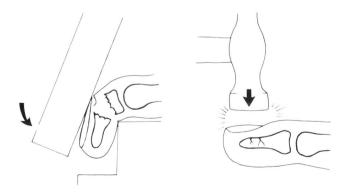

Fig. 34.11 A finger trapped in a door suffers a flexion injury with disruption of the nail bed and a displaced fracture. A hammer blow causes a subungual haematoma and an undisplaced comminuted fracture.

be identified, so that appropriate treatment can be undertaken and a full return of function achieved.

To the finger tip

If there is loss of tissue, some form of repair or terminalisation may be required (see p. 364).

Children frequently sustain a fracture when they trap a finger in a door. There is usually an element of angulation of the bone as well as crushing of the tissues. The epiphyseal plate may be distorted and the nail dislocated so that it lies on top of the nail fold. In adults the same injury causes a fracture of the terminal phalanx. In either case, the base or the whole of the nail should be removed, so that the fracture site can be well cleaned, and the nail bed reconstituted using a single mattress suture which draws the nail bed under the nail fold. This suture and a well-padded dressing are sufficient to stabilise the fracture. If there is no angulation involved in the crushing injury in adults, a comminuted fracture of the terminal phalanx results (Fig. 34.11). In this case the nail may be better left in place after trephining, and the hand elevated. Antibiotics should be given, however, because the nail fold is always potentially infected. The rate of recovery will depend on whether the joint surface has been involved or not.

To the middle or proximal segments

As with the finger tip, undisplaced ('subperiosteal') comminuted fractures of the proximal two phalanges are stable, and will heal rapidly without formal splinting. Recovery of function, however, will depend on the severity of the accompanying soft tissue injuries, which must be treated on their own merits. Open injuries should be referred for specialist attention.

The less severe closed crushing injuries of fingers may be supported by attachment to an adjacent finger — either by strapping or by a double elastic tube gauze. The latter is more convenient, as it can be readily removed for washing and for exercising the joints (Fig. 34.12).

The more severe crushing injuries should be splinted either singly on a flexible aluminium splint or jointly with other fingers on a plaster of Paris volar slab. In either case the fingers should be positioned with the metacarpophalangeal joints flexed and the interphalangeal joints nearly straight. The ridging of the plaster gives extra strength, whilst the use of the 'slab' (rather than a full plaster) allows the hand and fingers to be withdrawn at will for further examination and for exercising.

Direct blows to the fingers or hand may result in transverse fractures of phalanges or metacarpals. In the fingers these are potentially unstable and should be referred for specialist advice.

'End-on' injuries

When a finger is hit end-on (e.g. by a cricket ball) or is stubbed (e.g. when making a bed), the force may be transmitted longitudinally down the chain of phalanges which are held rigid by the tendons and ligaments. Alternatively, the distal joint may

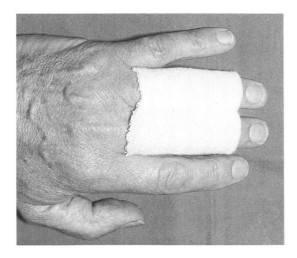

A

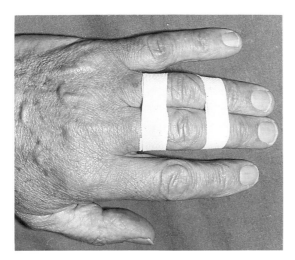

B

Fig. 34.12 A and **B** Neighbour elastic strapping or a double elastic gaiter are two ways of enabling an uninjured finger to give support to one which has been damaged. They should not be used for potentially unstable fractures or dislocations.

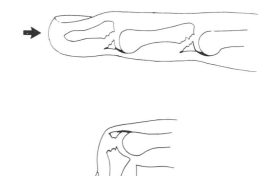

Fig. 34.13 End-on injuries. If the finger remains straight, the base of the middle or distal phalanges is split and a fracture subluxation results; if the terminal joint flexes abruptly, the extensor insertion, often with a fragment of bone, is avulsed from the distal phalanx, resulting in a mallet finger.

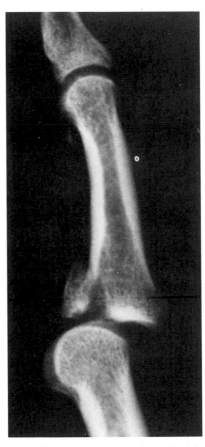

Fig. 34.14 An unstable fracture subluxation at the proximal interphalangeal joint, involving the intermediate phalanx.

be forcibly flexed, whilst the more proximal part of the finger remains straight.

Injuries to bone

When the whole finger remains straight, the base of the distal or middle phalanges may be split vertically by the rounded head of the more proximal phalanx. The major fragment usually subluxes from the interphalangeal joint (Figs 34.13 and 34.14). Such a patient should be referred for open reduction if a full return of function is to be anticipated. This fracture/subluxation is readily missed if the x-ray is not centred on the appropriate joint. The request to the radiographer must therefore indicate precisely which part of the finger has been injured.

Another common end-on injury is the boxer's injury to the neck of the fifth metacarpal. This is always an impacted fracture and

should not be disimpacted for correction of the angulation, unless this is extreme. Most transverse, spiral or oblique fractures of a single metacarpal also merit only supporting strapping and elevation. There are, however, some exceptions, and these include:

1. Multiple fractures of the metacarpals, which may require internal fixation.

2. A transverse fracture at the base of the first metacarpal (not involving the joint), which should be treated in the scaphoid plaster.

Injuries to tendon

When the tip of the extended finger is forcibly flexed, the extensor tendon may be avulsed — with or without a small fragment of bone (this is one example of an avulsion fracture). This has been described under the section on tendon injuries (see 'Mallet finger', p. 358).

Angulating injuries

Intra-articular fractures

An end-on blow to a finger may be accompanied by some lateral angulation. In children this commonly causes a fracture through the epiphyseal plate (Fig. 34.15). In adults the injury produces an intra-articular fracture, frequently associated with subluxation at the proximal or the distal interphalangeal joint. These are potentially unstable fractures and should be referred for specialist advice because some will require open reduction (Fig. 34.16).

These small triangular fractures may be readily missed unless x-rays are centred on the appropriate joint. One common example

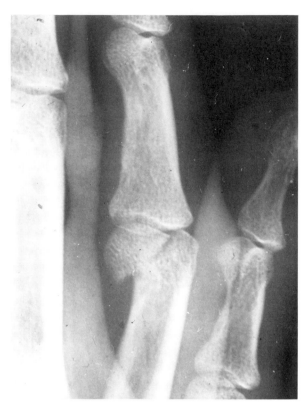

Fig. 34.16 Another unstable fracture subluxation at the proximal interphalangeal joint, this time involving the head of the proximal phalanx.

of this type of fracture is the Bennett's fracture/subluxation at the base of the first metacarpal. It is a difficult fracture to treat and may require internal fixation.

Oblique and transverse fractures of the shafts

An angulating force may produce a transverse or oblique fracture of the shaft of a phalanx or metacarpal — and this may be closed or open. All such fractures are potentially unstable and will therefore usually be referred for specialist advice. However, initial reduction and bandaging in the appropriate position can usually be achieved without much difficulty using a regional (digital) nerve block. Any rotation at the fracture site must be corrected and the finger bandaged in flexion and correct alignment in relation to the adjacent fingers. Ultimate recovery of function will depend on the degree of involvement of the soft tissues (such as flexor or extensor tendons) around the fracture site. These patients may therefore require prolonged physiotherapy and occupational therapy, and are better managed in a special hand clinic.

Dislocations of the proximal interphalangeal and distal interphalangeal joints

These may be easily reduced a few seconds after the accident on the sports field. If the patient decides to come to hospital for the manipulation there is often a delay of half to one hour, during which time swelling has developed around the joint, making

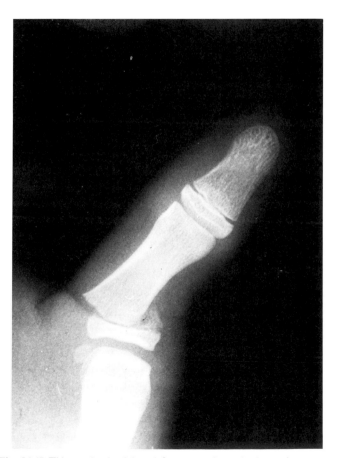

Fig. 34.15 This angulated epiphyseal fracture requires reduction and immobilisation for 2–3 weeks.

reduction more painful and more difficult. A radiograph should be taken to show that there is no associated fracture. The dislocation is then reduced under digital nerve block or a nitrous oxide-oxygen mixture (Entonox) and an adjacent finger attached to the injured digit by means of strapping or a double elastic tubular gauze bandage support for 10 days. Occasionally, however, dislocations of the interphalangeal or metacarpophalangeal joints cannot be reduced by this method. This is because the head of the phalanx or metacarpal has 'button-holed' the volar plate, and open reduction will then be required. Such patients should be referred for specialist care. Dislocation of the proximal interphalangeal joint is very likely to cause a rupture of the middle slip of the extensor tendon, an avulsion of the volar plate or a rupture of the medial or lateral collateral ligaments. These injuries should be sought in patients whose dislocations have been reduced prior to their arrival in hospital. They may also occur without complete dislocation.

Avulsion of the volar plate

This follows hyperextension injuries (Fig. 34.17). The proximal interphalangeal joint is most commonly affected and becomes distended with blood and spindle shaped. The front of the joint is tender, but the collateral ligaments feel stable when stressed. A good lateral radiograph centred on this joint will sometimes show a small fragment of bone which has been avulsed from the front of the base of the middle phalanx (Fig. 34.18). Immobilisation for two weeks on a padded aluminium splint, in slight flexion, followed by active use, results in rapid resolution of the pain and

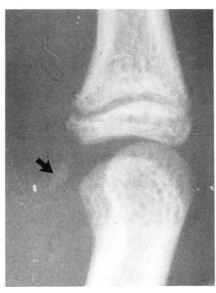

Fig. 34.18 A volar plate avulsion fracture. This type of 'sprained finger' should be rested in flexion until the pain subsides.

return of movement. The swelling, however, may take many weeks to resolve completely.

Collateral ligament injuries

In the proximal interphalangeal joint these present with asymmetrical 'spindling', tenderness on one side or the other, a feeling of 'give' when the ligament is stressed and, occasionally, a small avulsion fracture from the base of the affected side of the middle phalanx (see Fig. 34.19). The injured finger should be attached to the adjacent finger on the side of the torn ligament by strapping or double elastic tubular gauze bandage for three weeks. The pain usually subsides rapidly and movement returns, but the spindling may persist for several weeks. These injuries must not be confused with the intra-articular fractures which have been described.

Occasionally, the collateral ligaments of the metacarpophalangeal joints of the fingers may be injured, and avulsion fractures at this site may be mistaken for sesamoid bones (and vice versa). Whilst the collateral ligaments of the proximal interphalangeal joint should be examined and stressed with the finger extended, the collateral ligament of the metacarpophalangeal joint should be examined with the joint in the flexed position. The reason for this is that the flexed position the metacarpophalangeal collateral ligaments are normally tight. This anatomical peculiarity is also the reason for immobilising the metacarpophalangeal joints in the flexed position whenever possible.

One of the most commonly injured ligaments in the hand is the ulnar collateral ligament of the metacarpophalangeal joint of the thumb. To make the diagnosis, the ligament should be stressed by abducting the thumb on the metacarpal, which is fixed by the other hand (Fig. 34.20). The amount of movement should be compared with that in the other hand. Any excessive movement may be demonstrated with x-ray films of both thumbs in the

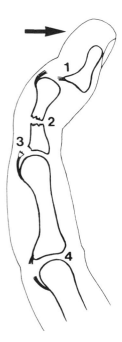

Fig. 34.17 Key: 1 — dislocation, 2 — transverse fracture, 3 — volar plate avulsion fracture, 4 — volar plate ligamentous injury. Hyperextension most commonly results in a volar plate injury, with or without avulsion of a fragment of bone and with or without dislocation. Alternatively there may be a transverse, unstable fracture in the mid shaft of the middle or proximal phalanges.

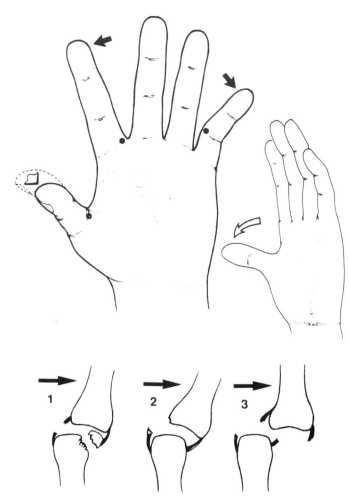

Fig. 34.19 Key: 1 — unstable fracture dislocation, 2 — collateral ligament avulsion fracture, 3 — dislocation with bilateral rupture of ligaments. These patterns of injury commonly affect the proximal interphalangeal joint.

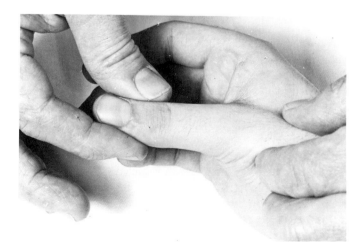

Fig. 34.20 To test the integrity of the collateral ligaments of the metacarpophalangeal joint of the thumb, grip the metacarpal to immobilise it and compare the range of abduction and adduction with that in the uninjured thumb.

stressed position. However, not infrequently a plain radiograph will show a small avulsion fracture at the base of the ulnar side of the proximal phalanx, which will confirm the diagnosis and obviate the need for stress films. Surgical repair may be necessary.

It will be seen, therefore, that critical scrutiny of the mechanism of the injury, of the physical signs and of carefully positioned radiograph will allow an anatomical label to be put on most so-called 'sprains' of the fingers. Only if this care is taken, will lesions which require active intervention be identified so that appropriate treatment can be undertaken early and a full return of function achieved.

FINGER TIP INJURIES AND AMPUTATIONS

Experience during the past decade has confirmed that the preferable method of treatment for amputations of the finger tip is to clean the wound (this may require a local anaesthetic), apply a non-adhesive sterile dressing and allow the tissues to regenerate. The results may be better in children than adults, but even older patients still have the ability to regrow a very acceptable finger end. The various plastic surgical procedures involving the advancement of skin flaps have no advantage over spontaneous tissue regeneration.

If the level of amputation is distal to the germinal area at the base of the nail, satisfactory regeneration will occur provided the process is not inhibited by primary skin closure or the application of a skin graft (Fig. 34.21).

When the injury has destroyed or devitalised the finger at the level of the base of the distal phalanx, terminalisation of the finger end is advisable. Even then the epiphysis of the phalanx should be preserved if possible, otherwise the flexor profundus sheath will be opened. If the flexor sheath is opened it will fill with blood resulting in swelling and limitation of flexion at the proximal interphalangeal joint, which may take weeks to resolve. Occasionally the detached profundus tendon retracts as a mechanical block to finger flexion and has to be removed later.

If the injury is at the level of the distal interphalangeal joint then the articular surface and condyles of the intermediate phalanx are resected. Whenever possible a volar skin flap is used to close over the end of the finger, thereby ensuring that the suture line lies on the dorsum of the finger. The flap must be firm, but not under tension, to give a pain-free, acceptable stump.

Amputation proximal to neck of intermediate phalanx

Preservation of remnants of fingers proximal to the neck of the intermediate phalanx seldom gives a satisfactory functional or cosmetic result. For the index or little finger, a cosmetic amputation in which half the metacarpal head is excised obliquely gives a good cosmetic result and satisfactory function (Fig. 34.22). When the surgeon has removed the index finger, the middle finger can take over all its functions; it has been like a reserve player waiting on the touch line for an opportunity to replace the first-choice finger. The only slight disadvantage is that, having only one extensor

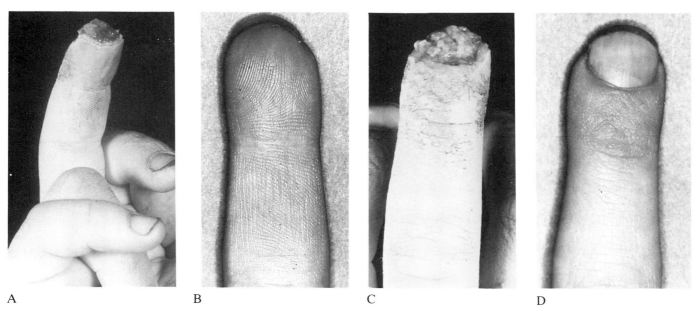

A   B   C   D

Fig. 34.21 A–D Treatment of a finger tip amputation by wound toilet and the application of a non-adhesive sterile dressing permitted regeneration of the pulp of the finger tip and also a new finger nail. Before and after photographs from the same patient.

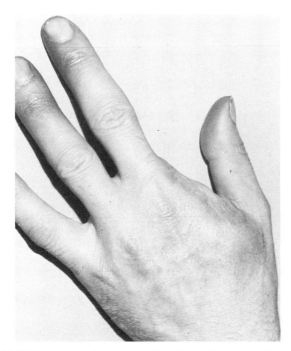

Fig. 34.22 Transmetacarpal amputation of the index finger in a skilled engineer enabled him to return to work with a cosmetically acceptable hand.

tendon, as compared with the two that serve the index, it is not quite as decisive when used as a pointing finger.

Amputation of the middle or ring fingers at the level of the metacarpophalangeal joint leaves a gap which is unsightly and a nuisance. A young patient in this situation should be referred to a hand surgeon with a view to excision of the distal two-thirds of the metacarpal so that the gap can be closed.

Thumb amputation

Partial amputation of an injured thumb needs careful consideration. In general, the level of amputation should be as far distal as possible, but the stump should be covered with viable full-thickness skin which retains its sensory innervation. Occasionally a neurovascular pedicle flap may be used, but it is usually more practicable to shorten the bone a few millimetres further, if this will allow a locally based skin flap carrying its own nerve supply to be used to cover the stump of bone. A thumb or finger tip which has poor quality of sensation will, in practice, be kept out of the way and never used.

OTHER HAND INJURIES

The severely mutilated hand which has been mangled by moving machinery or, for instance, crushed in a printing press, requires the attention of an experienced hand surgeon. Analgesia and a sterile dressing are the primary requirements in the A & E department.

High pressure injection injuries (grease or paint guns) need urgent surgical treatment. The pain is out of proportion to the visible signs of injury (Fig. 34.23). After a few hours the inflammatory response causes swelling and may result in gangrene of the fingers if decompression is not carried out urgently.

Patients occasionally arrive at hospital with amputated portions of the hands or fingers with a view to reimplantation. If the detached part has not been crushed, and particularly if more than one finger is involved, place it in a dry plastic bag and surround the bag with ice. Then contact a hand surgeon for further advice.

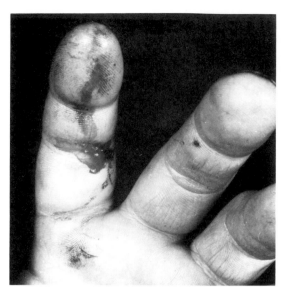

Fig. 34.23 Picture taken within an hour of the small, bleeding entry wound from a greasegun injury. In spite of its innocent appearance extensive exploration and decompression of the finger and palm were necessary for the eventual restoration of full function.

The problem of foreign bodies embedded in the hand is discussed in Ch. 39. Dressing and splinting is described in Ch. 38.

REVIEW CLINICS

The surgeon who manipulates or sutures an injured hand should ensure that the patient obtains the optimum result. If, after the initial visit, the patient is returned to the care of his general practitioner, the A & E surgeon has no means of monitoring the degree of success or failure of his work. The patient should be told to return at any time if the hand or finger becomes increasingly painful. If the circulation is in doubt, the patient should be seen again after one or two days. Non-absorbable sutures can usually be removed after 7 days and all patients with injuries confined to the skin or soft tissue should commence active movements after a week. Tendon repairs require 18–21 days immobilisation, but no finger should immobilised for more than 3 weeks.

REHABILITATION

For those patients whose fingers have become stiff or who are afraid to use their hand, a few days of 'wax and exercises' in the physiotherapy department in the second or third week after injury usually achieves rapid success. It is not acceptable practice to wait two or three months before starting treatment, for by this time the finger joints are stiff and rigid; weeks or months of treatment will be required and the result will be less than perfect. The maxim for hand rehabilitation is 'a treatment in time saves nine'.

Occupational therapy is indicated for those patients who find that their skill and dexterity have been impaired as a result of the injury. Close co-operation between surgeon, physiotherapist and occupational therapist can often achieve results far better than could be foreseen at the time of the initial injury.

FURTHER READING

The hand: diagnosis and indications Lister, G 1984 Churchill Livingstone, Edinburgh

Basic care of the injured hand Macnicol M F, Lamb D W 1984 Churchill Livingstone, Edinburgh

Musculoskeletal problems of the arm and leg

This chapter concerns musculoskeletal conditions of the limbs which may present to the A & E department. Although there are references to bony injuries, no attempt is made to cover the whole subject of fracture diagnosis and management. The reader is advised to consult a standard orthopaedic text for this aspect of emergency work (e.g. McRae 1981).

The chapter deals with the problems on a regional anatomical basis. However, a patient may have more than one lesion and it is important to appreciate that a problem in one part of a limb may have repercussions on the function of the limb as a whole.

At the end of the chapter is a short discussion of a few of the important points and problems of fracture management, the general treatment for soft tissue injuries and of peripheral nerve injuries. Related topics are discussed in Ch. 14 (The severely injured patient), Ch. 36 (Sports injuries), Ch. 27 (Limb pain) and Ch. 38 (Dressing and splintage). Hand injuries are reviewed in Ch. 34.

THE ACUTELY PAINFUL SHOULDER

Dislocation of the shoulder

The most dramatic presentation of the acutely painful shoulder is a dislocation at the glenohumeral joint, usually caused by a fall. The patient arrives at hospital in considerable pain and is unwilling or unable to move the affected arm. The humerus can dislocate in one of three directions.

1. **Anterior glenohumeral dislocation** (Fig. 35.1) is the commonest dislocation seen in the A & E department. It is common throughout adult life but the pathology and treatment are different at the two extremes of age. In young adults the labrum and capsule are stripped off the front of the scapula, whereas in the elderly the humeral head passes out of the joint through the anteroinferior or weakest part of the capsule. The diagnosis can be made by inspection since the normal rounded contour of the joint, formed by the greater tuberosity of the humerus and the overlying deltoid muscle, is lost (Fig. 35.2). The head of the humerus usually comes to lie in the subcoracoid position, where it can often be palpated from the axilla. It is wise to test for anaesthesia on the upper outer aspect of the arm in the distribution of the axillary nerve. This should be tested and recorded both before

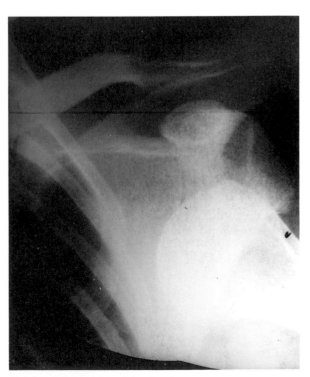

Fig. 35.1 Anterior dislocation of the shoulder

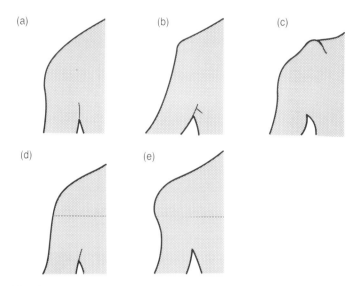

Fig. 35.2 The shapes of shoulders: a — normal, b — anterior dislocation, c — acromioclavicular dislocation, d — deltoid atrophy, e — fracture of the neck of the humerus.

and after reduction, to determine whether any nerve lesion was caused by the initial injury or by the manipulation.

2. **Posterior dislocation** (Fig. 35.3) is uncommon. The humeral head cannot displace medially behind the scapula and the arm becomes fixed in full internal rotation. There is often only slight incongruity of the humeral head and the glenoid articular surface in the AP radiograph yet the appearance of the humeral head seems odd. *Axial views* may be necessary to elucidate this easily missed condition.

3. **Luxatio erecta** (Fig. 35.4) is an extremely rare form of anterior dislocation in which the shoulder dislocates with the arm above the head.

Management of shoulder dislocation

Radiographic confirmation of the diagnosis should be obtained before attempting manipulation. If there is also a fracture of the neck of the humerus, manipulation will serve only to displace the fracture and not to reduce the dislocated humeral head. Where there has been associated avulsion of the greater tuberosity of the humerus, manipulation will reduce both this and the dislocation.

The favoured method of reduction of the uncomplicated subcoracoid dislocation is the *Milch technique* (Beattie et al 1986). This relies on a postural manoeuvre to achieve relaxation of all the muscles acting across the shoulder. Its advantage in the A & E department is that reduction can be effected without anaesthesia. The aim is for the patient to put his arm behind his head. With one hand steadying the humeral head in the axilla, the operator grasps the patient's wrist with his other hand and slowly and steadily abducts the patient's arm fully before gently applying external rotation and traction. Pressure on the humeral head is

maintained with the other hand until reduction is, silently, achieved.

When the Milch manoeuvre fails then *Kocher's method* can be applied. In an elderly patient Entonox can be used as analgesia, possibly with a titration of intravenous diazepam. In the younger subject a general anaesthetic with muscle relaxation may be necessary. In resistant cases the *Hippocratic manoeuvre* (traction against the counterpressure of the heel in the axilla) may be required. Very rarely closed reduction fails and operative reduction is then indicated.

Reduction of the posterior dislocation is usually easily effected by applying traction to the arm abducted to 90° and then externally rotating the arm. The reduction may be unstable and the arm may need to be immobilised in abduction.

In the elderly a broad arm sling outside the clothes for a week after reduction is all that is required, whereas in the young the joint should be immobilised in a sling under the clothes and the arm bandaged or strapped to the chest for three weeks to allow healing of the tear in the glenoid labrum. If this rigorous immobilisation is not enforced, recurrent dislocation is likely.

A *recurrent dislocation* is treated in the same way but the patient should be referred to an orthopaedic surgeon with a view to surgical reconstruction.

Acromioclavicular joint subluxation

This injury may, commonly, follow a fall on the point of the shoulder. There is tenderness over the acromioclavicular joint and, often, a visible or palpable step in the contour of the shoulder when the patient is upright. Conservative management with the arm supported in a broad arm sling for one week followed by strengthening exercises is all that is, usually, required.

Fractured neck of humerus

This is a common condition in elderly people following a fall. There may be an associated shearing fracture of the greater tuberosity. The shoulder will be swollen, bruised and stiff. The fracture to the surgical neck will be revealed on the radiograph and, frequently, the shaft will be seen to be impacted into the head in an abducted position. The majority of injuries are undisplaced and reduction is unnecessary, even when there is impaction. A sling is worn for three weeks with active shoulder mobilisation commencing after three days. The patient should be warned to expect extensive bruising in the arm.

In adolescents *fracture-separation of the upper humeral epiphysis* occurs. When there is severe displacement open reduction will be indicated.

Fractures of the clavicle

Most cases of collar bone fracture occur at its weakest point — the junction of middle and outer thirds — as a result of indirect force, usually from a fall on the outstretched hand. Healing is, usually, straightforward and no more is required than a broad arm

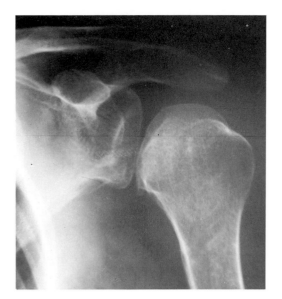

A

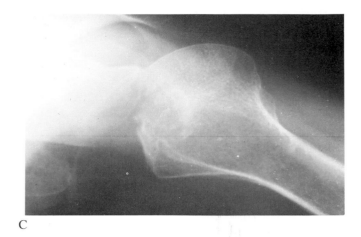
C

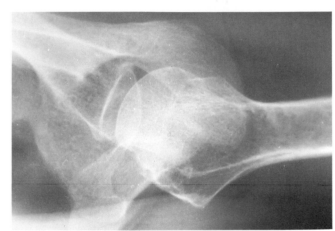
D

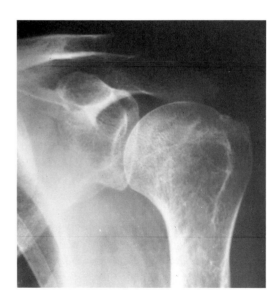

B

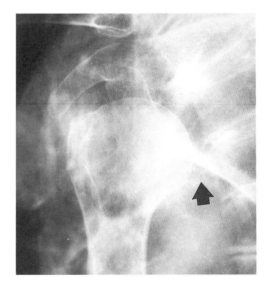
E

Fig. 35.3 Posterior dislocation of the shoulder. **A** The A-P view may look almost normal but is seen to be internally rotated when compared with **B** The postreduction view. **C** The axial view, the roughened area of the greater tuberosity is in contact with the glenoid. This reverts to its normal position after reduction — **D**. **E** The lateral view may be difficult to interpret. The head of the humerus comes to lie posteriorly in the glenoid fossa. There is a step (arrowed) in the normally smooth curve between humeral neck and margin of scapula.

sling worn under the clothes for three weeks. Where there is gross displacement, intolerable pain or a threat of damage to the overlying skin then the traditional treatment of 'figure of eight bracing' may be employed (ready made 'Macleod slings' are available). Felt rings encircling each axilla are held together at the back. As the link needs to be tightened twice daily and considerable pressure needs to be applied for the brace to be effective this form of treatment should be supervised in the fracture clinic.

Fractures at the end of the clavicle result from direct force, e.g. from a rugby or motor cycle accident, and are handled in the same way as acromioclavicular joint injuries. In extreme cases with displacement and rupture of the ligamentous complex open

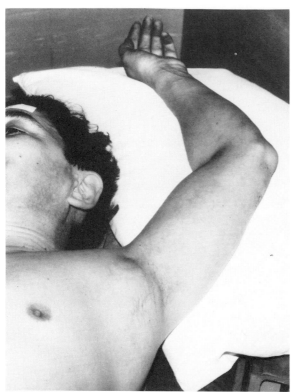

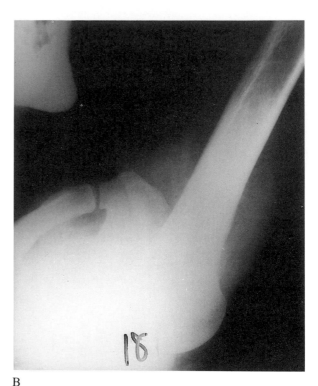

A   B

Fig. 35.4 A and **B** In the rare condition of luxatio erecta the arm is held vertically above the shoulder.

reduction and internal fixation with primary repair of the ligaments is sometimes preferred.

The painful stiff shoulder

A number of anatomical lesions in and around the glenohumeral joint are characterised by painful limitation of movement. The problem frequently follows trauma, in which there may have been damage to the rotator cuff muscles, or may arise spontaneously as a degenerative process. The shoulder is more likely than other joints to become stiff from disuse which may complicate and mask other shoulder disorders. Simple disuse stiffness responds well to exercises.

Rotator cuff tears

The tendons of supraspinatus, infraspinatus, teres minor and subscapularis all blend with the capsule of the shoulder and together constitute the rotator cuff. A fall on the arm, a jerking movement or physical violence to the arm in a road or sports accident may tear part of the rotator cuff. Typically, the patient gives a history of having lurched sideways, striking the upper arm, but the exact site of the tear depends on the direction of the force and the position of the shoulder at the moment of impact. A description of the accident and palpation for the point of maximum tenderness will help to determine which structure is mainly involved. The supraspinatus initiates abduction of the shoulder

and, together with the infraspinatus and teres minor, produces external rotation. The subscapularis tendon, which passes anterior to the joint, produces internal rotation. Testing active movements will confirm the anatomical site of the injury. A complete tear of the supraspinatus tendon is suggested by the patient's inability to initiate abduction accompanied by tenderness over the point of the shoulder. Rarely, this is amenable to surgical reconstruction. Incomplete lesions are more common. They usually respond to rest in a sling, analgesics and subsequent graded passive and active movements. If the pain persists despite rest then an injection of corticosteroid and local anaesthetic often results in dramatic improvement. An injection of 40 mg/ml methylprednisolone acetate combined with 1% lignocaine is commonly used. The injection often makes the pain worse for a day or so before improvement occurs. The patient should be warned about this, the shoulder rested in a sling and analgesics prescribed.

Supraspinatus tendinitis

This is essentially a degenerative condition. With the arm at the side the supraspinatus tendon is stretched over the dome of the head of the humerus where the fibres at its outer end become relatively avascular. Quite minor trauma may cause a small capsular tear in the ischaemic tendon. This condition occurs most frequently in middle-aged men. There will be a tender spot at the tip of the shoulder, close to the insertion of the tendon, and resisted movements of the muscle will be painful. Calcified material may

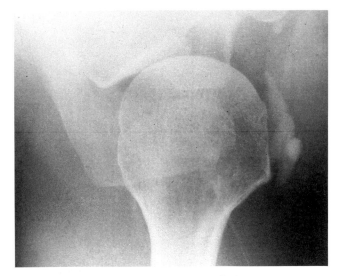

Fig. 35.5 Soft tissue calcification in the rotator cuff of a patient with an acutely painful shoulder.

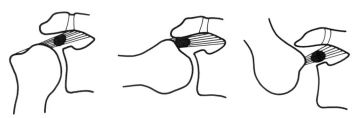

Fig. 35.7 The painful arc. As the arm is abducted the head of the humerus squeezes the subacromial bursa under the overlying acromial process. This produces symptoms between 60° and 120° of movement.

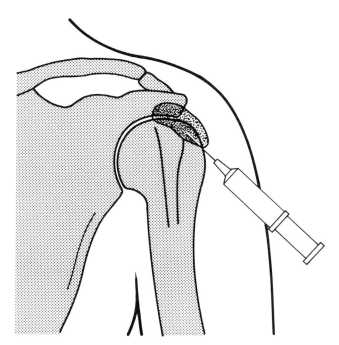

Fig. 35.6 Injection of a supraspinatus tendinitis.

be evident on radiographic examination (Fig. 35.5). The treatment is infiltration with local anaesthetic and a steroid followed by graded exercises (Fig. 35.6).

The 'painful arc'

With degenerative changes in the supraspinatus or in rotator cuff tears a 'painful arc' of movement may be demonstrated. Movements of the shoulder are full but on abduction there is pain as the arm passes through the arc between about 60° and 120°. The pain may be much worse as the arm is lowered when it may drop suddenly as it passes the horizontal position. It is due to the head

of the humerus squeezing the subacromial bursa under the overhanging acromial process (Fig. 35.7). The pain and inflammation is usually relieved by steroid injection into the bursa beneath the tip of the acromion process.

Acute calcification syndrome

Occasionally the heterotopic calcification in the rotator cuff leaks into the subacromial bursa producing a characteristic clinical picture. Pain is constant, present at rest and very severe. There will be very little active movement of the shoulder. Permanent relief should be obtained by a steroid injection into the subacromial bursa. Rarely, after repeated injections, curettage of this toothpaste-like material will be required, for which patients should be referred to the orthopaedic department.

Pericapsulitis (frozen shoulder)

This frustrating condition occurs mainly in elderly people. It sometimes follows minor trauma or prolonged use of the shoulder, as in house decorating. It can also occur after prolonged disuse, as after a stroke, a myocardial infarction or prolonged intravenous feeding. There is generalised constant pain which disturbs sleep and often depresses the patient. Movement in the shoulder joint almost disappears — though scapulothoracic movement is preserved. Pain may be relieved by analgesics but, as it may be some months before the patient is pain-free and even longer before movement returns, referral to an orthopaedic surgeon or a consultant in rehabilitation is advisable.

Brachial neuralgia

Neuralgia amyotrophia (p. 294) is an uncommon cause of pain and stiffness of the shoulder in men between the ages of 30 and 50. It is presumably due to a viral infection. Often there is a history of preceding illness, injury or operation. There is a sudden onset of extremely severe pain in the shoulder. The pain may limit shoulder movements. After the acute phase the patient may be left with a palsy of the long thoracic nerve which results in winging of the scapula but, occasionally other peripheral nerve roots or nerves are involved. The acute phase of severe pain may last up to three weeks during which strong analgesia is required. The neurological lesion recovers slowly over 12–18 months. Physiotherapy is required to restore power to affected muscles.

PAIN AROUND THE ELBOW

Dislocation

Dislocation of the elbow usually occurs posteriorly. It can be distinguished clinically from a fracture by noting the relationship of the three bony points (the olecranon and the two epicondyles). As with all severe injuries around the elbow, it is important to check the circulation and motor and sensory function in the forearm and hand. Before attempting reduction a radiograph is necessary to ensure that no fragments of bone (such as the medial epicondyle) have been pulled into the joint.

An uncomplicated dislocation of less than two hours old usually can be reduced under a nitrous oxide/oxygen mixture (Entonox). Otherwise a general anaesthetic will be required. A strong pull is applied in the line of the limb, with the elbow slightly flexed. Following reduction, the elbow requires support in a wool and crepe bandage and immobilisation for three weeks in a sling followed by gradual mobilisation.

Fractures around the elbow

A number of fractures occur around the elbow, their type varying with the patient's age and the mechanism of injury. For advice on diagnosis and management of the individual injury the reader is referred to a standard orthopaedic textbook.

In children the most important injury is the supracondylar fracture (see below). Another serious injury is the *fracture-separation of the lateral condylar epiphysis* which, without effective reduction, may fail to unite, leading to a valgus deformity and ulnar nerve palsy.

In the adolescent the *epiphysis of the medial epicondyle* may become avulsed following a fall on the hand.

In both children and adolescents it may be difficult to distinguish radiographically between a bony detachment and an ossification centre. X-ray films of the uninjured side can be obtained for comparison. A reference chart, held in the department, of growth centres with their fusion appearance at different ages is very valuable.

Injuries in the adult include the T-shaped and Y-shaped *intercondylar fractures;* the *fractured capitulum* and the *fractured olecranon.*

Elbow fractures with displacement at any age often require internal fixation, sometimes with open reduction, and should be referred to the orthopaedic department.

The childhood supracondylar fracture

This injury is given special emphasis because of its complications. The condition is an orthopaedic emergency. The patient with a displaced supracondylar fracture should be admitted to hospital and the fracture treated as a matter of urgency by an experienced surgeon. Following a fall onto the outstretched hand, the child with this injury will show a painful, swollen, motionless arm. Radiography will reveal the fracture with posterior displacement of the distal fragment and tilting or shifting of the fragment to

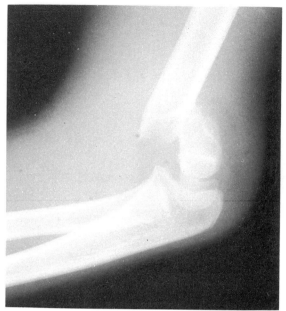

Fig. 35.8 Supracondylar fracture at the lower end of the humerus, a common childhood injury, is sometimes complicated by occlusion of the brachial artery.

one side or the other (Fig. 35.8). Vascular and nerve impairment of the forearm and hand should be looked for straightaway as damage to the brachial artery and/or median nerve occurs frequently when there is gross displacement. Operative manoeuvres seek to correct the displacement, the medial or lateral tilting of the fragment and rotational deformity about a vertical axis. After reduction a well-padded back-slab is applied in 60° flexion and half-hourly pulse, sensation and circulation checks are made over at least the next 24 hours. Again it is stressed that *this is a serious injury which demands expert care.*

Post-traumatic effusion

An effusion into the elbow joint may be detected most readily by comparing the hollows on either side of the olecranon from behind. Radiographically, an effusion will cause the anterior fat pad to become elevated from the front of the humerus and then the posterior fat pad to become visible (Fig. 35.9). Most post-traumatic effusions are accompanied by evidence of a bony injury such as a fracture of the head of the radius. Even when no fracture can be demonstrated the time to full recovery is increased (Smith & Lee 1978) and care must be taken in attempts to increase the range of movement. Any excessive passive manipulation may result in a local reaction and further loss of movement or the development of myositis ossificans (see below). Treatment is by analgesia if necessary and rest in a collar and cuff sling.

Myositis ossificans

After the thigh, the elbow is the second most common site for this condition. If, the elbow is not rested adequately after trauma repeated minor injuries lead to the formation of a haematoma in gentle active exercises under supervision. It may be weeks or even months before there is satisfactory resolution for a condition which should not occur if the initial treatment is correct.

Pulled elbow

'Pulled elbow' is a condition peculiar to young children aged from 1–4 years. It can occur when lifting the child up by the arm. After this the child refuses to use the arm which is held limply by the side. The condition frequently presents with pain in the wrist. The lesion is probably a subluxation of the head of the radius out of the annular ligament. Injury elsewhere in the arm should be excluded by gentle palpation of the shoulder (including clavicle), hand and wrist. Then, with the elbow flexed to a right angle and one of the examiner's thumbs on the head of the radius, the forearm is quickly supinated. If this does not produce a click, forced pronation should be applied. The child gives an extra loud cry, then eventually quietens down as the pain disappears and he can use the arm.

Radiology has nothing to offer in this condition except to exclude other injuries. The clinical presentation is so typical that the experienced doctor will proceed to manipulation without radiological examination. No immobilisation or further treatment of any kind is required other than to explain to the parents the nature of the problem.

Ruptured biceps

This lesion occurs most commonly in an elderly man doing manual work. He may have done the same job for many years but, one day, the strain proves too much for his ageing tissues and the muscle tears at the junction of the long head with the muscle belly. On examination it will be seen that the muscle still contracts, forming a prominent rounded mass in the arm (Fig. 35.10), but the strength of elbow flexion is seriously reduced. Unfortunately, the degenerating tissues are not amenable to surgical reconstruction and the disability has to be accepted. Rest and analgesics for a few days until the pain subsides is the only treatment.

Epicondylitis

Lateral epicondylitis ('tennis elbow') is common in adult life and may follow any activity involving prolonged gripping, such as

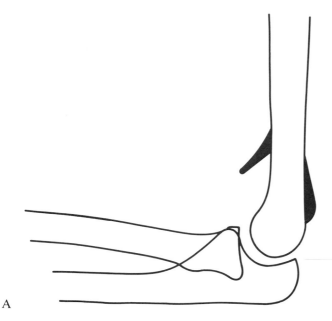

A

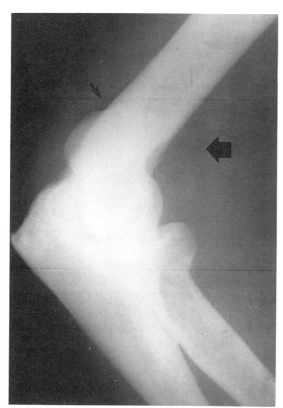

B

Fig. 35.9 A The 'fat pad sign' **B** Radiograph showing the posterior fat pad (arrowed) and the anterior fat pad (arrowed) pushed forwards from the lower end of the humerus by an effusion in the elbow joint of a patient with a fracture of the head of the radius.

the tissues surrounding the joint. Continued movement or, worse, forced passive movements result in this haematoma becoming calcified and the range of elbow movements diminishes even further. Never refer elbow injuries for physiotherapy. Treatment is by enforced rest for the joint until it is pain-free, and then by

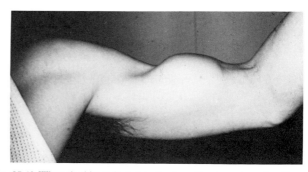

Fig. 35.10 When the biceps is ruptured, attempting to contract the elbow against resistance produces a characteristic bulge.

tennis, rowing, using a hammer or home decorating. Pain may spread from the elbow down the arm and tenderness is accurately localised to a point just in front of the lateral epicondyle of the humerus — the highest point of origin of the common wrist and finger extensors. Confirmation of the diagnosis may be had by eliciting pain on passive stretching (Mills's test; the elbow is straightened with the wrist flexed and the forearm fully pronated) or pain on active contraction against resistance (the elbow is held straight with the forearm prone and the fist clenched and the patient prevented from dorsiflexing his wrist). An injection of hydrocortisone into the tender spot often exacerbates the pain for one or two days following which the symptoms usually disappear. If this does not happen the injection may be repeated after a week but no more than two injections should be given. Ice and ultrasound therapy are beneficial for some patients. Occasionally surgical treatment is necessary.

Medial epicondylitis ('golfer's elbow') is much less common than tennis elbow. Treatment is similar.

Olecranon bursitis

A tiresome and incapacitating condition, this usually occurs in men with a manual occupation. It often responds to complete rest in a sling with firm crepe bandaging and a non-steroidal anti-inflammatory drug. Occasionally there is active infection in the bursa and antibiotic therapy is useful.

If the bursa is tense and painful, aspiration (approaching from above the elbow) followed by firm bandaging for a week will relieve the symptoms and may effect a permanent cure. If the aspirated fluid is cloudy or purulent benzyl penicillin 600 mg may be injected directly into the bursa and the aspirate sent for bacteriological investigation.

Permanent ablation of the bursa is indicated if a sinus develops or if there are repeated episodes of acute bursitis. The patient should be referred for such treatment.

Very rarely, *gout* may be the underlying cause of the symptoms.

FRACTURES OF THE FOREARM BONES

Fractured radius and ulna

There is no difficulty in recognising the fracture which runs through the mid-shafts of both forearm bones. This may be spiral or transverse depending upon the deforming forces. For spiral fractures reduction is usually achieved by traction and rotation and immobilisation provided by an above-elbow plaster cast. Transverse fractures may require internal fixation.

A fracture of only one forearm bone should raise the suspicion of an associated dislocation (Fig. 35.11) The entire forearm should be examined radiographically with views covering both elbow and wrist joints.

The Monteggia fracture-dislocation is a fracture of the shaft of the ulna with forward dislocation of the head of the radius. It follows a pronation fall onto the outstretched hand.

The Galeazzi fracture-dislocation follows a fall on the outstretched hand when the proximal carpus forces the forearm bones apart resulting in a fracture of the lower third of the radius and dislocation of the inferior radio-ulnar joint.

Both these injuries are problematic and should be referred for expert supervision.

Greenstick fractures

In the young child the bones are resilient and springy and accept a greater degree of bending or rotational deformity before they break. The subsequent fracture, therefore, shows the typical greenstick appearance. The fracture is angulated and incomplete with tearing of the periosteum and cortex on the obtuse side and preservation of these structures on the acute side as a 'hinge' (Fig. 35.12). Longitudinal compressive forces transmitted through the long axis of the bone which, in adults, result in impaction, produce, instead, the compression or buckle greenstick fracture (Fig. 35.13).

The obvious clinical features of swelling and point tenderness follow a fall onto the outstretched hand. The radiographic features should also be obvious to the doctor familiar with this type of injury (Fig. 35.14).

Treatment consists of support with a forearm slab, alloy splint or a firm bandage for up to three weeks. Manipulation is rarely necessary for the greenstick fracture in the centre of a long bone and has no place in the management of the buckle fracture.

The Colles fracture

In 1814 Abraham Colles described the commonest fracture seen in A & E departments:

> A transverse fracture of the distal end of the radius within 2 cm of the wrist joint with dorsal and radial displacement, dorsal and radial tilt and with impaction of the distal fragment. There may be a concomitant fracture of the ulnar styloid process.

The fracture follows a fall onto the outstretched hand in elderly women whose bones are osteoporotic and brittle. There is no mistaking the row of patients who present during the first frost, nursing their painful wrists in makeshift slings. There may be the classical 'dinnerfork deformity' (Fig. 35.15), visible swelling and bruising. There will always be localised tenderness over the fracture site. X-ray films show the degree of displacement and impaction — on the lateral view the normal 5° of forward angulation of the distal end of the radius is often reversed.

Unless there are compelling reasons to the contrary, most cases with impaction and/or more than 10° displacement should be reduced. Anaesthesia for reduction can be provided by a general aneasthetic, an intravenous regional anaesthetic or occasionally by direct injection of local anaesthetic into the fracture haematoma. (For anaesthetic techniques for fracture reduction see Ch. 9.) Reduction is achieved (Fig. 35.16) by:

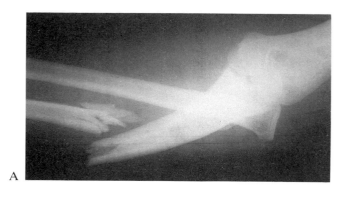

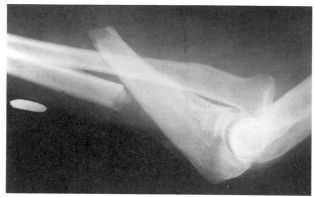

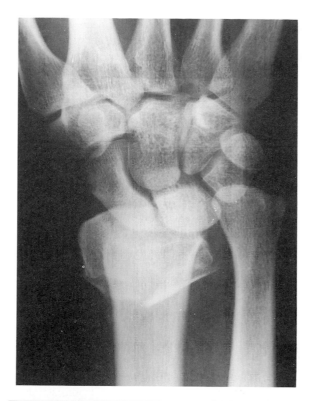

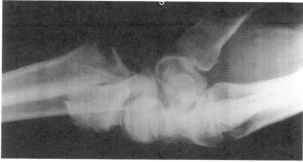

Fig. 35.11 Fractures of one forearm bone with associated dislocation. **A** and **B** The Monteggia injury is a fracture of the upper third of ulna with dislocation of the head of radius. **C** and **D** The Galeazzi injury is a fracture of the distal radius with dislocation of the distal radioulnar joint.

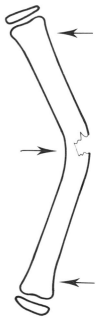

Fig. 35.12 A simple greenstick fracture.

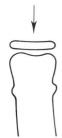

Fig. 35.13 A compression greenstick fracture.

1. Disimpaction of the distal fragment, usually by traction

2. Reduction by pressing the distal fragment in a volar direction followed by final flexion of the wrist (Robert Jones grip)

3. Locking the fracture by pronation, at the same time deviating the patient's wrist towards the ulna.

A forearm dorsal slab is applied to maintain the forearm pronated, the wrist slightly palmarflexed and with ulnar deviation. The

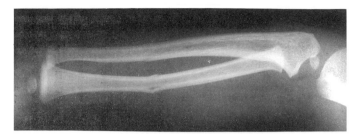

Fig. 35.14 A simple greenstick fracture of the radius.

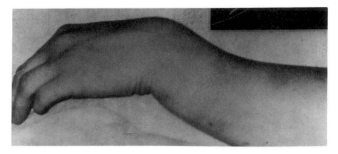

Fig. 35.15 The 'dinner-fork deformity' of the Colles fracture.

surgeon holds the limb in this position whilst the plaster is setting. Post-reduction radiographs are taken.

Commonly there is joint stiffness following this injury. The patient should be able to demonstrate shoulder abduction, elbow flexion and full finger movements — functions which may be rapidly checked by asking the patient to comb her hair.

The patient should be seen the next day so that the circulation and sensation in the limb can be checked. There should be no

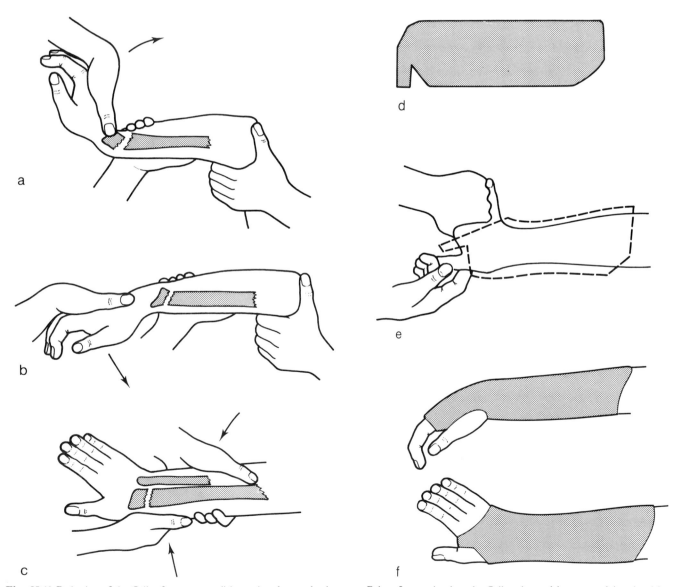

Fig. 35.16 Reduction of the Colles fracture: a — disimpaction, b — reduction, c — Robert Jones grip, d — the Colles plaster slab, e — applying the slab, f — the limb set in wrist-flexion, pronation and ulnar deviation.

hesitation in splitting the bandage if the fingers are blue, swollen and painful. The fracture usually unites in six weeks, during which time the patient will be supervised in the fracture clinic.

Fractures of the distal radius with anterior displacement

There are two main forms of fractures to the distal radius in which the fragment displaces forwards ('reversed Colles' deformity'):

1. **Smith's fracture** is a fracture of the lower end of the radius about 2 cm from the articular surface in which the lower fragments and the carpus displace anteriorly (Fig. 35.17). The fracture results from a fall on to the back of the wrist.

2. **Barton's fracture** is an anterior fracture-dislocation of the carpus in which a triangular fragment of the anterior margin of the lower end of the radius is shaved off and displaced proximally with the carpus (Fig. 35.18).

The Smith's fracture is reduced by disimpaction and is held, dorsiflexed in supination in an above-elbow plaster. The fracture-dislocation may be difficult to hold in a stable position and, usually, the preferred treatment is often open reduction with the fragment held by a small buttress plate.

Fracture-separation of the lower radial epiphysis

In children the force which, in an adult, would cause a Colles fracture, results in fracture-separation of the lower radial epiphysis. This is the juvenile Colles' fracture (Fig. 35.19). The injury is managed in the same way as in the adult.

THE ACUTELY PAINFUL WRIST

Following a sudden injury

Careful examination of the wrist following injury will usually reveal localised tenderness which indicates the anatomical source of the pain. A fracture of the scaphoid, the base of the first metacarpal

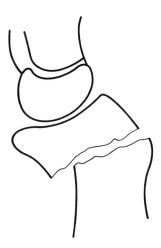

Fig. 35.17 Smith's fracture.

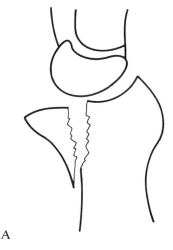

A

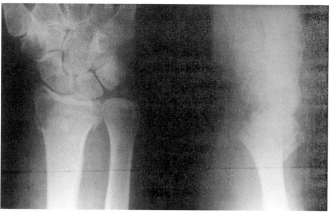

B
Fig. 35.18 A and B Barton's fracture.

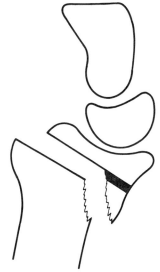

Fig. 35.19 The slipped lower radial epiphysis.

or the radial styloid are roughly similar on presentation. Similarly, confusion may also occur in the diagnosis of a fracture of the triquetral, the dorsal lip of the radius, the ulnar styloid or an effusion in the wrist joint. Accurate localisation of the tenderness will indicate the most probable site of the lesion. The precise anatomical diagnosis combined with an accurate history of the mechanism of the injury and its timing in relation to the onset of the pain will serve to differentiate between fractures, a carpal dislocation and other conditions such as arthrosis or tendinitis.

Accident doctors should be familiar with the normal features of wrist radiographs.

In the postero-anterior (PA) view (Fig. 35.20A):

1. The bones should appear of the right shape. For example the carpal lunate bone appears normally as a four-sided structure — with dislocation this bone assumes a triangular shape (see also Fig. 8.41).

2. The spaces of the three main joints (radiocarpal, midcarpal and carpometacarpal) should be clearly demarcated.

3. The midcarpal joint should be seen to form a 'C' around the proximal pole of the capitate.

In the lateral view (Fig. 35.20B):

1. There are two more 'C's; the convex proximal end of the lunate fitting into the distal end of the radius and the convex proximal end of the capitate fitting into the distal concavity of the lunate.

2. There is a straight line through the centres of the radius, lunate, capitate and the metacarpals.

3. The long axis of the scaphoid lies at 45° to the long axis of the limb.

4. Small avulsion fractures on the back of the wrist, usually from the triquetral (Fig. 35.21) are seen only on the lateral film.

If a fracture of a carpal bone or a carpal dislocation is suspected the four scaphoid views (including obliques) should be requested.

Dislocation of the wrist

This is rare. The force required to tear the surrounding ligaments is greater than that required to fracture the bones.

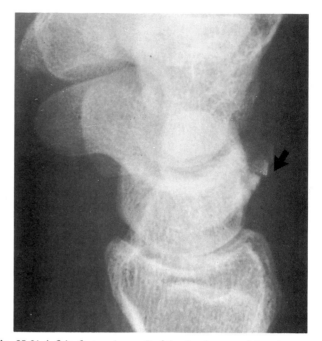

Fig. 35.21 A flake fracture (arrowed) of the dorsal aspect of the triquetrum following a forced dorsiflexion injury of the wrist.

Fracture of the carpal scaphoid

This fracture is common. In most cases, following a good history of a dorsiflexion injury, the indication by the patient of pain extending to both sides of the base of the thumb ('the clamp sign' — Kondoyannis 1982) and tenderness in the anatomical snuff box, a fracture line is visible on the original X-ray film. Nevertheless the original radiographs may show no fracture and, in suspicious cases, repeat radiographs should be obtained after two weeks. Isotope bone imaging may be used in doubtful cases. Meanwhile the wrist is immobilised in a scaphoid cast with the thumb and index finger in apposition and the wrist slightly flexed (Fig. 35.22). Non-union (and, in a small proportion of cases, avascular necrosis of the proximal pole) is the high price to be paid for failure to diagnose and adequately manage this injury.

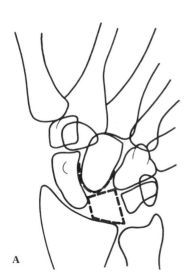 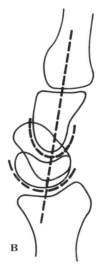

Fig. 35.20 Interpretation of the normal wrist radiograph: A — PA view, B — lateral view.

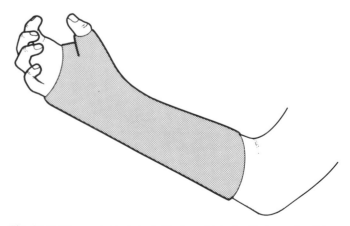

Fig. 35.22 The scaphoid plaster holds the wrist in dorsiflexion and radial deviation with the thumb in line with the index finger.

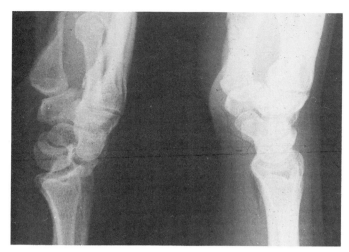

Fig. 35.23 Lateral radiographs of normal and abnormal wrists to show a perilunar dislocation of the wrist.

Lunate and perilunar dislocations (Fig. 35.23)

Following a dorsiflexion injury the hand and most of the carpus may be dislocated backwards leaving only the lunate in contact with the radius. This is the *perilunar dislocation*. Usually the carpus snaps back into position pushing the lunate ahead of it so that it remains dislocated *(dislocation of the lunate)*. When there is a concomitant fracture of the scaphoid and the ligaments responsible for maintaining the stability of the carpus are disrupted the proximal half of the scaphoid remains alongside the lunate in its displaced position *(trans-scaphoid perilunar dislocation)*. These dislocations of the carpal bones require expert management. Compression of the median nerve is very common and sensation must be checked and recorded. Urgent reduction is needed especially if the nerve is injured.

Following repetitive trauma

A prolonged bout of manual work, such as cutting a hedge with garden shears or painting a house, or starting a new job which involves constantly repeated movements of the wrists (such as typing, or wringing nappies) may cause pain on the radial side of the back of the wrist. The symptoms may present in one of two ways. The first is tenosynovitis of the wrist, the second stenosing tenovaginitis.

Tenosynovitis

In this condition, there will be a tender, often sausage-shaped swelling passing obliquely across the radial side of the back of the lower forearm. Crepitus is often felt when the patient moves the wrist or thumb. *Tenosynovitis* is the name usually ascribed to this very common, prescribed industrial disease. Strictly, however, there are two variants of the condition distinguished by their location: tenosynovitis proper affects the synovial sheaths where it is confined to the wrist and hand; the much commoner and more benign *peritendinitis crepitans* affects the

musculotendinous junctions which lie in the forearm well above the upper limit of the tendon sheaths. Both variants usually respond to immobilisation for 10 days — the former in a scaphoid plaster cast extended to include the interphalangeal joint of the thumb and the latter in a simple, proprietary wrist support. Non-steroidal anti-inflammatory drugs may be useful.

Stenosing tenovaginitis (de Quervain's disease)

This is commoner in women aged between 40 and 50 years. The retinaculum of the tendons of the abductor pollicis longus and extensor pollicis brevis muscles becomes inflamed. At a later stage it may be thickened and is felt as a hard nodule in the region of Lister's tubercle on the back of the wrist. There is a characteristic history of attempting to grip and lift a saucepan or a shovel of coal. The intense sharp pain makes the patient lose her grip and there is a danger of scalding. When not performing some such movement there is little or no pain. The pain may be referred proximally up the forearm but the tenderness is precisely located to the lateral aspect of the radial styloid. Palpable crepitus is absent. Pain is felt if the patient is asked to ulnar deviate the hand with the thumb clasped in flexion (Finckelstein's test) or if the thumb is passively adducted across the palm.

In the early stages the condition usually responds to an injection of hydrocortisone under the retinaculum followed by a week's rest. If this is unsuccessful, 14 days rest in a cast may suffice to relieve the symptoms. Once an obvious lump is present this is unlikely to give relief. Then surgical decompression of the tendons by incision of the retinaculum should be considered.

THE ACUTELY PAINFUL HIP

Age and hip pain

The hip joint suffers different pathologies at different ages. Congenital dislocation (Fig. 35.24) would never, one hopes, be diagnosed for the first time in the A & E department. Suppurative arthritis, however, may occur in the neonatal period. Like tuberculosis, though, it can be found at all ages.

Perthes' disease

From the age of 4–10 years, pain in the hip, or pain in the knee referred from the hip, may be due to avascular necrosis of the upper femoral epiphysis, known as Perthes' disease. The child has a limp and the radiographs show a dense flattened or fragmented epiphysis with an increased joint space.

Slipped upper femoral epiphysis

From the age of 8–15 years, similar symptoms accompanied by reduced range of hip movements (especially abduction and internal rotation) are frequently due to slipping of the upper femoral epiphysis. The first radiographic sign is the loss of the mound which normally rises above the superior surface of the neck of

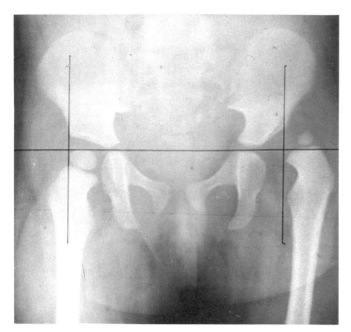

Fig. 35.24 Congenital dislocation of the hip confirmed radiologically by 'dropping' perpendiculars from the outer edge of the acetabulum and drawing a horizontal through the centre of the acetabuli (Perkin's squares). The normal femoral epiphysis will then lie in the lower medial quadrant. On the normal side note also the undersized epiphysis and the deficient acetabular roof.

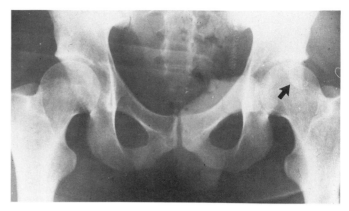

Fig. 35.25 In a head-on collision the patient's flexed hip was forced posteriorly, producing the fracture of the acetabular margin indicated by the arrow. This type of fracture is easily missed unless it is suspected from careful examination of the patient and of the radiograph. No X-ray film should be scrutinised until the patient has been examined.

the femur as one passes from neck to epiphysis on an AP film (see Fig. 8.45). The special 'frog view' will help in confirming the diagnosis. Early treatment is important if further slipping and long-term disability are to be avoided.

Irritable hip

Throughout any of these years, but especially between the ages of 3 and 8, a child may complain of pain, a limp and limited movement of the hip. If the radiographic appearance is normal, the child should be admitted to hospital under the care of an orthopaedic surgeon with the provisional diagnosis of 'transient synovitis'. If the symptoms resolve after a week's bed rest, then the diagnosis is confirmed. The differential diagnosis may be an infective arthritis such as tuberculosis.

Dislocation

Once the patient has reached the age of motor cycle riding or car driving, trauma becomes the main threat to the joint. *Posterior dislocation* or fracture/dislocation (Fig. 35.25) frequently result from head-on collisions, with the hip and knee flexed. It is particularly important to look for this injury in a patient who has another injury in the same leg, such as an open fracture of the tibia and fibula. For this reason, radiographs of the hip joint and pelvis should always be taken in patients with fractures lower down the leg. The sciatic nerve is sometimes damaged with posterior dislocation of the hip and this should be deliberately looked for. Reduction should be attempted with the patient deeply anaesthetised. It is more easily

effected with the patient lying on a mattress on the floor. *The anterior dislocation* is rare and may follow a weight falling onto the back of a miner or labourer who is working with his legs wide apart, knees straight and back bent backwards. The *central dislocation* is in reality a form of pelvic fracture with the acetabular floor disrupted and the femoral head thrust into the pelvis (see Fig. 8.44).

Degenerative hip disease

In the middle years of life, increasing pain in one or other hip joint, which may be exacerbated by a fall, may be due to degenerative changes in the hip joint or, at a younger age, to rheumatoid arthritis. Often by the time such patients are seen in the A & E department the rheumatoid changes have given place to advanced degenerative changes similar to osteoarthrosis. The radiological changes are reduced joint space, periarticular sclerosis and osteoarthritic outgrowths. Analgesia, local heat and rest will overcome the exacerbation of pain but referral to an orthopaedic surgeon may then be necessary.

Fractured neck of femur

Following a fall in the elderly, pain around the hip and clinical deformity with a shortened leg lying in external rotation is most commonly due to a fracture of the neck of the femur. Women suffer more commonly than men and this is associated with postmenopausal osteoporosis. Sometimes the condition follows a gradually developing stress fracture and may be regarded therefore as a pathological fracture. Occasionally the fracture occurs through an area of rarefaction due to bony metastases from carcinoma of the breast, bronchus, prostate or kidney.

An impacted fracture is less easy to diagnose, both clinically and radiologically. Good quality AP and lateral radiographs are required and the two joints should be compared. Even if the patient has a good range of movement (and may even be able to walk), she should be admitted to hospital for internal fixation.

Fractures with displacement are easily diagnosed. No splintage is required until the patient reaches the ward, but it is useful to take a chest radiograph because it is common for these patients to suffer pulmonary complications.

Finally patients may present with complications following a previous internal fixation or hip replacement surgery. The problem is usually clearly demonstrated by radiography and an orthopaedic opinion must be sought.

THE THIGH

Fractured shaft of femur

This is a serious injury and shock may be severe. Every patient with a femoral shaft fracture should have an intravenous infusion established and blood taken for cross matching even though, in the initial stages, there is no overt evidence of haemodynamic instability. If both femurs are fractured the probability of injury in the pelvis is high. The acute pain from muscle spasm and tissue damage can be abolished, often spectacularly, by the technique of femoral nerve local anaesthetic block (see Ch. 9 Anaesthesia and pain control). Early splintage (i.e. before radiographs are taken) on a fixed Thomas traction splint will help to reduce deformity and swelling and thereby control blood loss and pain. A number of emergency traction splints (some portable) are available which facilitate provisional traction splintage for first aid in the field or in the A & E department (Fig. 35.26). No patient with a femoral shaft fracture should leave the A & E department without traction splintage.

Quadriceps haematoma

After a direct blow to the thigh, e.g. a kick at football, a haematoma can develop in the muscle mass of the quadriceps. This is the most common site for the development of myositis ossificans (Fig. 35.27). A pressure bandage is initially applied. If at 72 hours there is less than 90° knee flexion then the risk of myositis is high and the knee should be immobilised for 14 days in a plaster of Paris cylinder. Expert supervision in a department of rehabilitation or physical medicine is needed.

THE ACUTELY PAINFUL KNEE

Examination of the injured knee

The assessment of a recent knee injury should take place with

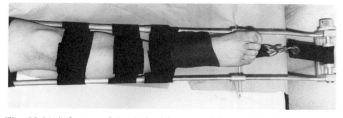

Fig. 35.26 A fracture of the shaft of femur receiving provisional immobilisation on a traction splint.

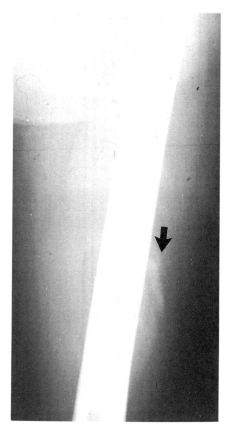

Fig. 35.27 Myositis ossificans of the thigh. Soft tissue shadowing (arrowed) in the quadriceps muscle of a patient who was kicked at football two weeks previously.

the patient undressed and on an examination couch. In most cases the diagnosis can be worked out from the history; examination merely confirms the doctor's suspicions.

Essential points in the history are the type of force involved: was it rotational, which might tear a meniscus, or was it direct violence, which might tear a collateral ligament? Has there been locking of the joint, i.e. has the patient been unable to straighten his knee fully? This would be evidence of a torn meniscus being trapped between the femoral condyle and the tibial plateau. If the knee is swollen, did the swelling appear within seconds of the injury (a haemarthrosis) or did it build up slowly (more likely a serious effusion)?

Inspection begins by comparing the injured with the uninjured knee. If there is an effusion, it will fill out the parapatellar fossae first, then the suprapatellar bursa. Any wasting of the quadriceps muscle, particularly vastus medialis, should be noted and quadriceps weakness checked by asking the patient to tense his leg with the foot inverted and the knee held straight. The pain of an acute meniscus tear may cause hamstring spasm to hold the knee in 10° of flexion.

Palpation may elicit specific areas of tenderness. Tenderness limited to the joint line suggests a torn meniscus. More widespread tenderness extending above or below the joint line on the medial or lateral aspects indicates a tear of the medial or lateral collateral ligaments.

Next, the integrity of the ligaments is assessed in turn:

The *collateral ligaments* are stressed by applying a valgus or varus strain with the knee in some 10° of flexion. If a collateral ligament is completely torn, the joint will open up and the bones then spring back into place as the pressure is released. As they do so, the examining hand will sense the moment when the tibial plateau impinges on the femoral condyle. A partial tear may produce a positive Apley's distraction test. With the patient prone, the flexed knee is pulled vertically when a pain will be experienced at the site of the tear.

The integrity of the *cruciate ligaments* is tested by examining the patient lying supine with the hip and knee flexed and the foot resting on the couch. If the tibia has sagged backwards in relation to the femur, as compared with the opposite knee, then the posterior cruciate ligament is torn. If the tibia can be drawn forwards from the femur (anterior drawer sign) the anterior cruciate, and, almost certainly, the medial collateral ligament are both torn.

The diagnosis of an *acute meniscus tear* is difficult to confirm in the presence of a large effusion. When the swelling has subsided, McMurray's test, rotating the knee in full flexion with the patient lying supine, may produce a click. Apley's grinding test, rotating the knee flexed to 90° with the patient lying prone, will be painful. Some loss of full extension, described above, is further strong evidence of a meniscus lesion.

Acute internal derangement of the knee

The femur and tibia contribute very little to the stability of the knee joint; the muscles of the thigh and leg make a small contribution but the main source of integrity and stability is in the ligaments, both those within the joint and those around it. A tear of one or more of these ligaments may have serious, permanent consequences.

Collateral ligament injury

A tear of the medial or lateral collateral ligaments of the knee follows a valgus or varus strain, respectively (Fig. 35.28). In a severe, disruptive injury the medial collateral ligament may be ruptured in association with the anterior cruciate ligament and the medial meniscus (O'Donoghue's unhappy triad). Most orthopaedic surgeons prefer to repair a completely torn collateral ligament, especially as the torn ends may be lying in the joint. A partial tear is sometimes treated surgically but more frequently it is treated by a plaster of Paris cylinder or a compression bandage and partial weight-bearing on crutches.

Cruciate injury tear

Injury to the cruciate ligaments may occur as an isolated event or in association with a major fracture around the knee (e.g. to the tibial plateau). Surgical reconstruction is the usual treatment.

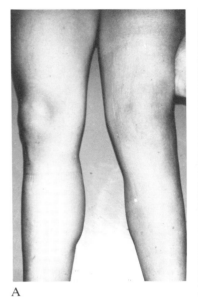
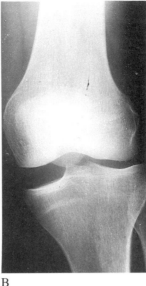

A   B

Fig. 35.28 A Rupture of the medial collateral ligament of the knee joint results in an abnormal range of abduction of the joint and is accompanied by an effusion which, in this patient, has filled out the normal hollow at the side of the patella. **B** An AP film of the same patient with the knee in forced abduction showing widening of the medial compartment.

Torn meniscus

A history of a twisting force to the bent, load-bearing knee should give the clue to the diagnosis of a meniscal tear. After 2–3 days rest in a compression bandage and/or knee immobiliser splint quadriceps exercises (see below) are commenced and the patient referred to an orthopaedic clinic for arthroscopy and excision of the torn portion. Very rarely the patient presents with a fixed locked knee. No attempt should be made to force the knee straight but the patient should be referred for an examination under anaesthetic and, occasionally, emergency meniscectomy. A cyst of the lateral meniscus presents as a slightly painful, bony hard swelling just below the lateral joint line. Treatment is surgical to remove the cyst and usually the lateral cartilage as well.

Osteochondritis dissecans

This condition usually presents insidiously, causing aching and a mild effusion in the knee joint in a teenager or young adult. Physical examination is not helpful unless a loose body is present. Radiological examination, including a tunnel view, will show an area of subchondral bone which is undergoing vascular changes or, at a later stage, a defect in the articular surface of one of the femoral condyles and possibly a piece of bone lying loose in the joint. Once the bone has become detached and formed a loose body, the patient may volunteer the information that a hard lump keeps appearing at various points around the knee joint. Occasionally the loose bone may become impacted between femoral condyle and tibial plateau and cause temporary locking of the knee. At whatever stage in the evolution of the condition the patient presents, he should be referred to an orthopaedic surgeon.

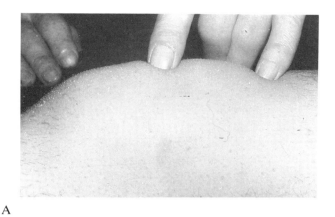

A

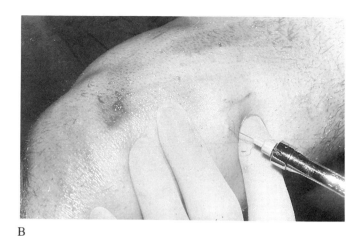

B

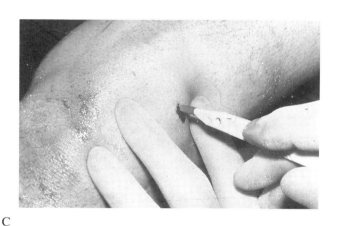

C

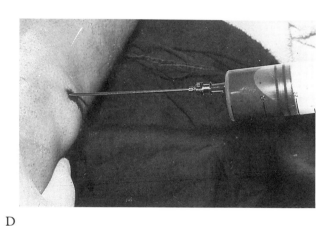

D

Fig. 35.29 Aspiration of the knee joint. **A** The examiner's right hand indicates the level of the patella. The examiner's left index and little fingers delineate the bulging suprapatellar pouch. The site of aspiration should be laterally (or medially) into this pouch — well away from the edge of the patella. **B** Using a 'no-touch' technique, the skin, subcutaneous tissue and synovium are infiltrated with local anaesthetic. **C** The skin should be punctured with a sharp pointed blade so that the needle is not gripped by the elastic tissue of the skin. **D** The needle then passes freely through the subcutaneous tissues until the operator feels the sudden loss of resistance as the point enters the joint.

Aspiration of the knee joint (Fig. 35.29)

Indications for aspiration include the relief of pain, haemarthrosis, a tense effusion, or for diagnosis. The procedure should be done with full aseptic precautions. After preparation of the skin and isolating the area with a sterile towel, inject 1–2 ml of local anaesthetic into the skin above and lateral to the patella. Then insert a wide-bore needle or intravenous cannula through this area into the joint. When the capsule is distended by fluid there is no difficulty in introducing the needle. Observe the fluid as it is withdrawn: is it serous or sanguinous and, if bloody, does it have fat in it which would indicate the presence of a fracture communicating with the joint? Record the quantity of fluid removed and, if there is any suspicion of infection, send a fresh specimen for bacteriological examination. The consequences of infecting the joint by a contaminated aspiration are so dire as to make aspiration of minor traumatic effusions unjustified. However, if carefully done, the risk of contamination is low. Aspiration gives instant relief and facilitates accurate examination for torn ligaments.

Problems of the extensor mechanism

Osgood-Schlatter disease

Young teenage children, usually boys who tend to be overweight, may come to the A & E department complaining of pain just below the knee at the insertion of the patellar tendon. They feel the pain when going upstairs and even more so as they come down and are relying on the extensor mechanism of the knee to take the whole weight of the body. This is a traction apophysitis (Osgood-Schlatter's disease) in which the tubercle at the upper end of the tibia is partially pulled off by the patellar tendon. Radiographic examination may show fragmentation or distraction of the apophysis but the diagnosis and management depend on the clinical condition, not the radiological appearance. The condition will respond to rest by immobilisation in a plaster of Paris cylinder.

Dislocation of the patella

This injury is a problem which arises most frequently in young

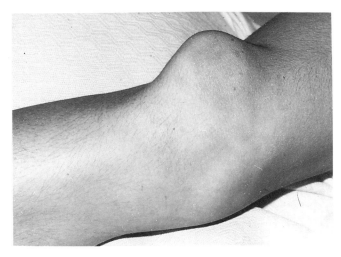

Fig. 35.30 Dislocation of the patella to the lateral side of the knee.

women. It is suggested that the width of the mature female pelvis imposes an oblique line of pull on the quadriceps and if, as seem to occur in these patients, they have a poorly developed lateral femoral condyle, then the patella is pushed laterally and dislocates to the outside of the knee (Fig. 35.30). After reduction a skyline patellar X-ray film should be obtained to exclude an osteochondral fracture which sometimes accompanies this injury. On the first occasion that dislocation occurs reduction should be obtained (under Entonox analgesia) and the knee rested for two weeks in a plaster of Paris cylinder. If recurrent dislocations occur surgical treatment is advisable and the patient should be referred to an orthopaedic surgeon.

Fractures of the patella

There are three distinct types of fracture of the patella which require different treatment. The *crack fracture* follows a direct blow to the bone but there is no displacement and, after aspiration of the accompanying haemarthrosis, the injury can be dealt with by compression bandaging followed by splintage. The *comminuted fracture* also occurs after direct force and is managed by patellectomy. The *transverse fracture* follows a sudden flexion strain. It may be managed by internal fixation, usually by circlage wiring.

Rupture of the quadriceps tendon

This is seen usually in elderly male patients — often resulting from stumbling over a kerb or an uneven paving stone. The patient falls to the ground and is embarrassed to find that he cannot stand up because the injured knee will not support his weight. Physical examination reveals a gap in the quadriceps tendon just proximal to the patella and straight leg raising is difficult or impossible. Prompt surgical repair is usually indicated and gives good results.

Swellings around the knee

Inflammations of the knee joint

Occasionally the cause of a swollen painful knee may be wrongly attributed by the patient to a minor injury. If such an effusion is warm it may be associated with an arthrosis (rheumatoid arthritis, osteoarthrosis or a crystal arthropathy) or with an infective arthritis (gonococcal or tubercular). Under these circumstances the joint should be aspirated and some aspirate sent for microscopy and culture. The osteoarthrotic knee frequently becomes swollen and painful after only minor trauma. The treatment is symptomatic with rest, warmth and analgesics.

Haemophilia

The haemarthrosis of haemophilia in children should not be treated by A & E department staff until the haematologist, the paediatrician or the orthopaedic surgeon (or all three) has been consulted.

Bursitis

Prepatellar bursitis ('housemaid's knee') and infrapatellar bursitis ('clergyman's knee') may develop as a result of kneeling or other minor trauma. The treatment is exactly the same as for olecranon bursitis (p. 374).

Semimembranosus bursa

This presents as a lump behind the knee, most easily palpable when the knee is in extension. Often, after some time, the normal communication with the knee joint opens up again and the swelling disappears. Failing this, the fluid can be aspirated or, if the bursa persists and continues to cause symptoms, the patient should be referred to an orthopaedic surgeon for its excision.

Rehabilitation of the knee

Injuries to the knee are followed by wasting of the quadriceps muscle. One essential part of treatment is to redevelop the power of the quadriceps. Three exercises are used:
1. Static contractions which move the patella but not the knee
2. Straight leg raising
3. Forced extension of the knee against resistance.

Patients should be carefully instructed in these exercises either by a physiotherapist or the examining doctor and advised to do them 4–6 times daily, starting with 1 minute and progressing to 5 minutes per session.

THE ACUTELY PAINFUL LEG

This section should be read in conjunction with Ch. 27 (Limb pain). Distinction between a minor tear of the calf muscles and a deep vein thrombosis in the calf is particularly important.

Pain at the back of the leg

Rupture of Achilles tendon

An acute, traumatic cause of pain at the back of the leg is seen most frequently in middle-aged patients. Sudden static contraction of the calf muscles to counteract forced dorsiflexion of the foot may cause a rupture of the Achilles tendon or a muscle tear at the musculotendinous junction at the middle of the calf. The moment of rupture of the tendon may be so dramatic that the subject looks round to see who or what has hit him. He then finds that he cannot rise onto his toes and he develops a painful tender swelling behind the ankle. The patient should be examined in the prone position with the foot over the edge of the bed. Squeezing the gastrocnemius (Simmond's test) causes plantar flexion in the normal patient but not so when the Achilles tendon has been ruptured. Incomplete rupture may be managed by immobilising the ankle in equinus in a plaster of Paris cast but, whether the tear is complete or incomplete, surgical repair may be required.

Gastrocnemius tears

A similar mechanism more commonly causes partial rupture at the junction of the gastrocnemius and its tendon. This produces localised tenderness in the centre of the calf and pain on dorsiflexion. Some ankle oedema may also develop after a day or two and such patients may be misdiagnosed as having a deep vein thrombosis. Supportive bandaging of the calf and partial weight-bearing on crutches is acceptable treatment for this condition, since the injury heals more quickly than tendon rupture.

Muscle tear or deep vein thrombosis?

The distinction between a muscle tear and deep vein thrombosis can usually be made from the history. The former results from a specific injury and the symptoms are maximal from the moment of injury. The symptoms of DVT develop more slowly over the course of an hour or two. Occasionally thrombosis of the deep veins may develop as a complication of a muscle tear or its treatment and should be suspected when there is an exacerbation of the symptoms some days after a traumatic incident. In doubtful cases the patient should be referred for venography (see Fig. 8.6, p. 66).

Achilles tendinitis

Pain in the lower part of the back of the leg, accompanied by tenderness deep to the Achilles tendon is sometimes seen in athletes or young girls who do a lot of dancing. It responds to rest, a raised heel and local electrotherapy.

Pain at the front of the leg

Anterior compartment syndrome

This is commonly seen in young people in the spring time following vigorous running with inadequate training. The pain on the outer aspect of the front of the leg between tibia and fibula can be temporarily incapacitating. Occasionally the pain is so severe that ischaemia should be suspected. If a patient develops any paraesthesia or numbness below the ankle or any weakness of dorsiflexion or eversion of the foot consideration should be given to urgent decompression of the deep fascia enclosing the muscles of the anterior compartment. Failure to do this may result in permanent foot drop and loss of sensation on the dorsum of the foot.

THE ACUTELY PAINFUL ANKLE

Sprains and fractures around the ankle following injury are very common. Some patients, however, may present in the A & E department with a vague history of injury but, when carefully examined, are found to have some other painful condition such as acute rheumatoid arthritis or gout, or an acute infection of bone, joint or soft tissues.

Pain of less acute origin following unusual exertion (often in athletes) may be due to peritendinitis, involving the tendon sheath of the tibialis anterior or posterior, or the peronei. This condition responds to rest, electrotherapy and gradual retraining.

Ankle fracture and fracture-dislocations

Ankle fractures can usually be differentiated by careful clinical examination. The physical examination must be carrried out with the patient on a couch with both legs exposed to the knees in order that swelling (or wasting) of muscles can be properly assessed and that a fracture of the proximal end of the fibula (associated

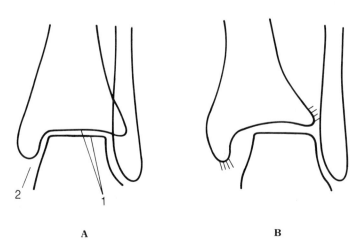

A   B

Fig. 35.31 A Diagram of the normal ankle radiograph: 1 — the surfaces of the tibia and talus are perfectly parallel, 2 — the normal distance between talus and medial malleolus. **B** With subluxation the talus is tilted and separated from the medial malleolus.

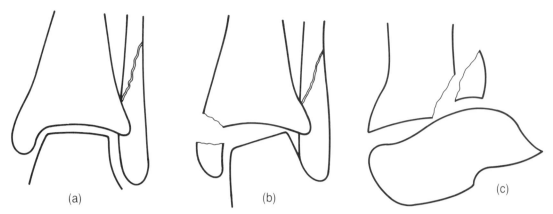

Fig. 35.32 Classification of ankle fractures: a — first degree fracture with no talar shift, b — second degree bimalleolar fracture, c — third degree trimalleolar fracture.

with a diastasis of the lower tibiofibular joint) should not be missed. The examination is not complete until the patient has been turned on the face so that the ankle joint can be seen and felt from behind and the calf and Achilles tendon palpated.

From a study of the fracture pattern on the radiograph the precise pattern of fracture–dislocation can be deduced. *The key to the diagnosis is the position of the talus.* In a stable injury (Fig. 35.31A) the surfaces of the tibia and talus are quite parallel and the medial malleolus is equally separated from the talus; with subluxation (Fig. 35.31B) the talus is tilted and separated from the medial malleolus.

The interpretation of ankle fractures is confused by the plethora of classifications and descriptive terminology. It is traditional to describe the severity of the injury according to the position of the talus (Fig. 35.32):

> 1. In first-degree injuries there is fracture without talar shift or tilt.
> 2. In second-degree injuries there is displacement of the talus.
> 3. In third-degree injuries there is, in addition, a fracture of the posterior mortise (the trimalleolar fracture).

It is better, however, to describe the injuries in terms of the deforming force. The widely accepted Lauge-Hansen classification groups the fractures under double-barrelled headings. The first word of each pair describes the position of the foot at the time of injury; the second refers to the direction in which the talus moves within the ankle mortise. (The common descriptive terminology is shown in brackets.) In order of frequency these fractures are listed as follows:

> 1. Supination/lateral rotation ('inversion' injury)
> 2. Pronation/abduction (abduction injury)
> 3. Pronation/lateral rotation ('eversion' injury)
> 4. Supination/adduction (adduction injury)
> 5. Pronation/dorsiflexion (vertical compression injury).

Figures 35.33–35.37 show the appearances of these different injuries and describe their evolution as increasing force is applied.

The management of ankle fractures is based on clinical examination and the degree of stability as assessed radiographically:

1. The simple sprain is treated by activity (see below).

2. The stable single malleolar fracture is treated symptomatically, much as for a sprain.

3. A potentially unstable fracture is treated in a well-moulded plaster cast. The pressure applied to the outer side of the foot must be below the lateral malleolus and the pressure applied to the inner side of the ankle must be above the medial malleolus (Fig. 35.38).

4. An unstable fracture with displacement or deformity would be admitted for treatment by internal fixation or manipulation and the application of a long leg cast under anaesthetic.

Ankle sprains

The sprained ankle is one of the commonest conditions seen in the A & E department. An inversion or adduction stress to the ankle is most likely to cause a partial tear of one or more of the fibrous components of the lateral ligament (Fig. 35.39). The commonest sprain is to the anterior talofibular ligament with extensions to the capsule of the ankle joint lying anteriorly and the extensor retinacular band over the dorsum. Resisted adduction forces may avulse the peroneus brevis tendon from the base of the fifth metatarsal bone (with or without a fracture). More severe forces disrupt the inferior tibiofibular ligament or fracture the ankle bones.

Careful clinical examination should pin-point the precise anatomical lesion in the majority of cases and tenderness should be elicited in the three specific sites shown in Figure 35.40. Occasionally clinical examination is rendered difficult by gross swelling. 'Posterior infilling' above the os calcis or beneath the medial malleolus implies an effusion into the ankle joint.

Where instability is suspected clinically the anterior drawer test is useful. With one hand supporting the leg at the ankle and the other holding the heel, the ankle is placed into 20° palmar flexion and attempts are made to draw the two examining hands away from each other. There should be no forward movement with a stable ankle joint.

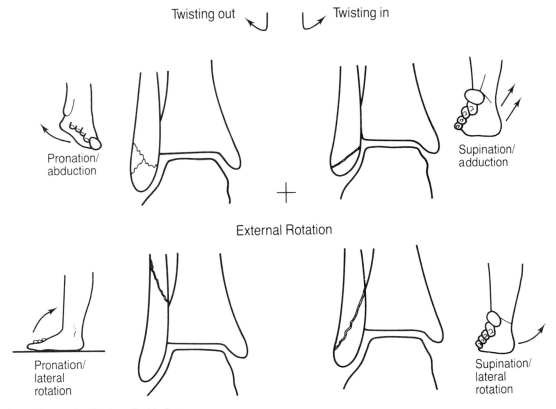

Twisting out   Twisting in

External Rotation

Pronation/abduction

Supination/adduction

Pronation/lateral rotation

Supination/lateral rotation

Fig. 35.33 The Lauge-Hansen classification of ankle fractures.

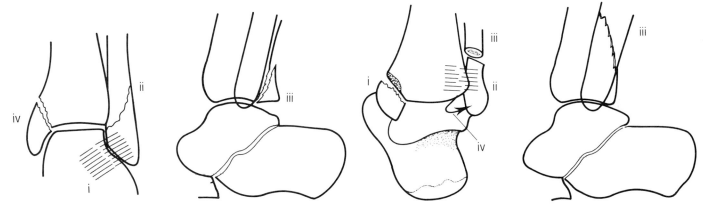

Fig. 35.34 Supination/lateral rotation injury: i — rupture ant. talofibular ligament, ii — spiral fracture of fibula, iii — posterior malleolar fracture, iv — fracture medial malleolus.

Fig. 35.35 Pronation/lateral rotation injury: i — fracture medial malleolus, ii — diastasis inf. tibio-fibular ligament, iii — fracture fibular shaft anywhere up to the neck, iv — dislocation of ankle.

Radiological examination is unnecessary for every case of sprained ankle, the indications, for exclusion of fracture, being

1. Where there is swelling hampering accurate palpation
2. Where there is point tenderness over a bone
3. Where there is clinical instability
4. In patients over 50 years of age in which clinical studies indicate a likely incidence of fractures of about 30%.

Management of the sprained ankle

1. The truly unstable injury is a rarity. Instability is defined as a positive anterior drawer test combined with 20° talar tilt shown on a lateral stress radiograph (see Fig. 8.47). (This could be performed under Entonox analgesia or general anaesthesia.) The complete, unstable ankle sprain should be referred for orthopaedic supervision.

2. The vast majority of ankle sprains should be treated by activity. Initially the I-ce, C-ompression, E-levation regimen used for soft tissue injuries (see below) combined with rest of the affected joint for 48 hours aims to reduce initial pain and swelling. Thereafter, immediate mobilisation and mobility is encouraged. The patient is advised to take little steps retaining normal heel–

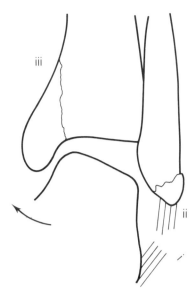

Fig. 35.36 Supination/adduction injury: i — partial tear lateral ligament or fracture fifth metatarsal if force resisted by peroneus brevis, ii — traction fracture lateral malleolus or complete tear lateral ligament, iii — vertical fracture medial malleolus.

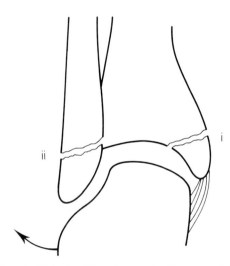

Fig. 35.37 Pronation/abduction injury: i — traction fracture medial malleolus, ii — fracture fibula at junction of shaft and malleolus.

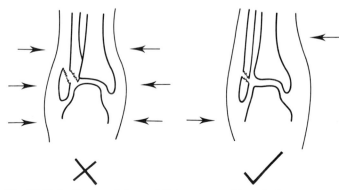

Fig. 35.38 Application of plaster of Paris to an unstable ankle fracture showing the position of moulding.

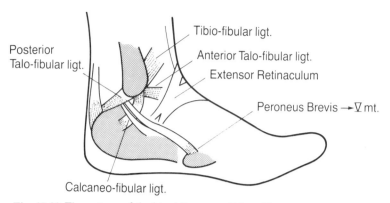

Fig. 35.39 The anatomy of the lateral ligaments of the ankle.

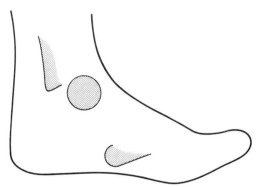

Fig. 35.40 The three sites which should be checked for tenderness when dealing with a suspected sprained ankle.

toe gait. Graded exercises should encourage proprioceptive mechanisms. This might include:

a. Describing the letters of the alphabet with the injured foot.
b. Balancing on the affected foot
   i) on the bottom step of a flight of stairs whilst the other foot touches the step and the floor,
   ii) on a soft pillow, and
   iii) on a 'wobble board' or its domestic substitute — the rubber hot water bottle.
c. Walking backwards.

At the completion of rehabilitation the fit patient should be able to walk normally; hop over a 30 cm foam block; effect a 180° jump turn and jump forwards and backwards off an examination couch (!).

3. Strapping should be considered only in special circumstances (e.g. the immediate need for completion of a specific task, such as a charity walk). Then the zinc oxide U-piece which prevents inversion yet allows dorsiflexion (see Chapter 39) can be applied. Figure-of-eight or other forms of strapping are not recommended.

THE ACUTELY PAINFUL FOOT

Fractures and dislocations of the foot

Fractures of the calcaneum

Following a fall from a height (often from a ladder) onto one or both heels, the calcaneum may be impacted against the talus and

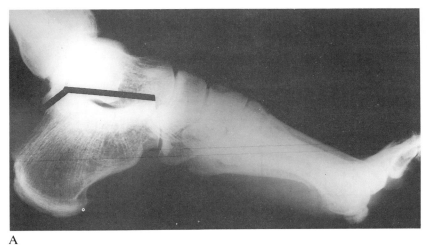

A

B

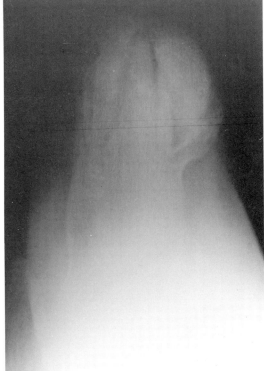

C

Fig. 35.41 A The normal lateral foot radiograph showing Bohler's angle. **B** In crush fracture of the calacaneum this is significantly reduced. **C** An axial view clearly shows the fracture.

crushed or split. The heel may appear squashed and tender and a D-shaped bruise may appear in the sole. Radiographic examination should include os calcis views with both lateral and axial projections. As the bone is cancellous, the fracture line of a crushing injury may not be visible. Instead Böhler's angle (anterior process-tuberosity-posterior border) should be sought on the lateral X-ray film; the normal obtuse angle of about 140° is considerably increased, sometimes to 180° (Fig. 35.41). Operation is seldom indicated for crush injuries. The heel is supported in a very well padded bandage of wool and crepe. The patient is non-weight-bearing whilst the swelling settles. In major cases with considerable pain and oedema the patient is best admitted to hospital for a few days.

Injuries of the talus

Though rare, these injuries are serious as they reflect the application of considerable violence applied to the foot. They are often associated with skin damage, avascular necrosis and degenerative changes within the subtalar joint and the functional prognosis is often poor. These patients should be admitted immediately under the care of an orthopaedic surgeon.

Metatarsal fractures

Crushing injuries to the foot, often compound, may cause fractures to the metatarsals, usually at the neck. Rotational forces may cause dislocation, fracture-dislocation and subluxation of the tarsometatarsal or mid-tarsal articulations. The foot is swollen and tender across the whole width of the foot. Pain is severe and walking impossible. Urgent reduction is required, the patient being referred for manipulation or, in some cases, open reduction.

The march fracture

Classically, this is an undisplaced stress fracture of the neck of the second or third metatarsal, resulting from unaccustomed overuse — such as a 'sponsored walk'. The patient complains of pain at this site and is tender to pressure on the central metatarsals. At initial radiographic examination it may be almost impossible to detect a bony lesion. The foot should be supported by a pad behind the metatarsal heads. The radiographs may be repeated after three weeks when a tell-tale swelling of callus (Fig. 35.42) will indicate the site of the fracture.

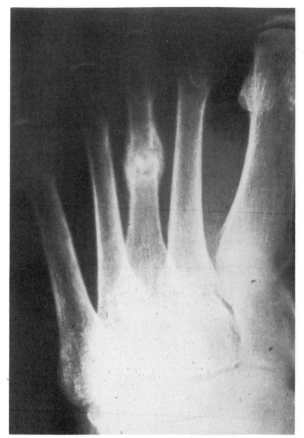

Fig. 35.42 The foot radiograph of a cross-country runner who developed pain in the forefoot three weeks previously. Callus around a stress (march) fracture of the third metatarsal is clearly seen.

Forefoot pain

There are a variety of conditions which cause pain in the foot for which patients sometimes seek advice in the A & E department. Most of them are more within the province of the orthopaedic surgeon than of the A & E doctor but this only becomes evident when the diagnosis is made.

Metatarsalgia

Clinically an attack of acute anterior metatarsalgia may be almost indistinguishable from a march fracture. The treatment is the same and only the second radiograph will definitely decide the diagnosis. If the symptoms have resolved by the second visit the distinction is of academic importance only.

Plantar fasciitis

This diagnosis is made for the patient who is acutely tender under the heel. A radiograph may show a calcaneal spur but this is not the cause of the pain. A soft heel pad in the shoe, an injection of hydrocortisone and local anaesthetic and ultrasound are all current lines of treatment, used singly or in combination. The condition is best managed in the orthopaedic clinic.

Calcaneonavicular fusion

This is a congenital anomaly in which a bar of bone joins the os calcis to the navicular (or, more rarely, the cuboid to the talus). As a consequence there is no effective mid-tarsal joint. Children do not complain but young teenagers find that their foot aches after walking over uneven ground. Treatment, if any, is by excising the bar. A patient with this condition should be referred to the orthopaedic department.

Osteochondritis

Avascular necrosis of a bone in the foot occurs in two classic sites. In children from 6–10 years the navicular may be affected *(Kohler's disease)*. The child limps and complains of pain. Physical examination is not very revealing but a radiograph will show a narrow, densely white, sclerosed navicular bone. The condition is self-limiting within a few weeks. A bandage and reassurance are the only necessary forms of treatment.

The other site is the head of one of the metatarsals — usually the second one *(Freiberg's infraction)* — and the condition occurs in adult life. The pain is similar to that of metatarsalgia but on X-ray films the metatarsal head is enlarged and the articular surface is flattened. Initial treatment using a metatarsal pad and analgesics may relieve the initial symptoms but the lesion is progressive and eventually many of these patients need to have the metatarsal head excised.

Afflictions of the toes

Hallux rigidus

This condition is described fully in Ch. 32 (Soft tissue infections). usually precipitated by walking on rough ground. Rest, a metatarsal pad or a metatarsal bar under the sole of the shoe will bring relief — until the next attack when the patient should be referred.

Gout

The first metatarsophalangeal joint in the foot is the most frequent site of gout. A dull, red swollen joint which is extruciatingly painful should always raise the possibility of this diagnosis. Radiographs will show gouty deposits and will demonstrate para-articular erosions and destruction of the joint surfaces in an advanced case, but it is usually early in the evolution of the disease that a patient presents to the A & E department. Blood should be taken to estimate the serum urate; by the time the result is available, a therapeutic trial of indomethacin will usually have relieved the symptoms.

Stubbed toe

This very common injury causes the patient pain and frustration. Unless there is clinical displacement, radiographs are unlikely to contribute to management, which should be by padded neighbour strapping and orthopaedic felt under the metatarsal head to raise the affected area off the floor.

Ingrowing toenail

This condition is described fully in Ch. 32 (Soft tissue infections).

INJURIES TO BONES

Because the bones give form to the skeleton and strength to the limbs, when they are broken or diseased the patient quickly presents in the A & E department.

Non-accidental injury

The vast majority of fractures are fully accounted for by some recent traumatic incident, but the A & E doctor must always be on the look out for 'non-accidental injury' If the explanation for a child's fracture is inconsistent with the injury, or if there has been more than one injury, then the local procedure for child abuse should be followed and the help and advice of a paediatrician sought to decide the immediate management (see Ch. 5 Social aspects).

Pathological fractures

In older patients, it is also important to have a high level of awareness of the possibility of a pathological fracture. Some malignant conditions first come to light when a secondary deposit results in a fracture (Fig. 35.43). Congenital anomalies such as osteogenesis imperfecta, or developmental anomalies such as fibrous dysplasia, or, in the elderly, osteitis deformans (Paget's disease) can all predispose a bone to fracture. In the fingers, enchondromas not infrequently predispose to fractures (Fig. 35.44). In the A & E department the fracture must be reduced and immobilised and, when appropriate, specialist care arranged for the underlying condition.

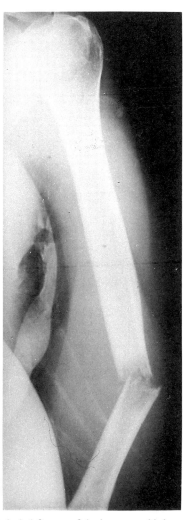

Fig. 35.43 A pathological fracture of the humerus with bone destruction above and below the fracture line due to metastatic breast carcinoma.

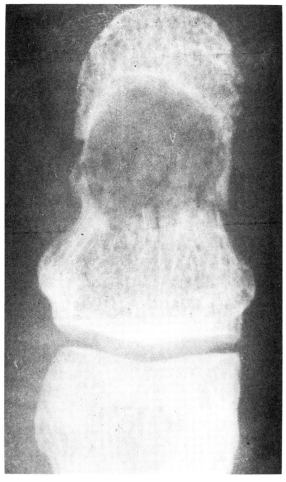

Fig. 35.44 This patient, who had been unaware of any abnormality in his finger previously, sustained a pathological fracture through an enchondroma following minor trauma.

Childhood fractures

There are a number of special features of fractures and dislocations in children. Childhood fractures are more common and heal more rapidly, sometimes with serious complications such as disturbed growth. Children's ligaments are strong and resilient and a diagnosis of a sprain in childhood should not be made until a fracture or joint injury has been excluded (for example, a fracture of the lateral aspect of the distal tibia is often misdiagnosed as a sprained ankle). The particular features of the greenstick injury have already been described (p. 374). In addition, children experience a special type of fracture: the bony injury involving the epiphyseal plate. Separation of the epiphysis from the metaphysis through the layer of calcifying cartilage of the growth plate is a common event. Salter and Harris (1963) describe five types of injury involving the epiphysis (Fig. 35.45). The commonest injury, a fracture-separation of the epiphyseal plate (type II) is, fortunately, fairly easy to manage. The type III and type IV injuries which extend into the joint and the type V lesion which follows a crushing force must be accurately diagnosed and treated to avoid permanent growth disturbance. The radiograph in the type V injury is often normal and reliance must be placed on the history.

Complications of fractures

When treating a fracture, it is wise to anticipate — and if possible prevent — complications which may be of more importance than the fracture itself:

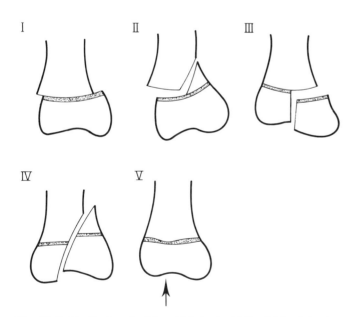

Fig. 35.45 Classification of epiphyseal injuries in childhood (after Salter & Harris):
Type I Complete separation of epiphysis without any fracture through bone. Good prognosis.
Type II Fracture-separation with triangular-shaped fragment of metaphysis. Most common variety. Good prognosis.
Type III Intra-articular fracture-separation. Poor prognosis with growth deformity if adequate open reduction and internal fixation not achieved.
Type IV As type III but fracture line extends through metaphysis.
Type V Crush injury. Rare and difficult to recognise. Poor prognosis.

1. Blood loss, either external or internal.
2. Impairment of the circulation distal to the fracture. This may be easily missed unless carefully sought.
3. Peripheral nerve damage:
   a. Axillary nerve at the shoulder
   b. Radial nerve at the arm
   c. Ulnar and median nerves at the elbow and wrist
   d. Sciatic nerve at the hip
   e. Common peroneal nerve at the fibular neck
4. Organ damage
5. Systemic complications, the effects of which may be reduced by skilled care and resuscitation at the reception of the patient. This category includes fat embolism, coagulopathies, infection, DVT and pulmonary embolus.

Some other long-term complications of fractures may not depend on the initial care, but it is wise to be aware of their possible occurrence. These include joint stiffness, growth disturbance, limb shortening, delayed union and, occasionally non-union and a pseudoarthrosis.

SOFT-TISSUE INJURY

Injuries to the soft-tissues (muscle, tendon, ligament) constitute a large part of the A & E department work load. Forces applied to the soft tissues of a limb may either be *compressive* resulting in contusion to skin or muscle, or *tensile* resulting in a strain to muscle or sprain of ligament. Sprains and strains are classified:

> 1st degree — 10% fibres involved
> 2nd degree — 11–99% fibres involved
> 3rd degree — complete tear.

All third degree soft-tissue injuries should usually be referred for primary repair.

The natural history of untreated soft-tissue injury is the production of fibrous union and scar formation (Fig. 35.46). The aim of treatment is to minimise scarring and reduce the occurrence of further injury by tackling the developing haematoma and rehabilitating the weakened tissues.

During the first two days after injury the I-C-E regimen is employed:

Ice packs to the limb (20 minutes application results in 45 minutes vasodilatation).

Compressive bandaging with crepe or elastic tubular bandage.

Elevation of the affected limb above the horizontal to permit gravity drainage of oedema fluid.

Thereafter a number of rehabilitation methods may be used to treat the soft-tissue injury.

1. **Rest and immobilisation.** This should be confined to the first 48 hours after injury unless immobilisation is required for the treatment of a specific injury.

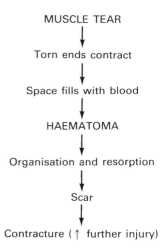

Fig. 35.46 The natural history of soft tissue injury.

2. **Heat and cold therapy.** This may be by the use of wax baths and ice packs respectively. At home *contrast bathing* can be employed (3 minutes of cold water followed by 1 minute of hot water). The way in which cold therapy influences healing is shown in Figure. 35.47.

3. **Electrotherapy.** Short wave diathermy is the electrical production of deep local heat allowing mobility to a specific area.

Ultrasound is particularly useful in breaking down haematoma. It should not be used near metal implants and care should be exercised in deep lesions near bone.

Pulsed electromagentic radiation ('Diapulse') is more effective than short wave diathermy in reducing oedema and stiffness. It appears to have a useful role in improving proprioception (e.g. in ankle sprains) and appears to hasten the regeneration of nerve fibres).

4. **Progressive exercise therapy.** This is the essence of physical therapy. The aim is to stretch and tone up individual muscles, to improve co-ordination of functional muscle groups and to reteach spatial orientation in the whole limb.

5. **Treatment with non-steroidal anti-inflammatory**

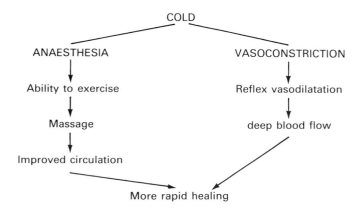

Fig. 35.47 The mode of action of cold therapy in rehabilitation.

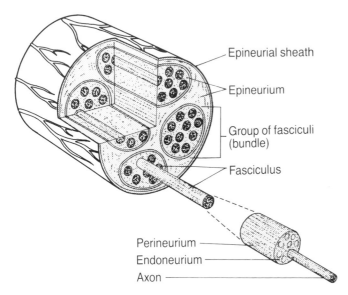

Fig. 35.48 Cross-sectional anatomy of a mixed peripheral nerve (reproduced with permission from Urbaniak J R 1982 Clinical Orthopedics 163:57).

the distal part of the nerve and, under optimum conditions, the nerve will regenerate at the rate of about 1 mm per day.

Grade 3 —*neurotmesis* is when the whole nerve is torn across and only surgical repair holds out any hope of eventual recovery.

It may be very difficult to assess the degree of nerve damage immediately following an accident, especially if the patient is unconscious. If necessary, the examination must be repeated when consciousness returns. A helpful sign, particularly in young children and drunks, is the loss of sweating in the territory of the injured nerve. This is described on p. 356. Conduction studies may be needed in assessing the nature and level of a nerve palsy. In open injuries, the only safe rule is to assume that every structure in the vicinity of a wound has been divided, until proved otherwise by adequate clinical examination or by surgical exploration. Altered sensation after a sharp cutting injury is almost always caused by division of nerve fibres and should not be attributed to 'contusion'.

The earlier a damaged peripheral nerve is repaired the better the results. For clean wounds, incised on a blade or by glass, most specialists in nerve or limb surgery now employ primary fascicular repair utilising the operating microscope. Open crushing nerve injuries should also be referred early to the specialist for microscopic assessment and preparation for secondary repair or nerve graft. About 75% of closed nerve injuries associated with fractures should heal spontaneously.

Traction injuries to the brachial plexus occur principally in motorcycle accident patients. The prognosis is poor. They often occur in the presence of other local injuries, e.g. 1st or 2nd rib fractures. Early repair can sometimes be successfully achieved and specialist assessment is essential.

REFERENCES

Apley A G 1947 The diagnosis of meniscus injuries: some new clinical methods. Journal of Bone and Joint Survery 29: 78-84

Beattie T F, Steedman D J, McGowan A, Robertson C E 1986 A comparison of the Milch and Kocher techniques for acute anterior dislocation of the shoulder. Injury 17: 349-352

Kondoyannis P N 1982 A clinical sign in suspected fractures of the carpal scaphoid. Journal of Bone and Joint Surgery 64A: 784

Lauge-Hansen N 1950 Fractures of the ankle. Combined experimental-surgical and experimental-roentgenologic investigations. Archives of Surgery 60: 957-985

Salter R B, Harris W R 1963 Injuries involving the epiphyseal plate. Journal of Bone and Surgery 45A: 587-622

Smith D N, Lee J R 1978 The radiological diagnosis of post-traumatic effusion of the elbow joint and its clinical significance; 'the displaced fat pad' sign. Injury 10: 115-119

FURTHER READING

Textbooks

Joint motion: method of measuring and recording American Academy of Orthopaedic Surgeons 1966 Churchill Livingstone, Edinburgh

The closed treatment of common fractures, 3rd edn. Charnley J 1970 Churchill Livingstone, Edinburgh

Textbook of orthopaedic medicine, vol 1, diagnosis of soft tissue lesions, 7th edn. Cyriax J 1978 Ballière Tindall, London

Radiological diagnosis of fractures Finlay D B L, Allen M J 1984 Ballière Tindall, London

A simple guide to trauma, 3rd edn. Huckstep T L 1982 Churchill Livingstone, Edinburgh

Joint disease: all the arthropathies, 3rd edn. Huskisson E C, Dudley Hart F 1978 Wright, Bristol

A practical guide to the care of the injured London P S 1967 E & S Livingstone, Edinburgh

Clinical orthopaedic examination, 2nd edn. McRae R 1983 Churchill Livingstone, Edinburgh

Practical fracture treatment, McRae R 1981 Churchill Livingstone, Edinburgh

Children's fractures, 2nd edn. Rang M 1983 Lippincott, Philadelphia

Fractures and dislocations in children Pollen A G 1973 Churchill Livingstone, Edinburgh

Care for the injured child Salter R B 1976 Williams & Wilkins, Baltimore

Injuries of the knee joint, 5th edn. Smillie I S 1978 Churchill Livingstone, Edinburgh

Apley's system of orthopaedics and fractures, 6th edn. Solomon L, Apley A G 1982 Butterworths, London

Watson Jones's fractures and joint injuries, 6th edn. Wilson J N (ed) 1972 Churchill Livingstone, Edinburgh

Journals

Neuralgic amyotrophy (paralytic brachial neuralgia) Aldren Turner J W, Parsonage M J 1957 Lancet ii: 209–212

Fractures of the shaft of the tibia Anonymous 1975 British Medical Journal 4: 4

Painful shoulders and painful arcs Anonymous 1977 British Medical Journal ii: 913–914

Traumatic tenosynovitis of the wrist Anonymous 1978 British Medical Journal i: 528

Injuries of the wrist Barton N 1983 Surgery 1: 57–62

Peripheral nerve injuries Burge P 1987 Hospital Update 7: 525–536

Multiple fractures in the long bones of infants suffering from chronic subdural haematoma Caffey J 1946 American Journal of Roentgenology 56: 163–173

The pulled elbow Corrigan A B 1965 Medical Journal of Australia ii: 187–189

Smiths and Bartons fractures Ellis J 1965 Journal of Bone and Joint Surgery 47B: 724–727

Tenosynovitis in industry; menace or misnomer Evans G 1987 British Medical Journal 294: 1569–1570

Tenosynovitis and tenovaginitis Griffiths D L 1952 British Medical Journal i: 645–648

Pulled elbow: a study of 100 patients Illingworth C 1975 British Medical Journal ii: 672–674

The fractured carpal scaphoid Leslie I J, Dickson R A 1981 Journal of Bone and Joint Surgery 63B: 225–230

Colle's fracture. A prospective study of treatment Pool C 1973 Journal of Bone and Joint Surgery 55B: 540–544

Anterior dislocation of the shoulder Rowe C F 1963 Surgical Clinics of North America 43: 1609–1614

Dislocation of the head of the radius associated with fractures of the upper end of the ulna in children Theodorou S D 1969 Journal of Bone and Joint Surgery 51B: 700–706

Colle's fracture. How should its displacement be measured and how should it be immobilised? Van der Linden W, Ericson R 1981 Journal of Bone and Joint Surgery 63A: 1285–1288

Skiing fractures Van der Linden 1975 Journal of Bone and Joint Surgery 57A: 321–327

Brachial plexus injuries Wynn Parry C B 1984 British Journal of Hospital Medicine 32: 130–139

Sports injuries

Sports injuries comprise about 4% of the new patients seen in an accident and emergency department in the United Kingdom. Association football produces about 40% and rugby 25% of these injuries.

The majority of sports injuries seen in the A & E department are contusions with the patient wondering whether they have a fracture. The other major group is ligamentous injury. There are few muscle and tendon injuries from sport presenting to A & E, although they are extremely common within sport itself. There are a few injury problems of which the doctor should be aware even though these are rarities in the department.

Many doctors do not like sports injuries because they are regarded as self-inflicted conditions in a young, healthy population. The athlete with a torn hamstring is as effectively disabled as if he or she had a fracture and should be helped to continue what is basically a healthy activity.

Sport injuries can be managed within the routine of the department providing the doctors are aware of the problems. The major requirement is for an early, active programme of treatment combined with complete rehabilitation up to the demands of that patient in their own sport.

Injuries to the head and neck

There are few particular problems in this area of injury. The athlete who has been even momentarily unconscious should avoid all contact sports for a minimum period of 10 days after he is free from headaches or other postconcussion symptoms (see Ch. 40). This time is the minimum period and most people would encourage the athlete to avoid contact sport for one month after injury. With two episodes in one season he should not play contact sport again that season.

Fractures of the facial bones are often seen, particularly from the rugby field. An abnormal bite, haematoma in the floor of the mouth and infraorbital anaesthesia all imply a fracture of maxilla or mandible. This can often be decided on the field of play without waiting for radiological examination. Injuries to the teeth are common and if a player arrives in the department with a tooth that has been knocked out, the tooth should be cleansed in saline,

replaced and held in position by a temporary splint before obtaining a dental opinion.

Injuries around the eye are frequent but injuries to the eye itself are less common. Unfortunately, penetrating injuries due to broken glass still occur; there really is no excuse for people playing squash in glass spectacles. The other important injury to the eye is hyphaema (haemorrhage into the anterior chamber of the eye) for which the patient should be admitted owing to the possibility of secondary haemorrhage and later development of glaucoma. This again is particularly seen in squash, which has the only ball in sport which can enter the orbit and it is important after an eye injury in squash that not only is the surface of the eye examined but also the retina. The larger, hard balls as used in golf, cricket and hockey can cause blow out fractures, the typical signs of which are diplopia, particularly on looking upwards and also infraorbital anaesthesia (see Ch. 43).

A 'cauliflower' ear is a haematoma between the perichondrium and the cartilage; this requires immediate treatment by drainage through multiple small incisions, using a careful aseptic technique.

Injuries to the cervical spine occur particularly in rugby, horse riding and gymnastics. The patient should be questioned carefully about the mechanics of injury and for even momentary symptoms in the arms. The athlete will often complain of a burning sensation in the arms rather than paraesthesia or weakness. Standard radiographs should be taken and then, the integrity of the odontoid having been verified, flexion and extension views may be required.

Injuries to the shoulder girdle

People with shoulder injuries frequently present at the A & E department and all too often the doctor shows a great deal of interest in the glenohumeral joint but forgets acromioclavicular and sternoclavicular joints. Examination should start with the sternoclavicular joint where the history of injury is usually that of a fall on the back of the shoulder. In subluxation or dislocation of this joint the clavicle usually moves anteromedially and is most easily recognised clinically rather than radiologically. Treatment consists of the shoulder being drawn backwards and the dislocation reduced by applying pressure over the medial third of the clavicle.

Occasionally this requires surgical intervention. Reduction is maintained with a figure-of-eight bandage or the use of clavicle pads.

Subluxation and dislocation of the acromioclavicular joint is usually distinctive. The history is of a fall onto the point of the shoulder. There is tenderness and swelling over the joint with pain on lateral flexion of the neck to the opposite side. A simple test is to have the patient standing with arms hanging by the side of the body and then for the examiner to pull down simultaneously on both wrists when the injured clavicle may be seen to ride upwards in relation to the acromion. The diagnosis is basically clinical but radiographs must be taken to exclude fracture of the lateral part of the clavicle. Treatment consists of a triangular sling worn under the clothes for one week then gentle mobilisation and finally strengthening exercises, the latter being particularly important in the athlete. The player should be off contact sport for about six weeks.

Dislocation of the glenohumeral joint is known to have a recurrence rate of approximately 80% in the young patient and if the injury occurs in the athlete it is important to have radiological confirmation of the diagnosis. He or she may have further dislocations and at some stage will arise the consideration of operative repair when the decision to operate will be based upon the number of proven dislocations. The injury requires adequate immobilisation with a sling and binder followed by a definite progressive rehabilitation programme. It is useless returning athletes to the more strenuous sports with inadequate strength around the joint because they will inevitably sustain further injury.

Injuries to the upper arm and elbow

Severe injuries to the upper arm are uncommon but spiral fractures of the humerus may occur in throwing sports and in arm wrestling. Repeated blows to the anterior surface of the upper arm, as can occur from tackling in rugby, may lead to the development of myositis ossificans in this area, so where this is a serious possibility the arm should be rested in a sling.

There are three groups of sports injury to the elbow joint:

1. Ligamentous injuries in contact sport which are commonly due to hyperextension.
2. The musculotendinous injuries associated with racquet sports
3. A variety of injuries associated with throwing.

The most common injury is 'tennis elbow' or lateral epicondylitis, a diagnosis which appears to include several indistinct pathological conditions. There is localised tenderness around the lateral epicondyle, difficulty in holding a heavy object and the most pronounced pain on resisted dorsiflexion of the wrist with the elbow extended. Initial treatment may involve the use of a sling for a short period, ultrasound or an injection of hydrocortisone accurately placed into the tender area. 'Golfers elbow' or medial epicondylitis is an apparently similar condition. Hydrocortisone injections in the athlete should not be given into tendon or ligament because the fibrinolytic activity will, under the stress of sport, predispose to rupture and it is better to avoid these injections in the lower limb.

Hyperextension at the elbow commonly injures the anteromedial aspect of the capsular ligaments and may vary from a partial tear to a complete tear or dislocation; these injuries are usually seen in rugby and judo. The elbow should be supported in a sling and full extension must be allowed to return slowly with no effort being made to force pace because of the danger of ectopic calcification, which is always a risk in the injured elbow. This is quite different from the situation in the shoulder where early activity can be undertaken.

Throwing produces a variety of conditions around the medial aspect of the elbow joint because most types of throwing place an overload on this area. Injury may consist of strain to the forearm flexors, avulsion of bone or tears of the medial capsule. A medial ligament sprain will be painful when tested by having the wrist flexed, the forearm pronated and then applying a valgus stress to the slightly flexed elbow. Treatment is primarily rest with some benefit from heat and hydrocortisone.

Injuries to the forearm and hand

Various strains of the forearm muscles occur but they are only a significant problem in sports such as weight lifting, canoeing and rowing, where the athletes have considerable hypertrophy of these muscles and a small amount of swelling in a tight fascial compartment can interfere with peripheral circulation. Tenosynovitis may occur with unusually prolonged activity and is often associated with a loss of style or technique due to tiredness. Treatment of tenosynovitis in the athlete is similar to that in the general population but a short initial period in POP is often helpful, for without it the athlete may be very reluctant to rest the tendon adequately.

Numerous fractures of the radius and ulna are seen in the child. The possibility of epiphyseal injury must always be borne in mind. Injuries to the wrist, particularly forced dorsiflexion which may occur during a hand-off in rugby or when landing in gymnastics, pose a diagnostic problem. Providing radiological examination does not show a fracture and there is no tenderness over the scaphoid bone, then a diagnosis of sprain may be made. Some would argue that there is a place for arthrography in these injuries. Ligamentous injuries in this area have a great tendency to chronicity and should be treated initially by being placed in POP for two weeks. A similar stress may damage the pisiform bone or its attachment which shows as a sharply localised tenderness and it can be treated as a sprain. An unusual injury is a fracture of the hook of the hamate in racquet players due to leverage of the butt end of the handle in players who are inclined to hold the racquet too near the base. There will be tenderness and pain in the hypothenar eminence and if this possibility is borne in mind then the radiographer can take special skyline views which show the hook of hamate. There is no specific treatment for this injury which may go on to a painful non-union and require surgery.

Fractures, dislocations and numerous ligamentous injuries of the hand and digits are extremely common. They are often treated with less care than their importance merits and should be treated as in the non-athletic patient (see Ch. 34).

Injuries to the trunk

There are few particular problems in this area. Blows to the abdomen and kidney region must be treated with normal care. Microscopic haematuria and albuminuria are common after endurance exercise and are not usually of great significance. Blows to the testicle are usually more distressing than medically serious, but cases do present where there has been considerable bleeding. Bedrest and the use of ice-packs are recommended, followed by a firm scrotal support for several days.

Mention should be made in this section of non-injury. Occasionally athletes are brought into the A & E department having 'collapsed' at the end of an endurance event. This problem may be difficult to resolve because the highly trained athlete often has a bizarre ECG with bradycardia, elevation of the ST segment, inversion of the 'T' wave and considerable cardiomegaly. These findings in the young athlete rarely imply a myocardial infarction; in the older athlete the patient should be admitted for observation and serial ECGs but with an awareness of the possible physiological interpretation of the results. There is a further problem in that the serum enzyme CK-MB is raised after weight-bearing exercise of over one hour's duration.

Injuries to the thigh

Muscular strains of the thigh occur in all sports but rarely present in the A & E department. When symptoms are sufficiently severe for the patient to attend, the possibility of a complete rupture or an avulsion fracture must be borne in mind. The latter is most likely to occur in the teenage athlete and involve the anteroinferior iliac spine or the ischial tuberosity. With an avulsion fracture, separation of the avulsed fragment by more than 1 cm requires an orthopaedic opinion; less separation than this requires relative or complete rest for the muscle and in this degree of separation callus will easily bridge the gap.

Contusion of the quadriceps muscle often occurs and it has the important complication of myositis ossificans. The patient with a large haematoma should be initially treated with a pressure dressing such as crepe and cottonwool bandage, he should go home and be told to rest. He should be re-examined on the second or third day and if there is more than 90° of knee flexion then he is unlikely to develop myositis ossificans. However, if there is less than 90° of flexion, immobilisation in a Robert Jones bandage or a plaster cylinder should be carried out, the patient being reviewed in two weeks with a repeat radiological examination to see if any calcification has developed.

Tears of the thigh musculature, most commonly the hamstring, occur in a variety of sports, particularly those with an explosive element. Usually these are partial tears. A small haematoma will form in the gap between the fibres, there will then be phases of non-specific inflammation, demolition, repair, scarring and contracture. The last is very important in the athlete because it leads to the problem where they have recurrent tears and to avoid this there has to be some gentle stretching during the rehabilitation phase, this requires intelligent physiotherapy.

Injuries to the knee joint

Injuries around the knee joint are less common that those to the ankle joint but are potentially more serious. In association football it is usually a painful contusion or a relatively minor ligamentous injury, but in rugby, where the whole of the opponent's body weight may be hurled at the joint, there is likely to be more serious damage. There is one condition, O'Donoghue's triad, with injury to the medial ligament, anterior cruciate ligament and medial meniscus, where the full diagnosis is often missed. In sport it is usually seen in rugby players or skiers but it is also seen in motorcyclists or pedestrians who have been knocked down.

It is essential to realise that examination for ligamentous injury of the knee joint must take place with the joint in full extension and in 30° of flexion. Instablility in full extension implies damage to the posterior cruciate ligament as well as to a collateral ligament. Complete rupture of the medial or lateral ligament as an isolated injury will only show in part flexion when the posterior capsule and the posterior cruciate ligament are relaxed. The complete ligamentous tear is usually associated with a tear of the capsule, consequently any haemarthrosis or effusion will leak out of the joint into the subcutaneous tissues. Consequently when a patient with a complete tear comes into the A & E department the knee will not obviously be swollen and the gravity of the condition may be overlooked. Early referral to an orthopaedic surgeon is essential for it is only in the first week after injury that the tissues are in a suitable condition for surgery. Doctors in the A & E department should have a high degree of suspicion and refer all doubtful cases within 48 hours. It is not good policy, when uncertain of the diagnosis in a knee injury, to place the joint in POP for two weeks and then re-examine; at this late stage it is not possible to suture the degenerating tissues.

The diagnosis of injuries to the meniscus requires a detailed history and a careful record of physical signs. The mechanics of injury usually involve weight bearing and rotation. Any loss of extension must be recorded. Care must be taken in localising as accurately as possible any tenderness, particularly in differentiating tenderness on the joint line, i.e. meniscus, from tenderness at other sites, usually ligamentous. Significant ligamentous injuries rarely occur in the adolescent in whom the possibility of an osteochondral fracture or epiphyseal injury must be suspected.

There are many other problems around the knee joint. Chrondromalacia patellae is common in athletes, particularly cyclists and runners. It is characterised by retropatellar aching pain which is worse on activity, particularly when going down hill and after prolonged sitting. The patient may be seen in the A & E department because of momentary giving way or locking, which usually occurs in the fully flexed position rather than in the true locking which is 30° short of full extension, this being typical of a meniscus lesion.

Subluxation and dislocation of the patella, common in the teenage girl, also occurs in the male athlete. Here again there is a history of giving way or the knee 'going out of joint' usually when turning to the side away from the knee joint involved. On examination there may be general tenderness and swelling around the joint, the patella is highly mobile, the skyline radiograph of the patella often shows a flat lateral femoral condyle. Visually the line of pull of the quadriceps muscle is usually at an angle to the line of pull of the patellar tendon, what the Americans refer to as a large 'Q' angle. The possibility of subluxation or dislocation must be appreciated early because all too often these unfortunate athletes end up with a lateral meniscectomy which only makes the condition worse.

Injuries to the lower leg

The teenage athlete occasionally comes in complaining of pain and swelling around the tibial tuberosity. This is often due to Osgood-Schlatter's disease which has been brought to their notice by direct trauma. Radiographs may show fragmentation of the tibial tuberosity. Treatment is restricted activity and the condition settles in about 3 months with time; POP is not necessary and leads to other problems from muscle weakness.

Stress fractures of the tibia and fibula may be seen as an acute problem in an athlete. There is a history of pain and tenderness localised to bone, not associated with direct trauma but with repetitive activity. There are rarely any radiological changes initially but the fracture itself, sclerosis or periosteal reaction, will show in two or three weeks. Initial treatment should simply consist of restriction of activity until the pain settles and, if it does not do so in two or three weeks, the athlete should return for further radiological examination.

The majority of athletes have a tense anterior compartment of shin and direct blows to this area with a resultant haematoma and increased pressure may pose vascular and neurological problems of considerable magnitude. Injuries in this area should be watched carefully for the possible development of these complications which may require admission to hospital for surgical decompression.

Injuries to the ankle and foot

Injuries to the ligaments around the ankle joint are the most common sports injury. Familiarity with this injury breeds contempt and it must be realised that the long-term results of a sprained ankle are extremely poor, not because the condition is difficult but because the treatment is inadequate.

The ankle is an easy joint to examine, with the principal structures being subcutaneous. There is little correlation between the amount of swelling and the severity of injury. One aspect of swelling which implies a more serious injury is when there is an effusion into the joint which is most easily seen with the patient standing. Anteriorly the effusion bulges over the surface of the joint extending up into the synovial reflection over the distal inch of the tibia. Posteriorly it fills out the normal hollows on either side of the Achilles tendon.

More serious ligament injuries include complete rupture of the collateral ligaments and tears of the tibiofibular ligament. Complete tears are usually of the lateral ligament and may be assessed by talar tilt or the anterior drawer test. Forced inversion is usually very painful and may require general anaesthesia, which is only justified if local orthopaedic practice would be surgically to repair complete ruptures. It is also very difficult to separate talar tilt from subtalar movement and therefore must be confirmed radiologically when only a tilt of greater than 20° is considered significant. The anterior drawer test is rarely painful and requires the foot to be placed in slight inversion and plantar flexion, pushing the anterior surface of the tibia backwards with the flat of one hand whilst the cupped fingers of the other hand placed behind the talus gently pull the foot forwards in the line of plantar flexion. Abnormal forward movement of the talus of greater than 5 mm is considered positive. Either or both of these tests may be positive in a complete rupture.

Standard radiographs of the ankle joint must include the distal third of the fibula. These may show various fractures but also, on the anteroposterior view, if there is widening of the joint space on one side of the talus, there being no malleolar fracture, there must be an increased gap between the tibia and fibula implying tearing of the tibiofibular ligament. This latter injury, together with complete rupture of the collateral ligament, do not require specific treatment but have a much longer recovery period than the common sprain of the lateral ligament.

In treating a ligamentous injury in an athlete, active physiotherapy is much more important than strapping or support bandages though these may be used if they give comfort and confidence. Proprioceptive function will be lost unless there is adequate stimulation within 10 days of injury. All too often there is a persistent abnormal gait with loss of ankle evertor strength. These two factors lead to recurrent sprains which are seen all too often and the essential feature of treatment is for an active, graduated exercise programme.

Rupture of the Achilles tendon occurs most typically in the older person taking occasional exercise, but may also be seen in the regular exerciser, particularly squash players. Swelling develops rapidly after the injury which may obscure a palpable gap in the tendon and the muscular development of the athlete may allow considerable plantar flexion of the foot by use of the accessory muscles. Because there is no obvious gap and plantar flexion is present, the doctor may be inclined to treat the injury as a sprained ankle. Testing plantar flexion requires firm pressure against the sole of the foot and the possibility of surgical repair should be considered in the younger patient.

The majority of foot problems are not acute although there may be various contusions and fractures, the only particular ones being: 1. a stress fracture of the metatarsal, which is usually seen in the occasional walker and 2. a stress fracture of the body of the navicular, which is particularly seen in the young athlete where there is a considerable impact, such as in hurdlers or long jumpers.

Summary

Many sports injuries are related to the repetitive stress of the training programme and do not present as emergencies, but others provide a significant number of patients in an A & E department. Some injuries are more common in this group and even simple injuries may be complicated by the excessive bleeding produced by the higher effective vascularisation resulting from training.

Burns

INTRODUCTION

The management of major burns is described in Ch. 14. This section deals with those burns which are not sufficiently extensive as to require resuscitation, i.e. burns of less than 10% body surface area in a child or elderly subject or less than 15% in the healthy adult. Remember *Wallace's rule of nine* for making a rapid assessment of the percentage surface area and that the patient's palm is equivalent to 1% of the surface area (see p. 186). If in doubt as to the extent of burning, it is wise to err on the side of caution and to proceed initially as for a major burn.

The great majority of patients who attend an A & E department can be dealt with on an outpatient basis. The *indications for admission,* in addition to the percentage area of burning listed above, are:

1. Respiratory burns
2. Deep burns of the scalp
3. Burns of the eyes
4. Crushing burns, especially of the hands
5. Burns of the buttocks and/or perineum
6. Full thickness burns, especially of the dorsa of the hands and fingers which will be suitable for early excision and grafting
7. Circumferential burns of the chest, which might impair respiration; or of a limb, which might embarrass the circulation
8. Severe electric shock
9. Patients whose home circumstances make it impossible for them to be managed as outpatients.

The problems of respiratory burns have been mentioned in Ch. 14 and smoke inhalation in Ch. 27. It is possible for a patient who has inhaled hot gases to walk into the A & E department and take his place among patients with minor injuries. It may be only after several hours that oedema builds up within the respiratory passages and causes difficulty in breathing.

> Any patient who has inhaled hot gases, been in an explosion, or in any way suffered the effects of blast on the lungs must be kept under close observation for the earliest signs of respiratory embarrassment.

PRINCIPLES IN THE MANAGEMENT OF BURNS

First aid

The first aid treatment for all external burns is immersion in cold running water. This has four beneficial effects: it puts out any smouldering clothing; it reduces the depth of the burn by cooling down the skin rapidly; it may numb the part and so reduce pain; but perhaps its main analgesic effect is to stop evaporation from the burned surface. In chemical burns its action is to dilute and remove the chemical. This treatment is easy to apply to the limbs but is more difficult when the trunk or head is involved. En-route to hospital the burned area should be covered with a sterile or freshly laundered sheet or towel. A sheet of polythene or a polythene bag is a reasonable alternative. If there is a considerable distance involved before reaching hospital commercial polyurethane foam burns dressings are available for the absorption of exudate and the isolation of infection. Creams or ointments should not be used as this makes the assessment of the burned area more difficult.

History and assessment

The history of the burning episode should be established and in particular the time since burning. The area of skin involvement and the proportion of partial and full thickness burning, as assessed by reaction to pricking with a sterile needle, should be recorded diagrammatically on the record card.

Relief of pain.

This is often achieved by preventing excess evaporation from the exposed burned surface. The patient should be received into a warm room without cold draughts, and the burns kept lightly covered. Intravenous analgesia or a sedative may be given in small doses and these may be supplemented by inhalational analgesia (see Entonox, Ch. 9) until the burn has been dressed. Table 37.1 gives age/weight related dosages for morphine sulphate and trimeprazine (vallergan) for use in children.

Table 37.1 Paediatric sedative dosages

Age	Average weight	Trimeprazine 6 mg/ml	Morphine 10 mg/ml
2/12	0 st 10 lb (4.5 kg)	12 mg (2.0 ml)	—
4/12	1 st 0 lb (6.3 kg)	18 mg (3.0 ml)	—
1 yr	1 st 7 lb (9.5 kg)	24 mg (4.0 ml)	1.5 mg (0.15 ml)
2 yr	2 st 0 lb (12.7 kg)	36 mg (6.0 ml)	2.0 mg (0.20 ml)
3 yr	2 st 4 lb (14.5 kg)	39 mg (6.5 ml)	2.3 mg (0.23 ml)
4 yr	2 st 5 lb (15.0 kg)	39 mg (6.5 ml)	2.4 mg (0.24 ml)
5 yr	3 st 0 lb (19.0 kg)	50 mg (8.0 ml)	3.0 mg (0.30 ml)
6 yr	3 st 4 lb (20.8 kg)	54 mg (9.0 ml)	3.3 mg (0.33 ml)
7 yr	3 st 8 lb (22.5 kg)	60 mg (10.0 ml)	3.6 mg (0.36 ml)
8 yr	4 st 0 lb (25.4 kg)	66 mg (11.0 ml)	4.0 mg (0.40 ml)
9 yr	4 st 4 lb (27.2 kg)	72 mg (12.0 ml)	4.3 mg (0.43 ml)
10 yr	4 st 10 lb (30.0 kg)	78 mg (13.0 ml)	4.7 mg (0.47 ml)
11 yr	5 st 4 lb (33.5 kg)	88 mg (14.5 ml)	5.3 mg (0.53 ml)
12 yr	6 st 0 lb (38.0 kg)	99 mg (16.5 ml)	6.0 mg (0.60 ml)

Antibiotic prophylaxis?

The use of prophylactic antibiotics is inappropriate for localised burns of the periphery. Burns of the perineum justify the use of a systemic antibiotic such as ampicillin or metronidazole as prophylaxis against infection from bowel organisms. Patients with minor burns require the same kind of tetanus prophylaxis as wounds (see Ch. 31).

Is there an underlying cause?

Burns and scalds can occur from a variety of causes. If no reasonable explanation is apparent look for an underlying physical cause, e.g. fit or faint, hypoglycaemia, drug or alcohol intoxication. In patients with cutaneous anaesthesia (from diabetic neuropathy, spinal cord injury, neurological disease, etc.) areas of deep, full-thickness burns can occur. In children, frequently occuring burns and scalds may indicate carelessness or lack of parental supervision and consideration should be given to involving the community services (particularly the health visitor) in further accident prevention. Similarly, self-neglect is seen in cases of alcohol abuse who may represent with full thickness burns to their fingertips from cigarettes or trunk burns from falling asleep against a hot radiator or fire. Rarely certain types of burns and scalds form part of the non-accidental injury syndrome (see Ch. 5).

MANAGEMENT OF THE BURN WOUND

Burns of the face

Initial treatment aims at reducing the pain and discomfort caused by the exposure of raw nerve endings. The application of cold saline packs has a soothing and relieving effect in the first hour or two after burning. Following this, facial burns are best left open to the air. Infection in this vascular region is rare, and the exudate quickly forms a crust if it is exposed to a warm, dry atmosphere. Full thickness burns of the face do not exude so copiously and also may be left open to the air prior to skin replacement by a plastic surgeon.

It is helpful to warn the patient and relatives that the face may become swollen on the day after the burn and the appearance may be very alarming, but the swelling will then resolve.

Burns of the trunk, arms or thighs (Fig. 37.1)

Scalds of limited extent on the chest, arms or thighs — particularly in children — are well suited to treatment by the application of a sterile adhesive vapour-permeable/waterproof film (e.g. *Op-Site* or *Tegaderm*), which serves to stop evaporation and to protect from further injury and contamination. The pain is thereby greatly reduced. Bulky dressings are avoided, so that normal clothing can

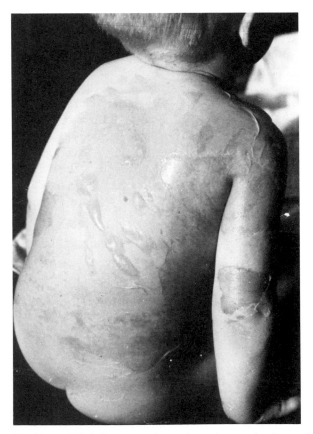

Fig. 37.1 Burns of limited extent on the trunk may be treated at home with protective dressings, provided there can be adequate supervision. More extensive burns such as this will require fluid replacement and admission to hospital.

be worn, and the patient can wash. As exudation continues beneath this type of dressing, it might need to be aspirated at appropriate intervals.

Burns of the buttocks, perineum and external genitalia

Patients will usually require to be admitted for supervision by a plastic surgical department. Early urinary catheterisation is often needed, before oedema makes the procedure difficult or impossible.

Burns near to joints

In the region of the shoulder, elbow, knee or ankle, a traditional bulky dressing will have the desired effect of resting or immobilising the joint in the optimum position. The dressing in immediate contact with the burn should be of a non-adherent porous material (one of the non-antibiotic impregnated tulles) which should then be covered with gauze and thick layers of wool to absorb the exudate. The whole dressing is then held in place by

bandaging so that the edges of the burn do not become exposed. Full thickness burns which involve flexor skin creases near a joint should be splinted in extension to prevent subsequent contractures; this can be achieved by a plaster of Paris slab outside the dressing.

Burns of the hands (Figs 37.2 and 37.3)

A patient with deep dermal or full-thickness burns should be referred immediately to a plastic surgeon. Even if the burns are initially only superficial, should they become infected, the finger joints may become ankylosed or contracted. One method of minimising the risk is to apply silver sulphadiazine *(Flamazine)* cream and then enclose the hand in a plastic bag or glove. This will prevent contamination, discourage infection and allow free movement of the fingers. The bag has to be changed frequently (often daily), however, because it fills up with exudate and the fingers tend to become macerated from repeated application of the cream. If the facilities for frequent changing of the bag and

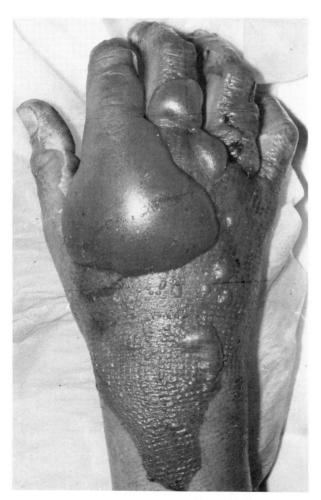

Fig. 37.2 Hand burns such as this (even if only partial thickness) should either be mobilised from the outset or immobilised for a brief period with the metacarpophalangeal joints in the flexed position. If immobilised in the extended position, permanent stiffness of the metacarpophalangeal joints may follow.

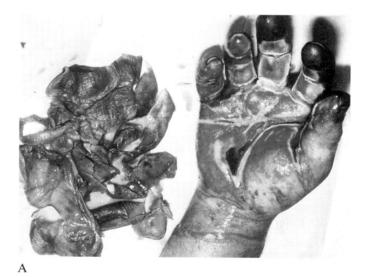

A

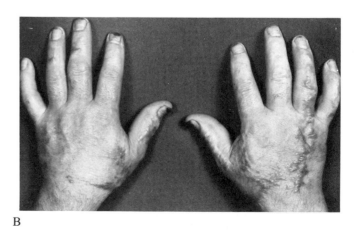

B

Fig. 37.3 A These petrol burns of the hands were treated by occlusive dressings. After three weeks the superficial epithelial layers of skin were peeled away leaving only small patches of deep skin loss. **B** The hands of the same patient, fully healed with no joint contracture at six weeks. The skin of the hand and face has remarkable powers of recovery.

reapplication of the cream are not readily available, or if only one or two fingers have been burned, the fingers should individually dressed with tulle, gauze and bandage and the whole hand and fingers then covered with sterile wool and bandaged with the fingers as nearly as possible in the optimum position for preventing contractures — that is with the metacarpophalangeal joints in 80° of flexion and the interphalangeal joints extended. (See Ch. 34.) The hands should be elevated in a high sling.

Treatment of blisters

Blisters form a biological dressing and protect the burn from contamination. They should be left intact until they burst or, if they become very large, they can be aspirated. 'Deroofing' blisters causes unnecessary pain, delays healing and increases the risk of infection.

SPECIAL TYPES OF BURNS

Substances which adhere to the skin

Bitumen (Fig. 37.4) usually produces only superficial burns, provided that the area is well washed with cold water immediately after contact. On no account should efforts be made to remove the bitumen immediately after the burning as this will result in removal of layers of undamaged skin resulting in a deepening of the burn wound. The area involved should be protected and the bitumen will eventually peel off spontaneously after a couple of weeks leaving healing partial-thickness burns. If, however, the bitumen is covering the face, or if it is surrounding a finger or limb and occluding the circulation, removal will be necessary. Liquid paraffin may be used to loosen the bitumen and allow gentle removal.

Burning polyethylene which has adhered to the skin is managed in the same way.

Chemical burns

There are very few chemicals which are absorbed through the intact skin. One of these is *phenol* and vigorous washing with cold water should take place as soon as possible after burning to minimise the absorption. Phenol burns may be pale and painless if nerve fibres are destroyed. Systemic phenol poisoning may occur; the first sign of this is grey-black discolouration of the urine. Renal failure may ensue.

Most strong chemicals will produce deep burns which may progressively become deeper over the course of the first 10–14 days. Vigorous immediate washing with cold water is once again the most important first aid measure and probably rates more highly than all the traditionally quoted antidotes.

A particularly nasty chemical burn is that caused by *hydrofluoric acid*, an extremely strong acid used in the glass etching industry. The burning process may continue long after the removal of contact. Treatment remains controversial: the one-time recommendation of the application of ice-cold 10% calcium

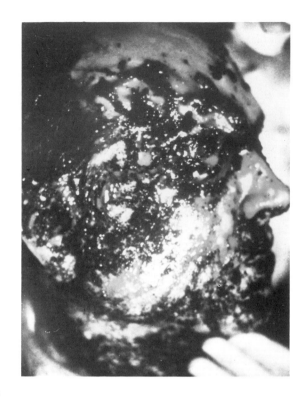

A

B

Fig. 37.4 Bitumen burns to the face **A** and both hands. **B** The only treatment applied was cold water and protection from across contamination. After three weeks the bitumen has separated spontaneously and healing followed without scarring.

gluconate jelly has recently been shown to confer no additional benefit over ice-cold water alone (Goodfellow 1985). If contact has occured beneath the fingernails, the nails should be removed. The risk of systemic fluoride poisoning achieves significance when an area greater than 2% is involved.

Many chemical burns involve only a small area and are therefore suitable for excision and grafting as soon as the full extent of the burn is apparent.

Contact burns

These are commonly sustained in the home (such as from touching a hot iron) and may heal spontaneously.

The child who grips the unprotected element of an electric fire sustains deep burns on the flexor aspect or the fingers and hand, which will often require early excision and grafting by a plastic surgeon to whom the patient should be referred.

Localised full thickness contact burns (e.g. from a live coal dropping onto the foot, from molten metal or from hot fat splashes) can be managed by early excision and grafting in the A & E department, provided the skills and facilities are available (Fig. 37.5).

Hot press burns combine physical injury with fairly prolonged application of very high temperatures and may result in amputation of the fingers. Clearly these injuries should be managed in a specialised unit (Fig. 37.6).

Friction burns

There may be two elements to the friction burn;
1. A *degloving wound*
2. The possibility of *ingrained dirt.*

Common modes of injury include the limb being run over or being caught between moving rollers (e.g. the 'wringer-injury'), or the skin sliding along a dirty uneven surface (e.g. the 'road-rash' known to cyclists and motor-cyclists). (Fig. 37.7)

Degloving may not be immediately obvious, if the skin is not disrupted. It will be anaesthetic to touch. If degloving is suspected from the nature of the injury (i.e. a tangentially applied force) or from the physical findings, the advice of a plastic surgeon should be sought. The skin is in jeopardy and appropriate early treatment will minimize the area of skin loss and provide an opportunity for early replacement of devitalised skin.

If the problem appears to be that of *ingrained dirt* then all the

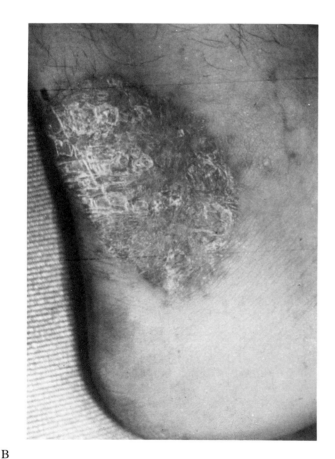

A

B

Fig. 37.5 A A live coal dropped into this man's boot which could not be removed quickly enough to avoid this obviously full thickness burn. Primary excision and split skin grafting were carried out within 48 hours. **B** At three weeks, sound healing has been obtained without admission to hospital, with a minimum of disturbance of function and early return to work.

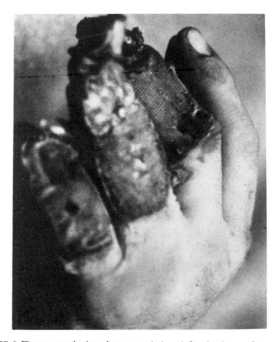

Fig. 37.6 Fingers caught in a hot press designed for shaping molten metal. All the fingers had to be amputated.

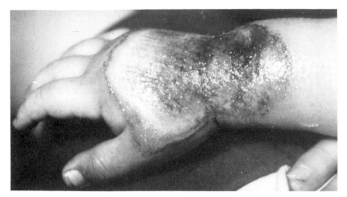

Fig. 37.7 This child's wrist was caught between the rollers of the wringer of a washing machine. The skin had to be removed and replaced with a skin graft.

dirt needs to be removed by the vigorous application of a scrubbing brush, assisted if necessary by the point of a knife. Adequate anaesthesia is essential and Entonox has proved useful in this application. Where large areas of skin are to be cleaned, a general anaesthetic may be required. The common practice of using lignocaine jelly is potentially hazardous, for toxic concentrations of the anaesthetic can readily be absorbed through the damaged skin. Scrubbing produces a raw bleeding area which can be dressed as for other burns (see 'Burns near to joints'). If ingrained friction burns are left untreated infection may follow (leading to full-thickness skin loss) or the dirt will remain as unsightly 'tattoo marks' in the skin. These marks are difficult to remove subsequently.

Beware *pressure burns* which are 'imprinted' on the skin, especially on the trunk. These should be regarded as a warning of possible underlying visceral injury (see Ch. 14).

Electrical burns (Fig. 37.8)

The effects of these burns have to be considered in two parts — general and local.

The general effects of electricity depend upon the voltage applied, the resistance of the body and the duration of application. The average resistance through the thickness of skin is 5000 ohm; this is reduced if the skin is moist or if there has been sufficient duration of contact for the skin and flesh to become coagulated. Nervous tissue is the least resistant to electricity and this accounts for the presence of neurological symptoms in the majority of cases: there may be alteration of consciousness and disturbance of higher function in varying degrees. Headaches are frequent. Abnormalities of motor function and balance are not unusual and, rarely, progressive spinal atrophy may develop. Cardiac manifestations are common with frequent abnormalities of conduction and cardiac rhythm. Cardiac arrest in ventricular fibrillation is often the terminal event.

Lightning burns are discussed in Ch. 27.

The local effects of electrical burns are, like those of chemical burns, often progressive during the first two to three weeks. Electrical contact produces an endarteritis and secondary necrosis.

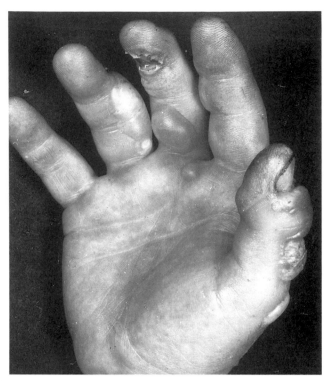

A

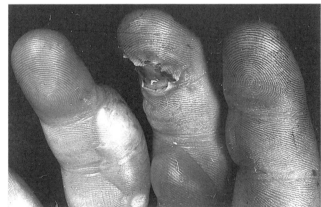

B

Fig. 37.8 A and **B** Contact burns from a domestic electric source. The blistered areas represent partial thickness flash burns. The area of broken skin represents a full-thickness burn where the finger was in contact with the live plug.

It is therefore wise to wait before excision and grafting of the affected area is undertaken.

The electrical contact burn should not be confused with the associated flash or heat burns, which are maximal in extent when first seen. Vapourisation of copper from electric terminals may cause a brown appearance from deposition of metal on the skin. This may look like a burn but there is no significant tissue damage.

Sunburn and burns from ultraviolet light (Fig. 37.9)

Patients who lie out in the sun on a hot day or who fall asleep under a sunlamp may suffer extensive burning. A cold shower

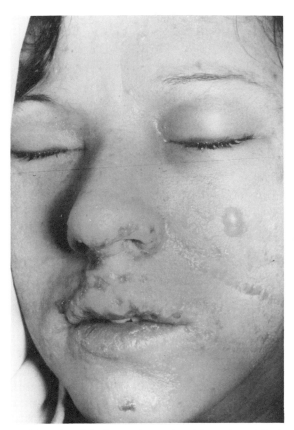

Fig. 37.9 This patient fell asleep under an ultra-violet sunlamp. The burn was treated by exposure.

followed by the application of calamine lotion may be sufficient. If blisters form they should be protected from abrasion; a sterile adhesive film is useful for this if the area burned is not too large. When extensive areas are involved, this dry heat burn can be managed by the 'open' method. The patient is confined to bed in a cool room and the burn is exposed so that a coagulum will form over any areas which are weeping serum. The coagulum seals the burn, stops infection and prevents any further fluid loss. If the patient is also suffering from sunstroke, fluid replacement will be required. This can usually be given as iced drinks to be taken in frequently repeated small quantities to avoid vomiting. The patient may be hyponatraemic and the ingestion of copious volumes of fluids without added salt may lead to water intoxication. The more severe cases with toxaemia, fever, nausea and weakness will require intravenous fluid replacement and more energetic cooling (see Ch. 28 Environmental emergencies and Ch. 45 Skin conditions).

A burn from an ultraviolet source is usually well localised and, if partial-thickness, can be treated by a protective dressing. Full-thickness ultraviolet burns should be referred for early excision and grafting.

Radioactive burns

See Ch. 28.

THE FOLLOW-UP MANAGEMENT OF BURNS IN THE A & E DEPARTMENT

All patients should be seen the day after their initial treatment. Patients treated with an adhesive film dressing, will have serum which has collected under the dressing aspirated using a sterile needle after cleaning the surface with cetrimide. A second sheet of the plastic may then be applied on top of the first. If serum has soaked through a tulle, gauze and wool dressing, bacteria will penetrate. The outer layers should be removed down to the gauze, and fresh sterile wool and bandages applied.

Depending upon the degree of attention required at the first revisit, the second visit can be planned for one or two days later. After 48–72 hours there should be no more leakage of serum and then, provided the dressing is in good condition, the patient does not need to be seen again until 10 days after the original injury. Changing the dressing too frequently is meddlesome and the hospital environment increases the risk of infection.

By the tenth day most superficial burns should be healed and a decision can be made about any areas of full-thickness burns. If these are small and in areas which have little importance from the cosmetic and functional point of view, they may be left to heal under a sterile dressing.

THE CONTAMINATED BURN

This can be a nuisance, delays healing and can lead to unpleasant scarring. A bacterial swab should be taken and the appropriate systemic antibiotic prescribed to prevent the colonisation leading to a septicaemia. The most frequently encountered contaminants are *Streptococcus pyogenes*, *Staphylococcus aureus* and *Pseudomonas* species. Frequent changes and variety of antiseptic dressings may be needed including chlorhexidine, povidone iodine, silver sulphadiazine and 'Furacin' dressings.

GRAFTING

Indications

Indications for grafting of burns treated in the A & E department are as follows:

1. Burns which are clearly full thickness when first seen. These will include contact with hot metal, electric bar injuries, hot press burns and some chemical burns (Fig. 37.10).
2. Deep dermal burns are now usually treated by tangential excision and grafting as soon as feasible after the time of burning. Such patients should be referred to a plastic surgeon.
3. Burns which at 10 days to 3 weeks after the injury are clearly seen to be full thickness or deep dermal burns. These will include some scalds and hot fat burns.

Except in the fingers and eyelids, burns which are less than 2.5 cm across will never be worth grafting. Burns which are extensive, or which involve flexion creases of the hand and fingers will usually be referred immediately to a plastic surgeon.

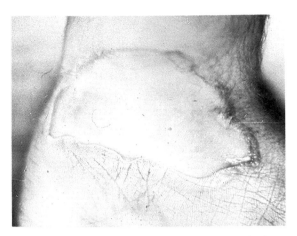

Fig. 37.10 An epileptic patient fell across a hot pipe and sustained an area of full-thickness skin loss across the wrist crease. This was excised and grafted as a primary procedure. The wrist was immobilised in a plaster of Paris splint.

Contraindications

1. Electrical burns and some chemical burns (e.g. hydrofluoric acid burns), in which further tissue loss may be expected, should not be grafted until demarcation is complete, some three or four weeks after the burn.

2. Obvious infection of the surface — as indicated by soggy, unhealthy looking granulations or the presence of slough. However, although there is inevitably some degree of infection on a granulating surface, a properly applied graft should 'take' provided that the β-haemolytic streptococcus is not present in the wound. This organism should be excluded by culture, or eradicated before such secondary grafting procedures are undertaken.

Technique of grafting

Dead skin, slough or granulation may be excised using a 22 scalpel or Silver's knife (for the small burns) or with a skin grafting knife with the blade in the fully opened position. Full-thickness free grafts should be considered outside the province of A & E doctors. Partial (split-) thickness grafts may be taken under regional or general anaesthetic. The graft must be carefully secured and firm pressure applied over a tulle dressing using Flavine wool or a sponge pad. This should be cut a little smaller than the graft and held in place with 'tie-over' crossing sutures.

REHABILITATION

Mention has been made of the importance of splinting joints in extension to prevent joint contracture as a burn heals. It follows that, as soon as possible, the joint should be put through its normal range of movement to prevent stiffness from prolonged immobilisation. For patients with superficial burns this will be by the 10th to 12th day. Patients treated by early skin grafting on the first or second day should start supervised active movements by the end of two weeks. Those patients who are to have delayed skin grafting should have a few days of active exercises between the 10th and 14th days before their limb is reimmobilised for a further 10 days after the skin grafting operation.

Once the burn has healed over, either by re-epithelialisation or by grafting, the skin will not be strong or supple. Massage two or three times a day with a lanolin cream will help to restore a normal texture to the skin.

Patients who have had burns to the hand or fingers will benefit from a few attendances at the physiotherapy department for 'wax and exercises'. In the case of infected hand or finger burns, active exercises with the extremity immersed in a jar of sterile silicone will speed up wound healing and improve joint function.

Occasionally, occupational therapy is useful in helping a patient with a hand burn to regain the maximum possible dexterity before returning to work.

REFERENCES

Goodfellow R C 1985 Hydrofluoric acid burns (letter). British Medical Journal 290: 937

FURTHER READING

Burns and their treatment, 3rd edn. Muir I F K, Barclay T L, Settle J A D 1987 Butterworths, London

Burns — the first five days Settle J A D 1987 Smith & Nephew Pharmaceuticals, Romford, Essex RM3 8SL

Dressings and splintage

DRESSINGS

The choice of dressing and dressing technique for the A & E department is a balance between what is considered scientifically ideal and what seems reasonably effective in practice. Cost is a significant and often the deciding factor.

Dressings may have several important purposes:
1. To *protect* the wound from interference during the healing process, from invasion by infecting micro-organisms and from dehydration.
2. To apply *compression*, which controls bleeding and reduces postinjury oedema and helps to prevent the formation of keloid scars.
3. To provide an environment which enhances *healing* with pH, temperature and humidity at optimum levels.
4. To *absorb* exudate whilst allowing gas exchange to continue.
5. To *remove pus and slough* from the wound, thus providing optimal conditions for healing.
6. To *relieve pain* by the exclusion of air from free nerve endings.
7. To provide an acceptable *appearance*.

These properties might be considered the ideal criteria for the use and choice of a dressing though not all may be important, or, indeed, necessary in the treatment of a particular wound. If none apply then the wound should be considered for treatment by exposure and left open.

Types of dressings

Table 38.1 lists the majority of primary wound dressings in

Table 38.1 Types of wound dressings

Gauze	BP
Synthetic gauze	Mesoft, Regal, Sofnet
Non-stick pads	Melolin, Perfron, Release, Telfa
Absorption pads	Surgipad
Island dressings	Airstrip, Bandaid, Mepore, Steripad, Primapore
Impregnated gauze	Paratulle, Bactigras, Inadine
Foams	Synthaderm, Lyofoam, Granuflex, Silastic
Gels	Vigilon, Geliperm, Scherisorb
Charcoal	Actisorb
Occlusive	Opsite, Tegaderm, Flamazine handbag
Biological	Sorbsan, Amnion, Porcine skin

common use. The most frequently used dressings in the A & E department are the non-adherent and impregnated gauzes. The use of topically applied antibiotics, e.g. fusidic acid or soframycin incorporated into tulle should be actively discouraged. They can stimulate the emergence of resistant organisms, sensitise the skin and are an unnecessary expense. Special dressings e.g. foams and gels are relatively expensive and their use should be restricted to those wounds in which the healing environment needs to be strictly controlled. However, quicker healing and fewer visits for redressing may make an 'expensive' dressing cost effective.

Method of primary wound dressing

At the patient's first visit the wound dressing will be applied by a member of the nursing staff as an aseptic procedure. Where it has been decided to treat the wound by exposure (e.g. wounds of the scalp and face) then a simple lotion (povidone-iodine paint is recommended) can be applied to the wound. The advantages of leaving a wound without a dressing include better observation of the wound, facilitation of washing or bathing and the absence of adhesives or allergens on the skin. Wounds which are oozing blood or serous fluid will require firm pressure applied over layers of gauze. All dressings require adequate fixation (see 'Bandaging' and 'Splinting' below).

Dressings for special areas

The scalp

Nearly all scalp wounds can be treated by exposure. Due to the extreme vascularity of the scalp, infection is uncommon. Injuries of greater complexity than simple scalp lacerations may require absorbent dressings secured by a compression crepe bandage (see below) with a corrugated or suction wound drain to prevent the development of haematoma. Such wounds would normally be treated by neurosurgeons.

The face

Wounds of the face heal quickly and should normally be left exposed to the air. Dressings are difficult to secure and tend to convert a dry, nicely knitting wound into a soggy mess.

The ear

'Cauliflower ear' (pp. 397 and 459) is a common complication of wounds to the pinna, especially when cartilage has been exposed. It should be prevented using a meticulous aseptic technique. Dressings should be compressed into the contour of the ear to prevent haematoma. Paraffin tulle gras and the traditional impregnated 'Flavine wool' are suitable dressing media.

The trunk

Large areas of abrasion or thermal injury to the trunk are quite a problem, chiefly because of the difficulty of securing them with bandages so that the dressings remain in place until the return visit. Initially, bulky dressings might be required to absorb exudate. Special outsize burns dressings should be used and admission to an observation ward considered. For outpatients consideration should be given to the use of *occlusive plastic dressings* which are tolerated well, are transparent — allowing inspection of the wound's progress — and are water resistant, thus allowing washing or bathing.

Digits

Many small wounds can be covered by island dressings and a patient who works in a dirty environment should be given a supply of patches. The dressing is changed if it becomes soiled. In a clean environment wounds of the fingers can be exposed. Non-adherent dressings, usually of impregnated gauze, retained in place with tubular gauze bandage (see below) are used for discharging or granulating lesions of the fingers and toes. Care should be taken to protect the webspace between the digits where friction and moisture can readily lead to a macerated 'intertrigo'. Unhealthy wounds can be 'improved' with dressings of gauze soaked in saline and changed half-hourly over a 2–3 hour period. After this a non-adherent dressing is applied. Fingertip injuries may be covered with silver sulphadiazine cream retained in plastic finger stalls.

Cavity wounds

Sinuses, deep wounds and those communicating with body cavities especially in the anorectal area are notoriously difficult to heal. Consideration should be given to employing a 'Silastic' *foam elastomer*.

Follow-up of wound dressings

If possible the dressing should be left undisturbed until such time as the wound would be normally expected to have healed. The reasons for disturbing a dressing are few. They include:

1. A suspicion of developing wound infection:
   a. discharge
   b. smell
   c. warmth, swelling, tenderness, pain
   d. lymphangitis/lymphadenopathy
   e. fever.
2. The removal of excess exudate. The dressing is only acting as a barrier against infection while it is clean and dry. Patients should be told to return should a stain of the exudate become visible on the bandage.
3. The removal of dead tissue, slough or eschar.
4. The local treatment of established infection.
5. The elective removal of sutures, etc.

It is useful to organise secondary wound management into review or dressings clinics conducted in a special area of the A & E department. There should be adequate medical and nursing staff for the number of patients attending and the work should be supervised by senior doctors and nurses. It is helpful to have a particular senior nurse with continuing responsibility in this area. If the patient is to make any follow-up visits, the first one is the most important when dressings and splints applied at the initial visit can be checked. Wounds which might be expected to bleed or produce exudate may need the outer covers changed but the inner dressing should only be removed on the second day if it is heavily soaked with blood.

The first follow-up visit is also the occasion to pick up any missed diagnoses such as a painful or stiff joint following an accident when at the initial visit the patient complained only of a laceration. Nerve and tendon function should be checked.

The functions of dressings applied at follow-up will overlap with those applied at the first visit, but may be conveniently described as follows:

1. As simple protection in the form of a dry dressing for those with clean wounds after suture removal or following the surgical treatment of abscesses (see Ch. 33). No further visit should be necessary for the majority of such patients.

2. For the clearance of necrotic or infective material from wounds which have become infected for other reasons. Irrigation and dressing with Eusol (a sodium hypochlorite solution) or saline is inexpensive and effective and may need to be repeated daily or

on alternate days, if appropriate, by the community or occupational health nurse, or by the patient. Small areas of slough can be managed by the application of a proprietary desloughing lotion, though once a definite slough has become established surgical excision will remove it far more quickly than any form of dressing.

3. For the control of soggy or exuberant granulations which are occasionally found in burns or wounds which have become infected. Simple astringent lotions such as zinc sulphate and mercurochrome are cheap and effective as is povidone iodine antiseptic solution; they carry less risk of sensitisation and drug resistance than topical antibiotic preparations. Silver sulphadiazine, applied daily, is effective in reducing small areas of granulations. Removal of excess granulation tissue may be achieved by touching with silver nitrate stick but occasionally surgical removal and cautery are required.

BANDAGES

The primary function of bandages is the retention of dressings (Fig. 38.1). However, bandages may have a role in applying even compression to a wound for the control of oedema and haemorrhage in a limb or on the trunk. By incorporating cotton wool, foam or gauze bandages may be used for the support and immobilisation of affected parts — in this way they function as splints. Slings are bandages used for the support and, usually, elevation of a limb.

Roller bandages

These are used for encircling of a limb. They vary from close-weave cotton gauze through open-weave conforming bandage (often crimped to permit one-way stretch) to elasticated crepe.

Tubular bandages

These include gauze bandages for digits and elasticated tubular bandages of various sizes. A shaped tubular bandage for the lower limb is available. Tubular bandages require the use of an applicator. The patient must always be given clear instructions and an explanation of the importance of elevation.

Triangular bandage

The triangular bandage was described by Esmarch in 1986 as a square of calico cut into two diagonally. Its major application is as slings for the upper limb:

The arm sling   (Fig. 38.2) is used to rest the limb with the elbow at right angles or the arm slightly raised. It is tied off at the injured side.

The elevation sling raises the limb with the hand held on the opposite shoulder. This is the sling chosen to elevate the upper limb after the dressing of a hand injury (Fig. 38.3). Venous blood and oedema fluid will drain away under gravity. The hand should never be allowed to dangle out of the end of the sling.

The collar and cuff sling made from a triangular bandage folded narrow or presented commercially as a padded foam strip is used to approximate the wrist to the neck allowing the elbow to sag at an acute angle. Whereas the broad and elevation arm slings are used for injuries of the shoulder, the collar and cuff sling is used for elbow trauma.

Bandaging for special areas

The fingers

Most finger dressings are secured with bandages of tubular gauze. This should be applied with even pressure. It may not be adequate

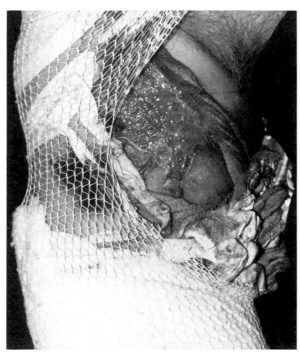

Fig. 38.1 An inadequately secured dressing in the groin.

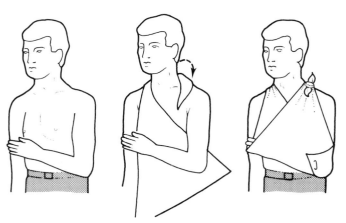

Fig. 38.2 The arm sling.

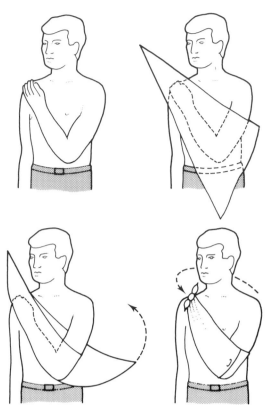

Fig. 38.3 The elevation sling.

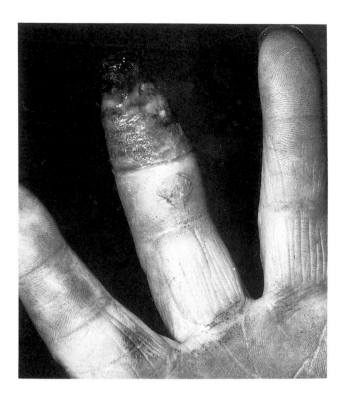

Fig. 38.4 This elderly man cut his finger and secured the dressing with a tight rubber band. The circulation was thus occluded and gangrene resulted.

to control bleeding when, for example, a tourniquet has been used, because of the reactive hyperaemia following its release. In this case the patient should be kept in the department for half an hour and a fresh dressing and bandage applied before discharge. Strapping used to secure bandages of the digits must not be allowed to completely encircle the digit lest strangulation of the blood supply occurs (Fig. 38.4). This is particularly likely to develop if bleeding occurs beneath the bandage. Slight overlap in the case of first-aid or island dressings does not matter, though care should be taken to avoid undue tension.

The lower limb

Bandages to the lower limb should be evenly applied from the toes upwards otherwise dependent oedema tends to form in the foot. Compression bandaging for the control of oedema, bleeding and inflammation may be applied, in varying degrees, by using crepe bandage, tubular bandage, elasticated crepe and the one-way-stretch 'Blue-line' bandage, respectively.

The knee

Firm support may be provided by a single or double layer of elastic tubular bandage. For the control of an effusion within the knee joint, or for the prevention of haemarthrosis following recent knee injury, a carefully applied double layer or orthopaedic wool and crepe bandage will give adequate short-term support; it is more

cost-effective than the classical *Robert Jones' knee bandage* of wool and domette which requires experience and skill to apply. The bandage can be reinforced by an extension splint of plaster of Paris or a proprietary 'knee immobiliser' splint (Fig. 38.5). Wasting of the quadriceps muscle occurs rapidly with an immobilised knee and so bandages should be applied only for a specified time and the patient taught quadriceps strengthening exercises (p. 384).

Impregnated bandages

Occasionally there is a place in the A & E department for bandages impregnated with lotions. For example, the proprietary bandage incorporating zinc oxide in an emulsifier base is an acceptable treatment for the inflamed lower limb, particularly in association with the varicose ulcer. Similarly, crepe bandages incorporating dressings soaked in coal tar derivatives, e.g. ichthammol, are helpful in reducing the inflammation from olecranon or prepatellar bursitis.

Strapping

Adhesive bandages are often used to provide immobilisation and support to an injured extremity. They may be elastic or non-elastic, zinc oxide plaster being the common form of the latter. Allergy to the adhesive material occurs occasionally and should be noted.

'Neighbour strapping' splints an injured finger or toe to its uninjured neighbour — adequate padding should be provided between the digits to prevent friction in the web space.

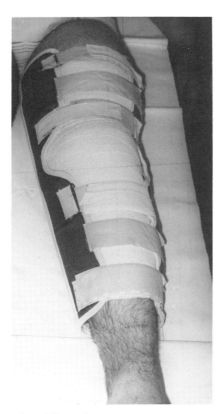

Fig. 38.5 A knee immobiliser splint.

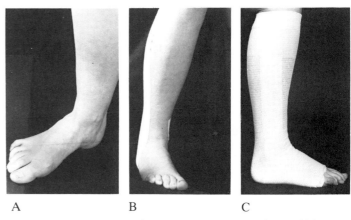

Fig. 38.7 U-shaped strapping for a sprained ankle. **A** The foot should be encouraged to take up the everted position with the toes resting on the edge of a stool set at an angle of 45° to the patient's chair. **B** A length of non-stretch strapping is then carried around the heel from medial to lateral side. **C** This is held in place with the minimum of elastic adhesive strapping, supported with elastic tubular bandage from toes to knee.

SPLINTS

Functions of splints

The functions of splints are threefold: the resting of an injured part; the maintenance of optimal position and the correction of deformity.

Rest

Pain can be caused by movement of injured, inflamed or infected tissues, tendons or joints. Immobilisation for the first few days after injury facilitates resolution of an acute inflammatory reaction and allows early movement of tendons and joints. This is particularly important in the hand (Fig. 38.8).

The *thumb spica* of overlapping turns of 2.5 cm bandage provides support to the injured thumb metacarpophalangeal joint (Fig. 38.6).

Occasionally *stirrup strapping* of the ankle is required where the inversion sprain is supported by the use of a stirrup of non-stretch 7.5 cm zinc oxide applied at the level of the ankle joint. The U-shaped stirrup is secured by one turn of adhesive bandage just below the knee and two or three turns to encompass the foot and ankle; the whole is enclosed in double tubular elasticated bandage from toes to knee (Fig. 38.7).

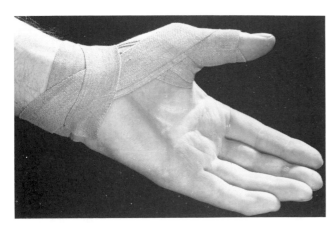

Fig. 38.6 A thumb spica may be applied in one length, as in this illustration, or in successive strips.

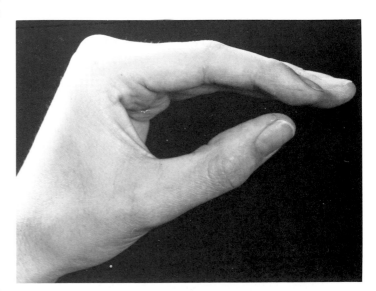

Fig. 38.8 Position of safe immobilisation of the hand.

Maintenance of optimal position

Splints are the main method of holding a fractured bone in an anatomical position after reduction. Repaired or injured tendons and nerves must be held in a relaxed position while healing takes place. This may involve immobilising a joint in a less than optimal position; for example, a digital extensor tendon which has been cleanly cut over a metacarpophalangeal joint may be sutured and the unaffected metacarpophalangeal joint immobilised in *extension* for three weeks when early return of function can be expected. However if the underlying joint has been injured as well as the extensor tendon (e.g. following a crushing injury or a human bite) then careful cleansing and excision should be followed by suture of the skin only and immobilisation of the metacarpophalangeal joint in the optimal flexed position of function. Once full passive movements have been regained, secondary suture of the tendon can be undertaken and the joint can then be safely maintained in extension during the healing period. If this precaution is not observed, the metacarpophalangeal joint will remain stiff in extension.

Correction of deformity

Splints may be used occasionally in the A & E department for treating an established deformity. A common example would be the boutonnière deformity of the finger. Corrective splints may be static or dynamic — in the latter case the *lively splint* incorporates a sprung coil of piano wire against which the patient can exercise the joint (Fig. 38.9). Most patients with corrective splints will be looked after by orthopaedic or hand surgeons.

Splintage materials

The use of bandages, slings and strapping as splintage materials has already been discussed. Permanent splints incorporate a firm but comfortable and preferably lightweight medium, e.g. polyethylene, light alloy and plastic. Such materials are usually padded with foam rubber.

Plaster of Paris

Plaster of Paris is still the most commonly used casting material in the A & E department. It is available as slabs or bandages.

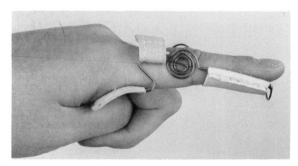

Fig. 38.9 A lively finger splint.

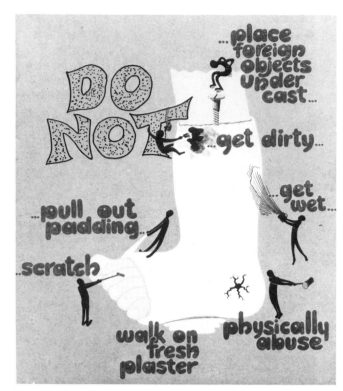

Fig. 38.10 Patient instructions in the care of plaster of Paris.

Techniques used in the application and removal of plaster of Paris are described in the specialist publications listed at the end of this chapter. The principles for the care of patients splinted with 'POP' must be instilled into every member of the A & E department staff (Fig. 38.10):

1. It is safer to effect primary splintage after the reduction of a limb fracture with slabs rather than encircling casts.

2. Every patient who has a cast applied must be warned to return immediately if the fingers or toes become blue or swollen or if there is increasing pain under the cast.

3. POP splints should normally incorporate the joints above and below a fracture; patients should be encouraged to mobilise surrounding joints (Fig. 38.11).

4. An upper limb cast must be supported in a sling for the first 24 hours until it is dry; a patient with a lower limb cast must be instructed in the use of crutches and ordered not to bear weight on the POP until it has dried out (this usually takes about three days) and a walking heel or plaster boot has been applied..

5. Patients are advised not to distort, deform or mutilate their cast; not to push anything between it and the skin, nor to scratch underneath it, however irritating it may feel.

6. Even if there are no untoward symptoms, the patient should be checked the day following the plaster application to confirm that the position is acceptable and that the circulation is satisfactory.

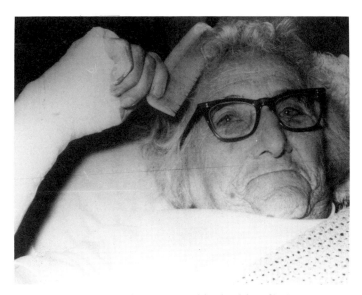

Fig. 38.11 A patient in a Colles cast exercising her joints. She is able to raise her arm above her head in order to comb her hair.

Synthetic casting materials (Baycast, Cristona, etc.)

These materials are enjoying an increasing popularity in A & E departments. Though more expensive than Plaster of Paris, they are lighter and more durable. They do require considerable skill in correct application. In particular, unless carefully moulded to the limb, they have a tendency to spring back into the shape of a cylinder and compromise the circulation.

Complications of plaster of Paris and synthetic casting

A limb enclosed in plaster, if not carefully supervised, may develop one or more of the complications of casting: swelling, plaster sores, impaired venous circulation, impaired arterial circulation, nerve entrapment. Though these conditions are preventable, the A & E doctor should know what to do if something does go wrong. The most important complication is impairment of the arterial circulation recognised when there is pain, pallor, coldness of the digits and reduction of capillary flow. The cast should be split immediately down the whole length of the lateral aspect with a plaster saw. The split is gently widened with plaster spreaders. If this does not relieve the pressure the patient should be referred to the orthopaedic department for removal of the cast and admission to hospital for limb care. Occasionally, with synthetic casts, the patient may experience discomfort from its sharp edges digging in. In the case of thermoplastic materials, e.g. Hexcelite, these can be softened and remoulded by applying a hot air stream from a hairdryer.

Splintage for particular areas

The use of splints for major fractures, e.g. Thomas's splint has been mentioned in the first section of this book. The rest of this chapter is concerned with the application of splints to particular areas.

Finger splints

Neighbour strapping or the commercially equivalent Bedford splint is the simplest way of resting an injured finger. When used to immobilise a phalangeal fracture control is achieved by holding the metacarpophalangeal joint at 90° as in the position of function: *padded aluminium splints* (Zimmer splints) are adequate when one finger only is involved (Fig. 38.12). The relatively new California splintage system appears to be a satisfactory alternative.

Splinting of extensor tendons which have been cut and repaired in the hand or proximal part of the finger should include wrist, metacarpophalangeal joint and interphalangeal joints and should be maintained in extension for three weeks. Damage to the extensor mechanism over the proximal interphalangeal joints of the fingers is difficult to treat and the patient should be referred to a hand surgeon.

The commonly contused ulnar collateral ligament of the thumb can be supported in the thumb spica strapping described above. A complete rupture or division of this ligament should be referred for surgical repair.

The common 'mallet' finger deformity at the distal interphalangeal joint requires splinting in extension for 6–8 weeks without interruption (Fig. 38.13). The choice of mallet splint is wide — indicating that none is entirely satisfactory! Indeed there is some evidence to support the suggestion that there are two types of mallet fingers — those that will recover with no treatment, and others that will never recover whatever the length of splinting.

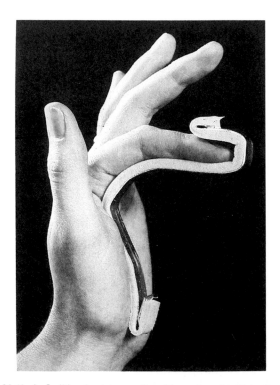

Fig. 38.12 A flexible aluminium splint. The splint should be bent twice around the finger tip to avoid pinching. The sharp ends should be bent back and protected with strapping.

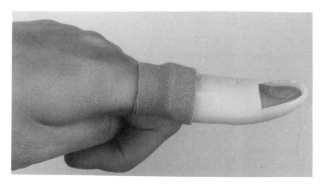

Fig. 38.13 Plastic mallet finger splints such as this are supplied in several sizes. The size chosen should allow flexion at the proximal interphalangeal joint.

Hand and wrist

When more than one finger is involved or when hand, wrist and thumb need to be splinted (as for various forms of tenosynovitis around the wrist) a ridged plaster slab — *the volar slab* — applied to the volar surface (Fig. 38.14) is cheap, easy to apply, relatively light, can be modified for many different purposes, and can be removed to allow inspection, change of dressing, or periodic movement of all the joints. The ridge in the splint provides extra support — a principle not unlike that of the T-girder in the construction industry. When the volar aspect of hand or fingers is wounded it is possible to use a similar splint on the dorsal aspect. Dressings and inspection of the wound are possible without removing the splint.

When a wrist or hand splint is likely to be required for a longer period of time a polyethylene or alloy splint secured with Velcro straps may be more appropriate (Fig. 38.15).

Lower limb splints

After a recent injury to the lower limb it may be necessary to supply crutches to prevent or relieve the pain of weight bearing. Before such a patient leaves the hospital a nurse or physiotherapist should provide a few minutes instruction to avoid the possibility of the patient falling and reinjuring himself when trying to use the

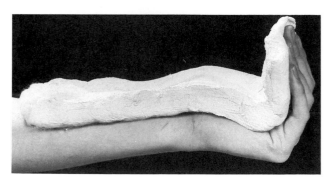

Fig. 38.14 The strength of a volar slab is in the ridging. This principle can be adopted for any posture or indeed for any joint. It should be carefully secured — particularly in the palm.

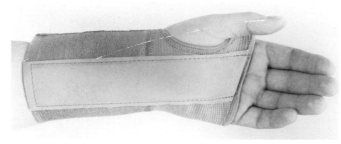

A

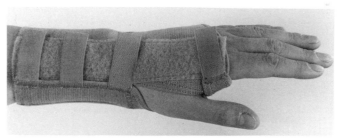

B

Fig. 38.15 A and **B** A ready to wear splint made of canvas or moulded plastic will provide relief for an acutely painful joint, whilst allowing easy removal by the patient for washing.

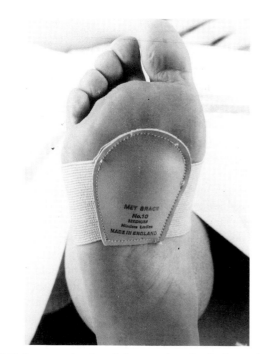

Fig. 38.16 A metatarsal pad applied to ease the pain of a fractured toe.

crutches. Instruction in the use of a walking stick, held in the hand opposite to that of the injured leg, should be given as soon as the patient can be persuaded to discard the crutches.

An injured knee may be rested in a knee immobiliser splint with or without the addition of compression bandaging (see above).

The toes may be splinted with neighbour strapping or by the

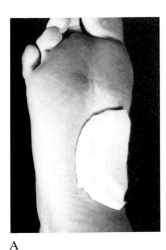 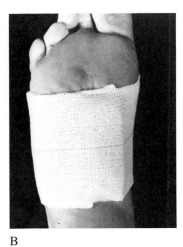

A   B

Fig. 38.17 A and **B** Insole applied for the relief of anterior metatarsalgia and for some other painful conditions in the foot.

use of a *collodion* enveloping bandage. Many fractures of the distal phalanx of the toe will heal, if well padded and protected by a large strong shoe. The weight may be taken off the toes by applying a transverse pad of thick orthopaedic felt under the metatarsal heads (Fig. 38.16).

Patients with acute forefoot pain (anterior metatarsalgia), march fracture or an avulsion fracture of the base of the Vth metatarsal may obtain some relief by the application of a thick orthopaedic felt insole or a commercially available *metatarsal pad* within the arch of the foot and behind the metatarsal heads (Fig. 38.17).

FURTHER READING

Dressings for leg ulcers Anonymous 1986 Drug & Therapeutics Bulletin 24: 9–12

A colour atlas of nursing procedures in accidents and emergencies Bache J B, Armitt C R, Tobias J R 1985 Wolfe Medical Publications, London

Wound management. A comprehensive guide to dressing and healing David J A 1986 Martin Dunitz, London

A colour atlas of plastering techniques Mills J, Page G, Morton R 1986 Wolfe Medical Publications, London

Techniques with elastoplast bandages and **plaster of Paris technique** (Handbooks for students). Smith and Nephew Ltd, Welwyn Garden City, Hertfordshire, AL7 1HF

Foreign bodies

INTRODUCTION

The majority of foreign bodies entering body cavities do so by 'design' — either by the psychiatrically disturbed adult or as the result of the exploring activities of a child. On the other hand, the majority of foreign bodies entering the soft tissues from without do so by 'accident', and are usually (but not always) accompanied by a visible puncture wound. These two groups are discussed separately, and the latter (the soft tissue foreign bodies) is further subdivided into those which do not require removal and those which do.

INTRACAVITARY FOREIGN BODIES

Swallowed foreign bodies

Fish bones may stick in the hypopharynx or lower in the oesophagus, or may be inhaled and stick in the larynx. Removal of these is discussed in detail in Ch. 44. Most foreign bodies which reach the stomach and successfully negotiate the pylorus will pass spontaneously (Fig. 39.1). It may be safer, however, to remove open safety pins from the stomach of a child, particularly if the point of the safety pin is facing distally. Even razor blades (swallowed by prisoners to secure a period in hospital) will usually pass spontaneously without incident. So also will the majority of pins and needles. A few of the latter, however, will migrate outside the gut and remain embedded in the soft tissues — again without causing any untoward symptoms. The risk of migration into the blood stream is so remote that early surgery is not justified. Patients who have swallowed smooth foreign bodies (like coins) may be reassured and discharged. All patients who have ingested sharp foreign bodies, however, should be reviewed on alternate days as outpatients for a few days and again at the end of 7–10 days. The child's parent should be asked to examine the faeces. Radiological examination should only be repeated if a foreign body has not been recovered at the end of this time, or if the patient develops symptoms. The presence of tenderness or guarding or the onset of abdominal pain or vomiting are indications for admission to a surgical ward.

Recently button batteries, such as are used for digital watches and calculators, have emerged as a somewhat special type of danger. If they get held up in the oesophagus or elsewhere in the gut, they can cause tissue destruction. Perforation of the oesophagus and even of the aorta have been recorded. If the battery casing splits, the child may absorb mercury and develop mercury poisoning. However, the great majority of batteries are small, and pass right through the gut with no symptoms and no damage.

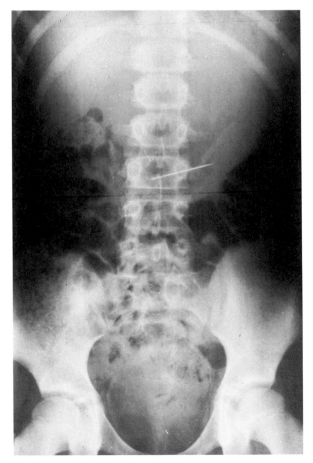

Fig. 39.1 A needle in stomach of a child. This may pass naturally but will require careful monitoring.

Where a child presents with a history of swallowing such an object, radiographs must be taken, especially for the scrutiny of the oesophagus. If nothing is found there, the neck, lungs and abdomen should be similarly examined. Should the radiographs reveal a battery in the oesophagus, the child should be admitted to hospital with a view to removal of the battery via an oesophagoscope. Should the radiographs reveal splitting of the battery admission is necessary for measurement of blood mercury levels, and treatment of mercury poisoning should it occur. An inhaled battery calls for bronchoscopy. All other cases should be monitored carefully as outpatients until the battery is passed.

Recent advances in the techniques of fibreoptic endoscopy are making it possible to remove many of the dangerous or impacted foreign bodies without resorting to open surgery.

Inhaled foreign bodies

This is discussed fully in Ch. 11 (p. 125).

Foreign bodies placed in orifices.

Ears and nose

Children presenting with a snuffly nose or a discharging ear should be carefully examined for the presence of a foreign body (Fig. 39.2). This will often be a bead or a piece off a plastic toy. Such foreign bodies (Fig. 39.3) should be removed only with the help of adequate sedation or anaesthesia and with the appropriate instruments (including blunt hooks) (see Ch. 44).

Rectal foreign bodies.

These are often bizarre and are usually inserted from below by psychiatrically disturbed patients or homosexuals. The patient shown in Figure 39.4 is a good advertisement for Coca-Cola — the foreign body was removed without permanent harm to the patient (or to the bottle) using obstetric forceps.

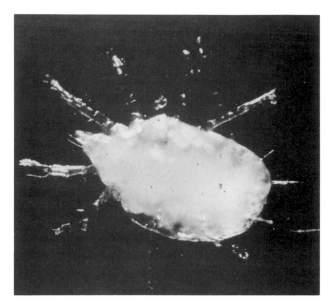

Fig. 39.3 This was removed from the ear of a child!

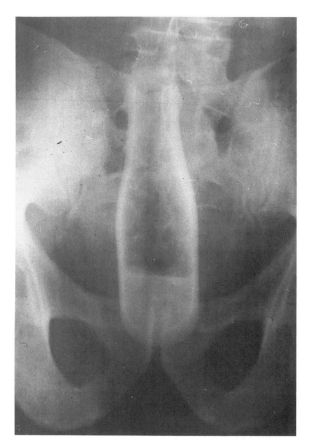

Fig. 39.4 This inmate of a mental hospital complained of constipation!

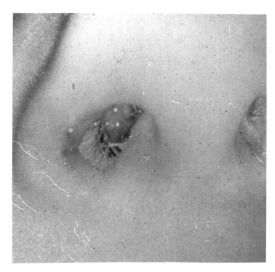

Fig. 39.2 Glass bead in the right nostril of a small child. This is not as easy to remove as it looks.

Vaginal foreign bodies.

Young girls may conceal the fact that they have inserted a foreign body into the vagina. This may only come to light when the mother notices the vaginal discharge. Some teenage girls with tight hymens may insert tampons which expand and then cannot be removed. Once again, adequate sedation or anaesthesia is necessary before examination or removal can be attempted.

SOFT-TISSUE FOREIGN BODIES

Patients are often worried by the presence of foreign bodies, particularly those that show up as dense shadows on radiographs. Removal may be difficult and it is a tragedy when such an operation causes an injury to an important structure or results in infection. The A & E doctor should spend time reassuring those patients whose foreign bodies do not require removal — and these will be discussed first. It should be remembered that these foreign bodies enter the body through a wound, and the risk of tetanus should be considered and appropriate prophylaxis given (see Ch. 32).

Foreign bodies not requiring removal

Small foreign bodies away from pressure sites

Small metallic or glass fragments which become embedded in fleshy or muscular parts of the body where they are not exposed to undue pressure, soon become encapsulated in fibrous tissue and cause no harm. For example, fragments less than 1 mm in size may be safely left in the back of the hand or the dorsum of the foot, but much larger fragments up to 1 cm in size may sometimes be safely left in the muscles of the arm, forearm, back, buttock, thigh or leg. It should be noted that most glass is opaque to X-rays, using good soft-tissue technique.

Early infection foreign bodies

In the case of a foreign body which has been present for more than 12 hours and is showing some signs of infection, one has the option of early removal without suturing the wound, or waiting in the hope that the inflammation will settle down when excision and suturing is possible.

Small superficial foreign bodies

Sometimes rose thorns or prickles and fine wood splinters (such as those of the sea urchin becoming embedded in the sole of the foot — Fig. 39.5) are often best left to work their way out spontaneously. There are many homely remedies which may be used as first aid measures (such as passing urine on the sole of the foot — but not in the A & E department!).

Occasionally, however, thorns may penetrate joints or tendon sheaths, causing severe infection (see Ch. 33).

Foreign bodies which do require removal

Impaling or transfixion injuries

The removal of these foreign bodies should only be attempted when full surgical and anaesthetic facilities are immediately available to

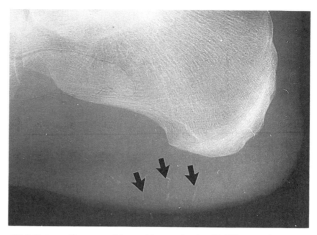

Fig. 39.5 Spines of a sea urchin trodden on in the Caribbean and presented for removal in England three days later.

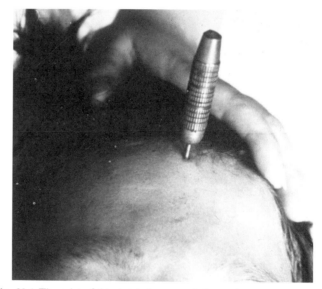

Fig. 39.6 The point of this dart had penetrated the meninges.

deal with any injured structures, such as major blood vessels or the involvement of viscera (brain, intestine or lung). Such injuries may carry infective material into the meninges (Fig. 39.6), the pleura or the peritoneum, or into the synovia. All such wounds (even the relatively innocuous ones in fleshy parts of the limbs and trunk) should be treated by excision of entry and exit wounds and thorough cleansing, followed by elevation of the part, antibiotics and delayed primary closure. This will minimize the risk of serious infection.

Severe local reaction

Foreign bodies which cause severe local reaction, or whose presence might result in absorption of toxic substances should be removed. In practice, however, the removal of multiple lead pellets following shotgun injuries is not indicated because lead poisoning very rarely occurs under these circumstances (Fig. 39.7).

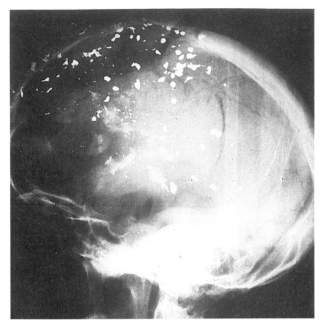

Fig. 39.7 Self-inflicted 12-bore gunshot wound of the head. The patient died three days later.

However, it is essential to remove at the earliest possible opportunity the fine, widely dispersed globules of oil, grease and paint which may be injected by industrial high pressure guns or sprays (Fig. 39.8). These injuries usually affect the hand. If the track is not widely laid open and the fascial spaces decompressed within two to three hours of the injury widespread oedema, necrosis and even gangrene of the fingers may follow. The initial puncture wound may seem trivial but the pain is excruciating and this should warn the A & E doctor that he is dealing with a serious condition, which warrants immediate referral to a hand surgeon.

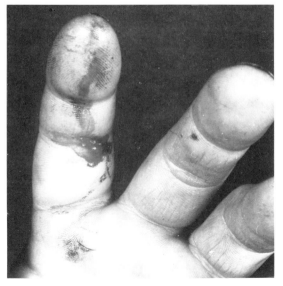

Fig. 39.8 Grease gun injury of finger tip. The finger and palm were widely laid open within two hours of the injury, and full recovery resulted.

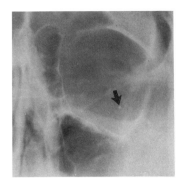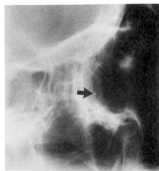

Fig. 39.9 If sight is to be retained in this eye, the fragments of metal must be removed at the earliest opportunity.

Foreign bodies which may cause disturbance of function

Penetrating wounds of the eye by a small metallic fragment

This injury is surprisingly easy to miss because the entry wound may pass unnoticed by the doctor and by the patient (who may have been using a hammer and chisel at the time) (Fig. 39.9). Radiological examination of the orbit in the posterior-anterior plane with an eye up and down lateral view will reveal the fragments and lead to its early removal by an ophthalmologist. Precise radiological localisation within the globe can be made if required. Failure to make this diagnosis early enough may result in permanent loss of vision (see p. 453), and this in turn may result in an action for negligence.

Foreign bodies in the joints or synovial sheaths

Small foreign bodies (usually metallic fragments or needles) which traverse or lodge in joints or synovial sheaths, warrant exploration and removal. Such procedures should be carried out under general anaesthesia with full aseptic precautions, a bloodless field and additional facilities such as radiographic control and a powerful magnet.

Needles

Whilst needles which lodge in the fleshy parts of the body (such as the muscles of the trunk or proximal limbs) may usually be left alone as indicated at the beginning of this section, needles which lodge in the fingers or toes or in the palm of a hand, or sole of a foot, will usually give rise to pain or limitation of function and should therefore be removed. This operation may easily be accomplished in the fingers or toes under digital nerve block and using a tourniquet, but may present considerable difficulties in the palm of the hand or sole of the foot. Nevertheless, provided the following precautions are taken, all such foreign bodies can be removed in a properly equipped A & E theatre.

1. Adequate anaesthesia or analgesia, a bloodless field, appropriate fine instruments (including fine hooks and retractors) and a surgeon with some experience are essential. Such operations should not be performed by the new senior house officer at 0100 hours with

a queue of patients waiting to be seen, but should be carried out at a prearranged time next morning.

2. Marker films should be taken at right angles to each other (Fig. 39.10(A) and 39.10(B)), and the marker (which should be rigidly strapped to the skin) should only be removed when the surgeon is about to clean the skin, and then only after the incision has been carefully planned by reference to the radiographs.

3. The incision should be at right angles to the needle in two planes (Fig. 39.10(C)). Whilst important structures such as digital nerves should be avoided by careful retraction, this incision should be continued in the same direction by sharp and blunt dissection until the needle is felt. The needle is then grasped firmly in an artery forceps (Fig. 39.10(D)), which should not be released until the needle has been extracted.

4. The tissues are cut or teased from one end of the needle to allow its removal (Fig. 39.10(E)). However, if the needle is deeply seated it may be pushed outwards through the hand or foot until close under the skin, and removed through a small counter-incision.

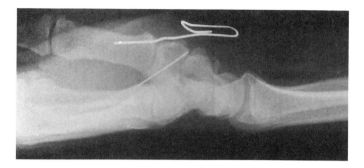

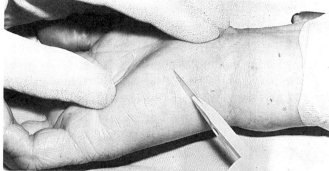

Fig. 39.10 C The incision must be planned to pass at right angles to the centre of the needle.

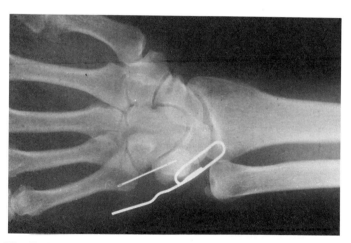

Fig. 39.10 A Marker radiographs taken at right angles to each other revealing a needle buried deeply in the hypothenar eminence.

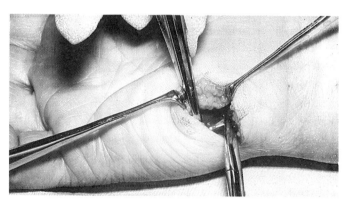

Fig. 39.10 D The incision has been deepened, fine retractors introduced, the needle has been located and grasped with an artery forceps.

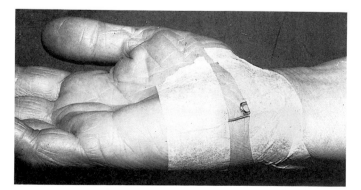

Fig. 39.10 B The tip of the marker should be placed on an identifiable mark or crease on the skin so that when it has been removed, the incision can be planned in relation to the X-ray films.

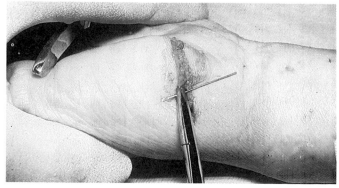

Fig. 39.10 E One end of the needle was first released and the needle then removed. It is shown here in the axis in which it lay within the hypothenar eminence.

Glass wounds in soft tissues

These may cause pain in the foot or hand or may leave unsightly scars in the face (Fig. 39.11). *Radiographic examination of all glass wounds is essential* since most glass will be visible provided the tissue in which it lies is not too thick or too dense. Thus a large piece of glass may be overlooked in the buttock whereas even fine slivers of pipette glass will usually be visible in the pulp of a finger provided radiographs are taken in two planes at right angles to each other. There should be no hesitation in postponing removal of such small fragments of glass if they cannot be readily found at the initial operation. Being transparent, such slivers of glass are often invisible in a fresh wound, whereas after several weeks they become embedded in scar tissue, which can then be carefully delineated and excised together with its contained glass fragments.

Barbed hooks in the skin

These may be dealt with under local or regional analgesia in one of two ways.

1. The hook is grasped in an artery forceps and passed onwards until the point comes through the skin. Either the point or the shaft is then cut off with wirecutters and the rest removed.

2. A small incision is made from the entry point onto the hook, which then falls out.

Bullets

These are discussed in detail in Ch. 14. After removal of these foreign bodies, a decision must be made as to whether primary

or delayed primary closure is appropriate. This will depend on the considered risk of infection, which in turn will depend on the delay before operation, the amount of dirt on the foreign body itself or on any object which may have been in contact with the wound.

Complications and sequelae

Infection

This can usually be avoided by clean surgery, delayed primary closure and the judicious use of systemic antibiotics. Neglect of contaminated foreign bodies may lead to sinus formation. A gentle exploration of sinuses anywhere in the body with a fine angled probe may sometimes reveal the unexpected presence of a foreign body which may have come from within (such as a piece of dead bone or a stone) or from without.

Tender scars

These will be less likely if early removal is carried out and infection avoided (see preceding paragraph).

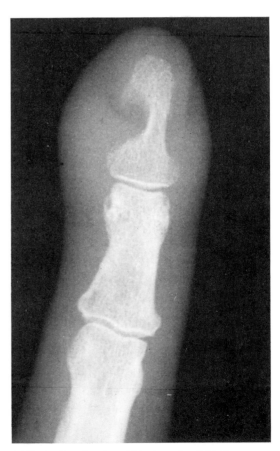

Fig. 39.12 The implantation dermoid in the pulp of this finger was unusual in that it had been present so long that it had produced this indentation in the distal phalanx.

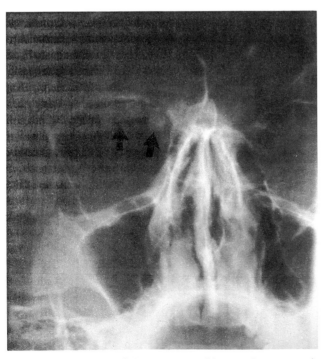

Fig. 39.11 These fragments of glass were removed because they were causing pain in the distribution of the supraorbital nerve.

Damage to nerves, arteries and viscera

All of these structures will need reparative surgery and rehabilitation if they have been damaged.

Implantation dermoid cysts

Small pieces of epithelium may be carried down with a foreign body into the subcutaneous tissues and may there form an implantation dermoid cyst (Fig. 39.12). These may develop in the palms of the hands or elsewhere, and may require excision at a later date.

Concussion

INTRODUCTION

The problems of patients with severe head injuries are discussed in Ch. 14. However, many patients are brought to hospital with head injuries which do not appear very severe.

Minor head injuries may involve five different areas:

1. The brain (concussion)
2. The facial bones (see Ch. 42)
3. The skin of face and scalp (see Ch. 32)
4. The eyes (see Ch. 43)
5. The ear, nose and throat (see Ch. 44)

This chapter deals with the first of these.

CONCUSSION

The term 'minor head injury' though widely used is not entirely satisfactory as it is too easily confused with minor injury to the head, which means something different. Minor brain injury would be preferable, but the word concussion is succinct and, if clearly defined, satisfactory. Concussion may be defined as an acceleration/deceleration injury to the head almost always resulting in amnesia and followed by a characteristic group of symptoms such as headache, dizziness and defective memory.

It used to be said that in concussion there was no structural damage. In recent years special histology and also magnetic resonance imaging both clearly demonstrate lesions. However, the doctor in the A & E department will have to make a diagnosis on the clinical presentation and from this point of view amnesia combined with the history and signs of trauma to the head are the crucial factors. Concussion is sometimes described as a minor head injury. However, it is both difficult and unhelpful to divide head injuries by setting an arbitrary limit on the amnesic period, for some patients above that limit will make an excellent recovery while some below the limit will have protracted and severe symptoms. The mechanism of the injury, the pathology and the prognosis vary from the mildest to the very severe with no obvious intermediate dividing line.

The patient may describe his condition in many ways — that he was knocked out, that he had a black-out, that he was unconscious, etc. To establish whether he had concussion, it is necessary to prove first, trauma directly or indirectly to the head and second, either amnesia immediately following (and sometimes also preceding) the moment of trauma, or else confusion short of full amnesia yet followed by the symptoms which are characteristic of concussion.

The pathology of concussion

A blow to the brain — or coup — will result in a 'primary brain injury'. The severity of this is related to the severity of the blow with damage to nerve tracts and localised areas of bruising and tearing of brain substance. The force of the blow may be transmitted across the skull producing a collision between the soft brain and the opposite, unyielding calvarium. The resulting injury is known as a 'contracoup' lesion. Initial shaking of the brain — concussion proper — will disturb the reticular activating system and produce problems of awareness and amnesia (see The amnesia of concussion, below).

The lethal factors in head injury are more often the secondary intracranial events; the development of an intracranial haematoma, brain swelling or cerebral hypoxia. These conditions are compounded by extracranial events — hypoxia, haemorrhage, pain, vomiting and chest injury. The 'classical' description of an acute extradural haematoma with a blow followed by a lucid interval is the exception rather than the rule. Acute subdural haematomas and bleeding from the surface of the brain are as important causes of intracranial space occupation as middle meningeal artery tears. Subdural haematomas in particular may be confused with drunkenness or stroke in elderly people.

In this Ch. concussion is dealt with in three main sections:

1. Arrival in the A & E department
2. Care in the observation ward
3. Subsequent care at review clinics.

THE CARE OF PATIENTS WITH CONCUSSION ON ARRIVAL IN HOSPITAL

Differential diagnosis

Almost any condition which causes sudden loss of consciousness can be mistaken for concussion. The most common conditions which give rise to difficulties in diagnosis are as follows.

Alcoholic intoxication

A drunk patient with wounds, abrasions or brusies in the scalp or face may be confused and uncooperative. This may be due to a distended bladder or stomach, hypoglycaemia or hypoxia. These should be sought and, if present, treated. It is often very difficult to know whether he is behaving aggressively from cerebral irritation or alcoholic intoxication. It is very easy to suspect intoxication even when there is no alcohol in the blood, and to think there is no alcohol where there may be 200–300 mg/dl. A breath or blood alcohol test is valuable in establishing the amount of alcohol present, and this test is probably much underused. However, one needs to remember that the presence of a high blood alcohol does not in any way exclude concussion — they may well coexist. The patient should be asked whether he has memories of the accident taking place and of the subsequent few minutes. If such memories exist, concussion is unlikely. Often the patient refuses to, or is unable to, answer clearly and has to be treated as a suspected case of concussion until proved otherwise.

Vasovagal syncope ('faint')

This may be preceded by feelings of weakness and dizziness. As the patient falls he may sustain a bruise or wound to the head. Concussion is assumed to have complicated the syncope if the period of amnesia is longer than 10 minutes.

Hysteria

Patients involved in road accidents or other serious accidents often are terrified by the experience. They may shiver and shake, they may weep and be obviously upset. Such terror may cause hysteria and this is usually associated with a period of amnesia. Patients with concussion do not usually look or feel emotionally upset. Where the possibility of hysteria is remembered and assessed, it is usually identifiable, though it must be admitted that in some hysterical patients who have obvious external head trauma it may be difficult to exclude the possibility of an element of concussion.

Epilepsy

Epileptic attacks are associated with amnesia. If the patient falls he may at the same time injure his head. The usual way of separating epileptic attacks accompanied by superficial head injuries from attacks complicated by concussion is by the length of the amnesic period. Where the amnesic period is very similar to that which the patient has experienced in other attacks it is likely that this is a simple epileptic attack. With amnesia of an hour or longer concussion becomes more likely. One cannot separate the two conditions with complete certainty, and for practical purposes the amnesia is presumed to have been caused by the epilepsy unless there are strong reasons for believing otherwise.

Hypoglycaemia

Most patients with, hypoglycaemia collapse gently and do not look like head injured patients. However hypoglycaemia may be precipitated by drinking alcohol, and where patients are confused it is probably wise to measure the blood glucose level.

Cerebrovascular accident

These often occur in elderly people who may live alone. If the patient is upstairs, falling downstairs is not uncommon. Signs of one-sided weakness should be sought. In a cerebrovascular accident the blood pressure is often raised. In simple concussion the plantar reflexes are usually flexor, and in cerebrovascular accidents extensor.

Chest compression

Sustained compression of the chest may cause cerebral anoxia, resulting in a short period of amnesia not dissimilar to that occurring in breath-holding attacks of small children. The pressure may be caused by a safety belt. If the mechanism is remembered, the correct diagnosis can usually be made.

As well as these conditions being possible alternative diagnoses to concussion, any of them may be complicated by concussion.

Concussion with no signs of head injury

With motor cyclists wearing crash helmets or people in mining or construction work wearing safety helmets, a severe blow to the head may cause concussion without leaving any external mark on the scalp or face. A fall from a height on the ischial tuberosities may cause a shock wave to be transmitted through the spine to the head, causing concussion. Apart from these exceptions, one should be slow to diagnose concussion unless there is clear evidence of a blow of considerable force to the outside of the head.

Examination

A full neurological examination is unnecessary in the vast majority of cases of concussion. However, neurological testing is important for the exclusion of differential diagnoses and a thorough examination of the body is undertaken to identify any other injuries.

First the level of responsiveness of the patient should be established and recorded. The Glasgow Coma Scale is used for this purpose (see p. 154).

Baseline pupil size should be accurately measured with a pupil gauge and any pupillary irregularity noted (see p. 169 for interpretation of pupillary signs). The pupillary reaction to light should be recorded. The ocular movements should be checked. Traditionally the fundi are examined although papilloedema is exceedingly rare in minor head injury.

The scalp should be scrutinised for any wounds or bruising — in particular linear bruising behind the pinna (Battle's sign) might indicate a fracture of the petrous temporal bone in the base of the skull. The ear drums should be examined for a tear or a haematoma behind the drum. The presence or absence of blood or CSF from the nose should be noted.

The power and tone of the limbs on either side should be compared — and initial weakness is a serious sign which might indicate brain haemorrhage (see p. 163) A thorough examination of the body is undertaken to identify any other injuries and any coexistent illness.

Radiographic examination of the skull
(Figs 40.1, 40.2, 40.3, 40.4)

There is now a general concensus that skull radiographs are usually advisable for head injured patients in the following circumstances:

1. Loss of consciousness or amnesia at any time.
2. Neurological symptoms such as diplopia, vertigo, confusion or vomiting.
3. Neurological signs such as irritability or altered level of consciousness.
4. Cerebrospinal fluid and/or blood from the nose or ear.
5. Suspected penetrating injury.
6. Suspected alcohol or drug intoxication.
7. In all but the most minor bruising of the scalp and forehead.

A scalp wound which has been carefully examined by inserting a finger and palpating the skull to exclude a fracture does not merit radiographic examination.

It is important that films of good quality should be obtained. This may be difficult or impossible in a restless patient. Unfortunately, this is the patient in whom information from a good radiograph may be very valuable. A blurred film taken under these circumstances may be misleading if the fracture is missed and the patient is sent to the police cells as a drunkard. On the other hand, it is not justifiable to send a patient to the police cells without attempting to exclude a skull fracture by radiographic examination. It is usually wise, therefore, to detain such a patient for a short period within the department (if necessary with police surveillance) until he is able to co-operate or at least remain quiet. In a very irritable or violent head-injured patient the airway should be checked and oxygen administered, and if this does not relieve the situation it may be necessary to give a small intravenous does of

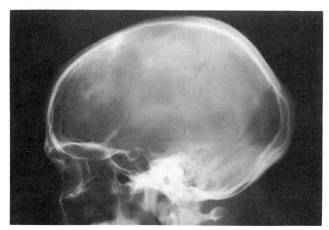

A

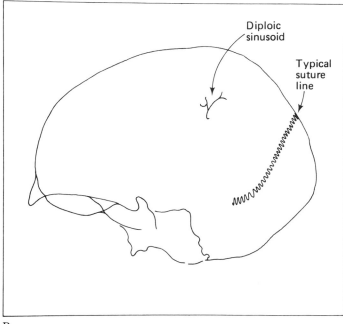

B

Fig. 40.1 A Lines in normal skull radiographs which should not be mistaken for fractures — diploic sinusoid and suture lines. **B** Outline drawing of radiograph.

diazepam to allow adequate assessment and radiological examination — despite the difficulties in monitoring the level of consciousness.

The following views should be taken routinely when radiographs of the skull are requested following a head injury:

1. Posteroanterior — to show fracture of the frontal bone.
2. Brow-up lateral — to show fractures of the vault, fluid levels in the sinuses and intracranial air. Where the injury is limited to one side, a single radiograph is enough, the X-ray plate being positioned on the injured side.
3. Towne's view — to show the occipital bone and to demonstrate a shift of a calcified pineal (calcification is present in about 50% of adults).

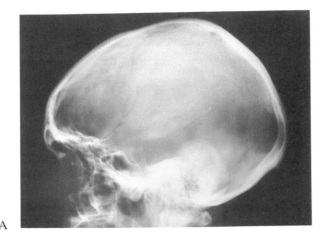

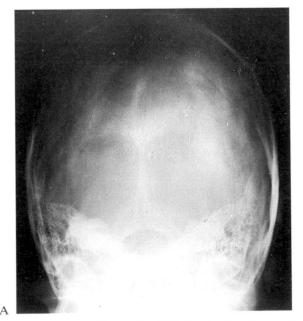

The A & E doctor may ask for the following additional films, either initially or after seeing the first series of films:

1. Tangential views at the site of a depressed fracture.
2. The other lateral if there is difficulty in deciding on which side a fracture is located.

Radiographs of the cervical spine should always be requested in an unconscious head-injured patient.

Radiographs taken days after the acute episode are unlikely to yield information which will influence clinical management and should not therefore be taken for 'medicolegal reasons' only. Clinical management may be affected as a result of the radiological finding in the following ways:

1. Antibiotics may be needed if a fracture involving a paranasal sinus is accompanied by a CSF leak into the nose.
2. Patients with skull fractures should be admitted because 90% of intracranial haematomas occur in the presence of a vault fracture.
3. A patient with a depressed fracture of the skull may require elevation of the bone fragments, special precautions to avoid intracranial infection and possibly anticonvulsants. Discussion with or referral to a neurosurgeon is necessary.
4. The presence of intracranial air, fluid levels in the sinuses or intracranial foreign bodies point to a high risk of intracranial infection for which special measures may be required.

Fig. 40.2 A Lines in normal skull radiographs which should not be mistaken for fractures — middle meningeal artery and diploic vein. Note also pineal gland. **B** Outline drawing of same radiograph.

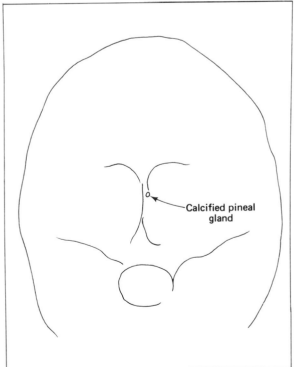

Fig. 40.3 A Calcified pineal in Towne's view. **B** Outline drawing of same radiograph.

especially valuable in hospitals without facilities for CT scanning, where it may be performed routinely with the skull radiograph in those patients who meet the criteria for admission to hospital (see below) or in doubtful cases. A probe is placed on the side of the head (see Fig. 40.5) and ultrasound waves transmitted. They are bounced off the falx and other mid-line structures. Repeat estimations of the mid-line distance are charted and the examination then repeated from the other side. The value for the mid-line is taken as the median of at least 30 readings — recording stops after the 15th reading of the same value on each side. Automated versions of this device are now available. A single 'mid liner' result is of little value — where there is continuing concern a repeat estimation after 4 hours (or earlier) should be undertaken on the observation ward.

Is admission to hospital necessary?

There are three reasons for suggesting that routine admission of patients with concussion is advisable. Firstly when patients arrive in hospital it is frequently not possible to make a clear diagnosis. The initial diagnosis is often inaccurate, many cases being falsely

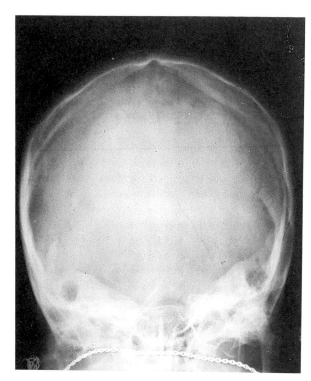

A

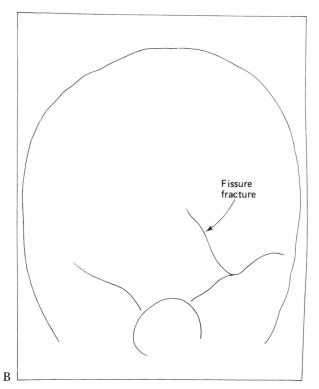

B

Fig. 40.4 A Fissure fracture of occiput — sharp edges and relatively straight. **B** Outline drawing of same radiograph.

Computerised ultrasound

This cheap, non-invasive test is increasingly being found to be a useful, sensitive and specific method of screening for initial, or developing, mid-line shift of the intracranial structures. It is

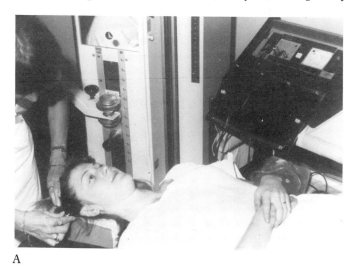

A

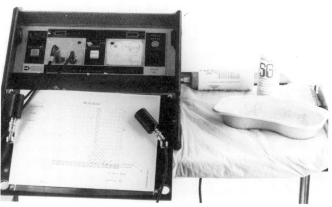

B

Fig. 40.5 A A computerised ultrasound investigation being performed on a patient with a head injury. **B** The equipment and an example of the read out.

diagnosed as having concussion. It is to the advantage of both the patient and his doctors that a correct diagnosis is established at an early stage both to ensure the patient gets good care and advice and also for medicolegal purposes. It is true that this could be performed by reviewing all such patients within 24 hours, but in practice many would fail to attend for such appointments.

The second reason for admission is to minimise the number of patients in which a diagnosis of extradural haemorrhage or subdural haemorrhage is missed. It must be admitted that overnight admission does not guarantee that there will be not mishaps, but the likelihood is undoubtedly less where admission is the rule. Those who advocate a policy of non-admission are not usually those to be blamed when such mishaps occur.

Thirdly concussion is not just an abnormality of consciousness or memory. After consciousness has been regained and memory returned the brain functions at less than its usual efficiency for a period of about three months in most patients. During this period symptoms are common. Some patients continue to complain of symptoms which may still be present for as long as 10 years or more in a few patients. The incidence of symptoms can be reduced by good advice, explanation and support, and the foundation of this aftercare needs to be laid in the early days following the injury. In an illness of this length and severity an overnight admission to an observation ward is a reasonable price to pay for good care.

It is true that a minority of patients can be cared for reasonably well at home. Where the post-traumatic amnesia is less than 5 minutes and there is no severe headache or vomiting this may be considered. Such a patient should not be allowed to go until he or she has been fully orientated for at least 2 hours. There must be some reliable relative or friend prepared to take responsibility for the first 24 hours who should be given printed instructions indicating how to care for the patient. The most important feature of these instructions is repeatedly speaking to the patient, especially through the night hours, to ensure that the level of consciousness is not deteriorating. It is advisable to record in the notes that such instructions have been given.

Patients allowed to go home should be called for review the following morning and should be examined in the same way as the patients who have been observed in hospital. Arrangements for further follow up should be made and advice about work and sport given.

Should a neurosurgical unit be consulted?

Consultation is advised if any of the following conditions exist.

1. A fracture of the skull in combination with confusion, altered level of consciousness, focal neurological signs or fits.
2. Focal neurological signs and confusion for more than 12 hours.
3. Failure to improve from deep coma within 3 hours after adequate resuscitation.
4. Suspected cerebrospinal fluid leak or intracranial air.
5. Depressed fracture of the skull.
6. Neurological deterioration.

CARE OF CONCUSSION PATIENTS IN THE OBSERVATION WARD

The purpose of observation

The chief reason for monitoring the progress of people with head injuries is to identify those patients with extradural or subdural haemorrhages and increasing intracranial tension. This is no easy task, for these complications are only likely to arise in 1% or 2% of patients being observed. Nurses are liable to be lulled into a false sense of security, feeling that, by writing down lists of figures on a chart, they have done something for the patient. It is important for doctors to keep educating nurses about the purpose of the observations and the indications for reporting to a doctor any change in observation findings.

The factors to be noted in observation

A good policy is to monitor quarter-hourly for 1 hour after injury, half-hourly for 4 hours, then hourly — at least until the following day. A number of detailed head injury monitoring scales have been developed for the recording of the levels of response of patients

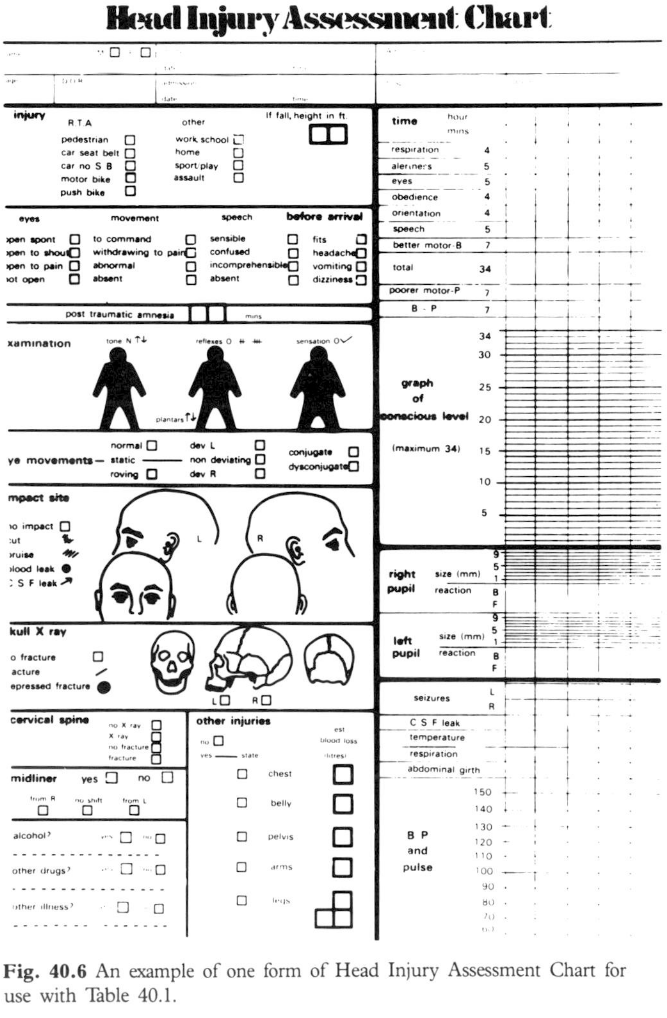

Fig. 40.6 An example of one form of Head Injury Assessment Chart for use with Table 40.1.

Table 40.1 Assessment of conscious level

Respiration
4. Normal spontaneous and regular
3. Hyperventilation or shallow but regular
2. Cheyne Stokes (periodic) or variably irregular support
1. Inadequate spontaneous ventilation requiring support

Alertness (A measure of rousability shown by flinching, facial, respiratory or limb movements)
5. Fully alert — immediately responds to name
4. Drowsy but easily roused by speech or gentle shaking
3. Rousable by shout or firm shaking
2. Unrousable by shout but rousable by superficial pain
1. Rousable by deep pain only
0. Unrousable

Eyes
5. Spontaneous eye-opening and looks at people
4. Spontaneous eye-opening but not looking at people
3. Opens eyes in response to normal speech
2. Opens eyes to shout
1. Not looking at people and only opens eyes to pain
0. No eye-opening even to pain

Obedience
4. Obeys complex commands
3. Immediate appropriate response to simple commands
2. Delayed response to repeated simple commands
1. Doubtful or inappropriate response to simplest commands
0. No obedience to simplest commands

Orientation
4. Fully orientated in all respects with good memory of today's events
3. Aware of who he is and where he is but has poor memory of today's events
2. Moderately confused and uncertain as to where he is
1. Very confused and even unsure of who he is
0. Too drowsy to assess

Speech
5. Spontaneous conversation — answering all questions with quite elaborate answers such as, 'I am all right apart from my headache'
4. As above but with no spontaneous conversation
3. Answers only simple questions with several appropriate words
2. Answers simple questions with monosyllabic and often inappropriate words
1. Incomplete sounds (in response to speech or pain)
0. No sounds in response to speech or pain

Better motor response (BMR)
(Stronger side)
7. Brisk movement with full power or if less conscious, localising immediate purposeful and useful responses (against resistance to pain)
6. Impaired postural maintenance, or some weakness, or if less conscious, sluggish localising purposeful response to pain with effective withdrawal
5. Non-localising effective withdrawal from pain
4. Abnormal flexion with non-purposeful response to pain
3. Brisk extensor posturing without either purpose or effective withdrawal
2. Sluggish extensor posturing without effective withdrawal
1. Only a flicker of pain
0. None

Poorer motor response (PMR)
(Weaker side)

BMR minus PMR
This gives a measure of the severity of hemiparesis

TOTAL SCORE 34

admitted to hospital with concussion. One example is given in Figure 40.6 and Table 40.1. These have been shown to be more specific than the initial Glasgow Coma Scale performed on arrival.

'Head injuries' on the second day

At the time of admission it is not always possible to make a definite diagnosis as to whether a patient has been concussed or not. Once the patient has recovered fully from the initial confusion, clear decisions about the diagnosis become much easier. The differential diagnosis is the same as listed on p. 428.

The amnesia of concussion

An attempt should always be made to record the length of the amnesic period on the morning after full consciousness has been recovered. It is made up of two components: retrograde and post-traumatic.

Retrograde amnesia. It is common to have a brief period of amnesia (about 1–10 seconds) for events immediately before the accident. The man falling from a roof remembers just leaving the roof but has no memory of the end of his fall. The pedestrian remembers the car when it was 15 yards away, after which all is blank. So common is this retrograde amnesia that, where it is absent, special care should be taken in making a firm diagnosis of concussion. Occasionally a patient remembers the impact and, even more rarely, the events immediately following this, before he develops an amnesia which seems to be due to the concussion.

In about 95% of cases there will be retrograde amnesia for a few seconds, and in 5% it may be as much as 2–3 hours. The patient may find it very upsetting to realise that he walked and talked and now has no memory of it. One can explain the phenomenon as being similar to a photograph which was correctly taken but spoiled in the developing. In minor head injuries a patient sometimes remembers the incident if questioned within a few minutes yet next day there may be typical retrograde and post-traumatic amnesia.

A long period of retrograde amnesia may become less over the first few days. Short periods are usually permanent.

Very occasionally a head injury of relatively minor severity may be associated with retrograde amnesia of months or even years. Some people believe that such cases occur only against a background of psychological or psychiatric abnormality. However, this is not always evident. Over two or three months the period of retrograde amnesia shrinks, but usually the patient is left with at least a week or two of permanent retrograde amnesia.

Post-traumatic amnesia.   Post-traumatic amnesia is usually continuous with a period of retrograde amnesia. Most typically it is total at first, the patient having no memory at all of his surroundings. A patient who can remember pain and awareness that he was hurt does not have complete amnesia. Figure 40.7 is a diagrammatic representation of the way memory often recovers after concussion. Between the area of complete amnesia and the area of clear memory there is an intermediate zone of partial memory. Often recovery does not proceed in a direct linear fashion, but with waves and troughs. A woman has a fleeting memory of her child beside her in the car after the crash. Next she is aware that she is in an ambulance which is moving. She is confused as she comes into hospital but her memories become clear from the time the wound in her forehead is being sutured. Post-traumatic amnesia is measured from the moment of the accident until the memory is clear and continuous.

The length of the amnesic period is a good general guide to the severity of the concussion. However, some patients with a long amnesic period have no continuing symptoms and some with a short amnesic period have severe and long-lasting complaints.

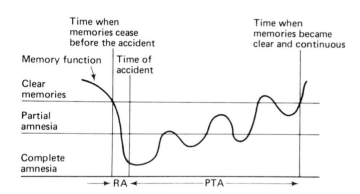

Fig. 40.7 Diagramatic representation of a common pattern of retrograde and post-traumatic amnesia. RA = retrograde amnesia, PTA = post-traumatic amnesia.

Symptoms of concussion on the second day

Headache

This is common, and is present in about 75% of cases, although sometimes it lasts only a few hours. There are a few patients with concussion who never have a headache at any stage. As with many other symptoms, the headaches may clear up in a few days or continue for weeks, months or years.

Nausea and vomiting

Nausea occurs in about 50% of adults with concussion, and vomiting in about 25%. Among children, vomiting is more common. Children are sometimes brought to hospital with vomiting when it may not have been realised that they have suffered a head injury. It is also not uncommon for young children to be brought by parents with a history of a fall and vomiting. In most cases this is due to an infection (especially of the middle ear). It seems that young children with infections are prone to falls. Before accepting a diagnosis of 'head injury' the temperature should be taken and the ears examined. In adults vomiting usually clears up within 6 hours of the end of amnesia, and nausea is usually gone within 12 hours, though it may last 24 hours.

Drowsiness

This is another symptom almost always confined to the first 24 hours. Many head injuries occur late at night and are followed by a considerable period in transport, diagnosis and treatment in the A & E department, and then frequent disturbance by nurses making observations. Their drowsiness may be due largely to tiredness. Alcohol is a concomitant factor in many cases. Nonetheless, patients often complain of being drowsy, and observation usually corroborates their statement. Drowsiness is also common after head injuries sustained in the morning and afternoon and in patients who have not taken alcohol.

Dizziness

This most commonly occurs immediately the patient is aware of his surroundings. It may continue till the next day and occasionally it is a persistent symptom.

Fatigue

Even more than drowsiness, it can be hard to know when fatigue is the natural reaction to pain and sleeplessness. However, in many patients the sensation of fatigue does not pass away even after adequate rest. It is a very characteristic feature of the period when a patient is attempting to return to work.

Epilepsy

This is a very rare early complication of mild concussion unaccompanied by skull fractures. The possibility that epilepsy preceded or even caused the head injury should be considered.

Symptoms from associated or pre-existent illness

It is well to ask about pre-existent illness and medication when examining a patient on the day following the accident.

Symptoms from associated injuries

Systematic questioning should probe the possibility of injuries to the other structures of the body. It is often evident next morning that too many radiographs were taken on admission, but now and then fractures which were overlooked on admission will be found. A special watch should be kept for malar fractures and blow-out fractures of the orbit. The great majority of patients with concussion will have an associated neck sprain. In most cases this is mild and settles down without any treatment. More severe sprains may need the support of a cervical collar.

Traumatic subarachnoid haemorrhage

This may arise as a complication of concussion. It may also occur after a blow on the head where there has been no amnesia at any time. The headache is abnormally severe and persistent. In the early stages it is often felt behind the eyes, in the forehead and up over the top of the head. After 12–24 hours the pain seems to settle down towards the occipital region and neck and to be associated with neck stiffness. There may be photophobia. With rest, analgesics and reassurance the condition usually resolves, but where the symptoms are severe a neurosurgeon should be consulted.

Other injuries

The assessment and care of all other injuries is very similar to that practised in the admission area. However, the situation has altered since admission. The patient is usually more co-operative, and a slower and more careful examination is possible. At admission an unco-operative patient will not allow good quality radiographs to be taken. Next day one should take any omitted views or repeat views if a poor radiograph cannot be read.

Advice on discharge from hospital

When patients who have sustained a minor head injury are discharged home they should be provided with a printed card indicating possible complications for which an immediate return to hospital is necessary. The instructions on this card would presuppose some degree of supervision at home and it is therefore necessary to ensure that the patient will not be alone and that the home circumstances are suitable. One should also make sure that the patient or relative can read English. In addition, the patient should be advised as to the period of rest and given mild analgesics. If he is not to be followed up in the hospital, he should be given a letter for his general practitioner. The fact that he has been given a head injury card should be recorded on the notes.

There is great variation in the length of time during which symptoms persist after concussion. Some cases will be symptom-free within 24 hours, some within a few days, while some patients will continue to have symptoms for weeks or months. Symptoms will be more likely to settle quickly if the patient is not under too much strain until symptom-free. Once a patient feels well he or she may start to think about returning to work. However, neurophysiological and psychometric testing have shown that even patients with no symptoms may still have depressed brain function. It is not uncommon for the patient when he or she starts work, to feel greatly fatigued by evening and this may be followed by irritability and headache. A very noisy work environment and a high degree of responsibility mitigate against an early return to

work. A patient who is allowed to return to work too early may be unable to cope. This may even lead to the patient losing his or her job. Those who have sustained their concussion in a contact sport need to be advised to avoid playing again for four weeks (see Ch. 36).

CARE OF CONCUSSION PATIENTS IN REVIEW CLINICS

The review of patients with concussion is not widely accepted as an essential responsibility of A & E doctors. However, in many centres no other hospital specialty regularly follows them up and general practitioners may not have sufficient interest or experience. The rest of this chapter gives guidance to A & E doctors who may wish to undertake the responsibility.

While a very few patients are asymptomatic from the moment they recover consciousness and a fair number symptom-free within 1 week, at 6 weeks after the accident 50% of patients with mild concussion still have some symptoms. Of these, about a third will have only 1 symptom, but some will have 2, 3 or 4 symptoms and a few have as many as 10 symptoms.

As time passes, more and more patients become asymptomatic, but after a year about 15% of patients who have been treated for concussion in the observation ward still have some symptoms.

Common late symptoms of concussion

Headache

This is the most common symptom. There are three different forms of headache which can often be distinguished as different in cause and significance.

1. A post-traumatic neuritis in the scalp is caused by a crush injury of the skin and its nerve supply. The pain is localized at the site of the trauma. The skin, if it can be seen, may appear red. The area is often sensitive, and pain may occur in cold weather or when the hair is combed. This recovers slowly but some sensitivity may last for a year or more.

2. Pain referred up the back of the head, secondary to an injury to the neck. Neck sprains are very common in concussion and cervical spondylosis may have been present prior to the injury. Treatment will concentrate on the neck where this appears to be the cause of the headache.

3. Whether all the remaining concussion headaches have a single cause is not certain; however, in the absence of any evidence for a system of classification, it seems best to treat them as a single group. About a quarter of patients with mild concussion complain of headaches at six weeks. By one year fewer than one-tenth of concussion patients still have headaches.

About 50% of those who have headaches suffer from them daily, in both the earlier and the late phases. The headaches usually last for less than an hour and only rarely over six hours. Some patients take no tablets for their headaches, but when tablets are taken some relief is usually obtained. About half the patients complain of headaches across the forehead but the pain may be generalised or localised to any point in the head. In about 50% of patients the headaches occur at a fairly regular time of day, usually in the morning or afternoon.

Irritability

Sometimes the relatives are aware that the patient has become irritable but he may be acutely aware of it himself. A happily married man is distressed to find himself shouting at his wife. A man who looked forward to playing with his children finds he has no patience with them. Some patients are particularly sensitive to noise. If they work in a noisy environment, this may prevent a return to work.

Anxiety

Anxiety is complained of by about a fifth of mild concussion patients at six weeks but by very few at one year. It is difficult to know how much of the anxiety is due to the brain trauma and how much to the emotional stresses and strains of the accident and its aftermath. Some patients develop nervousness which is specifically related to the type of accident they were involved in. A person knocked down on a pedestrian crossing may develop an excessive fear of crossing the road. Other patients will develop non-specific nervousness. Both of these types of nervousness may develop after accidents in which there is no trauma to the head and at present it is not known whether the postconcussion anxiety and the post-traumatic anxiety are one and the same.

Depression

Like anxiety, depression may follow injury to any part of the body but it is more common following injury to the head. It may be mild and transient, or severe and long lasting.

Insomnia

The common insomnia after concussion is different from the insomnia of depression in that it nearly always upsets the ability to go to sleep, and rarely makes the patient wake in the early morning. Should early morning wakening develop it may be a sign that the patient is becoming depressed.

Fatigue

This is a non-specific symptom, but can be a considerable disability, especially to patients who were energetic prior to their accident. It may affect the ability to work and prevent various social activities.

Difficulty in concentration

This complaint is much more likely in patients whose daily life and work demands a high degree of concentration. There are various methods for measuring the ability of patients to add a series of random numbers, or to react to the position of flashing lights on a screen. Such tests reveal a diminished capacity of the brain to process information for about six weeks following a minor head injury. There has recently been considerable development of such testing and it is possible to compare the patient's performance with known standards. This can be useful in elucidating and quantifying the disability.

Poor memory

As with difficulty in concentration, this may be quantified by psychometric testing. Although deterioration in memory is something which many people have to face with increasing age, there is no doubt that concussed patients find it very distressing that suddenly they cannot remember the names of their friends, where they put things away in the house, or why they went out shopping.

Deterioration in memory and concentration often occur together. This is not surprising because unless what is read on one page is remembered there is very little point in reading the next page.

Dizziness

At six weeks about 12% of patients with minor head injuries complain of dizziness. By one year, fewer than 5% of patients complain. The typical history is of a sensation of rotation of the head provoked by alterations in the posture, and lasting for a few seconds. Often it is felt on awakening and getting out of bed, and also at night when lying down. It may also occur on bending down to put on or take off shoes, or on looking to the left or right. Patients sometimes describe quite different types of dizziness. Some of these sound like vasovagal attacks, and many appear to be hysterical.

Epilepsy

This is uncommon in mild head injuries where there has been no fracture of the skull and only a short period of amnesia. However, sometimes seizures, usually of the temporal lobe type, develop after relatively minor concussion.

Sensitivity to alcohol

This is quite common in severe head injuries but rarely occurs in patients with mild concussion at six weeks after the accident. By a year almost all cases have recovered from this symptom.

Other symptoms

Patients occasionally complain of anosmia, diplopia, visual defect and deafness. These are probably due to injuries to the cranial nerves sustained at the time of the head injury. Such patients should be referred to a neurosurgeon.

The evolution of symptoms after concussion

The symptoms which patients complain of at six weeks differ from those complained of during the first day or two after injury. Nausea and vomiting, are common in the first 24 hours but unknown later on, and drowsiness is a very uncommon late symptom. On the other hand, irritability, anxiety, depression, insomnia, difficulties in memory and concentration are complained of at six weeks but not immediately. It is possible, however, that all these symptoms and the underlying pathology which causes them are present from the beginning. It takes some days and the experiences of coping with the environment from day to day, to make the patient realise that he is irritable, anxious, depressed or lacking in his powers of memory and concentration.

Of the patients with symptoms at one year, about half have symptoms which were among those they complained of at six weeks. The other half now have some new symptoms, not reported at six weeks.

Pathogenesis of the 'post concussion syndrome'

There have been two main schools of thought. The first, forcefully advocated by Miller of Newcastle-upon-Tyne, considers the symptoms which follow concussion to be a neurosis. Miller believed that the more trivial the head injury, the greater the incidence — caused largely by the strains of litigation. The opposite view is that the symptoms are caused directly by the trauma to the brain. We know that repeated trauma to boxers' heads causes a condition called 'punch drunk'. In this condition the patient develops a spastic gait and becomes irritable, with a marked change of personality. At autopsy marked brain atrophy is found. Microscopic axonal damage can also be demonstrated after single concussive episodes. It is therefore logical to expect some deterioration in cerebral function following trauma.

It has recently been demonstrated that the symptoms following a concussive injury at six weeks and at one year correlate both with positive neurological findings on the morning after the injury and with the patient's feelings about who was to blame for the injury. This suggests that both organic and psychological factors contribute to the pathogenesis. Concussion probably always results in the distraction of a certain number of axons. The patient's symptoms will depend on exactly which circuits are knocked out. With time the brain learns to use new pathways, and symptoms may abate. As both the public and many doctors feel that the patient should have recovered when consciousness returns, the patient finds it difficult to understand why he or she is experiencing symptoms. Fatigue, poor concentration and memory, headache and irritability may make work impossible. This situation leads to many social problems and resulting stress. The patient's self image deteriorates and depression may supervene.

One obvious form of emotional strain is that connected with involvement in a law case. It is sometimes thought that everyone who seeks compensation following a head injury will complain of symptoms. This is not so. In one study it was found that at the time of writing legal reports 43% did not claim to have any symptoms directly connected with their head injury. However, these reports were written about a year after the injury, and the symptom rate was roughly the same as was found at six weeks in a follow up study of unselected patients, that is to say approximately half complained of symptoms.

Another common belief is that no improvement occurs as long as the process of litigation continues. This was also found to be a myth, almost 20% of patients becoming symptom free between the time of the report and the time of settlement. The third widely held belief is that settlement will bring a rapid resolution of symptoms. However, in this series only 5% of patients improved in the year following settlement, and at the end of this period 34% of patients still complained. The time from injury to final follow up was a little over three years, yet the symptom rate was well over twice the symptom rate found after one year in an unselected series. The great majority of patients in the litigation series had contacted their solicitors within two months of the accident and presumably were discussing this option from very early days. There was no evidence that cases involved in litigation were the more severe cases.

It would seem that the strains and stresses of being involved in litigation greatly slow down the healing process after concussion, although some healing does slowly take place. However, if the litigation process goes on for one or two years, relatively little improvement can be expected later on.

Treatment

Treatment follows from pathogenesis. There is little that can be done about the organic damage which has occurred. It is interesting to see how frequently symptoms (such as memory loss) in patients with no apparent neurosis improve with the passage of time. It is possible that the brain in time finds alternative pathways to those which were broken, in a way not dissimilar from the development of collateral circulation after vascular injuries.

It is difficult to know whether the symptoms due to organic damage of a mild head injury would always heal if there were no emotional stress. It is probable that few patients with mild concussion will have symptoms at one year unless there are some such factors are involved.

A few weeks after injury, the patient should be called for review and should be told the nature of his complaint and the great likelihood of his making a complete recovery. It also seems sensible that patients with symptoms should not undertake any stressful responsibilities which they can avoid. Knowing that symptoms are not unusual is often reassuring.

The second step is to discuss with the patient at an early stage the possibility of emotional stress complicating the course of the illness. This may not be necessary in cases with one or two symptoms which seem to be diminishing. It is probably necessary in cases with three or more symptoms at six weeks, especially if there is a likelihood of litigation. As in other stress illnesses, considerable tact and sympathy are required to be able to explain the situation without arousing resentment. If the patient can be helped to gain insight into his own condition, the outlook improves greatly.

As litigation is the most obvious stress factor in many cases, every attempt should be made to obtain a settlement in as a short a time as possible. Where judgement is postponed for some years there is a danger that the neurosis may become so deep seated that resolution is unlikely. In some cases liability may be denied by the opposite party and an unfavourable judgement may leave the patient deeply resentful. This is a potent cause of a continuing resentment and emotional upset.

Symptoms may require treatment on a symptomatic basis. Most headaches respond to simple analgesics. Anxiety and depression can be helped with drugs given symptomatically. Patients who have dizziness must avoid heights, and certain occupations are impossible until dizziness resolves.

Once patients are symptom-free, they usually remain so. Patients clear of symptoms immediately after their accident may start work at once. Those with symptoms usually return to work after the symptoms have cleared or become very mild. Some patients feel depressed because they are off work. If the patient is anxious to return to work and the responsibilities are not too heavy this may do good rather than harm. Should the condition deteriorate the decision can always be reversed.

A special sphere of interest

There is a strong case for the A & E doctor taking a special interest in the care of minor head injury patients who have suffered concussion but are unlikely to require major surgery. This is a common accident and may result in a disability lasting months or years. In many centres neurosurgeons do not feel that they can or should provide a service for these patients. Some patients are looked after by general practitioners, but few general practitioners see sufficient to become expert in their management. In general surgical wards, their care is often left to junior staff whose main interest is in those patients requiring operative treatment. In the great majority of cases early treatment consists of observation in hospital for one or two nights or discharge home with a review visit in 24 hours. A & E doctors working closely with their neurosurgical colleagues are well placed to give this care. If they continue this with special review clinics they can build up a very useful expertise in a common injury and, by their efforts, prevent much unnecessary long-term morbidity. Ideally the A & E doctor should be one of a team. The medical social workers and occupational therapists can help patients both in their return to a job and also in gradually undertaking more home and social activities. Contact with employers to arrange gradual return to full work is important. For patients with severe or prolonged symptoms neurophysiological assessment may be helpful. The A & E doctor will find it helpful usually to work with the same neurologist, neurosurgeon or psychiatrists. Concussion is a relatively common injury which has till recently been paid little attention. There is probably much unrecognised morbidity in the community which with proper care and attention could be considerably reduced.

REFERENCES

Fee C R A, Rutherford W H 1988 A study of the effect of legal settlement on post-concussion symptoms. Archives of Emergency Medicine 5: 12–17

Millar H 1968 Accident Neurosis. British Medical Journal I: 991–998

Rutherford W H, Merret J D, McDonald J R 1977 Sequelae of concussion caused by minor head injuries. Lancet I: 1–4

Rutherford W H, Merret J D, McDonald J R 1978 Symptoms at one year following concussion from minor head injuries. Injury 10: 225–230

FURTHER READING

Le devenir du syndrome post-commotionnel Amphoux M, Gagey P M, LeFlem A, Pavy F 1977 Revue de medicine du travail 5: 53–75

Persisting effects of minor head injury observable during hypoxic stress Ewing R, McCarthy D, Gronwall D, Wrightson P 1980 Journal of Clinical Neuropsychology 2: 147–155

Delayed recovery of intellectual function after minor head injury Gronwall D, Wrightson P 1974 Lancet ii: 605–609

Duration of post-traumatic amnesia after mild head injury Gronwall D, Wrightson P 1980 Clinical Neuropsychology 1: 51–60

Post-traumatic syndrome; another myth discredited Kelly R, Smith B N 1981 Journal of the Royal Society of Medicine 74: 275–277

Mild head injury Levin H S, Eisenberg A L, Benton A L (eds) 1988 Oxford University Press, Oxford

Measurement of reaction time following minor head injury McFlynn G, Montgomery E A, Fenton G W, Rutherford W H 1984 Journal of Neurology, Neurosurgery and Psychiatry 47L: 1126–1331

Microscopic lesions in the brain following head injury Oppenheimer R D 1968 Journal of Neurology, Neurosurgery and Psychiatry 31: 299–306

Disability caused by minor head injury Rimel R W, Giordani B, Barth J Y, Bell T J, Jane J A 1981 Neurosurgery 9L: 221–228

Subtle neuropsychological deficits in patients with good recovery after closed head injury Struss D T, Ely P, Hugenholz H, Richard M T, La Rochelle S et al 1985 Neurosurgery 17 (i): 41–47

A follow-up study of accident neurosis Tarsh M J, Royson C 1985 British Journal of Psychiatry 146: 18–25

Post-traumatic neurosis Trimble M R 1981 John Wiley, Chichester

Time off work and symptoms after minor head injury Wrightson P, Gronwall D 1980 Injury 12: 445–454

Attitudes to concussion in young New Zealand men Wrightson P, Gronwall D 1980 New Zealand Medical Journal 92: 359–361

Sprained neck

INTRODUCTION

The cervical region is the most mobile area of the spine, allowing flexion, extension, lateral flexion to left and right and rotation to left and right.

Extreme force applied to the neck may result in fractures or dislocation, with or without damage to the spinal cord. A lesser degree of trauma may result in soft tissue injury. The resulting pain and disability may last for months or even for years.

MECHANISM OF INJURY

The neck is occasionally injured by direct trauma, but usually by forces acting either on the head or the trunk. Any closed head injury which is sufficiently severe to cause concussion (see Ch. 40) is likely to cause some degree of neck sprain. However, in the great majority of these cases the neck pain disappears within a week or two without any special treatment. Those few cases with severe symptoms and spasm of the muscles may be treated like the other form of neck sprain, to which the rest of this chapter is devoted.

By far the most common type of accident is where the forces are applied primarily to the trunk in road traffic accidents. The classical example is of a motorist in a stationary car which is hit from behind by another vehicle. The seat back propels the patient's trunk rapidly forwards and the inertia of the head causes extension of the neck which may continue until the occiput comes to rest against the interscapular area of the thoracic spine. Within a few seconds the vehicle comes to an abrupt stop. At this point the trunk rapidly decelerates, especially if restrained by a seat belt, and the head is thrown forward, flexing the neck. Crowe in 1928 coined the term 'whiplash' to describe this movement.

It is often emphasised that when the head is violently thrown forward in a head-on collision, the chin impinges on the chest

before the neck has passed its normal anatomical limits of movement. Similarly, in side on crashes the ear impinges on the shoulder. However, in practice it is found that sore stiff necks result from accidents with impacts from all directions. It is certainly true that hyperextension is the movement which seems most likely to result in rupture of ligaments and muscles. Sometimes a tear of the anterior ligament extends into the end plate of a vertebral body with separation from the intervertebral disc. Coned radiography may demonstrate damage to posterior ligaments in flexion injuries as well as damage to anterior ligaments in extension injuries. Certainly the rear-end crash is the one with the highest incidence of neck pain. However, in a recent series of patients, rear impact accidents formed less than 25% of the total. As it is not possible by clinical examination to distinguish different types by the direction of impact, and as there is no evidence that the prognosis is dependent on the direction, it seems better to use the term 'neck sprain' to describe all these injuries. 'Whiplash' is certainly a dramatic term but it is applicable to a certain mechanism which accounts for some neck injuries rather than to the injury itself. Classical experiments by McNab causing acceleration injuries to monkeys, killing the animals and dissecting their necks, revealed tears in ligaments and muscles. The best term to describe such a soft tissue injury seems to be 'sprain of the neck'.

It has been mentioned already that neck sprain may arise in an accident where the primary injury is concussion. Before the widespread wearing of seat belts in cars it was not uncommon for patients to sustain both hyperextension neck injuries and head injury with concussion as the head struck the windscreen or the front rim of the roof. With seat belts patients may sustain a concussive brain injury even when there is no external impact to the head. The brain stem is anchored at the foramen magnum. Severe rotatory forces acting on the brain are sufficient to cause concussion with resulting amnesia. Such patients may suffer the after effects, not only of their neck injury, but also of their concussion (see Ch. 40).

PRESENTATION

Patients with neck sprain secondary to a head injury do not usually complain of neck pain on arrival at hospital yet often have pain the next day. The pain is usually mild, and a cervical collar is rarely needed unless there was pre-existing cervical spondylosis.

Acceleration/deceleration neck injuries are usually due to road traffic accidents. Following such accidents, 60% or more of car occupants, who present at hospital develop neck pain, but about half of them may have no pain immediately (Deans et al 1987). Because neck pain is so common patients who report immediately after such an accident who appear to be fit to go home and who have no neck pain should be warned that it may develop, and if severe they should report back to hospital.

While all patients with neck sprain complain of neck pain, other symptoms may also occur. Foremost of these is headache, which may be due either to pain referred along the greater or lesser occipital nerves, or to accompanying concussion. Dysphagia may occur associated with tears in the paraspinal muscles which may cause an increase in the prevertebral soft tissues seen on the lateral radiograph. Disphonia also occurs, though less frequently. The patient may complain of weakness in the arms or paraesthesia. Visual symptoms, auditory symptoms and vertigo are probably due to accompanying concussion.

The movements of the neck should be carefully examined and the exact position of any tenderness noted. Areas of anaesthesia or hypoaesthesia should be sought. These are most common at the C6 or C7 dermatomes. The most usual weakness is in elbow or wrist flexion. Occasionally the biceps jerk may be absent.

Radiographs of the cervical spine should be taken. The most useful views are the lateral and AP open mouth view of the odontoid peg. The AP view of the remaining spine rarely gives additional information. As well as excluding any dislocation or fracture, one should note whether the normal lordosis is present and whether there are any signs of cervical spondylosis.

EXAMINATION

You must make a careful examination of the undressed patient if you wish to determine the anatomical cause. Examination should include inspection, palpation, movements of the neck plus a brief check on the neurology of the upper limb.

Notice the way the patient holds his neck and observe posture, wasting or colour change in the arm. Feel the soft tissues and in particular the muscle masses for tenderness and the triangles of the neck for lymph node enlargement.

Tenderness due to a neck sprain is usually found at one of three sites:

1. In the mid-line at any level from C1 to the mid-thoracic region.
2. At C5, C6 and C7 level to the upper bodies of the trapezius muscle.
3. To one side of the mid-line in the paravertebral musculature. Often this is accompanied by nerve root irritation.

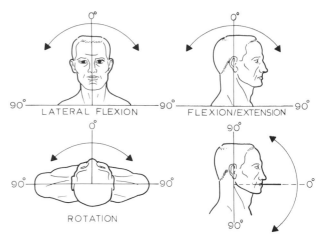

Fig. 41.1 Measurement of range of movement in the cervical spine: flexion and extension, lateral flexion, rotation to left and right.

Check the main movements of the neck. A spatula held in the patient's teeth will allow a precise measurement of the range of movements (Fig. 41.1).

Make a quick check of upper limb neurology. An assessment of root involvement requires examination of segmental motor and sensory groups and the reflexes. An absence of biceps jerk (C5) with a pronounced triceps or supinator jerk (C6) — the 'inverted supinator response' is strongly suggestive of nerve root involvement from the neck (Fig. 41.2).

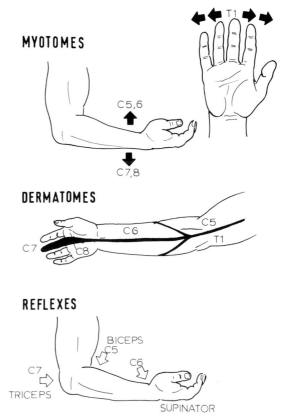

Fig. 41.2 Dermatomes and reflexes in upper limb.

Radiography

Standard views are anteroposterior, lateral and open-mouth views to show the dens. The lateral film is usually of most value and should be checked systematically for:

1. *The normal cervical curve*

Loss of normal cervical lordosis (the 'splinted spine') indicates muscle spasm protecting organic disease.

2. *Relationships of the vertebrae*

Angulation implies ligamentous rupture — not necessarily in association with a fracture.

Forward or backward subluxation suggests rupture of the vertical ligamentous complexes, with one facet fractured if the displacement is greater than one-third vertebral body width and two facets if two-thirds vertebral body width. Oblique views may be required in doubtful cases (see Ch. 8).

3. *Relative positions of the atlas and axis*

The normal arch/atlas distance should not exceed 4 mm. A greater distance implies transverse ligament laxity (as in rheumatoid arthritis) or fracture of the odontoid peg.

4. *Vertebral bodies and processes*

Look for collapse, fusion, osteophyte formation, cystic change, fractures of transverse or spinous processes (e.g. the clay-shoveller's fracture).

5. *The soft tissues of the neck* (Fig. 41.3)

The pharyngeal soft tissues may be displaced by a tumour or a haematoma following recent injury — the interval between the cervical spine and the trachea on the lateral radiograph may be increased as a result of tears in the paraspinal muscles.

MANAGEMENT

On clinical grounds the patients can be divided into three groups. The first group consists of those cases in whom, although the neck is sore, neck movements are still full. The second group have demonstrable limitation of neck movement and one can often feel muscle spasm. In the third group, as well as reduced neck movements there are positive neurological signs — hypoaesthesia, anaesthesia, muscle weakness or absent jerks.

Most of the patients in the first group can be managed without the use of supporting collars. Analgesics or anti-inflammatory non-steroidal drugs may help. Only if symptoms are not settling within two or three weeks should a soft collar be used.

Patients in the second group should be fitted with soft cervical collars from the start. However, they should be encouraged to take

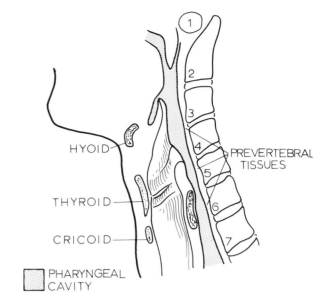

Fig. 41.3 Soft tissues of the neck.

the collar off before and after each meal for a few minutes when the neck should be deliberately exercised within the range of painless movement. If it is possible, exercises should be taught and supervised in the early stages by physiotherapists. The collar may also be disposed of in most cases in bed at night.

Patients with very severe neck pain and spasm, especially if there are positive neurological signs, should initially be referred to an orthopaedic surgeon for admission and follow-up.

PROGNOSIS AND THE PROBLEMS OF CONTINUING PAIN

When seen some weeks or months later at a review clinic patients often complain of difficulty with reading, knitting, typing or swimming. It seems that flexion of the neck accompanied by arm use provokes pain. When driving, turning the head to look over the shoulder may be difficult. The patient may complain of clicking sensations on the neck, though this cannot be confirmed on examination. Even with careful assessment and conscientious treatment, the prognosis for sprains of the neck is not good. In one recent series 42% of patients still had pain 1 year after the accident, in another 66% still had pain at final assessments 18 months to 2 years after injury. Some of these patients have moderate intermittent pain, but in others the pain is severe and continuous. This is a devastating result for such an apparently simple injury. Some people have sought to explain this on the basis of a neurosis which is culturally based. The problem is common in advanced developed countries, whereas in the developing countries the condition is rare. It is suggested that the high prevalence is linked with the expectation of financial gain from litigation. There are two reasons for doubting whether accident neurosis is a complete explanation. Firstly the more severe the original injury the higher the likelihood of persistent pain.

Thus, while in group 1 about 40% of patients may have late pain, in the case of group 3 patients 90% are likely to do so. Secondly, even when litigation is finalised, 50% of patients in group 1 show no further improvement, and 75% of patients in group 3, show no further improvement.

There seems therefore little doubt that physical factors are involved, not merely in the immediate but also in the late pain. However, as is the case with concussion symptoms, it seems likely that the picture is compounded by an element of accident neurosis. In the eyes of the law, the driver of a stationary car is usually considered to be the innocent party. Therefore anyone with neck pain as a result of being in a motionless car struck by another vehicle has a legitimate cause for claiming damages. It has been shown in the case of concussion that involvement in such litigation raises the likelihood of persistent symptoms. Litigation is often protracted, and even when the claim is settled, it is far from certain that an accident neurosis will then regress. As with concussion, one would like to know the effect of early settlement of claims on a no-fault basis.

Attention has been drawn to comparisons between the late sequelae of neck sprains and of concussion. It should be remembered that many patients sustain both conditions simultaneously.

THE PREVENTION OF NECK SPRAINS IN CAR ACCIDENTS

The advent of aircraft carriers, where aeroplanes were catapulted from the deck at very fast acceleration, caused severe neck pain in a large number of pilots. It was soon realised that this was an extension sprain, and the seats were modified to include a neck and head rest. Neck sprains were completely prevented by this measure.

When surgeons and accident scientists gradually became aware of neck sprains as a common and debilitating injury after road accidents, it was thought that it would be possible to eliminate these in a similar way. In practice, head rests in motor cars have proved much less satisfactory than in aircraft.

The reason for the difference in the relative effectiveness of head rests in cars as compared with aircraft probably lies in the difference in the forces involved. In aircraft acceleration is rapid but steady, continuing over a period and then gradually decreasing as a desired velocity is reached. In motor accidents a sudden violent acceleration is followed almost immediately by deceleration. Even with a head rest in position, the whole body of the driver or passanger is propelled forwards away from the seat. The neck will begin to extend. In unbelted occupants, extension may increase as the forehead strikes the windscreen. In belted occupants extension is replaced by flexion as the seat belt holds back the trunk as the car decelerates. With inertia reel belts there will be sufficient movement of the trunk away from the seat back and head rest to allow considerable extension. Car accidents, even from the rear, will rarely occur in a perfect anteroposterior alignment, so there is often an element of rotation as well as extension or flexion.

Although the efficacy of the head rests is limited, a small improvement is better than none. There is also another possible line of research. It is known that if the seat back breaks, neck sprains are rare. It would seem worth investigating whether a sensor operated by a rear impact, which would allow the seat to move to a reclining position, might not be more effective than head rests.

Accident neurosis is at least a partial contributor to late morbidity. No-fault compensation, if it could be completed within three months of the accident, might substantially reduce the persistence of symptoms.

REFERENCES

Deans G T, McGalliard J N, Rutherford W H 1987 Neck sprain — a major cause of disability following car accidents. Injury 18: 10–12

MacNab I 1964 Acceleration injuries of the cervical spine. Journal of Bone Joint Surgery (Am) 46A: 1797–1799

FURTHER READING

The anatomy and pathophysiology of whiplash Bogduk N 1986 Clinical Biomechanics 1: 92–101

Survey of one hundred cases of whiplash injury after settlement of litigation Gotten N 1956 Journal of the American Medical Association 162: 865

Cervical spine injuries; epidemiological investigation, medical and social consequences Juhl M, Seerup K K 1981 Procedings of the 6th International Conference on Biomechanics of Impacts, Bron, France, 49

The 'whiplash syndrome' MacNab I 1971 Orthopedic Clinics of North America 2(2): 389–403

The prognosis of neck injuries resulting from rear-end vehicle accidents Norris S H, Watt I 1983 Journal of Bone Joint Surgery 65: 609

Injuries to car occupants — some aspects of the interior design of cars Nygren A 1984 Acta Otolaryngologica 395: 105

Neck injury to women in auto accidents Scutt C H, Dohan F C 1968 Journal of the American Medical Association 206 (12): 2689

Soft-tissue injuries of the neck Skates J D 1975 Society of Automotive Engineers, Warrendale Paper no 790135

Orofacial problems

FACIAL FRACTURES

The immediate management of gross facial injury has already been described (see Ch. 14).

Fractures of the facial skeleton include fractures of the orbit, considered in Ch. 43, and nasal fractures, considered in Ch. 44.

This section deals with fractures of the malar complex, the middle third of the face and the mandible.

Facial fractures are usually accompanied by swelling which may mask deformity. A fracture should be suspected if the occlusion is abnormal. The teeth meet in a precise manner when the mouth is closed and a displaced fracture alters the biting position. A step deformity may be seen in the level of the teeth (Fig. 42.1).

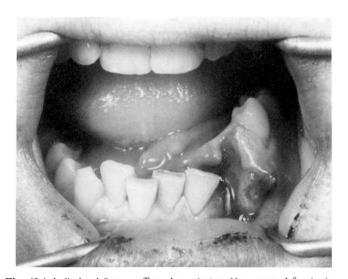

Fig. 42.1 A displaced fracture affects the occlusion. Here a step deformity is seen.

Radiographic views at right angles to each other will be needed together with an *orthopantomograph* (OPT) view which demonstrates the relation of the teeth to any fractures (Fig. 42.2).

All fractures should receive expert review within 48 hours of occurrence and displaced fractures require to be seen and treated within a few hours to control pain and bleeding. Fractures involving the tooth-bearing area should be considered as compound fractures likely to become infected and antibiotic prophylaxis is needed. (Most facial infecting organisms are penicillin-sensitive.)

Fractures of the malar complex

The malar bone, which provides the skeletal foundation for the prominence of the cheek, is a solid piece of bone. For diagnostic purposes it is helpful to picture it as a stool with a seat and three legs. The seat of the stool — the body of the bone — is thick and heavy. Of the three legs, the first two are fairly thick — the frontal process running upwards and the zygomatic arch running backwards from the lateral side of the body. The third leg, which is formed by the part of the maxilla which adjoins the malar bone, appears much the thickest when seen in a skeleton. But it is a hollow leg with the maxillary antrum forming its hollow centre. In an AP radiograph it appears as two plates of bone — the floor of the orbit and the lateral wall of the maxillary antrum.

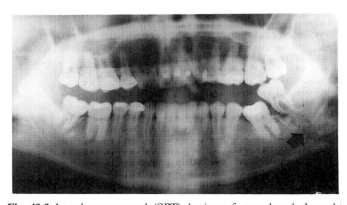

Fig. 42.2 An orthopantomograph (OPT) showing a fracture through the angle of the mandible on the left.

In a 'malar fracture' it is not the bone itself — the seat of the stool — which breaks: the fractures occur in the legs or bony processes and plates. Points of tenderness may be identified over the prominence of the cheek where the tissues are bruised and over fractures in each of the three legs. Obvious tenderness will be found over fractures of the frontal process and the zygomatic arch. The fractured maxillary leg will be tender both at the infraorbital margin and in the sulcus above the upper molar teeth. To feel this a gloved finger is placed in the mouth. When all three processes are fractured the condition may be referred to as a *'tripod fracture'* of the malar complex.

If the force is severe, the body of the malar bone will be driven downwards and backwards. This can best be detected by inspection from behind the patient, looking down over the forehead. The cheek depression cannot be appreciated shortly after injury if there is marked overlying swelling. The back of the indriven malar bone may obstruct forward movement of the coronoid process of the mandible, thus preventing mouth opening. With lesser degrees of violence malar fractures may not be accompanied by any bony displacement.

When the infraorbital margin breaks, the usual site of the fracture is the infraorbital foramen. The infraorbital nerve is bruised and the cheek, lip and upper teeth on the injured side are numb. It is often possible to feel a step in the infraorbital margin at the point of the fracture. If the floor of the orbit is markedly depressed, diplopia may be present, particularly in upward and downward gaze.

When the orbital floor is disrupted bleeding occurs and blood may track forward into the subconjunctival region to give a bright red area in the white of the eye. This extends to the posterior limit of the sclera, unlike the haemorrhage from a 'black eye' when white sclera is present posteriorly.

In summary, a malar fracture may show the following features:

1. Tenderness over the body of the malar, the zygomatic arch, the frontal process, the infraorbital margin and in the sulcus.
2. Anaesthesia or hypoaesthesia of cheek, upper lip and upper teeth on the affected side.
3. Depression of the prominence of the cheek, masked at first by overlying soft tissue swelling.
4. A palpable step in the orbital margin.
5. Diplopia.
6. Subconjunctival haemorrhage with no posterior limit.
7. Incomplete opening of the mouth.

The first of these features is always present, together with some or all of the other findings.

The diagnosis is confirmed by radiographs of the face taken with the head tilted backwards (occipitomental views) so that the shadows of the petrous bones do not obscure the fractures through the walls of the maxillary antrum (Fig. 42.3). In the radiograph the maxillary antrum may be opaque, either from overlying soft tissue swelling or from blood in the antrum. The fractures can

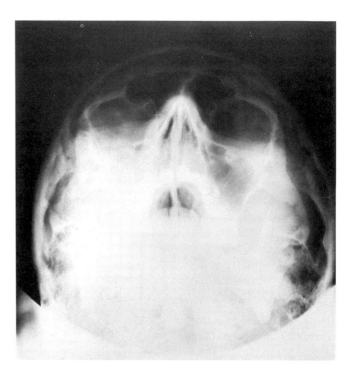

Fig. 42.3 A 30 radiograph of facial bones showing a fracture of the right malar complex. Note the opacity in the antrum, step in intraorbital plate and fracture of lateral wall of antrum.

be seen at the expected sites, the radiographs serving only to confirm what is strongly suspected from clinical examination.

Undisplaced fractures of the malar bone do not require treatment. If displacement can definitely be excluded it is unnecessary to make any referral; if there is displacement the patient should be referred to a maxillofacial surgeon. The ideal time for treatment is when the soft tissue swelling has resolved and before new bone formation has started — usually between the fifth and eighth days.

Diplopia present after trauma to the eye but with no clinical or radiographic evidence of fracture, may be due to orbital blow-out injury (see Ch. 43) or bruising of the extraocular muscles. Monocular diplopia is a serious symptom denoting either lens dislocation or retinal detachment.

Fractures of the middle third of the face

The face is divided into upper, middle and lower thirds by the orbits and the mouth: above the orbits bony damage causes skull fractures, below the mouth bony damage causes mandibular fractures. In the middle third, fractures rarely involve only one bone but run through the whole collection of bones which surround the nasal cavities and support the teeth. It is sufficient to know the common fractures. The low transverse is known as *Le Fort I*, in which palate, alveolus and upper teeth are separated from the rest of the upper jaw and facial bones. The high transverse, *Le Fort III*, which involves orbits and nasal bones, is in effect a craniofacial disjunction. The *Le Fort II* is a pyramidal fracture of the central part of the face, the base of the pyramid being the upper teeth and palate and the apex being the nasoethmoidal region. Fracture of the cribriform plate of the ethmoid in Le Fort II and III injuries may give rise to cerebrospinal fluid rhinorrhoea (Fig. 42.4).

In normal use, the facial bones are subjected to vertical forces while food is being chewed. There are few, if any, horizontal forces applied normally. Most of the bony box which comprises the middle third is made up of thin sheets of bone with a few strong vertical buttresses. If the face is struck horizontally, either from before backwards or from one or other side, the bone structure is unable to provide resistance: a punch, a kick or a ball or stone thrown with force will rarely cause fractures elsewhere in the body yet these forces are quite sufficient to cause fractures of the middle third of the face. Most commonly, fractures result from forces applied in an anteroposterior direction. Because the floor of the skull is a plane inclined at 45° to the horizontal, as the facial bones are driven backwards they also move downwards. The downward movement produces lengthening of the face and backward movement produces the 'dished in' appearance.

Examination of middle third fractures

Inspection. There may be profuse bleeding from the nose and mouth. The face may show *dish deformity* and elongation resulting from downward and backward displacement of the maxilla. The mouth may be wedged fully open with only the posterior teeth in contact. Mouth movement may be further limited by painful muscle spasm. Where the impact has been high on the maxilla flattening of the nose and spreading of the orbits may be present. Gross swelling of the eyelids occurs and examination of the globes may be impossible. (Fig. 42.5).

Tenderness. With a knowledge of the common fracture lines, it is possible to test for tenderness at these sites. This is most significant when the tender area is not directly under the point at which the main impact has been taken by the soft tissues.

Anaesthesia. In many fractures there is damage to the infraorbital nerves and to the sensory nerves to the teeth and palate. The cheek and lips should be examined in an area where they are not too swollen.

Percussion of the teeth. When the teeth are firmly tapped with a metal object such as a dental mirror or other instrument handle a characteristic dull note is produced if a fracture lies above the level of the tooth roots.

Diplopia. Disruption of the orbital floor may produce a change in ocular level or disturbance of globe position due to trapping

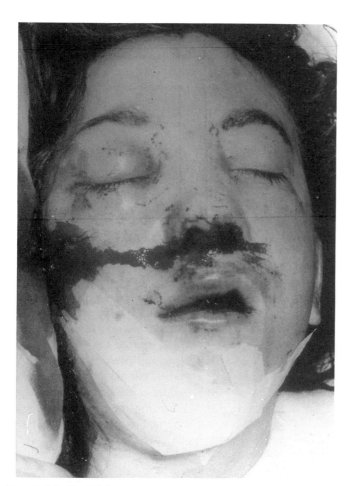

Fig. 42.4 Le Fort III fracture. CSF rhinorrhoea showing as a persistent blood-stained fluid running from the nostril.

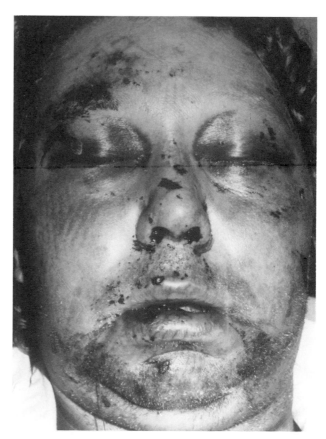

Fig. 42.5 Dish deformity with nasal flattening, increase in intercanthal distance and gross swelling of the eyelids.

of the extraocular muscles. Testing will be difficult if the eye is damaged or if the lids are grossly oedematous.

Mobility of alveolar margin. The upper teeth and gum can be grasped and an attempt made to move them. Any movement is readily appreciated if the bridge of the nose is steadied by the thumb and fingers of the other hand.

Radiographic appearances.   Clinical examination should give a good indication of where the fractures will run. It is then easier to inspect the exact site under suspicion. An opaque maxillary antrum will usually be present, though may sometimes be due to overlying soft tissue swelling. The orbits may appear to have been moved laterally and to have become oval in shape as a result of the downward displacement of the maxilla carrying with it the orbital floors (the so-called *Mickey Mouse orbits)*. Lateral radiographic views demonstrate facial elongation with a fully opened mouth and posterior tooth contact only (Fig. 42.6).

Fracture of the mandible

Gross comminuted fractures have already been discussed (Ch. 14); this section is concerned with fractures which might possibly be overlooked, at least in the initial examination of a patient who may have several other serious injuries or who may appear merely to be drunk or bruised. Where a fracture of the lower jaw is suspected, careful clinical examination will usually detect a mobile fracture. Radiographic examination will be necessary to exclude stable fractures. If one fracture of the mandible is found, other fractures should be looked for since the mandible is often broken in two or more places.

Examination of mandibular fractures

Inspection of the face.   Fractures of the angle and of the body are most likely to lead to displacement and deformity. The amount of deformity depends on the site of the fracture and its plane of inclination. Where there is obvious deformity a fracture is certain; where there is none it is not immediately excluded. A fracture may be visible inside the mouth if the periosteum and mucosa over the fracture are torn. Lingual ecchymosis is always highly suggestive of a fracture. There may be a broken or displaced tooth in the fracture line. Blood may be seen at the external auditory meatus and may indicate a fracture of the neck of the mandibular condyle and tympanic plate and not necessarily a fracture of the floor of the skull.

Palpation.   The fracture site will be tender. Tenderness is most significant at a point distant from the point of impact of the force, e.g. tenderness over the necks of the condyles where there has been

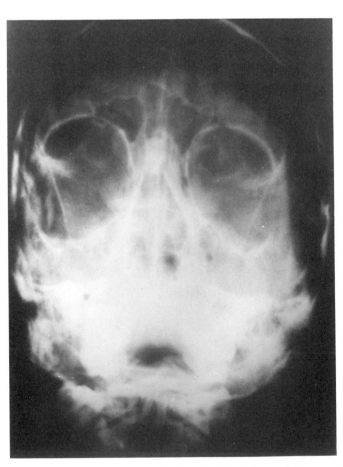
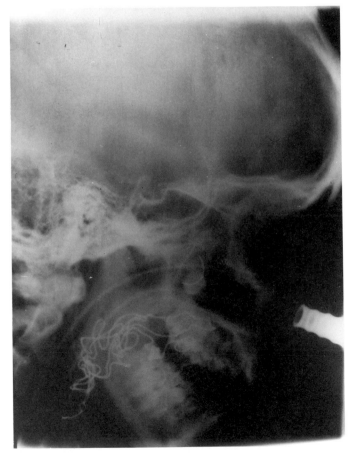

Fig. 42.6 Anteroposterior and lateral radiographs of a middle third fracture. Note the 'Mickey Mouse' orbits and the elongated face.

a blow to the chin. Condylar tenderness may be elicited by palpation from the external meatus. With fractures of the body, angle or ramus, tenderness elicited from the lingual aspect of the mouth is more significant than external tenderness.

The dental occlusion.   The dental occlusion is altered by even minor degrees of displacement of a mandibular fracture. It is useful in diagnosing fracture of the neck of the condyle where overlap at the fracture site causes shortening and early contact of the teeth on the injured side

Sensation.   Absence of feeling in the area of the front of the chin should raise a high suspicion of a fracture involving the inferior dental nerve.

Radiography.   Radiographs of the mandible can be difficult to interpret, especially in the region of the temperomandibular joints. Lateral and posteroanterior radiographs are necessary to avoid missing a mandibular fracture. In the tooth-bearing area it is clinically important to detect undisplaced fractures as well as those showing displacement. An OPT will be helpful.

Treatment of mandibular fractures

If the tooth-bearing area of the jaw is involved an antibiotic should be given. Penicillin or erythromycin (250 mg q.d.s.) will provide adequate prophylaxis against infection entering the fracture from the periodontal membrane of any tooth in the fracture site. Immobilisation of an unstable fracture will be required, but in the emergency situation little can be done other than allowing the patient to adopt the most comfortable jaw position. Bandages passed beneath the jaw and over the head may increase displacement and lead to airway problems. Definitive treatment is by direct fixation at the fracture sites or immobilisation of one jaw to the other (or a combination of both forms of treatment). General anaesthesia will often be necessary with close airway supervision during the recovery period.

INTRA-ORAL SOFT-TISSUE WOUNDS

Wounds may arise from entry of an external object such as a stick or pencil being held in the mouth at the time of a fall. Alternatively, the teeth can lacerate the oral soft tissues, particularly the tongue, when a violent blow forces the mouth shut unexpectedly. Most small oral wounds including soft palate perforations do not require suture. Larger wounds which give rise to troublesome bleeding, bone exposure or obvious deformity should be sutured. Except in the very young, local anaesthesia can be used. Suitable suture materials are 2/0 or 3/0 silk or soft catgut. The synthetic resorbable materials do not perform well in the mouth. A generous bite of tissue is necessary to prevent the suture cutting through the mucous membrane. When closing tongue lacerations haemostasis of the muscle layer is necessary to prevent the development of a

haematoma. The tongue may swell to such an extent after injury and suture that the airway may be obstructed.

DISLOCATION OF THE JAW

The anatomy of the jaw only permits dislocation of the condyle in an anterior direction and this requires over-riding of the articular eminence. The head of the condyle is then free to move upwards under muscle pull. Only the posterior teeth make contact and the mouth is fixed partly open with the chin prominent. Dislocation may be unilateral or bilateral. The method of reduction is the same in each case. Standing behind the patient with the thumbs on the lower posterior teeth apply a firm, downward pressure for a minute or two. This is to fatigue the elevator muscles so that the condyle head can be brought below the articular eminence before being pushed back into the fossa. If reduction can be achieved without sedation or anaesthesia there is little likelihood of a repeat dislocation within the immediate postreduction period. If reduction cannot be achieved without analgesia or sedation the following approach is useful. Commence by infiltrating local anaesthetic into the masseter muscles either intraorally or extraorally. If using the intraoral route, the medial pterygoid muscles can also be infiltrated. Two or three millitres of plain lignocaine (1%) on either side will suffice. In nervous patients this may be supplemented by intravenous diazepam, though one must be wary of producing disorientation and protestation leading to repeat dislocation. Similarly, whilst the relaxation produced by general anaesthesia makes reduction easy, repeat dislocation during recovery can occur. Since dislocation is produced by wide mouth opening the patient must be warned to avoid this or reminded by the application of a restraining head bandage. Remember that those drugs such as phenothiazines which can produce dystonic reactions may predispose to recurrent dislocation.

INJURIES TO TEETH

Injuries to the teeth require accurate description when medicolegal reports are prepared and it is helpful if the standard dental terminology is used in the initial description of the injuries in the A & E department. The teeth are numbered 1–8 in each quadrant in the full permanent dentition and from A to E in the deciduous dentition (Fig. 42.7). The teeth present are charted for convenience into quadrants. Left and right appear as if the observer is looking at the patient from the front. Where a tooth is missing, the appropriate number will also be missing from the charting. For example, if a patient has received damage to the left upper jaw and the left central incisor, canine, second premolar and third molar are missing the charting would show:

87654321	2 4 6 7
87654321	12345678

In describing actual damage to the crowns of the teeth, the part of the crown nearest to the mid-line is referred to as the mesial

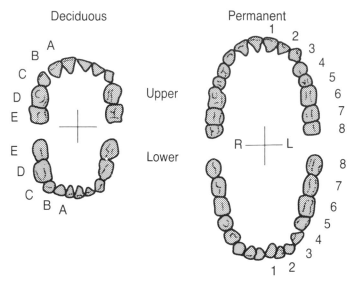

Fig. 42.7 Schematic representation of the teeth (plan view).

aspect and that furthest from the midline as the distal aspect. The tooth surface adjacent to the lip and cheek is the labial or buccal surface whilst that adjacent to the tongue is the lingual surface. The biting surface is referred to as the occlusal surface. (Damage to artificial teeth, whether fixed or removable, is similarly described.)

Chipped teeth and dislodged artificial crowns are not an emergency. Teeth damaged to the extent where the dental pulp is visible as a small bleeding area within the crown give rise to a very severe pain and warrant emergency dental care.

Where the injury involves loosening or even avulsion of teeth particular care is needed to ensure tooth survival. The objective is to replace the tooth into an approximately correct position within the socket as soon as possible. There may be difficulty in closing the mouth if teeth are displaced backwards. With or without local anaesthetic the teeth can usually be manipulated into place and will remain adequately fixed pending the arrival of expert help.

When teeth have been knocked from the mouth they must be managed in such a way as to preserve the vitality of the delicate periodontal membrane surrounding the root. The tooth may be gently washed in cold water and should then be kept moist. A tooth allowed to dry out for more than 20 minutes will not survive. With co-operation of the patient, the ideal place to store an avulsed tooth prior to replantation is in the buccal sulcus bathed in saliva. Specialist help will be needed for fixing a replanted tooth. Antitetanus precautions should be applied and an antibiotic combination such as ampicillin and metronidazole or erythromycin and metronidazole should be prescribed. Teeth of the primary dentition are not reimplanted.

When a tooth cannot be accounted for and the patient has a history either of unconsciousness or of coughing after an accident the possibility of inhalation of the tooth must be considered and excluded by chest radiography. Ingested teeth do not seem to cause any problems.

POST EXTRACTION HAEMORRHAGE

Fresh bleeding from extraction sockets should cease within 15 minutes of extraction, although blood staining of saliva may persist for a number of hours. If a number of teeth are extracted at one visit and bleeding is from all sockets then a systemic factor should be suspected. When the bleeding is from an isolated socket, in the absence of a significant medical history the source of bleeding will be either the soft tissues around the socket or the bone within the socket. Pressure from a gauze swab may be applied by the simple expedient of the patient biting down onto the pad. If, after 10 minutes of undisturbed pressure, the bleeding persists then this method of control should be abandoned. To discriminate between bleeding from bone or soft tissue the socket should be squeezed between finger and thumb. This procedure will arrest soft tissue bleeding; continued haemorrhage is strongly suggestive of bleeding from bone. In the former case the definitive treatment is to infiltrate local anaesthetic with vasoconstrictor on either side of the socket and then insert an horizontal mattress suture in the manner of a purse string to compress the soft tissue against the bone. If the bleeding is from bone a resorbable haemostatic agent can be pressed into the socket beneath the suture.

Notes on local anaesthesia in the oral cavity

The vascularity of the mouth and jaws means that plain local anaesthetic without vasoconstrictor has a very short duration of activity. The local anaesthetic is carried into the circulation and adequate anaesthesia may never be obtained. Lignocaine with adrenaline 1:80 000 and prilocaine with felypressin are both highly effective. Infiltration of anaesthetic into and around the affected area gives acceptable anaesthesia for soft tissue work. Nerve blocks are excellent and easily mastered with tuition from any dental department. For treatment to the jaw bone, block anaesthesia is advantageous, but for wound closure and socket suture infiltration anaesthesia is adequate.

NON-TRAUMATIC OROFACIAL PROBLEMS

Bleeding gums

Chronic bleeding from the gums on brushing the teeth or eating hard foods is not an emergency. The patient should be advised to consult his dental practitioner.

Spontaneous bleeding indicates either a haematological disorder or a severe gingival infection. Disorders of haemostasis include excessive anticoagulation therapy, thrombocytopenia and, rarely, a fresh presentation of an acute leukaemia. The commonest gingival infection is due to a fusospirochaetal symbiosis with similar tissue-destructive properties to that found in cancrum oris. The condition is commonly known as *trench mouth* or *'Vincent's acute ulcerative gingivitis'*. It produces a marked halitosis, pyrexia, constitutional upset and painful lymphadenitis. The organisms are invariably sensitive to either penicillin or metronidazole. Treatment with one of these antibacterials should be commenced without delay lest irreversible gum destruction occur.

Dental pain

Pain originating from the teeth may be severe and require analgesia in effective doses. When a tooth becomes very tender to pressure, an abscess is probably developing and antibiotic therapy (ampicillin, metronidazole or erythromycin) may retard and lessen the severity of the problem.

Dry socket (Fig. 42.8)

This is the name given to a condition of postextraction pain without swelling. It usually comes on four to eight days after tooth extraction and is usually due to loss of blood clot from within the socket. The exposed bone is extremely painful and dressing of the socket should be carried out. The aim is to cover exposed bone and prevent food packing into the socket. A dressing of zinc oxide mixed with eugenol on gauze is particularly effective, for the eugenol exerts an anodyne effect as well as binding the dressing to the cavity. Premixed proprietary products with a long shelf life are available.

Trismus

Trismus is an inability to open the mouth. It may be due to spasm of the masticatory muscles or, rarely, to displacement of the cartilaginous disc within the temperomandibular joint. Some drugs, such as metoclopramide and members of the phenothiazine group, may be associated with dystonic contractions of the masticatory muscles. Tetanus is the only cause of trismus requiring emergency action. Recent dental injections may produce bleeding into the masticatory muscles followed by trismus, which may take up to three months to resolve. Infection around an erupting wisdom tooth or a peritonsillar abscess (quinsy) may limit opening. After an episode of forced wide mouth opening painful jaw stiffness is common. Remember that the main sign in dislocation of the jaw is inability to close the mouth — not restricted opening. An attempt to manipulate the lower jaw to improve opening may be painful and may lead to an exacerbation of the condition. Careful diagnosis must precede any treatment.

Dental abscess

An acute dental abscess requires both antibiotic therapy to limit the spread of infection and the surgical drainage of pus.

Particular attention should be given to cellulitis of the upper face in the 'danger area' around the nose (see Ch. 33 on Soft tissue infections) for the risk of developing cavernous sinus thrombophlebitis.

Attention too should be paid to a lower jaw abscess producing elevation of the tongue with trismus. Any lower jaw abscess starting unilaterally and becoming bilateral means that the anatomical planes within the floor of the mouth and neck are opening up to infection. The end result can be rapidly developing neck swelling with respiratory obstruction (Ludwig's angina, Fig. 42.9). Numbness or paraesthesia of the lower lip in the presence of infection indicates the presence of inflammatory exudate around the inferior dental nerve within the mandible and warns of developing osteomyelitis and severe swelling. A patient with some or all of the above symptoms and signs should be admitted to hospital.

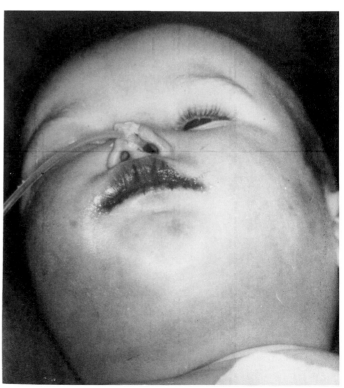

Fig. 42.9 Ludwig's angina developing after infection following minor trauma to the lower jaw. This baby required emergency endotracheal intubation and surgical drainage.

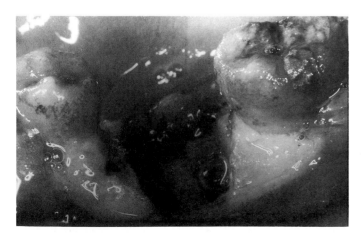

Fig. 42.8 Dry socket.

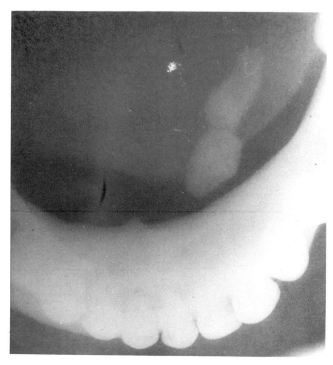

Fig. 42.10 A calculus in the submandibular duct.

Salivary gland swelling

Any of the salivary glands can show swelling, which may be simple retention or may take the form of retention followed by infection. Swelling related to meal times, which subsides after the meal, is characteristic of an obstructive lesion. This is most commonly a salivary calculus. It almost always affects the submandibular gland. A stone may be found on bimanual palpation with one finger in the mouth over Wharton's duct and the other over the gland in the neck. Radiographs of the lateral oblique view and floor of the mouth may show a calculus, provided that minimal exposure is used — as the stones are not very radio-opaque (Fig. 42.10).

When infection is present, pain and swelling persist beyond meal times and pus may be seen exuding from the salivary ducts. In the case of infection, rigorous antibiotic therapy with metronidazole combined with ampicillin or clindamycin is needed. Surgical drainage may be required and must be by the intraoral route because of the risk of salivary fistula to a skin surface. The commonest cause of salivary swelling remains endemic parotitis (mumps) which can present atypically affecting a single submandibular salivary gland.

FURTHER READING

Handbook of dental local anaesthesia Evers H, Haegerstom G 1981 Schultz, Copenhagen

Simple dental care for rural hospitals 4th edn. Halestrap D J 1981 Medical Missionary Society, 6 Canonbury Place, London N1 1NJ

Fractures of the mandible 2nd edn. Killey H C 1974 John Wright, Bristol

Fractures of the middle third of the facial skeleton 3rd edn. Killey H C 1977 John Wright, Bristol

Dental, oral and maxillofacial surgery — a guide to hospital practice Poswillo D, Babjens A, Bailey M, Foster M 1986 Heinemann, London

Emergency dentistry Watt D G 1975 Clausen Publications, Weybridge, Surrey

Eye conditions

INTRODUCTION

Trauma now ranks as one of the most common causes of ocular morbidity and loss of vision. Injuries due to domestic causes and direct assault have increased over recent years, but there has been some reduction in industrial injuries due to the introduction of various protective measures. More recently, since the introduction of compulsory seatbelts, injuries from road traffic accidents have decreased. It should be remembered that the eye is a complex and delicate optical structure which tolerates only slight injury without loss or alteration of function. Most serious injuries require the expertise of an experienced ophthalmic surgeon because techniques of repair are difficult and require specialised microsurgical instruments and an operating microscope.

Medical emergencies such as loss of vision, diplopia and pain in the eye can also pose difficult diagnostic and management problems to the doctor in the A & E department and it is necessary for him to know which cases he can reasonably treat and which require immediate referral for specialised ophthalmic attention.

It is essential in managing patients with ophthalmic complaints to establish good channels of reference between the A & E and ophthalmic departments. It is also important that the A & E department have a room allocated for the examination of ophthalmic emergencies, appropriately equipped with basic ophthalmic diagnostic equipment and therapeutic agents (Fig. 43.1). The basic essentials to permit an adequate evaluation of the eye in the accident and emergency department are the following.

1. A Snellen test type to assess visual acuity at 6 metres. If the room is less than 7 metres in length, a reverse Snellen type with a mirror at 3 metres is quite adequate. There is no substitute for an accurate evaluation of central visual function and each patient attending the A & E department with an eye complaint or suspected ocular abnormality must have visual acuity documented. The use of a pin-hole corrects most refractive errors that may be present.

2. A fully operational ophthalmoscope. The +10 to +12 lenses may be used in examination of the anterior segments of the eyes. It should be checked at frequent intervals to keep it in good working order.

3. Magnifying spectacles or a magnifying loupe may be used for inspecting the anterior segment of the eye to exclude foreign bodies or perforating injuries.

4. A slit lamp microscope. This not only makes it possible for the patient to have a specialized consultation in the A & E department, but also is a worthwhile instrument for training resident A & E doctors to examine the eye in detail and to learn the fundamentals of ocular pathology.

5. A source of good focal illumination, preferably fixed to a movable stand. Good illumination is essential for accurate evaluation of the anterior segment of the eye and for carrying out minor ocular procedures, such as the removal of a corneal foreign body. A cobalt blue torch light is useful to show up corneal lesions in conjunction with fluorescein.

6. Cottonwool-tipped applicators for the removal of superficial conjunctival and corneal foreign bodies; a fine hypodermic needle (21G green) fixed to a special holder or a 2 ml syringe, may be necessary if the foreign body is fixed in the corneal epithelium or has penetrated to a slight deeper level.

7. Glass rods or fine wooden spatulae for eye lid eversion (Fig. 43.2).

8. Irrigation solutions, for example Ringer's solution, normal saline or balanced salt solution, should be immediately available

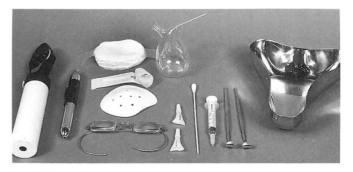

Fig. 43.1 Basic diagnostic and therapeutic equipment.

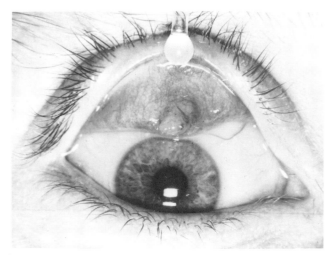

Fig. 43.2 Everted upper lid. Meibomian granulation tissue is shown.

in the event of chemical burns of the eye lids, cornea or conjunctiva. Chelating agents such as ethylenediaminetetra-acetate (EDTA) are particularly useful for the treatment of specific chemical injury (e.g. lime or acid burns).

9. Desmarres' lid retractors are essential for adequate examination of the conjunctival fornices, particularly when the eye lids or conjunctiva are swollen, infected or ulcerated.

10. Eye pads, crepe bandages and plastic eye shields are necessary for dressing purposes and for providing some measure of protection to an eye which has been lacerated.

11. Eye-drops in minim form are useful for both diagnostic and therapeutic purposes. There are many sterile single-dose disposable eye-drops and the following are recommended:

a. Tropicamide drops for rapid dilatation of the pupil without significant cycloplegia.

b. Cyclopentolate (Mydrilate) 1% eye-drops to dilate the pupil and produce cycloplegia in those instances where it is essential to relieve ciliary spasm (e.g. corneal abrasions and ulcers).

c. Pilocarpine 1% or 2% drops may be required occasionally to constrict a pupil after dilatation.

d. Local anaesthetic drops such as amethocaine 1% or oxybuprocaine 0.4% are essential for a wide variety of ophthalmic investigative procedures, and for the removal of conjunctival or corneal FB's.

e. Chloramphenicol (Chloromycetin) 0.5% is a good multipurpose topical antibiotic effective against a wide range of pathogens and is only rarely the cause of sensitivity reactions.

f. Sterile fluorescein-impregnated strips (Fluorets), which may be discarded immediately after use, are employed for staining the cornea to highlight abrasions and superficial ulcers.

Common eye complaints will be described under two main headings: trauma and non-trauma emergencies.

TRAUMA

Multiple system injuries

Injuries to the eye lids and orbit, unaccompanied by injuries to other parts of the body, do not pose an immediate threat to life and their management must be subordinate to the resuscitation of the seriously injured patient. Major emergency operative procedures (e.g. neurosurgical explorations) take precedence and the immediate management of ocular and orbital wounds in such cases is limited to achieving haemostasis and protecting the eye with a firm plastic or metal shield taped to the orbital rim.

When injuries are limited to the face and do not involve the intracranial cavity, perforating eye injuries take priority and, if at all possible, repair should be carried out in an ophthalmic theatre. It must be remembered that swollen eye lids and periorbital tissues may conceal serious underlying ocular injuries, and care and patience should be exercised during the examination. For the examination of a child or apprehensive adult, either local or general anaesthetic may be required before adequate exposure for a proper inspection and evaluation is obtained. When blepharospasm is severe, it may be necessary to instil a drop of local anaesthetic to relieve discomfort. In those instances where blepharospasm persists despite local anaesthetic drops, it may be necessary to produce facial paralysis by injecting lignocaine 2% along the course of the facial nerve.

Injuries to the globe, lid, lacrimal apparatus and orbit

Globe and conjunctiva

Foreign bodies.   Using magnification and good illumination, surface foreign bodies of the conjunctiva and cornea may be removed with a moistened cottonwool-tipped applicator following the instillation of one or two drops of oxybuprocaine 0.4% or amethocaine 1%. Deeper or more adherent corneal foreign bodies may be removed with a fine hypodermic needle (no. 21 green) on a holder or syringe. Slit lamp microscopy is necessary in these latter cases so that the depth of the foreign body in the cornea can accurately be assessed. This is particularly important when a foreign body involves the axial cornea so that manipulation and resultant scarring can be kept to a minimum. Rust rings remaining after the removal of a ferrous foreign body should be meticulously removed to prevent a chemical keratitis and corneal ulceration. This may most easily be accomplished after two or three days. The involved area of impregnated cornea can then be removed in toto. Following removal of the corneal foreign body, a drop of cyclopentolate 1% and an antibiotic such as chloramphenicol 0.5% is instilled and the eye covered with a pad. Follow up at the eye department is recommended.

Arc flash.   Flash burns or 'welder's flash' which involve the cornea are quite common in industrial societies and cause severe pain, epiphora and blepharospasm. The discomfort characteristically occurs several hours after exposure to the ultraviolet radiation, and often the patient presents in the A & E department at night. 'Snow blindness' has a similar aetiology. Instillation of anaesthetic drops affords immediate relief and permits adequate evaluation of the anterior segments of the eyes. Antibiotic and cycloplegic drops are prescribed and the eyes covered with a firm pad. The patient should be provided with sufficient analgesic tablets (e.g. paracetamol) to relieve discomfort once the effects of the local anaesthetic have worn off. It should be emphasised that local anaesthetic drops have no place in the management of corneal disease because their prolonged use may retard epithelial healing. Most flash burns of the cornea heal within 24–28 hours and it is only necessary for the patient to return to an ophthalmic outpatient clinic if he is having further symptoms.

Corneal abrasions.   Corneal abrasions give rise to severe discomfort, foreign body sensation, pain and watering of the eye. Diagnosis can be facilitated by staining the cornea with fluorescein, easily executed by touching the inside of the lower eye lid with a Fluoret. (The abraded or ulcerated area of the corneal epithelium stains green.) This shows up best with a cobalt blue light. Corneal abrasions and ulcers are treated by instilling a cycloplegic and antibiotic drop and covering the eye with a firm pad and bandage for 24–48 hours. Treatment is continued until the corneal epithelium has completely healed and no staining is present. Occasionally, imperfect epithelialisation of the cornea occurs, leading to a 'recurrent erosion', which is particularly painful and requires specialist management. In the majority of cases follow-up should be carried out in an eye department.

Chemical burns.   Chemical burns of the conjunctiva and cornea are ocular emergencies and require immediate treatment. The cornea and conjunctival sacs should be immediately and copiously irrigated with water or normal saline from a drip set. Appropriate neutralising solutions are valuable but immediate irrigation should not be delayed. Any solid chemical particles, such as lime or cement, which may be present or entrapped in the conjunctival fornices should be meticulously removed irrespective of their size. Both upper and lower fornices and the inside of the upper and lower eye lids should be carefully examined using a Desmarres retractor after instillation of an anaesthetic drop. All A & E doctors should be able to evert the upper eye lid deftly and quickly without undue discomfort to the patient. This is most easily accomplished using a glass rod, matchstick or applicator to depress the upper tarsal plate. Once irrigation and debridement of the cornea and conjunctival sacs are complete, cycloplegic and antibiotic drops should be instilled, the eye covered and the patient referred immediately for specialist management.

Corneae which become opaque following a chemical burn are particularly difficult to treat, and corneal grafting is much less successful in such patient. If the chemical penetrates the anterior chamber, a violent intraocular inflammation ensues which may lead to severe disorganisation and secondary glaucoma. These serious complications emphasise the need for immediate irrigation, debridement and specialist management.

Perforating injuries.   Perforating injuries of the eye comprise the most important ocular emergency and require immediate ophthalmic evaluation and repair. Corneal or scleral lacerations may be associated with prolapse of intraocular tissues such as iris, ciliary body, choroid or vitreous. The pupil is characteristically

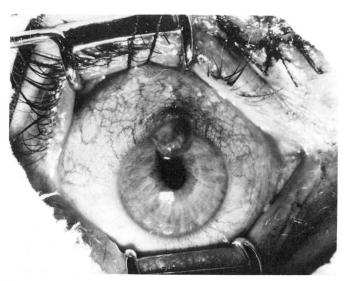

Fig. 43.3 Perforating injury with prolapse of iris, updrawn pupil and shallow anterior chamber.

irregular and blood is frequently present in either the anterior chamber or vitreous (Fig. 43.3). The anterior chamber of the eye is usually shallow if the laceration involves the anterior segment (cornea, limbus) and deep if the posterior segment (sclera) is involved. In extensive lacerations of the eye the lens is frequently damaged, causing cataract, dislocation or even expulsion from the globe. Careful evaluation should be carried out without exerting pressure on the eye or causing the patient to close his eyes forcibly.

Following examination, the eye lids should be gently closed and a plastic shield taped to the orbital margins and the patient immediately referred to an ophthalmic surgeon. Excessive manipulation of the eye lids or globe may precipitate further loss of intraocular contents, increase the incidence of complications and seriously influence the final visual outcome. If there are coexistent facial lacerations, they should not be sutured until the ocular lacerations have been repaired. All faciomaxillary or dental manipulations should be avoided or postponed until the integrity of the globe has been established.

Intraocular foreign body.   Intraocular foreign bodies may be difficult to diagnose, but if there is a history of a hammer and chisel injury, grinding or welding or an explosion or windscreen injury, they should be suspected and an anteroposterior and lateral X-ray of the orbit taken prior to seeking an ophthalmic consultation. A small perforating corneal or scleral laceration or a low intraocular pressure should alert the A & E doctor to the presence of a retained intraocular foreign body. This may be assessed by gentle digital pressure with the forefingers through the closed lids. Other signs may be a localised tear of the iris, lens opacity, vitreous opacity or intraocular haemorrhage.

Contusion injuries.   Contusional injuries of the globe and conjunctiva are common and vary from mild subconjunctival haemorrhage to severe hyphaema (blood in the anterior chamber), dislocation of the lens or haemorrhage into the posterior segment of the eye (vitreous, retina, choroid). All cases with intraocular involvement or reduced vision should be referred immediately for an ophthalmic opinion. Most hyphaemata spontaneously resolve. In some instances secondary haemorrhage occurs, producing the sudden onset of a secondary glaucoma. It is a good policy to admit patients with significant hyphaemata for a few days' bed rest and observation. Immediate treatment is then available should there be any secondary haemorrhage or rise in intraocular pressure.

Severe contusional injuries may result in rupture of the globe. Tears or lacerations of the globe may present with extensive subconjunctival haemorrhage and loss of vision. Thus, every patient who gives a history of injury to the eye and has subconjunctival haemorrhage or ocular hypotony should be examined carefully to exclude the presence of a scleral rupture and the appropriate treatment immediately instigated.

Ocular contusions are often complicated by long-term complications such as glaucoma and retinal detachment. Patients with significant trauma therefore should be referred to an ophthalmic department for careful long-term observation. A guarded prognosis for vision should be given to patients with substantial ocular contusion injuries. Even though the globe remains intact, small macular scars may reduce the visual acuity to counting fingers or less.

Lids and lacrimal apparatus

Imperfectly repaired eye lid lacerations may cause long-term discomfort, corneal damage and loss of vision. All full-thickness lacerations of the lids require suturing by an ophthalmic or plastic surgeon.

Superficial lid lacerations in adults, not involving the margins, may be carefully sutured in the A & E department using local anaesthetic (1% lignocaine with 1:200 000 adrenaline). Wound edges must be meticulously cleaned, aligned and closed with interrupted sutures of 0.5 metric gauge (6/0) silk or nylon. Eye lid skin is thin with relatively little subcutaneous fat, and mattress sutures are often required to prevent inversion of the skin edges. The sutures should be removed about the fourth or fifth day.

Severe lacerations and partial or complete avulsion of the lids may result in corneal exposure. In such cases the anterior segment of the eye should be meticulously protected, either by saline soaks or, in the longer term, using a soft 'bandage' contact lens until the appropriate corrective surgery has been carried out.

Lacerations of the medial aspect of the lower eye lid may involve the drainage apparatus of the lacrimal system and a torn canaliculus may be present. If there is any suspicion that the lacrimal canaliculi or sac are involved, the patient should be referred immediately for ophthalmic evaluation. The re-establishment of the integrity of a torn or lacerated canaliculus is difficult and requires an ophthalmic microscope and specific lacrimal instruments. Failure to recognise a lacrimal tear may make subsequent corrective surgery difficult and may mean that the patient is left with a chronically watering eye.

Orbit

Fractures of the orbit are common in contusional injuries and should be suspected where a subconjunctival haemorrhage or periorbital swelling is present. Palpation of the orbital rim should be carried out and any crepitus or surgical emphysema noted. Impaired skin sensation in the region of the lower lid and cheek usually indicates the involvement of the intraorbital nerve in an orbital floor fracture. Blow-out fractures of the orbit usually involve the floor. They are caused by objects generally over 3 cm in diameter, such as a cricket ball or fist, directly impinging on the eye and orbital rims (Fig. 43.4). The orbital rim generally remains intact and the orbital floor is forced or prolapsed into the superior maxillary antrum. Characteristic symptoms and signs include vertical diplopia (Fig. 43.5), usually maximal on looking up, loss of upwards ocular movement, depression and enophthalmos of the globe and skin hypoanaesthesia in the distribution of the infraorbital nerve. Oedema and ecchymosis may be such that these signs cannot be elicited immediately and the patient should be reviewed over a few days to exclude a blow-out fracture. X-rays may help to establish the diagnosis. A plain radiograph can only suggest a fracture, usually by the presence of blood resulting in an opaque antrum, and special tomograms are necessary to illustrate the fracture and possible prolapse of soft tissue.

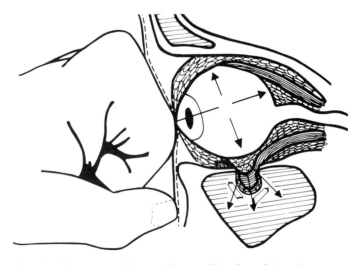

Fig. 43.4. Mechanism of 'blow-out' fracture of the floor of the orbit.

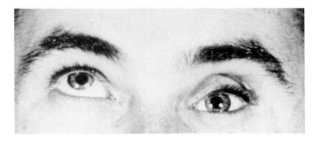

Fig. 43.5. 'Blow-out' fracture illustrating depression, enophthalmos and loss of elevation, left eye.

Indications for immediate reparative surgery are relatively few because spontaneous resolution of swelling and improvement in oculomotor function is the rule. Gross enophthalmos and persistent diplopia are the two major indications for surgery, which can usually be delayed for a period of several weeks.

NON-TRAUMATIC EMERGENCIES

Red painful eye

The doctor in the A & E department may be presented with a patient who complains of a red painful eye with or without loss of vision. Such eyes may only have minor lesions; for example, mild conjunctivitis. Alternatively, they may harbour a severe intraocular inflammatory process or have suffered an acute rise in intraocular pressure. The doctor should be aware of the causes of a red irritable eye and be capable of identifying those patients with significant ocular disease which require specialist management.

Conjunctivitis

The maximum injection of blood vessels is usually in the fornices or palpebral conjunctivae. A discharge is characteristically present and by its nature gives vital clues as to the aetiology of the disease process. Bacterial conjunctivitis is accompanied by a mucopurulent discharge and the offending organism can be readily identified, either by direct microscopic examination or following culture on appropriate media. Viral conjunctivitis is usually associated with a minimal watery discharge and sometimes a foreign body sensation in the eye. In allergic conjunctivitis the main symptoms are itching and irritation and the discharge is also clear and watery. Visual acuity is generally not significantly affected. However, if the cornea is involved or excessive mucopurulent discharge is present, the vision may be disturbed. Uncomplicated conjunctivitis is not an emergency and may be referred to an eye outpatient clinic. Treatment is not necessary in the A & E department, but a swab report taken at the time may be useful for specialist follow-up.

Keratitis and corneal ulcer

Vascular injection is usually ciliary in type (i.e. circumcorneal) and photophobia, watering and foreign body sensation may be present. Vision may be reduced if the inflammatory process involves the axial cornea. Loss of epithelial integrity is best identified by staining the cornea with fluorescein and examining under high magnification (e.g. slit lamp microscopy). When such an instrument is not available a magnifying loupe is helpful, used with good focal illumination. The pupil should be dilated and the ciliary body paralysed using a cycloplegic. An antibiotic drop or ointment is instilled, a pad and bandage applied and the patient referred to an eye department.

A branching or dendritic ulcer is pathognomonic of herpes simplex infection. Complete debridement of affected corneal epithelium generally is sufficient to combat the disease. Alternatively, specific therapy with acyclovir (Zovirax) or vidarabine (VIRA A) is often effective. Specific antiviral drugs are particularly effective in children in whom multiple dendritic ulcers are present. These cases, when recognised should immediately be referred for specialist management.

Acute iritis

The principal symptoms are pain, photophobia and blurring of vision. The signs include ciliary injection, a small irregular pupil and accumulation of cells and protein in the anterior chamber. Untreated iritis may result in severe long-term complications with loss of vision and should be referred immediately for an ophthalmic opinion. The accumulation of pus at the bottom of the anterior chamber (hypopyon) may complicate either acute iritis or fungal or pneumococcal ulcers of the cornea. All hypopyons require investigation and treatment and patients should be admitted to an ophthalmic ward.

Acute closed angle (congestive) glaucoma

This condition, which is an ocular emergency, typically occurs in elderly patients with shallow anterior chambers and developing lens sclerosis. Loss of vision and acute pain in the eye, occasionally accompanied by nausea and vomiting, are the common symptoms. Circumcorneal injection, a shallow anterior chamber, a fixed dilated pupil which is often oval in shape, and a hazy cornea are the usual signs. The eye is hard on palpation and on applanation tonometry the pressure often measures in excess of 60 mmHg (8 kPa). This level of pressure is easily recognised as a very hard eye on digital pressure.

The patient should immediately be admitted to an ophthalmic ward so that medical therapy can be instituted. The intraocular pressure can be immediately reduced by intravenous hyperosmotic agents such as mannitol 25% solution (1.5 g/kg body weight) and acetazolamide (Diamox) 500 mg by intravenous injection. Pilocarpine 4% drops are used intensively to constrict the pupil and facilitate drainage through the outflow passages of the eye.

Episcleritis and scleritis

These conditions usually present with pain and a local patch of redness on the white of the eye (episcleral injection). Vision is not usually affected and the patient need only be given a routine ophthalmic appointment.

Miscellaneous

Acute infections of the eye lids or central face should be treated energetically or at least carefully reviewed. Rarely, they may lead to a cavernous sinus thrombosis.

Hordeolum or stye. This acute, usually staphylococcal, infection of an eye lash follicle is best treated initially by epilating the appropriate lash. Hot bathing gives symptomatic relief and helps small abscesses to point. Recurrent multiple styes may require a course of appropriate systemic antibiotics.

Infected meibomian cyst.   In the acute phase this may be confused with a stye. Once the infection has resolved, the residual chronic granulomatous lesion is easily recognised as a firm pea-sized swelling of the lid. There is no urgency and the case may be referred for incision and curettage under a local anaesthetic.

Orbital cellulitis.   This is an emergency because it may give rise to orbital thrombophlebitis, central retinal vein occlusion and loss of vision. Less commonly, cavernous sinus thrombosis may occur. The patient should immediately be admitted to the ophthalmic ward and intensive antibiotic therapy initiated. At a later date, if an abscess develops or pus becomes localised and points subcutaneously, the lesion should be explored and drained. An X-ray of the paranasal sinuses is indicated in children because sinitis is one of the most common causes.

Acute dacryocystitis.   This condition presents as a tender red swelling of the tear sac, which lies below and medial to the medial palpebral ligament. Watering of the eye and retrograde discharge of pus from either the lower or the upper punctum may be present. These cases should be referred for an ophthalmic opinion and given a prescription for a course of appropriate systemic antibiotics.

Herpes zoster ophthalmicus.   The vesicular lesions are acutely painful in the early disease and postherpetic neuralgia is a common complication. Relief of pain is important and strong analgesia may be required. The eye itself is often involved if the nasociliary branch of the fifth nerve is implicated. This is clinically evident when vesicles are present on the side of the nose. Eye complications include blepharitis, conjunctivitis, keratitis, iridocyclitis, secondary glaucoma, optic neuritis and ophthalmoplegia. If the eye is involved, inpatient treatment is usually necessary in view of the intense swelling of the eye lids which makes instillation of drops and ointment into the eye particularly difficult.

Sudden loss of vision

Sudden loss of vision may be painful or painless, transient or permanent, unilateral or bilateral. The following are the important causes of visual impairment.

Acute closed angle glaucoma

See page 455.

Temporal or giant cell arteritis

Temporal arteritis should be suspected in all elderly patients who present with a sudden loss of vision in one eye. Affected patients frequently complain of loss of weight and malaise, and the ESR may be markedly raised. Loss of vision is secondary to infarction of the distal optic nerve and is clinically apparent as a pale swollen optic disc, often with a few splinter haemorrhages in the papillary region. Temporal arteritis is considered an ophthalmic emergency and immediate admission to the ophthalmic ward is advisable so that the patient can have the diagnosis confirmed and large doses of systemic corticosteroids started. The principal aim of treatment is to prevent involvement of the second eye by the disease process, with total loss of vision (see also Ch. 19).

Optic neuritis and retrobulbar neuritis

This condition is associated with ocular discomfort and tenderness and typically pain is present during ocular movement. Often, however, loss of central visual acuity is the only symptom and sign. If the inflammatory lesion (usually a demyelinating plaque) is placed anteriorly in the optic nerve head, the optic disc may be swollen. However, if the retrobulbar portion of the optic nerve is affected, the optic disc looks normal in the early stages of the disease, although it may become atrophic two or three weeks later. The pupil on the affected side is generally dilated and reacts poorly to direct light. It does, however, retain good consensual reaction. Generally no treatment is necessary and good recovery of visual function can be anticipated. An ophthalmic or neurological opinion, however, should be sought to exclude other conditions that might present with a central scotoma. This condition may be a presenting episode or occur during the natural history of multiple sclerosis.

Central retinal artery occlusion

Occlusion of the central retinal artery causes complete or almost complete painless loss of vision. The common causes are thrombosis or emboli. The pupil on the affected side dilates and does not react to a direct light stimulus (conduction defect). The fundus of the eye is pale, oedematous and demonstrates a 'cherry red' spot at the fovea. Occasionally, if there is severe vascular stasis, movement of the red cell column can be appreciated in the retinal vessels (cattle trucking).

Recovery of vision after a central retinal artery obstruction is unusual. However, if the occlusion is of short duration and caused by an embolus, it may be possible to retrieve some visual acuity by rapidly reducing the intraocular pressure either by massage or paracentesis, thus encouraging an impacted embolus to move into smaller retinal vessels. The patient should therefore be immediately referred to an ophthalmologist.

The A & E doctor should also recognise that the vast majority of emboli arise from the common carotid artery just proximal to its bifurcation into the internal and external carotid arteries. Most obstructions are caused by atheromatous plaques which ulcerate and disseminate small microemboli to the blood vessels of the eye and brain causing attacks of amaurosis fugax and/or transient cerebral ischaemia. Localised atheromatous plaques are amenable to therapy in some circumstances and, if suspected, the patient should be referred to the appropriate specialty.

Central regional vein occlusion

Obstruction of the central retinal vein presents a pathognomonic fundal picture of extensive intraretinal and preretinal haemorrhage, distension of the retinal veins and severe loss of vision. No treatment is available for this condition and the patient should be referred to the next ophthalmic outpatient clinic. Branch retinal vein occlusion with haemorrhage involving the maculae may also present with visual loss.

Vitreous haemorrhage

Severe vitreous haemorrhage may cause sudden loss of vision in one eye. Smaller degrees of haemorrhage, however, are apparent to the patient as multiple floaters or a 'smoke' sensation before the eye. Non-traumatic vitreous haemorrhage should alert the A & E doctor to the presence of a retinal tear, of preretinal neovascularisation which may be secondary to diabetic retinopathy, central or branch retinal vein obstruction or indeed any condition associated with widespread ischaemia. In the absence of retinopathy, any patient with a vitreous haemorrhage should be assumed to have a retinal tear and/or detachment and should be admitted immediately to an ophthalmic ward for bed rest until the vitreous haemorrhage has subsided to a degree which permits clear visualisation and evaluation of the fundus. Vitreous haemorrhage secondary to neovascularisation can be treated by laser photocoagulation and the patient should be referred to an ophthalmic outpatient clinic for immediate attention.

Retinal detachment

Retinal detachments may be preceded by a sensation of flickering lights, which usually indicate the presence of a posterior detachment of the vitreous or multiple floaters which indicate a vitreous haemorrhage. A history of trauma or high myopia may be obtained. If the detachment is substantial, the patient will volunteer a visual field defect; if the macula is involved, there will be a sudden and severe loss of central vision. All patients with retinal detachments require immediate admission to an ophthalmic ward for evaluation prior to surgery.

Migraine

Severe migrainous attacks may be preceded by unusual and alarming visual aura or visual field defects. Both sensations are characteristic and are generally followed by severe headache, nausea and sensory disturbances and the diagnosis is often obvious. The patient should be referred to a neurological outpatient clinic for evaluation and long-term management (see also Ch. 19).

Maculopathies

Painless loss of central vision may be due to a wide variety of conditions which affect the macula. Macular changes are often subtle and involve alterations in both the retinal pigment epithelium and the retinal receptors. They may be associated with accumulation of fluid in the outer retina. The precise diagnosis is often difficult to establish, and requires detailed and sophisticated electrophysiological techniques. There is, however, no emergency with such patients and they should be referred to a routine ophthalmic outpatient clinic.

Toxic retinopathy or optic neuropathy

Certain drugs such as methyl alcohol and quinine can cause sudden loss of vision. A careful history will generally elicit whether toxic substances have been ingested. The treatment is the treatment of poisoning with the drug implicated.

Cortical blindness

Sudden loss of vision affecting one or both eyes may be due to damage to the posterior visual pathway. The most appropriate test is evaluation of visual fields, which will indicate where in the visual pathways the lesion or lesions lie. If both pupils react briskly to light, the lesion either involves the lateral geniculate bodies or is posterior to them. Sudden cortical blindness is generally vascular in nature and usually emergency treatment is of no avail. The patient should be referred for neurological evaluation to exclude a demyelinating disease, a tumour or other clinical entity which may affect the visual pathways.

Functional

Functional loss of vision (hysteria) is relatively common. The most common complaint is of peripheral constriction of visual fields which cannot be accounted for on structural grounds. Patients may be referred to a neurological or psychiatric clinic for evaluation.

Diplopia

Diplopia may be uniocular or binocular. Uniocular diplopia is generally secondary to opacities or irregularities in the media, e.g. cataract, keratoconus, dislocated lens or a tumour or oedema affecting the macula. Such conditions are rarely emergencies and require routine ophthalmoscopic examination and treatment.

Binocular diplopia is either secondary to an abnormality of the third, fourth or sixth cranial nerves or a lesion which restricts ocular movements (e.g. orbital tumour, abscess, endocrine exophthalmos or adhesions). The A & E doctor should be capable of categorising the type of diplopia and referring the patient to an ophthalmic outpatient clinic. Sudden diplopia associated with headache in young individuals should raise the possibility of intracranial aneurysm and the patient should be immediately admitted to hospital.

CONCLUSION

In conclusion, it can be stated that eye trauma and disease form a small but important part of accident and emergency medicine. The doctor in this situation can quite quickly learn to deal with minor trauma, such as lid lacerations and foreign bodies. Major injuries must be recognised so that they can quickly be referred for specialist treatment.

The repeated evaluation of medical eye problems should make examination of both the anterior and posterior segments of the globe familiar procedures. This, in turn, will lead to earlier recognition of many medical and neurological diseases.

FURTHER READING

The unquiet eye: a diagnostic guide 1983 Flaxo Laboratories Greenford, Middlesex

Atlas of ophthalmology Glasspool M G 1982 MTP Press, Lancaster

Modern concepts in ophthalmic casualty management McKinlay R T, Cohen D N 1973 Annals of Ophthalmology 5: 1221–1247

Ophthalmology: principles and concepts, 3rd edn. Newell F W, Ernest J T 1974 C V Mosby, St Louis

Concussive and penetrating injuries of the globe and optic nerve Runyan T E 1975 C V Mosby, St Louis

44

Michael J. Cinnamond and Alan G. Kerr

Ear, nose and throat conditions

INTRODUCTION

Patients frequently present in the A & E department with problems related to their ears, noses or throats. Ear conditions are often accompanied by severe pain; bleeding noses and foreign bodies in the throat are frightening. Unfortunately, many junior staff in A & E departments lack understanding of otolaryngology and tend to refer all cases for specialist care. This is not necessary and many can be dealt with fully without referral to the otolaryngology department.

Although the ability to use a head mirror, or head light, is an asset in that it leaves both hands free, this is not imperative. The list of essential instruments is small: for examination one needs an auriscope, pen torch, tongue depressor, nasal speculum and tuning fork, and much can be achieved with a blunt hook, ear syringe, nasal forceps and suction apparatus.

THE EAR

The auricle and external auditory meatus

There are three common conditions of the auricle and external auditory meatus seen in the A & E department: haematoma auris, lacerations of the auricle and foreign bodies in the meatus.

Haematoma auris

Haematoma auris is a collection of blood deep to the perichondrium of the auricle and results from blows to the ear. Failure to drain the haematoma may result in organisation of the blood clot and the development of an ugly deformity known as 'cauliflower ear' (see p. 410).

The haematoma can be evacuated under local anaesthesia but full sterile precautions must be taken because of the risk of perichondritis, which can lead to even greater deformity. A small incision is made into the most dependent part of the swelling, blood clot is evacuated and a pressure dressing applied. Unless pain or pyrexia suggest the development of infection, the dressing may be left undisturbed for several days. Antibiotics are not required unless infection supervenes

Lacerations of the auricle

Perichondritis is a risk in all lacerations involving the auricle and, therefore, wounds should be thoroughly cleansed and dead tissue excised. It is desirable to retain all viable tissue to minimise the problems of secondary cosmetic surgery.

When lacerations involve the greater part of the circumference of the meatus, there is always the risk of the development of meatal stenosis and the patient should be referred to an otolaryngology department.

Antibiotic treatment is desirable in most cases of severe trauma to the auricle and meatus.

Foreign bodies

Foreign bodies in the ear are found most often in children. Since damage from the foreign body itself is rare compared with damage from clumsy or ill-advised attempts at extraction, it is unwise for those without experience to undertake removal. This need never be rushed and it is essential that all preconditions are met.

First, the patient must be co-operative, quite still and unlikely or unable to move suddenly. If this condition cannot be met it is better to postpone removal and arrange for general anaesthesia.

Secondly, good lighting is essential. A superficially situated foreign body may be removed using direct lighting, but more often a head light, or a mirror with reflected light, will be necessary.

Finally, the correct instruments must be available. A blunt, right-angled probe is usually most satisfactory. It can be passed beyond the foreign body and gently withdrawn. With this method, sudden movement is unlikely to result in anything more serious than scratching of the meatal skin; there is no risk of the foreign body being driven into the middle ear as there is when using forceps. When these conditions cannot be met, the *judicious* use of syringing will sometimes dispose of a foreign body (see note on syringing on p. 463).

After removal it is important to ensure that the tympanic membrane has not been damaged and to check that there is not a second foreign body in the other ear or in the nose. Children with 'glue ear' (see below) are more inclined to interfere with their ears and there is evidence to suggest that the incidence of aural foreign body is higher in such children.

The tympanic membrane

Traumatic perforation

Rupture of the tympanic membrane may result from sudden changes in air pressure, as from a blow on the ear or exposure to blast; from fluids, as in syringing; from injury by solid objects, such as hair clips or sparks of hot metal in welding; or from a fracture involving the base of the skull.

Management. Most traumatic perforations heal spontaneously. The two main factors influencing the prognosis are infection and loss of tissue. The more severe the infection and the greater the loss of tissue, the less likely is the perforation to close spontaneously. The prognosis is best, therefore, with small perforations in uninfected ears.

The main principle of management is to avoid contamination of the middle ear and, therefore, in most cases the best approach is one of inactivity. The ear should not be cleaned out unless there is contaminating material in the meatus or there is evidence of active infection. Systemic antibiotics or antibiotic ear-drops are unnecessary in the absence of overt infection unless there is good reason to believe that the ear has been contaminated. The patient must be advised to keep water out of the ear canal. Cottonwool alone is insufficient; it must be smeared with petroleum jelly to make a watertight seal.

Patients with traumatic perforation of the tympanic membrane should be referred to an otolaryngology clinic.

The inner ear

Inner ear damage may result from abnormal stimulation, barotrauma, head injuries and surgical trauma. Barotrauma and head injuries are dealt with later in the chapter. Surgical trauma to the ear is not relevant to this textbook.

Stimulation injury of the inner ear

Stimulation injury of the inner ear may result from exposure to blast, gunfire or noise.

In blast injury or report trauma the patient may be severely deaf initially with a gradual improvement in hearing with the passage of time. This improvement in hearing often occurs rapidly over the first few hours after the injury. In mild or moderate cases, non-urgent referral to an otolaryngologist is adequate. Where the deafness is severe, urgent referral, probably with admission to hospital, is indicated because of the possibility of helping the deafness by some of the numerous regimens which have been advocated, although not proven to be of value. These include the use of vasodilating drugs, corticosteroids, intravenous low molecular weight dextran, anticoagulants and carbon dioxide inhalations.

Tinnitus is a common complaint in these patients and many require strong and repeated reassurance. The severity of the tinnitus tends to reflect the degree of sensorineural deafness. Tinnitus tends to decrease with the passage of time and even in those cases where it does not disappear entirely, the patient usually comes to terms with it.

Patients with noise-induced deafness should be given a routine appointment to see an otolaryngologist.

Temporal bone fractures

Fractures of the temporal bone are broadly classified into longitudinal and transverse, depending on the relationship of the fracture line to the long axis of the petrous bone. These fractures do not always show on routine skull radiology and often the diagnosis must be made on purely clinical grounds, such as bleeding from the ear or delayed 'bruising' over the mastoid (Battle's sign).

Longitudinal fractures

About 80% of temporal bone fractures are longitudinal and result from blows to the temporal or parietal areas. The fracture line begins in the squamous temporal bone and extends along the roof of the bony external auditory meatus, crossing the roof of the middle ear and running into the petrous temporal bone anterior to the labyrinthine capsule, through the carotid canal to end near the foramen lacerum. As the skin of the external auditory meatus and tympanic membrane are frequently torn, there is usually bleeding from the ear. In the absence of any other obvious cause, bleeding from the ear following a head injury is pathognomonic of a fracture of the base of the skull.

The middle ear is always involved in longitudinal fractures although the conductive component of the deafness is usually mild. Inner ear involvement is usually restricted to high tone sensorineural hearing loss. Facial nerve injuries are uncommon and when they occur are usually delayed in onset.

Transverse fractures

Transverse fractures, resulting from frontal or occipital blows, occur in approximately 20% of temporal bone fractures. The fracture line extends transversely across the petrous bone, passing through the vestibule of the inner ear. In a pure transverse fracture there is blood in the middle ear behind an intact tympanic membrane. Consequently, there is no bleeding from the ear. There is usually complete and permanent sensorineural deafness on the affected side, accompanied by tinnitus. As there is also severe damage to the vestibular apparatus in the inner ear on the affected side, the patient experiences marked rotatory vertigo with nausea and vomiting. Horizontal nystagmus is present, with the fast component towards the contralateral ear. Facial nerve injuries occur in about 50% of these patients and the onset is frequently immediate.

Management of temporal bone fractures.   Obviously the management of the head injury is the most immediate and important aspect of these cases. From the otological view point, three things must be established when the patient is first seen. Is there any leakage of cerebrospinal fluid from the meatus? Is there any nystagmus? Is the facial nerve functioning normally?

In uncomplicated cases of leakage of cerebrospinal fluid from the meatus, no treatment is required. Where the risks of ascending infection are deemed to be high, however, such as in the presence of pre-existing otitis media or otitis externa, a broad-spectrum antibiotic should be used. Nystagmus suggests severe vestibular damage and a record of its presence or absence at the time of admission can be of considerable significance in subsequent management and litigation. The presence of an immediate facial paralysis indicates direct damage to the nerve that will probably require early surgical attention.

In view of the importance of avoiding the introduction of infection into the middle ear, it is better to leave untouched any blood clot in the external meatus unless there is evidence of active infection.

The deafness and dizziness resulting from temporal bone fractures can be investigated by an otolaryngologist after the patient has recovered from the acute effects of the injury. However, when there is facial paralysis, especially if it was known on admission, it is important to seek the opinion of an otolaryngologist within 24 hours for exploration of the nerve to be considered.

Otitic barotrauma

Otitic barotrauma (aerotitis) results from the development of a pressure difference between the middle ear and the environment. This may occur following flying, during diving or in a hyperbaric chamber.

Otitic barotrauma is seen most often following air travel. The patient is aware of impaired hearing and discomfort, often increasing to severe pain. The tympanic membrane becomes retracted, the middle ear mucosa oedematous, and there is a transudate of fluid into the middle ear. Tinnitus may also be present.

The negative pressure in the middle ear will be reduced by the production of the transudate and in a matter of hours the pain is replaced by discomfort, although the deafness persists or may even increase. The deafness resulting from the fluid is always conductive in nature but, in addition, sensorineural hearing loss has, very occasionally, been reported.

Management.   Usually the pain is decreasing in severity by the time the patient reaches the hospital. Although immediate relief can be given simply by puncturing the tympanic membrane with a hypodermic needle to relieve the negative pressure, this should be done only by an experienced otolaryngologist. If there is persistent severe pain, urgent referral to an otolaryngologist is indicated.

Underwater divers can experience the same pressure difficulties as those who fly, although immediate return to the surface usually eliminates the problem. However, vertigo, which is rare in aerotitis, is not uncommon among divers and specialist investigation is required. (For further discussion of barotrauma see Ch. 28, p. 302).

Pain in the ear (otalgia)

Pain in the ear can be primary, when the lesion is in the ear itself, or secondary, when the lesion is elsewhere and the pain is referred to the ear. Up to 50% of cases of otalgia are referred in type.

In the vast majority of patients with primary otalgia the cause is readily seen on examination of the ear. Most of these can be diagnosed and treated without specialist training and do not require referral to an otolaryngologist.

In secondary otalgia the ear is usually normal on examination; the cause must be sought elsewhere and specialist examination is often required to exclude serious underlying disease such as pharyngeal or laryngeal cancer. In view of the complicated nerve supply to the ear, with contributions from the fifth, seventh, ninth and tenth cranial nerves and the cervical plexus, the upper air and food passages need to be examined in these cases.

Primary otalgia

External otitis.   External otitis is a common condition which usually begins with itching in the external auditory meatus, often associated with a scanty serous discharge. However, in severe cases, the itching rapidly gives way to pain, often with a change in the nature of the discharge from serous to purulent and sometimes with the development of a mild degree of conductive deafness due to occlusion of the meatus. Occasionally there is no history of itching and the first complaint is of pain in the ear. A boil in the external auditory meatus may occur in association with external otitis or as an isolated condition. Because of the close attachment of the skin to the underlying perichondrium and periosteum of the ear canal, there is little room for inflammatory swelling and the ear may become extremely painful.

The diagnosis is usually straightforward. A furuncle occurs in the outer third or hair-bearing area of the external ear canal and can usually be seen. In diffuse external otitis the whole ear canal is inflamed and oedematous and the inflammation may well spread out onto the concha. Usually the discharge is scanty. Movements of the ear canal will be painful so that gentle traction on the auricle produces pain, as does opening and closing of the mouth. The tympanic membrane, if it can be seen, will be normal or simply injected. Sometimes a diagnostic problem arises when the meatus is closed by oedema and discharge so that the tympanic membrane cannot be seen. In these cases there is the possibility of an underlying otitis media and prompt referral to an otolaryngologist is required.

Management.   Acute external otitis usually responds promptly to treatment. Simple analgesics will be required to provide symptomatic relief of the pain. If the condition is severe with inflammation extending onto the concha and the involvement of pre- or postauricular lymph nodes, a wide-spectrum systemic antibiotic such as ampicillin should be prescribed. Usually, however, local treatment is adequate for this condition. The patient should be advised to clean out the ear with cotton buds, as best he can, and instil antibiotic/anti-inflammatory drops twice daily. The most commonly used drops contain neomycin and hydrocortisone. The patient must be advised to keep water out of the ears for some months after the attack.

If the condition does not settle within a week or 10 days, or if there have been many previous attacks, the patient should be referred to an otolaryngologist.

Viral infections of the outer ear

Viral infections may result in severe otalgia due to involvement of the outer ear. This occurs in bullous myringitis, frequently due to the influenza virus, and in herpes zoster oticus due to the zoster virus. In bullous myringitis there are blood-filled vesicles on the tympanic membrane. The treatment of this condition is purely symptomatic; rupturing of the vesicles does not relieve the pain. Similar bullae are sometimes seen in the early stages of acute otitis media and, for this reason, the ear should be examined again within 24 hours to confirm the diagnosis.

In herpes zoster oticus the pain is often accompanied by or followed by, facial paralysis sometimes associated with deafness and dizziness the (Ramsey Hunt Syndrome). While the vesicles are most often seen on the ear-drum or in the skin of the ear canal or concha, they may also be seen on the mucosa of the soft palate or side of the mouth, or on the skin of the scalp or neck. There is evidence that acyclovir improves the prognosis in these cases and they should be referred without delay to an otolaryngologist.

Middle ear

Pain from the middle ear may accompany the development of negative pressure, infections or malignant disease. The pain due to negative pressure usually lasts only for a matter of hours because a transudate develops which relieves the pain by filling the vacuum. However, in some of these cases, the condition progresses to an acute suppurative otitis media.

Suppurative otitis media. Middle ear infections can be classified broadly as acute or chronic.

Acute otitis media is common in children and is frequently associated with an upper respiratory tract infection. This develops rapidly with increasing pain over a matter of hours and is associated with pyrexia and malaise. There is an associated conductive deafness and throbbing tinnitus but, it is rare for children to complain of these symptoms and, even in adults, pain is usually the dominant feature.

The findings on examination depend on the stage of the disease. Initially there may simply be a retracted tympanic membrane. There is a progression in stages through an intensely congested and thickened membrane, a full bulging membrane and, in some

cases, a perforation with a pulsating purulent discharge. Because the pain is due largely to pressure in the middle ear, perforation of the tympanic membrane results in a dramatic improvement in the pain and, in addition, a fall in temperature.

Acute otitis media is a common condition which ought to be treated in most cases without any specialist help. It should be emphasised that ear-drops have little or no place in the management. A systemic antibiotic, such as ampicillin, is adequate for most cases. However, because the infection drains through the eustachian tube, it is desirable to treat nasal infection and obstruction where this is present. In the past it has been considered important to attempt to decongest the eustachian tube even in the absence of nasal obstruction. However, there is increasing evidence that neither local nor systemic decongestants influence the outcome.

It is essential that the patient is referred to the care of his general practitioner to ensure that the tympanic membrane and the hearing return to normal. Failure of complete resolution of acute otitis media in children is a cause of secretory otitis media ('glue ear').

Acute mastoiditis

Acute otitis media usually involves the whole middle ear cleft but when the infection progresses to osteitis, acute mastoiditis is said to be present. Initially there is an increase in the clinical features of pain and pyrexia. The mastoid area becomes tender, eventually becoming red and oedematous as the outer plate of bone is eroded (Fig. 44.1). Acute mastoiditis does not occur without a preceding middle ear infection.

These patients should be referred immediately to an otolaryngologist.

Chronic suppurative otitis media

Uncomplicated chronic suppurative otitis media is usually painless

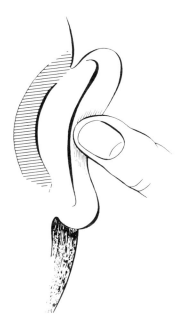

Fig. 44.1 Area of tenderness behind the auricle in acute mastoiditis.

and is characterised by long-standing discharge associated with hearing loss. The most common complication is the development of acute or chronic infection with pain in the ear and an increase in the volume of discharge. However, the development of pain in chronic otitis media is an ominous sign, which may herald intracranial infection for which urgent treatment is required. This is an especial risk in the presence of a cholesteatoma. The importance of urgent referral to an otolaryngologist cannot be overemphasised when pain develops in long-standing chronic suppurative otitis media.

Malignant disease of the ear

Malignant disease of the middle ear or external auditory meatus is rare. Most cases develop in ears with a long-standing history of middle ear infection and pain is a common manifestation. Once again, urgent referral to an otolaryngologist is indicated.

Referred pain in the ear

Pain referred to the ear is common and the external auditory meatus and tympanic membrane are usually normal in appearance. It is common practice, although completely valueless and to be condemned, to prescribe ear-drops for patients with referred pain.

Dental

The commonest causes of pain referred to the ear are in the teeth or temporomandibular joint. Usually dental caries is obvious and the patient should be referred to a dentist. Pain secondary to temporomandibular joint dysfunction is not quite so obvious. There is often a history, if sought, of dental work having been done in the previous month or two. A slightly high dental filling can upset normal occlusion and precipitate temporomandibular joint dysfunction. The pain in these cases takes the form of a vague ache, usually (but not always) maximal just in front of the ear, spreading into the lower jaw or up into the temple. It is aggravated by eating. Many of the patients and their spouses will be aware of grinding their teeth. There is tenderness, often severe, over the temporomandibular joint. In addition, there are often tender areas in the muscles of mastication.

Instruction in avoiding grinding the teeth and explanation of the cause of the symptoms is often sufficient to overcome the pain but referral to the patient's dentist or a specialist in dental prosthetics may be required.

Glossopharyngeal neuralgia

Glossopharyngeal neuralgia is a rare condition which may cause a person to attend at the A & E department, often with a history of having been given drops for undiagnosed ear pain. The symptoms are dominated by short-lived shooting and extremely severe pain in the ear extending into the throat. The pain may be precipitated by moving the lower jaw or by swallowing. In a full-blown case the patient is the picture of misery. He is loath to talk and even more loath to swallow, and consequently may have a mouth full of saliva. Otherwise, examination is normal. The treatment is similar to that of trigeminal neuralgia, with the prescription of carbamazepine (Tegretol).

Malignant disease of the throat

One of the presenting features of malignant disease of the throat is referred pain to the ear. The neoplasm may be in the postnasal space, the pharynx, the tonsil, the base of the tongue, the hypopharynx or the larynx. Sometimes the pain, usually in the form of a dull ache, is limited to the ear without any throat symptoms. The diagnosis may be obvious on direct examination of the throat but often requires mirror examination. Any undiagnosed earache, especially in the elderly, must be referred to an otolaryngologist to exclude underlying malignant disease.

Bleeding from the ear

Bleeding from the ear usually causes alarm in the patient and prompt attendance at the nearest A & E department. When it is due to trauma, there will be a history of injury, and the management will depend on the cause and the other findings.

Other than trauma, the most common cause is granulation tissue due to chronic otitis media, especially where there is an underlying cholesteatoma. Most of these cases will require specialist care and routine referral to an otolaryngologist is indicated. It is rare for the amount of bleeding to be of any serious significance but in these cases emergency referral to the otolaryngology department must be undertaken.

Sudden deafness

Wax

Sudden deafness is almost always unilateral and the serious causes are always sensorineural. However, wax in the external auditory meatus may swell — usually following exposure to water — and occlude the meatus, causing sudden conductive deafness. In these cases the diagnosis is obvious and the treatment is straightforward. Syringing the ear restores the hearing immediately.

The syringing of ears is a routine procedure in general practice. There is no necessity to refer these patients to the otolaryngology department and it will rarely be performed in A & E departments. In those few cases where syringing *is* to be done, however, it is important to establish that there is no history of a persistent perforation, which is a contraindication to the procedure. The irrigating solution — tap water or normal saline — should be at body temperature to avoid stimulating the vestibular apparatus and should be directed along the posterior wall of the external auditory meatus (Fig. 44.2).

Sensorineural deafness

Sudden sensorineural deafness may be of viral, vascular, traumatic

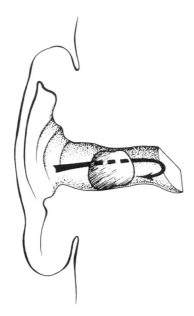

Fig. 44.2 Syringing wax or a foreign body from an ear.

or toxic aetiology. In many cases there will be an obvious history of preceding viral illness or trauma such as exposure to noise or blast, or pressure changes as in the skin-diving and strenuous exertion. When it is due to ototoxic drugs, both ears are usually affected. Occasionally an acoustic neuroma presents with sudden onset of unilateral deafness.

There is considerable doubt as to whether or not treatment influences the course of the deafness but most otologists feel constrained to treat these patients promptly and energetically. The current management often requires admission to hospital. For this reason, emergency referral to an otolaryngologist is recommended in all these cases.

Functional deafness

The malingerer may try to simulate unilateral deafness but the hysterical patient usually complains of bilateral deafness. Often, hysterical deafness is profound and the most striking feature is the lack of concern about what would be seen as a tragedy to the normal person. Referral should be to an otolaryngologist in the first instance to confirm that there is no organic cause. The hysterical patient will require psychiatric treatment.

Vertigo

Broadly speaking, patients with vertigo can be divided into two distinct groups: those with and those without additional neurological symptoms or signs other than deafness. When neurological aspects are present, referral should be to a neurologist. Otherwise, it is probable that any severe rotatory vertigo is of labyrinthine origin and the patient should be referred to an otolaryngologist. Mild cases may be referred to their general practitioner.

Many cases of labyrinthine vertigo are episodic in nature, the attacks rarely lasting more than a few hours. In a patient presenting with episodic vertigo, the best management is the prescription of a labyrinthine sedative drug such as cyclizine (Valoid), by injection, accompanied by bed rest. The patient can then be referred to an otolaryngologist when the acute attack has resolved. There is little advantage in referring the patient during the acute attack, apart from the opportunity of observing any nystagmus.

An acute destructive lesion of the vestibular labyrinth, resulting from trauma, infection (either viral or bacterial) or vascular disturbance, causes sudden failure of one labyrinth with acute vertigo accompanied by nausea and vomiting. Horizontal nystagmus is usually present with the quick phase towards the contralateral ear. In these cases the vertigo will persist for days or longer and it will be weeks or months before the patient is able to go out and about unaided. When the acute attack does not resolve in a matter of hours, referral to an otolaryngologist is indicated. In most cases the treatment is purely symptomatic but, when there is underlying chronic suppurative middle ear disease, urgent exploration and drainage of the middle ear and mastoid may be required.

There are many other forms of vertigo which may present at the A & E department but, in nearly every instance, there will be a history of previous episodes and referral to an otolaryngologist is the suggested management. There is one important form of vertigo which is only rarely seen in the A & E department but which should be borne in mind. This is in the patient who is receiving injections or irrigations of ototoxic drugs, such as gentamicin or neomycin, as an outpatient. He will present with vague but increasing unsteadiness and the first and the most important step in these cases is to discontinue the use of these drugs.

FACIAL PARALYSIS

As with vertigo, facial paralysis due to a central neurological lesion is usually accompanied by other obvious neurological symptoms and signs. The most common is the facial paralysis associated with hemiplegia. An upper motor neurone paralysis usually affects only the lower face because of the bilateral representation of the forehead in the central nervous system. However, in the absence of any other neurological signs, facial paralysis usually indicates a lesion of the facial nerve in its course through the temporal bone.

Facial paralysis may be due to trauma, inflammation or malignant disease, or may be idiopathic.

Traumatic facial paralysis

In these cases there will be a history of trauma. The paralysis may be immediate in onset, or delayed. Paralysis of immediate onset indicates either tearing or entrapment of the facial nerve. Cases of immediate traumatic facial paralysis should be surgically explored and, therefore, urgent referral to an otolaryngologist is indicated.

In delayed traumatic paralysis the onset is usually between the fifth and the tenth day. The prognosis in these cases is very much better but the management is best undertaken by an otolaryngologist.

Inflammatory facial paralysis

Facial paralysis due to inflammatory lesions may be viral or bacterial. Viral paralysis results from herpes zoster infection, frequently known as the Ramsay Hunt syndrome. In these cases the facial paralysis is usually accompanied by pain in the ear or face and the development of herpes zoster vesicles. There may be involvement of hearing and balance. These cases should be referred urgently to an otolaryngologist. Treatment with acyclovir is recommended.

Bacterial facial paralysis is almost always a complication of otitis media. While it can occur in acute otitis media, it is more common in chronic otitis media in the presence of a cholesteatoma. Emergency admission to the otolaryngology department is required as surgical exploration will probably be necessary.

Idiopathic facial paralysis (Bell's palsy)

This is probably the commonest cause of facial paralysis in patients presenting to the A & E department. The patient may have had some pain in or about the ear for a few days before the abrupt onset of facial weakness, which usually becomes maximal in 24–48 hours. It may amount only to a slight facial asymmetry or to complete paralysis associated with inability to close the eye properly and difficulty with eating and drinking. Diabetes and hypertension should be excluded in the general examination. Spontaneous and complete recovery is the rule when the paralysis remains incomplete, but a poor prognosis may accompany a complete paralysis, especially if there is marked pain or the patient is elderly. In cases of complete paralysis the prognosis is assessed on the basis of the response of the facial nerve to electrical stimulation.

There is continued controversy about the value of various treatments, which include the administration of steroids and surgical decompression of the facial nerve. Some experts recommend that all patients seen within 2 days of the onset should have a course of prednisone, starting with 80 mg daily for 5 days and tapering the dose off over the next 4 days. All cases of facial palsy should be referred promptly to an otolaryngologist for diagnosis, investigation and management because the diagnosis 'idiopathic' can be made only after exclusion of other possible causes, such as cholesteatoma, and this requires the expertise of an otolaryngologist.

THE NOSE

Examination

Whilst most doctors in training are taught the use of the auriscope, few indeed ever master the art of using the head mirror, much less the use of the nasal speculum and nasopharyngeal mirrors. Although we strongly recommend that every doctor who works

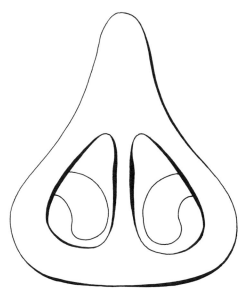

Fig. 44.3 Examination of the nose.

in an A & E department should be able to use these instruments, much valuable information can be gleaned with the aid of a pen torch alone.

To examine the interior of the nose, lift the nasal tip with the thumb, pressing inwards, illuminating the interior with a pen torch held as close as practicable to the axis of your eyes. In this way it is possible to see the anterior ends of the inferior turbinates and the anterior portion of the nasal septum (Fig. 44.3). By packing the nose with either 1.25 cm (0.5 inch) ribbon gauze or elongated pledgets of cotton wool, wrung out in an equal parts mixture of 4% lignocaine and 1:1000 adrenaline, it is possible, by shrinkage of the nasal mucosa, to see at least to the midpoint of the nasal cavity and often beyond.

Nasal trauma

It has been said that the nose is the most outstanding feature of the face — this is obviously more true for some faces than for others! However, by virtue of its outstanding position, the external nose is particularly susceptible to trauma (either accidental or intentional).

Lacerations

Lacerations of the nose should be treated with the same care as lacerations elsewhere on the face — perhaps more so because many people are peculiarly conscious of the appearance of their noses.

Nasal bone fracture

This is not always obvious. The nasal bones, particularly in children, may not be displaced by a force sufficient to fracture them. By very gentle palpation of the nose it is often possible to elicit slight 'give' in the nasal bones, sometimes accompanied by a sensation of crepitus. Remember that displacement of the external nose does not always imply a fracture of the nasal bones: deviation of the septum and fracture of the nasal cartilages may also cause external nasal deformity. The best method of detecting minor degrees of nasal bone displacement is to stand behind the sitting patient and look down his nose from above (Fig. 44.4). Minor degrees of deformity may be masked by overlying oedema and bruising, and it is often wise to arrange for review of such a patient.

X-ray examination of the nasal bones is of no value clinically and does not assist in the management of these injuries. There are, however, two associated injuries which must be excluded and where X-ray examination is essential. These are fractures of the other facial bones and cerebrospinal fluid rhinorrhoea due to fractures involving the anterior cranial fossa. These two conditions are dealt with fully in Chapters 14 and 42.

In primary management of nasal bone fractures, consideration must be given to the following categories:

1. Obvious displacement of the external nose with misalignment of the nasal bones to one side, or depression of the nasal bridge. These cases should be referred to the next otolaryngology clinic, preferably the following day and certainly no later than 10 days from the date of injury. Where the injury is more than 10 days old, the nasal bones are likely to have become fixed, making subsequent reduction of the fracture difficult or impossible.

2. Gross swelling of the nasal tissues obscuring the true shape of the nose. These patients should be advised to apply icebags or cold compresses frequently to the nose and should be referred to the otolarngology clinic in two to three days time for further assessment.

3. Obvious fracture of the nasal bones but with no displacement. Having ascertained that there is no septal deformity (see below) these patients can be reassured that the nasal bone fracture will heal rapidly and spontaneously within 10–14 days. Any pain or tenderness remaining in the nose after this time will eventually settle.

4. Very recent fracture. If the patient is particularly stoical (or especially where he or she is partially anaesthetised by alcohol), and where the injury is no more than a few hours old, it is sometimes possible to achieve a satisfactory (and satisfying) reduction of the fracture by applying steady, firm pressure, with the thumbs, to the outwardly displaced nasal bone. There will often be a sharp click and the nasal bone will snap back into position. A word of warning, however, choose your patient carefully and do not try too hard or you may acquire a fractured nose yourself!

Nasal cavity

It is mandatory that every patient receiving a nasal injury should have the interior of the nose examined to rule out the presence of a nasal septal deformity.

Uncomplicated fracture or deviation of the nasal septum does not require any immediate or emergency treatment but the patient should be referred to an otolaryngology clinic.

In those cases, however, where a nasal septal haematoma or abscess is present, or even suspected, the patient should be immediately referred to the otolaryngology department for further management. Such patients are recognised by their complaint of gross nasal obstruction, often accompanied by pain in the nose and forehead, and by the finding on examination of a boggy inflamed swelling of the septum to one or both sides (Fig. 44.5).

Failure to manage this condition correctly may lead to dissolution of the septal cartilage, with subsequent falling in of the nasal dorsum leading to a characteristic and ugly deformity known as saddle nose (Fig. 44.6).

Nasal foreign bodies

As with aural foreign bodies, these are much more common in

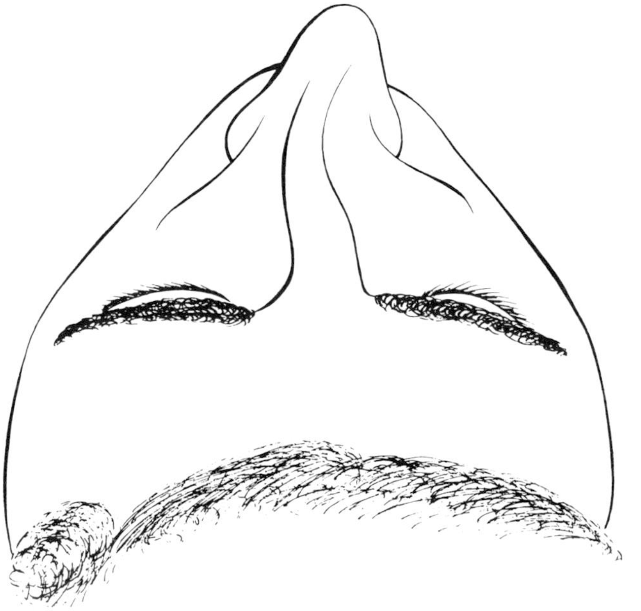

Fig. 44.4 Detection of minor degrees of nasal bone displacement.

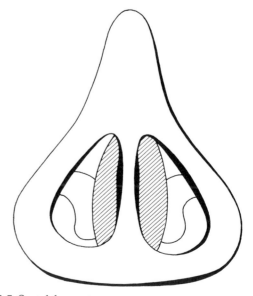

Fig. 44.5 Septal haematoma.

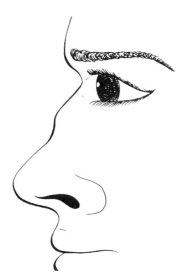

Fig. 44.6 Saddlenose.

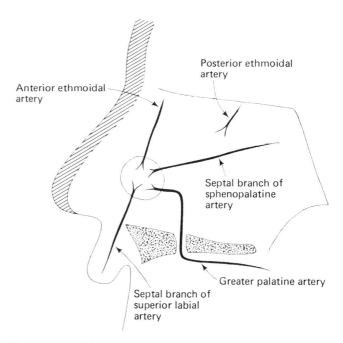

Fig. 44.7 Little's area.

children. Just about everything that will fit into the nasal cavity has been placed there at one time or another! It is convenient, however, to consider two classes of foreign body:

1. Soft and often porous materials quickly become infected, leading to a characteristic foul-smelling unilateral nasal discharge. The commoner materials here are bits of rolled up tissue paper or pieces of foam rubber or plastic. Examination of the nose will reveal an obstructing mass hidden by exudate.

2. Hard, smooth surfaced objects. These do not become infected but will often lead to a local tissue reaction in the nasal cavity with much production of mucus. Common examples are pieces of stone, plastic or beads. In these cases, the foreign body itself is usually fairly easily seen on examination.

Management

Remember that the first attempt at removal of a nasal foreign body in a distraught child is the one most likely to succeed without recourse to general anaesthesia. Forcible nose blowing may, on occasion, be effective, but otherwise, unless the foreign body is very easily seen and grasped, do not attempt removal in the A & E department; instead refer the child directly to the otolaryngology department. Foreign bodies in the nose may become dislodged posteriorly and be inhaled, constituting a definite risk to the child; all such cases, therefore, should be referred immediately rather than waiting until the following morning.

Epistaxis

The nasal mucosa is liberally supplied with blood from many different sources. Most of the supplying vessels form an anastomosis on each side of the anterior portion of the nasal septum in an area known as Little's area (Fig. 44.7). The vast majority of nasal bleeds, especially in children and young adults, occur from this site. In the elderly, however, the bleeding is more often from the

posterior regions of the nasal cavities and is, hence, more difficult to deal with. Remember that, although most cases of epistaxis are minor in nature and of little consequence, some nasal bleeding may be catastrophic and life-threatening. Do not, therefore, dismiss epistaxis as a trivial complaint.

Observe or ask the patient which side has been bleeding. Enquire about the degree of blood loss and whether or not this has been a recurrent problem. Do not forget that epistaxis is sometimes a sign of more generalised disease, such as hypertension or a haematological disorder.

Management

First aid.   Sit the patient up and leaning slightly forwards so that blood will flow from the front of the nose rather than down the back. Apply even and firm pressure to the anterior nasal septum by pinching the nostrils closed between thumb and forefinger, and keep the pressure on for several minutes. Cold compresses to the nasal bridge sometimes result in reflex vasoconstriction and may be of additional value.

If the bleeding continues or restarts following this, pack the nose gently with 1.25 cm (0.5 inch) ribbon gauze or pledgets of cotton wool, soaked in 4% lignocaine and 1:1000 adrenaline mixture. Leave these in for 5 minutes and remove. Inspection of the nasal cavity may then reveal an obvious bleeding point or dilated vessel, particularly in Little's area. In children, the vessel should be cauterized by the application, for 10–15 seconds, of either a stick tipped with fused, solid silver nitrate, or a small pledget of cotton wool wrung out in 40% silver nitrate solution. In adults the hot wire cautery may be used instead.

If the bleeding point cannot be seen and bleeding continues then the nose should be firmly packed using 1.25 cm (0.5 inch) ribbon gauze. Do not use the lignocaine/adrenaline mixture for this; the gauze will quickly dry out and become adherent to the nasal mucosa, causing fresh bleeding on removal of the pack. Rather, soak the ribbon gauze in an oily paste such as bismuth iodoform paraffin paste (BIPP). It is very undesirable that a patient with a nasal pack in situ should be allowed to go home; the posterior portion of the pack, particularly if inexpertly applied, may slip over the soft palate and be inhaled.

The proper technique of nasal packing is to build up successive layers of pack from the base to the roof of the nasal cavity (Fig. 44.8). Do not try to pack too far back in the nose: 6–7 cm is far enough in most adults, because the pack which is too far back is liable to become dislodged with movement of the soft palate. Fortunately, children's noses rarely need to be packed. If anterior nasal packing does not control the bleeding, contact the otolaryngology department immediately.

Headache

Headache is probably the commonest symptom in medicine and sinus headache the most misapplied diagnosis. Frontal pain, especially, is prone to be wrongly designated as being due to sinusitis whereas, in fact, most frontal headaches are due to migraine or tension. Headache, of any sort, due to sinus disease is relatively rare.

Headache is dealt with fully in Ch. 17.

Facial pain

Like headache, facial pain often forms a trap for the unwary (or uninformed) diagnostician. Many doctors overlook the fact that

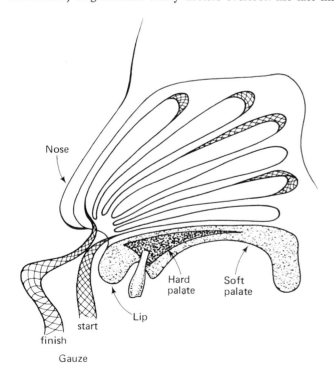

Fig. 44.8 Packing the nasal cavity.

a considerable proportion of cases of facial pain are due to dental disease. It is imperative, therefore, that a careful examination of the teeth, including percussion, should be carried out in every patient complaining of facial pain. Do not forget that even the edentulous patient may have retained root fragments which can give rise to trouble.

The other causes of facial pain are many and varied. The A & E doctor can best deal with these cases by sorting out those requiring emergency treatment, those requiring admission because of the severity of the pain and those which can be dealt with by simple means.

Acute infections of the nose and sinuses

Most infections of the nasal cavities, such as acute coryza, are of a relatively minor nature and do not require any emergency management.

Nasal furuncle

As with the previously described aural furuncle, furunculosis occurring in the nasal vestibule gives rise to intense pain and discomfort. The patient must be warned not to attempt to squeeze the furuncle lest infective thrombi are liberated into the angular vein, resulting in cavernous sinus thrombosis. Treatment consists of orally administered cloxacillin or flucloxacillin, and mild analgesics.

Acute frontal sinusitis

This usually follows an upper respiratory tract infection and is characterised by severe frontal headache, often periodic in nature, tending to increase in severity up to mid-day and then easing off towards evening. It is usually made worse by stooping. Marked tenderness is always present on applying pressure to the floor of the sinuses (i.e. the orbital roof, medial to the supraorbital notch) and on percussion over the anterior wall. Oedema and inflammation may occur around the eyebrow and upper eyelid. Pus may be noted in the nose. X-rays of the sinuses may confirm the diagnosis, often revealing the presence of a concomitant maxillary sinusitis.

Management. The risk of a serious complication, such as osteomyelitis, meningitis or frontal lobe abscess, is high and most patients should be admitted to the otolaryngology ward. Treatment consists of the administration of appropriate antibiotics, in high doses and preferably by the intravenous route, plus nasal decongestants, both topical and systemic.

Acute maxillary sinusitis

This also usually follows an upper respiratory tract infection, but may occasionally be of dental origin, arising from an apical root abscess or following dental extraction. Pain may be felt in the cheek but is more often referred to the frontal region or to the upper teeth. There may be tenderness over the cheek but swelling and inflammation are rarely present: the latter are much more likely to be due to dental disease or neoplasia affecting the sinus. The presence of a fluid level, on straight and tilted plain radiographs, or opacity of the maxillary antrum, will confirm the diagnosis.

Management. Treatment is commenced with antibiotic and both topical and systemic nasal decongestants to promote drainage. Rarely, the patient may require admission and surgical drainage of the sinus.

THE THROAT

Acute laryngeal obstruction

This is dealt with in Ch. 10 (p. 118).

Laryngeal trauma

Trauma to the larynx may be caused by external or internal injury.

External injury

Where the cause is external the larynx may be the sole organ injured, as in hockey stick injuries, or may be but a part of the total injury, as in road traffic accidents.

In severe cases the laryngeal injury will be obvious and life threatening. It may be found impossible to pass an endotracheal tube because of disruption of the larynx, and emergency tracheotomy will then be required to secure the patient's airway. In less severe cases the laryngeal injury may be overlooked owing to other severe injuries elsewhere. In such circumstances, it should be borne in mind that increasing laryngeal oedema and haematoma formation may gradually but seriously compromise the patient's airway. In addition, the laryngeal injuries may be compounded by passage of an endotracheal tube for anaesthesia, necessitated by the patient's other injuries.

In the milder cases, it may be sufficient to observe the patient in hospital for 24 hours to ensure that the airway remains satisfactory. Steroids may help to reduce glottic oedema, thus obviating the need for more drastic action. In all cases where there has been gross disruption of the larynx, the patient should be referred, as soon as possible, to the otolaryngology department for further assessment. Failure to do this may result in subsequent total laryngectomy and a permanent tracheostomy.

Internal injury

Internal injury to the larynx may arise as a result of the accidental ingestion of strong acid or alkali, the aspiration of hot gas or liquid, or the inhalation of a foreign body.

Corrosive poisoning

This is dealt with in Ch. 16.

Foreign bodies

Airway — see p. 118.

Digestive tract

Pharyngeal and oesophageal foreign bodies do not usually present in a life-threatening fashion but must, nonetheless, be regarded as potentially serious in nature. In young children especially, a foreign body impacting in the upper oesophagus may compress the relatively soft trachea from behind, leading to obstruction of the airway. The cricopharyngeal sphincter is the narrowest point in the digestive tract and any foreign body which passes through the sphincter, unless it has sharp points or is irregularly shaped, will usually pass on into the stomach and be voided in the faeces some days later.

All patients who give a history of ingestion of a foreign body should have anteroposterior and lateral plain X-ray examination of the chest and upper abdomen carried out. Where ingestion has taken place very recently and a smooth foreign body (such as a coin) has been observed, at the first X-ray examination, to be in the pharynx or oesophagus, it is worth waiting for an hour and then repeating the radiographic examination as the foreign body may have, meanwhile, moved on into the stomach. Fish bones often stick in the tonsil crypts or into the base of the tongue and can be removed directly. In many instances, pointed foreign bodies, particularly bones, will scratch the pharyngeal or oesophageal mucosa, giving rise to a feeling that the foreign body is still present, even though the bone itself has passed on into the stomach. Despite this, however, all patients who give a history of having ingested a foreign body, unless it is definitely in the stomach, should be referred to the otolaryngology department without delay.

Acute infections of the throat

Acute throat infections presenting in the A & E department vary from trivial cases of pharyngitis to life-threatening emergencies such as epiglottitis. Management of the more severe causes only will be given here.

Ludwig's angina

Ludwig's angina is a severe form of acute non-specific pharyngitis in which there is brawny swelling of the floor of the mouth, sometimes leading to airway obstruction (see Ch. 42). Such patients should be admitted for observation and treatment with appropriate antibiotics.

Acute tonsillitis

Acute tonsillitis is characterised by severe pain in the region of the angles of the jaw associated with dysphagia and a peculiar 'plummy' character to the voice. Inspection of the throat will reveal a bilaterally symmetrical enlargement of the tonsils with acute inflammation. There will often be small flecks of pus on the surface of the tonsil (follicular tonsillitis) and in severe cases, particularly in the young child, the tonsils may meet in the midline, causing respiratory embarrassment.

Management. In small children (up to about the age of 5 years) the responsible organism is usually *Haemophilus influenzae*, while in older children and adults the *Pneumococcus* or haemolytic *Streptococcus* is more often found. In small children, therefore, ampicillin is the antibiotic of choice, whilst older children and adults are best treated with penicillin V or G.

In severe cases, treatment should be commenced with parenterally administered antibiotic; such patients are best dealt with by admission to either an isolation ward or infectious diseases unit.

Peritonsillar abscess

Acute peritonsillitis or peritonsillar abscess (quinsy) is an acute bacterial infection of the tissues surrounding the tonsil. It normally follows an acute tonsillitis but is almost always unilateral. The patient will complain of severe or agonising pain in the region of one or other angle of the jaw, often with radiation of the pain into the ipsilateral ear. He or she will usually be almost totally dysphagic, unable even to swallow his or her own saliva, and there is often marked trismus, making examination of the mouth difficult or impossible. The appearance of the mouth and pharynx is typical, with unilateral swelling of the soft palate and faucial pillars. The tonsil will appear to be grossly enlarged and the swollen uvula will be deviated and pointing to the opposite tonsil (Fig. 44.9).

Management. If pus is present then immediate relief may be afforded to the patient by making a stab incision, with a guarded scalpel, either at the site of maximal swelling or at a point midway between the third upper molar tooth and the base of the uvula.

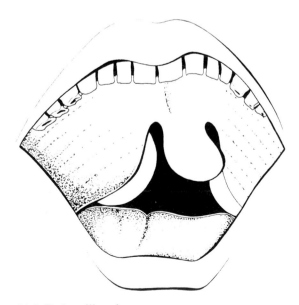

Fig. 44.9 Peritonsillar abscess.

The patient should be sitting up during this procedure so that blood and pus, if released, can be spat out easily. Where actual pus formation has not occurred, i.e. (peritonsillitis), surgical intervention will not be necessary. Whether or not an abscess is present, the patient should be started on large doses of parenterally administered penicillin and, in most instances, admitted to an isolation ward or an infectious diseases unit. Subsequently, such cases should be referred to the otolaryngology department for further management.

Acute retropharyngeal abscess

Acute retropharyngeal abscess is caused by suppuration in the retropharyngeal lymph nodes, which become infected from the nasopharynx or oropharynx. Occasionally the abscess may arise following penetration of the posterior pharyngeal wall by a sharp foreign body. It occurs almost exclusively in small children and presents as a boggy, red, obstructive swelling of the posterior pharyngeal wall. Feeding and breathing difficulties may ensue, and rapid progress to complete respiratory obstruction is not uncommon.

Management. Incision and drainage of such an abscess should not be attempted by the inexperienced as there is a serious risk of pus being inhaled. It is essential that suitable airway protection, in the form of a cuffed endotracheal tube, is used. All cases, except in extreme emergency, should therefore be referred immediately to the otolaryngology department.

Parapharyngeal abscess

Parapharyngeal abscess forms in the areolar space lateral to the pharynx. It is due to spread of infection from the tonsils, peritonsillar tissues or the lower wisdom teeth. It may occur at any age, but is commonest in adolescents or adults. It presents as a swelling in the neck or pharynx. In the latter presentation, the tonsil may be pushed medially, mimicking a quinsy; in parapharyngeal abscess, however, the bulk of the swelling tends to lie posterior to the tonsil. The abscess may spread upwards to involve the base of the skull or downwards into the superior mediastinum.

Management. All cases should be referred immediately to the otolaryngology department for management.

Acute epiglottitis

See Ch. 10 (p. 121).

Laryngotracheobronchitis (croup)

This is primarily a disease of children and is due to a viral infection of the larynx, trachea and bronchi. It affects a slightly younger age group than does epiglottitis, occurring mainly in 1–4 year olds.

The disease is usually of slow onset and there are many clinically mild cases. On occasion, however, this disease can be fatal and severe cases must be admitted for careful observation. Typically, the child presents with a harsh, barking cough of a few days' duration which progresses to the onset of inspiratory stridor: in severe cases, further progression may lead to increasing and serious respiratory distress. Dysphagia is not a prominent feature and there is no toxaemia.

Management.   Most cases will settle over a few days with treatment consisting of sedation, humidification and, occasionally, steroids. A few will require airway management, either by endotracheal intubation or tracheotomy.

Tonsillar haemorrhage

Despite the large number of tonsillectomies performed annually, serious secondary haemorrhage following the operation is, fortunately, rare. Massive and rapidly fatal bleeding does, however, occur and all patients presenting with tonsillar haemorrhage must be treated with caution.

Management

In most cases it is sufficient, having made the diagnosis, to refer the patient immediately to the otolaryngology department. Where bleeding is very profuse, however, it may be necessary to take immediate steps to control it. This is best done by sitting the patient upright and applying to the tonsil fossa a tightly folded gauze swab held in a pair of forceps and soaked in an equal part mixture of 4% lignocaine and 1:1000 adrenaline. This should be held in place firmly for several minutes. Attention should also be given, of course, to the patient's general condition, any hypovolaemic shock being treated in the normal way.

Miscellaneous causes of acute upper airway obstruction

Allergic glottic oedema

Hereditary angioneurotic oedema.   This is dealt with in Ch. 15 (p. 204).

Neoplasms

Acute obstruction may occur in patients with neoplastic lesions of the larynx, trachea and surrounding structures. In most instances, obstruction will be of slow onset but, occasionally, bleeding into a degenerating growth will cause rapid swelling with encroachment on the airway. Tracheotomy may be necessary in some cases.

Emergency tracheotomy

The technique is described in Ch. 10 (p. 119).

Skin conditions

Dermatological emergencies are not usually life-threatening. Furthermore, if there is a good dermatological service in a city it is likely that such patients will present to the skin department rather than an A & E department. Nevertheless, patients do present to casualty with acute, or semiacute and at times chronic, skin conditions. A & E doctors may give initial treatment, some simple conditions may then be referred to general practitioners for continuing care, others will require further management by a dermatologist.

Other texts on this topic have often classified the urgencies as diseases. This is not the way the patient presents to the emergency clinic. The patient comes along with specific symptoms and signs and consequently the complaints are discussed in alphabetical order.

BLEEDING

Bleeding due to dermatological disease into or onto the skin is unusual. Bleeding from the lips can be due to *hereditary haemorrhagic telangectasia*. The patient often knows the diagnosis but may present to the A & E department with nose bleeds and females may have menorrhagia. The treatment required is cautery of the lesions but topical epsilon aminocaproic acid may help.

Localised bleeding of the finger can often occur at the site of a fleshy *pyogenic granuloma*. This may arise as a result of recent trauma, although this may have been so insignificant not to have been remembered. The lesion, some 5–20 mm, red, fleshy and raised from the surface, has usually been present for a few weeks. Firm pressure may stop the bleeding. Cautery of the granuloma may be necessary and, even then, it is sometimes difficult to stop the bleeding and tying of the feeding vessel may be necessary.

A *malignant melanoma* may bleed; the history is usually longer and there may, but not always, be a history of a preceding mole. If in any doubt, excision of the lesion and urgent histological examination are required. A pyogenic granuloma is normally much more pedunculated than a melanoma, but remember, not all melanomata are pigmented. Feel for enlarged glands; they may be found in melanomata but never in pyogenic granuloma.

Bleeding may occur from a *cavernous haemangioma*. The bleeding is usually slight yet may make the patient anxious, and superficial ulceration may develop. Simple pressure with a sterile dressing is required.

BLISTERING DISEASE

There are many reasons for a bullous eruption. A *localised* bullous eruption, occurring usually on an erythematous background, is suggestive of *papular urticaria*. These lesions can be found, usually, on the exposed parts of the body and are often in groups (Figs. 45.1 and 45.2). They are due to flea bites and

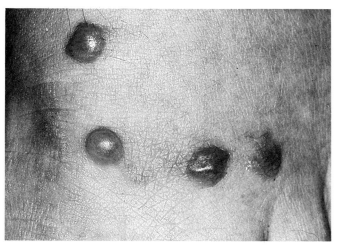

Fig. 45.1 Shows the group of blisters in a patient with *papular urticaria*.

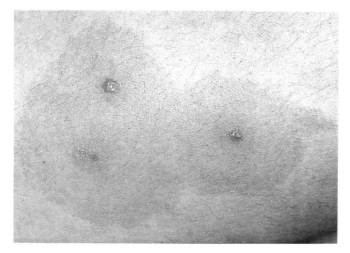

Fig. 45.2 Shows other lesions in a patient with *papular urticaria*. These lesions showed intense erythema and the development of small blisters in the centre.

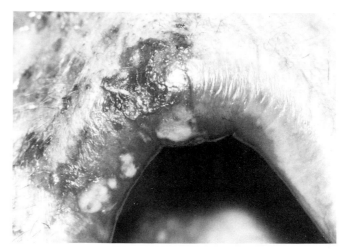

Fig. 45.4 *Herpes zoster*. Close up of the patient shown in the previous figure. The superficial ulcers arose from vesicles.

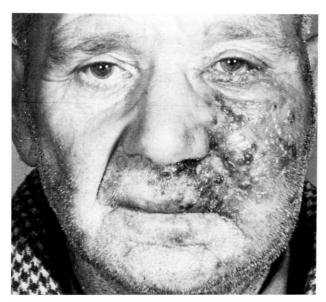

Fig. 45.3 *Herpes zoster*. This patient suddenly developed a painful blistering eruption in the second division of left cranial nerve.

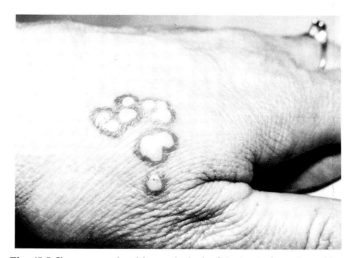

Fig. 45.5 Shows grouped vesicles on the back of the hand of a patient with *herpes simplex*. An unusual site.

there may have been obvious contact with animals. The patient may give a past history of similar trouble. The treatment consists of popping the blisters with a sterile needle and applying a steroid-antiseptic combination such as Betamethasone C cream twice daily and, if itchy, oral antihistamines such as triprolidine 1.25–2.5 mg twice a day.

A localised but painful form of blistering is *herpes zoster* (Figs. 45.3 and Fig. 45.4). The patient may present initially with pain and this may confuse the doctor. A simple trick to aid the diagnosis of a suspected herpes zoster is to run a needle over the area of pain and if the patient notices an area of hyperaesthesia it is quite likely that, within 24 hours, the multilocular blisters will arise. Within a few days they will become confluent, necrotic and pustular. Usually herpes zoster affects only one dermatome but it can, especially in immunocompromised people, become quite

widespread producing a varicelliform eruption. Treatment consists of relief of pain with adequate analgesia. If the diagnosis is made early — within 2–3 days — Acyclovir 800 mg/four times a day for 5 days and Acyclovir cream topically (four times a day) can help considerably; antibiotics are usually given, especially erythromycin 250 mg q.i.d. for 5 days, to control any secondary infection. If there is much oozing, potassium permanganate baths 1:100 000 dilution is helpful.

Localised small blisters (vesicles) may be seen in patients with *herpes simplex*; patients with herpes simplex will only present at the A & E department if lesions are at an odd site. The vesicles are grouped and itchy (Fig. 45.5).

Localised blisters on the palms and soles are usually due to constitutional eczema — the so-called *pompholyx*. The onset is sudden with itchy multilocular blisters. The patient may have a long history of previous eczema either widespread or localised. The A & E physician should prescribe Betamethasone C ointment and triprolidine 1.25–2.5 mg twice daily.

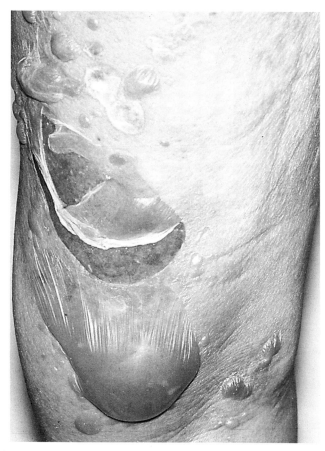

Fig. 45.6 The thigh of a patient with *toxic epidermal necrolysis*. Notice the blisters, one in particular shows the ease with which the blister ruptures producing tender denuded areas of skin.

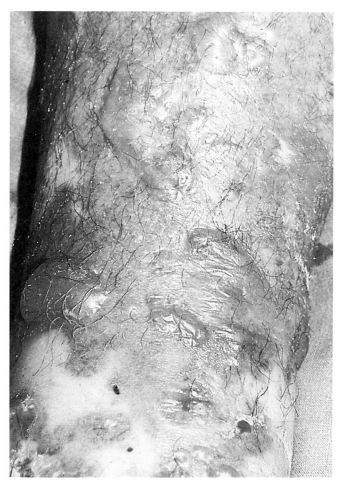

Fig. 45.7 The thigh of a patient with *bullous pemphigoid*. The blisters are tense and have occurred on urticated oedematous red background.

Painful, *widespread* blistering should alert the physician to the possibility that the patient has *toxic epidermal necrolysis* (TEN). This can be a life-threatening condition, especially if drug induced. Onset is usually sudden, the patient complaining of painful tender skin (Fig. 45.6). Within hours of the onset, the skin may come off, even when touched, producing widespread denuded areas. Hospitalisation is essential. Up to the age of 14 or 15 years, the likeliest cause is a *Staphylococcus aureus* infection which produces an epidermolytic toxin. Look for a source of infection such as impetigo. In older people, drugs are the cause. Virtually every drug in use has, at some time or another, caused this potentially fatal condition. Care in the dermatological ward is essential.

A similar but slower onset of widespread blisters and denuded skin is seen in *pemphigus vulgaris*. This is often associated with a history of mouth ulcers for some weeks before cutaneous involvement. It is unusual in pemphigus to see intact blisters as the split in the skin is within the epidermis and so the presentation is usually that of raw tender areas. The patient is usually in the mid-50s or older and often Jewish. Admission to hospital and confirmation of diagnosis by biopsy (both routine and immunofluorescent) are essential as well as checking for pemphigus antibodies. Therapy is with oral steroids, 60 mg/day, often combined with azathioprine 100 mg/day. Therapy is for life.

A patient with blistering for a few weeks may present to casualty because of the sudden deterioration or persistence of their symptoms. The onset of tense blisters, at times haemorrhagic, at times serous, occuring on a red background showing some features of urticaria, should alert the physician to *bullous pemphigoid* (Fig. 45.7). The rash is normally quite widespread, although it can begin in a localised area. Mouth lesions normally do not occur. The age affected is 55 years and over. The patient requires admission to a dermatological ward for diagnosis by biopsy and examination of the blood for pemphigoid antibodies. Therapy, as with pemphigus — for life, is initially with oral steroids (60 mg/day), possibly plus azathioprine (100 mg/day).

Widespread blistering in infancy is very uncommon but usually signifies one of the several variants of *hereditary epidermolysis bullosa* (Fig. 45.8). At least half of such patients have a poor prognosis and may die early in infancy. The onset is usually with a few hours of birth. The presentation is that of tense blisters and raw areas which arise wherever the skin is touched. Mucosal lesions may occur. Referral to a dermatologist is necessary.

DISCRETE, BUT WIDESPREAD, RED SPOTS

Such a patient will usually present with a history of a rash present for a few days or even a few hours. It is necessary to note whether

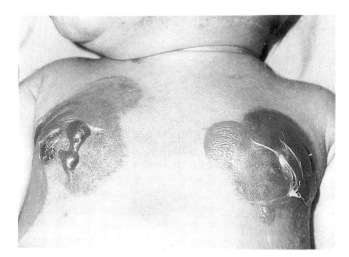

Fig. 45.8 Shows the chest of a neonate with *hereditary epidermolysis bullosa*. The blisters arise as a result of touching the child's skin.

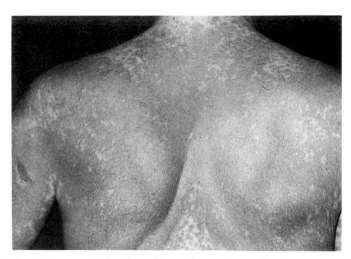

Fig. 45.9 *Drug rash*. A patient with macular-papular eruption due to penicillin.

the rash is *scaly or* not scaly. If *scaly* it could well be that this is an acute *guttate psoriasis*. There may be a family history of psoriasis, and a history of a (streptococcal) sore throat. The lesions vary in size from 1–20 mm, are usually non-itchy, but at times can be quite itchy. Removal of a scale will usually demonstrate bleeding points because of the irregular nature of the epidermal-dermal junction in psoriasis. Look at the nails, there may be pitting and onycholysis (separation of the distal end of the nail). There may also be scalp involvement.

Pityriasis rosea usually presents in the 15–30 year age group with the sudden onset of non-itchy widespread spots. A careful history may reveal that the patient has had a spot, the so-called herald spot (a single plaque — up to 5 cm in diameter) for two to three weeks beforehand. The rash usually affects the trunk in a fir tree-like distribution. It may affect the upper arms and in atopic individuals can be more widespread and more itchy. Reassurance is required and a prescription of oily cream. Admission for both these diseases is not required and the general practitioner can adequately manage such patients.

If the *red rash is not scaly*, then consider that the patient may have one of the many exanthemata or drug rashes. Most drug rashes are macular-papular, and are not further described since most A & E physicians are good at diagnosing these disorders (Fig. 45.9). However, if infection is suspected, it is important to know the immunisation status of the individual, known exposure, distribution of the rash, spread pattern, associated symptoms and, in order to distinguish a drug rash, known allergies and any associated therapy. It is important to note that even the commonest of diseases can be atypical and extensive in immunocompromised patients and that such a patient may also be an adult. In addition to the *well recognised viral causes* of an exanthema one has got to consider the *enteroviruses*, the *Epstein Barr virus* and the *parvoviruses* and the *paramyxovirus* — the rashes being usually macular-papular. It is also important to ask whether the patient has been to any other part of the world — not necessarily to exotic parts of the world. For example, *Rocky Mountain spotty fever* is a virus contracted from a tic bite. It is seen particularly in eastern USA,

but could be seen in Great Britain because of intercontinental travel. Such a patient may present with a fever, arthralgia, a macular-papular rash and a characteristic feature is gangrene of the genitals. Treatment is tetracycline if the patient is over the age of 8 years, otherwise chloramphenicol. Most exanthemata are associated with some constitutional upset but this may be mild. In *hand, foot* and *mouth* disease there are oval vesicles, usually occurring in an area of mild erythema on the hands and feet with superficial ulcers in the mouth. The condition is self limiting and needs no treatment.

Under this heading of 'Discrete red spots' need to be included *erythema nodosum*, which is discussed under 'Tender Skins', and *erythema multiforme*. Patients with the latter complain of an acute rash being present for a matter of a few hours up to 72 hours. The rash, characteristically, is more evident on the extensor aspect of the limbs, although it can be widespread; the individual lesions have a target-like appearance and may show central vesiculation (Figs 45.10 and 45.11). In more extreme cases there may be involvement of the mucous membrane and the genitals, the eyes and mouth producing the so-called *Stevens-Johnston syndrome*. The physician should look for a cause such as preceding herpetic simplex infection, streptococcal sore throat, mycoplasma infection, drugs; radiation of a pre-existing tumour may also induce erythema multiforme. Potent topical steroid creams may be indicated but treatment is not usually started in the A & E department. A dermatological referral is usually appropriate.

FLEXURAL RASHES

The patient may come to casualty complaining of discomfort in the groin or axilla. This could be an exacerbation of a pre-existing and perhaps more widespread rash, such as psoriasis or eczema, but one should consider *hidradenitis suppurativa* (see Ch. 32), *intertrigo* or, especially in the groin, *candidiasis*. Intertrigo simply refers to friction between two opposing surfaces and this therefore presents as a problem in individuals who are overweight, in whom it may also affect the breasts. The skin is normally of a glazed

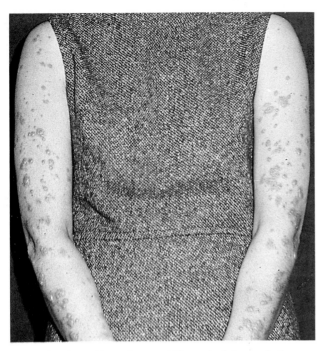

Fig. 45.10 A patient with *erythema multiforme*; the lesions typically occurring on the extensor aspect of the forearm.

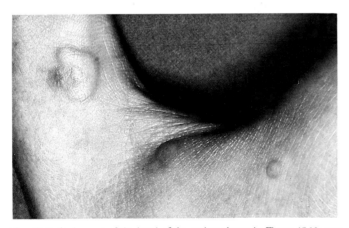

Fig. 45.11 A close up of the hand of the patient shown in Figure 45.10; note target-like lesions.

appearance and may show superficial ulceration. Bacteriological culture often grows a mixed colony of organisms including, maybe, *Candida albicans*. Immediate treatment is to keep the adjacent skin apart with simple dressings or, in the case of the breasts, good fitting bra, the topical application of clioquinol paste or, if moist, Betadine spray and, if dry and cracked, Betadine or Bactroban ointment. The diagnosis of *Candida* should be suspected especially if the patient has some pre-existing factor such as diabetes; the physician should look for the so-called peripheral satellite lesions, which occur as small red papules — usually with a little scaling or vesiculation. A satisfactory treatment for candidiasis is miconazole (Daktarin) or econazole cream (Ecostatin) or, if the area is a little moist, use the lotion. If the physician considers that the rash is, in addition, possibly eczematised then a good therapeutic bet would be the use of steroid antimonalial combination such

as Vioform-hydrocortisone cream. Remember, if there is any itching prescribe appropriate antihistamine therapies. Follow up by the general practitioner or dermatologist is necessary.

INFECTIONS

The combination of acute, pustular, crusted, tender lesions may be associated with systemic symptoms and is suggestive of infections. Infections can be divided into primary and secondary. Secondary infections usually consist of impetiginisation of such conditions as scabies and pediculosis. More often than not, impetigo occurs as a disease entity in its own right, presenting with a few days history of superficial, golden-coloured crusts, initially on one part of the body but frequently spreading to other parts. Impetigo tends to affect the less fortunate members of the society and close relatives and friends may be affected. Occasionally in children, impetigo may become bullous. A swab will usually grow a *Staphylococcus aureus*, occasionally a haemolytic streptococcus. The treatment is with an oral antibiotic such as erythromycin for 5 days, chlorhexidine (Hibitane) as a wash or for use in the bath, a palmful of the solution being placed in a basin full of warm water and applied to the whole of the skin, kept on the skin for a minute, before the patient baths or showers. In less extensive cases povidone-iodine (Betadine) ointment or mucopirocin (Bactroban) ointment can help tremendously in conjunction with chlorhexidine baths. It is always useful, if possible, to swab the nose of other members of the family. If this is not possible, provide other members of the family with chlorhexidine for washing purposes and to apply naseptin (chlorhexidine and neomycin) cream to the nostrils to reduce the nasal carriage of *S. aureus*. All patients and, where relevant, family contacts should use this routine for one week.

ITCHING CONDITIONS

Although many dermatological problems may itch, there are some which are particularly more itchy than others and a good dividing point is those that will keep the patient awake at night. In such situations consider dermatitis, eczema, scabies and urticaria. Consider *scabies* particularly where there has been a recent onset of itching — not just in the patient himself but in other members of his family or non-relatives, such as girlfriends/boyfriends. As with almost all dermatological problems, it is essential to examine the whole skin. Look for small burrows — these are lesions 1–3 mm long occurring particularly between the fingers and in the axillary fold; nodules on the scrotum is a diagnostic sign of scabies. There may be secondary impetiginisation and one parasite goes with another so always look for pediculi. If in doubt, you could always scrape the lesion with a blunt scalpel and 10% potassium hydroxide; place a smear beneath a microscope and look for the mites doing a breast-stroke on the glass slide. Most A & E physicians are quite good at diagnosing scabies because they have a high index of suspicion — whatever the walk of life of the patient. The treatment consists not just of treating the patient and family but all close contacts, even if they have no symptoms whatsoever.

The doctor must ensure that:

1. Patients and contacts are treated at the same time.

2. They have a bath/shower on the first night of treatment and apply the therapy, i.e. 25% benzoyl benzoate, gamma benzene hexachloride (Lorexane), to the whole of the affected area from the neck downwards, including the genitalia.

3. During the next 48 hours when the individual washes they must reapply the therapy, which must be in constant contact with the skin for 48 hours. At the end of 48 hours, if the skin is still itchy, they can be given steroid cream such as flurandrenolone (Haelan) cream and antihistamines may be needed to control the residual (non-infectious) itch.

4. After 48 hours, they must wash all clothes, including bedlinen, and press with a hot iron articles such as anoraks and trousers which are not easily washed.

Some patients will deny that there is any way they could have contracted scabies, so it is useful to remember that occasionally animal scabies can affect the human and, if this is a useful way out, then tell them to buy some antiscabetic powder to treat their pet.

Eczema is the most likely diagnosis in the patient with a long-standing, or relatively long-standing, history of an itchy rash, especially if he/she or any relative has asthma or hayfever, or when a relative has eczema. In young children eczema classically affects the flexures, especially of the arms and the legs, although it can become very widespread and so loses its original localisation. Patients with widespread disease and bleeding from excoriated lesions might need hospitalisation. Secondary infection with *S. aureus* is common even though there may be no frank impetiginised lesions. In the treatment of such patients, prescribe:

1. Adequate does of antihistamine — telling the patient to adjust the dose of the antihistamine to find that which will control the itch without them feeling drowsy.

2. Oil substitutes, such as oilatum in the bath are helpful.

3. If such a patient has presented at A & E department, it is almost universally true that they will be colonised with *S. aureus* and so a 5-day course of erythromycin is well worthwhile giving.

4. A potent topical steroid combined with an antiseptic such as Betnovate C or Betnovate N as an ointment, not as a cream, applied twice daily should control the patient's symptoms until they can be seen by a dermatologist.

Children with atopic eczema may contract from their mother or other relative widespread herpetic lesions. This is called Kaposi's varicelliform eruption and is characterised by the presence of many vesicles (Fig. 45.12). The child is usually ill and admission is needed. Acylovir cream and tablets are of considerable benefit.

The term 'eczema' usually refers to a non-infective inflammation of the skin such as constitutional eczema as just described, with the term dermatitis being reserved to a non-infective inflammation of the skin caused by external factors. *Contact dermatitis* may be irritant or allergic in origin. Both types are usually itchy and the dermatitis often occurs at the site of contact with a chemical causing the problem — although in the case of an allergic reaction the dermatitis can spread to other parts of the body by an ill-understood immunologically mechanism. The back of the hands and fingers

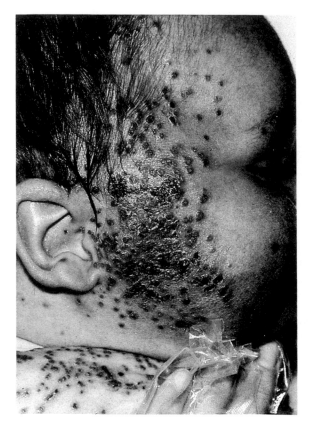

Fig. 45.12 A child with *Kaposi's varicelliform eruption*. This child's mother had a small cold sore. Note the multiple papular vesicular lesions. The child was unwell and admission was necessary.

are a common site for an irritant and contact dermatitis. The face is frequently the site of involvement also in contact dermatitis. Sometimes the offending antigen is obvious (Fig. 45.13), i.e. an acute dermatitis due to a hair dye may produce sudden facial swelling or great concern to the patient; an acute reaction to eyedrops may also induce enough anxiety to warrant a visit but sometimes ingenuity is required to identify the antigen. Who would think that the man's acute lip dermatitis is due to his wife's lipstick? Therapy consists of withdrawing the offending agent and thus a careful history is required to determine what the patient may have applied to the skin, including medicaments given by another doctor. A potent steroid such as Betnovate cream or ointment is required, plus oral antihistamines and, in the severe widespread cases of an acute allergic dermatitis, oral steroids (40 mg reducing over 6 days).

The sudden onset of a widespread itchy rash in crops — each crop lasting for several hours — is diagnostic of *urticaria* (Fig. 45.14). Many patients with urticaria may attend the A & E department because of the associated facial oedema, the so-called angio-oedema. The swelling of the face may involve the eyes and the lips and, at times, can be very severe. There are many reasons for acute urticaria but, in particular, the physician should ask the patient whether he has taken any certain foods (in particular shellfish, strawberries, bananas), or drugs, (in particular codeine and aspirin). Physical factors such as sunlight, heat and cold can

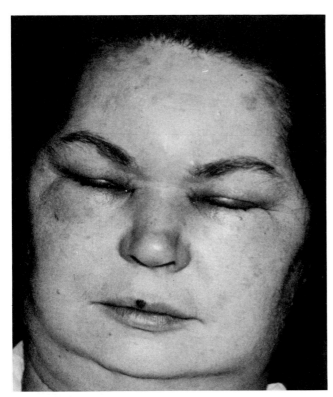

Fig. 45.13 The patient with an *acute contact dermatitis*. Note the considerable oedema and vesiculation. This reaction was to hair dye.

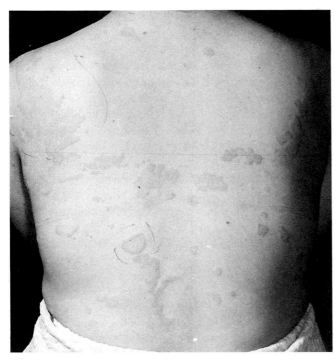

Fig. 45.14 This patient has *urticaria*. Note the widespread weals.

induce urticaria. Certain dyes (such as azo-dyes) and preservatives in foods can precipitate intermittent attacks of urticaria, so the patient may present with an acute episode based on a chronic background of a long history. Rarely a patient with urticaria may

have swelling of the tongue, difficulty with breathing and difficulty in swallowing. Any of these signs warrant admission at least for observation. If any of these coexist and if there is also abdominal pain, then it is mandatory that blood is taken for C1 esterase inhibitor to exclude the potentially fatal hereditary angio-oedema. A reduction in this factor can be associated with acute dyspnoea resulting in sudden death. Fortunately, most district hospitals can now perform this test and if such a patient is suspected of having this disease they must be kept under observation until either the symptoms disappear and/or the test comes back as normal.

The treatment of urticaria includes reassurance as the condition to the uninitiated can be quite frightening. Intramuscular antihistamines such as chlorphreniramine maleate 10 mg may be given. Intravenous steroids, if severe, 100 mg hydrocortisone succinate and 1:1000 adrenaline subcutaneously 0.2–0.5 mg may be required. In the case of hereditary angio-oedema, resuscitation may be required; steroids do not help this condition. Anabolic steriods, Stromba 5 mg b.d., can prevent the symptoms; in an acute attack, fresh plasma may be needed and, at times, tracheotomy will be required. The patient must be given a Medic-Alert necklet or bracelet and relatives should be checked for the same condition.

PURPURIC RASHES

Purpuric rashes are characterised by the relatively sudden onset of a very florid rash, particularly on the lower legs. At times the purpuric rash can become papular, vesicular and may ulcerate — even over a matter of 48 hours. A purpuric rash has many aetiological factors and for practical reasons can be divided into those which are purely of the cutaneous variety — for which the reader is referred to standard textbooks of dermatology — and the systemic variety. The most likely to be encountered in A & E department is *Henoch Schoenlein purpura* (Fig. 45.15). The term purpura in this eponym is a little misleading as many of the lesions are, in fact, papular and may show vesiculation. The patient will often give a history of a polyarthropathy and there may be haematuria and melaena with abdominal pain. The cause is often a preceding streptococcal sore throat, although in the older age group frusemide is a recognised cause. In some patients no cause is discovered. Hospitalisation is often required and treatment is usually symptomatic.

Purpura along with vesicular and pustular lesions can also be seen in *chronic gonococcocaemia, meningococcaemia* and acute *Gram-negative septicaemia*. In the former two there are usually few lesions and in the gonococcal patient the lesions usually occur on the palms, fingers and soles. However, acute Gram-negative septicaemia and meningococcaemia may be associated with variable widespread lesions. Admission is necessary. Skin cultures and blood cultures are necessary as may be other investigations including cervical, prostatic and urethral smears. Meningococcaemia is usually associated with positive blood culture but negative skin culture. There may be evidence of disseminated intravascular coagulation. If there is any suspicion of meningococcal infection then immediate treatment with parental penicillin is necessary.

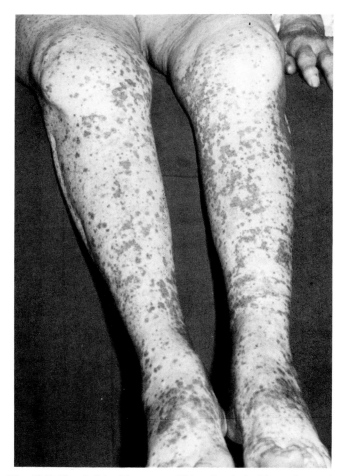

Fig. 45.15 Henoch Schonlein purpura. This patient had widespread purpuric lesions some of which become papular and nodular. This patient presented to the A & E department with acute abdominal pain and at laparotomy was found to have a haemorrhagic small intestine.

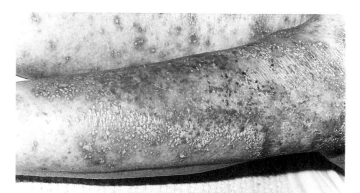

Fig. 45.16 Patient with *generalised pustular psoriasis* — within a matter of hours many small creamy yellow pustules developed.

PUSTULES

Since pustules erupt fairly quickly, it is not surprising that patients with pustular lesions may present at an A & E department. The pustules may be *infective* or *non-infective*. The infective pustular disorders have been described in other sections here.

There are several non-infective skin diseases which may present relatively acutely. Three will be discussed. *Pompholyx* is described in more detail on p. 474, but in addition to the classical tense sago-grain vesicles a few, and sometimes many, pustular lesions may develop. *Pustular psoriasis* can present either as a localised or generalised variety. It is unlikely that localised pustular psoriasis, which is associated with no constitutional disorder, will present to the A & E department.

Specialist advice must be sought in patients who have widespread pustular psoriasis. Such patients present with the rapid onset of pustules. In a matter of a few hours the patient may be covered with hundreds of many small, creamy, yellow pustules — 1–2 mm in size (Fig. 45.16), often associated with superficial scaling of the skin, which is intensely red, hot and uncomfortable; the patient is unwell. Such patients are usually in hospital for several weeks and require intensive, specialised dermatological management. If no dermatologist is immediately available, oral antihistamines and topical therapy with half strength Lassar's paste (BNF) is reasonably adequate.

SUN-INDUCED PHOTODERMATOSES

It is not surprising that a patient may present to casualty with an acute photodermatosis and most patients should be referred to a dermatologist for investigation and treatment. The reaction could be a flare-up of a *pre-existing* skin trouble such as *rosacea* or *discoid lupus erythematosis* but is unlikely that such a patient will come to casualty. The most likely reason for a patient presenting is either the development of pain in the skin or a rash following exposure to sunlight. Patients with *erythropoetic porphyria* may be diagnosed as being hysterical and sent home again — only to reappear on the next sunny occasion. Examination of such a patient's skin reveals usually very little, but there may be some oedema. The patient will complain bitterly of tenderness on exposure to the sun. The A & E doctor should be aware of the condition and refer the patient to a dermatologist for analysis of the red cells for porphyria.

Porphyria cutanea tarda presents with slightly itchy small tense blisters especially on the hands. Detailed investigation of the urine and faeces are necessary, plus the help of a dermatologist.

A common reason for a patient attending casualty with a photodermatosis is due to the interaction of u.v. radiation with either a topically applied drug or an oral medicament. Patients who sunbathe and apply oil of Bergamot are at risk of developing an *acute contact photodermatosis*. Likewise some drugs may cause a *toxic or allergic photodermatosis*. Such drugs include sulphonamides, nalidixic acid, Negram and chlorpromazine (Largactil) and thus a careful drug history is required. Treatment consists of the use of oral antihistamines and a potent topical steroid such as Betamethasone cream or Betamethasone ointment and, of course, stopping the relevant drug.

A clue to the diagnosis of a photodermatosis is the localisation of eruption affecting the exposed areas, especially the prominences of the forehead, the tips of the ears, the upper cheeks and the chin. The shaded areas are spared. Such patients may be aware of their problems. They must be strongly advised to use adequate sun protection creams when in the sun, such as those with a factor of 15, available from most chemists.

TENDER, PAINFUL SKIN

A patient may attend the casualty department complaining that their skin is painful or tender. Under such situations one should consider if the problem is widespread, *toxic epidermal necrolysis* (see p. 474); if localised to a dermatome *herpes zoster* (p. 473); *cellulitis* (Ch. 33, p. 345); or if localised to the legs, especially both legs, and on the shins, *erythema nodosum*. To the non-dermatologists this is often thought of as being very well defined circumscribed nodular lesions — this is not so. The skin usually has a red, bruised appearance with some superficial oedema, there being anything from 1 to up to 12 lesions. Occasionally, the condition is more widespread. Aetiological factors to be considered include streptococcal sore throats, sarcoidosis, tuberculosis, drugs (including the contraceptive pill), pregnancy and inflammatory bowel disease (such as ulcerative colitis and Crohn's). Immediate treatment consists, if necessary, of bedrest, analgesia such as aspirin or non-steroidal anti-inflammatory drugs, a cradle to reduce pressure from the bedlinen. As the disease is an immune reaction, topical steroids such as betamethasone cream four times a day are necessary and, occasionally, oral steroids or ACTH will be given.

Cellulitis (Ch. 33) may be confused with erythema nodosum.

ULCERS

Three features may precipitate a visit to A & E department — pain, bleeding or chronicity. Severe intractable *pain* is usually associated with arterial rather than venous ulcers. Arterial ulcers tend to be deeper, venous ulcers more superficial. Arterial ulcers tend to occur more on the shins and toes whereas venous ulcers favour the malleoli. Venous ulcers stimulate a local inflammatory reaction, arterial ulcers do not (Fig. 45.17). *Bleeding* is rare from arterial ulcers (Fig. 45.18). Treatment of this complication consists simply of elevation of the leg and a firm bandage, but it is important to feel all the peripheral pulses before a firm occlusive bandage is applied. The treatment of pain may involve the use of powerful therapies such as the opiates and hospitalisation may be required for local management of the leg ulcer which, in turn, should help the pain. The third reason for attendance at the A & E department is that the *chronicity* of the leg ulcer has driven the patient to distraction. Something needs to be done and a visit to the A & E department was the obvious choice.

There are further reasons why ulcerated lesions may be the cause of attendance at the A & E department. Patients with *cutaneous vasculitis* may develop, as well as purpuric and nodular lesions, multiple ulcers (Fig. 45.19). The ulcers are usually on the lower legs small and painful. A patient who has a cutaneous vasculitis and presents to the A & E department may have systemic disease such as Henoch-Schoenlein purpura, rheumatoid arthritis or polyarteritis nodosa. Patients with the latter two diseases may have a patchy, mottled appearance on the leg — the so-called livedo reticularis.

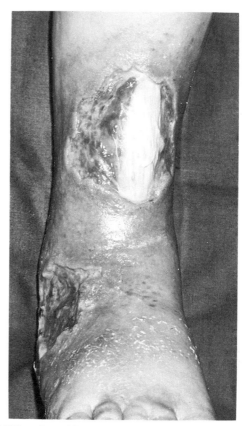

Fig. 45.17 This patient with an *arterial ulcer* presented to the A & E department because of severe pain.

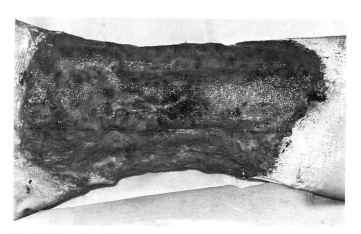

Fig. 45.18 A patient with a very extensive *venous ulcer*. The patient presented to the A & E department with superficial oozing of blood. The patient's haemoglobin was 6.2 G.

An ulcer at an unusual site, such as on the upper thigh, arm or chest, and in particular of sudden onset should raise the possibility of *pyoderma gangrenosum*. These lesions are quite large, up to several centimetres in diameter, and may initially present with multiple small vesicles or pustules, the lesion rapidly breaking down to form a large ulcer. Such patients may have or may subsequently develop ulcerative colitis, Crohn's disease or, occasionally, leukaemia. Specialist advice is necessary but

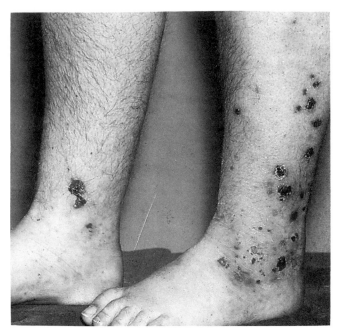

Fig. 45.19 A patient with multiple small vasculitic ulcers. This patient had rheumatoid arthritis.

symptomatic therapy of the pain will help. Oral steroids and Azathioprine are frequently required.

The onset of an ulcer on one side of the forehead or scalp, usually with a 2–14 day history, should raise the suspicion of *temporal arteritis*. Additional features include headache and impaired vision on the same side as the ulcer. The temporal artery may possibly be tender and there may be papilloedema. It is essential, even if the diagnosis is in doubt, to treat immediately with oral steriods (60 mg/day) to prevent blindness. Admission is necessary.

An ulcer at an unusual site may also suggest *dermatitis artefacta*. Such an ulcer is often round, oval or square (Fig. 45.20). The patient may have a long complicated medical history and may not give away the clue of previous psychiatric referral. The patient usually does not look ill. Referral to a dermatologist is necessary.

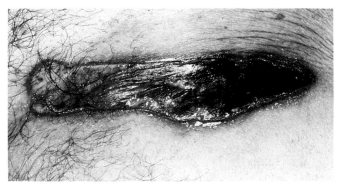

Fig. 45.20 *Dermatitis artefacta*. This patient presented to the A & E department with malaise and a rash. The rash proved to be deliberately, chemically induced. Eventually her hospital records revealed a very complicated psychiatric history.

THE WIDESPREAD RED PATIENT

Such a patient is usually referred to as *erythrodermic*. Occasionally scaling may be more of a feature and dermatologists will then call this an *exfoliative dermatitis* (Fig. 45.21). This latter title may lead the non-initiated into assuming the rash is due to a contact factor. The terms exfoliative dermatitis and erythroderma are frequently used — interchangeably, depending upon whether the skin is more red or more scaly. Such a patient is usually very unwell and needs hospitalisation. In all but 10% of cases, the cause can be found. Usually it is due to a flare of already pre-existing psoriasis (25%), pre-existing eczema (42%), drugs including allopurinol, gold, sulphonamides and penicillin (10%). Eight per cent of subjects will be found to have underlying reticulosis. Patients with erythroderma have considerably deranged skin physiology which may result in hypothermia, hyperthermia, dehydration, prerenal kidney failure. Secondary infection of the skin is common.

Treatment requires hospitalisation and management by a dermatologist.

ADDITIONAL NOTES

Cutaneous features of systemic disease

A patient who presents with an acute fever, polyarthropathy and

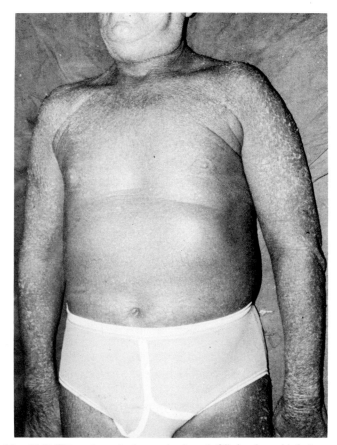

Fig. 45.21 This patient who has *erythroderma/exfoliative dermatitis* had a long history of constitutional eczema: this rapidly deteriorated producing virtually total skin involvement with redness and scaling.

Raynaud's phenomenon may have the butterfly erythematous rash of *systemic lupus erythematosis*. A patient may present to casualty with proximal muscle weakness; close examination of the skin reveals a violaceous appearance around the eyelids and the 'v' of the neck, and a linear pattern running down the backs of the hands and fingers — *dermatomysitis* should be considered. The patient may present with an epileptic fit — examination may reveal on the cheeks the fleshy coloured papules of *adenoma sebaceum*. Alternatively, the patient may be noted to have the fleshy multiple skin tumours of *von Recklinghausen's disease*; such patients have freckling in the axilla — virtually never seen in any other situation — plus café au lait spots; six or more of 1.5 cm or greater in diameter are required usually to support the diagnosis. Patients with von Recklinghausen's disease may have a meningioma, phaeochromocytoma or spinal pressure problems. A patient may present to casualty with profuse arterial bleeding from the mouth, clearly emanating from the gastrointestinal tract. A careful look at the skin may reveal the plucked chicken appearance of the patient with *pseudoxanthoma elasticum*. A patient with profuse nose bleeds may be noticed to have telangectasia on the lips — as part of the *hereditary telangiectasia* syndrome.

Babies

Babies deserve special attention, especially the first born. It is not unusual for their parents to bring their child with only mild *atopic eczema* simply because the general practitioner's therapy is not doing too well.

Seborrhoeic eczema is possibly a variant of atopic eczema. Usually such children are not driven to distraction with itch. The rash, which occurs particularly on the face, the upper trunk and the scalp, has a dry or scaly appearance. Therapy with an intermediate strength steroid such as flurandrenolone (Haelan) ointment, oilatum bath oil and referral to a dermatologist is all that is required. Diagnostic confusion may occur with the so-called *psorasiform napkin dermatitis*; such a child is relatively well and has a widespread rash starting in the nappy area, spreading particularly to involve the flexures and sometimes much of the body. The rash resembles psoriasis and is usually non-itchy. An intermediate steroid such as Haelan ointment will help, as too will a referral to a dermatologist.

Napkin dermatitis is of great concern to parents, particularly as they usually blame themselves when no blame should be placed on them (Fig. 45.22). Treatment with clioquinol paste, Haelan C cream and elixir of trimeprazine tartrate (Vallergan) usually helps. If necessary, hospitalisation could be arranged and the baby nursed without nappies.

Therapeutic principles

To teach a non-dermatologist the therapeutic principles of

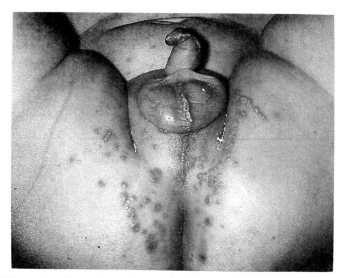

Fig. 45.22 A baby with a typical napkin 'ammonicial' dermatitis.

dermatology is difficult, but some success can be achieved if each time you see a patient with a rash you ask yourself certain questions:

1. Ask yourself, 'should I use oral antihistamines?' Become familiar with one or two therapies rather than many. A standard therapy is triprolidine (Actudil) 2.5 mg twice daily, the dose being adjusted to find that which will control the itch without making the patient drowsy.

Youngsters up to the age of about 4 years tolerate much larger doses of antihistamines than adults. In children, elixir of Vallergan (forte) is a very useful preparation and many youngsters can often tolerate 30 mg at night and 10 mg in the morning — this dose would make you or me totally incapable of carrying out a day's work.

2. Ask yourself, 'should I use a topical steroid?' and, 'should it be combined with an antiseptic such as clioquinol or neomycin or not?'.

3. Ask yourself, when you give that preparation, 'should it be used as an ointment or a cream?' — if the skin is dry use an ointment, otherwise a cream will suffice. The choice of base is clearly important for now well established pharmacological reasons.

4. Ask yourself, 'what advice should I give the patient for bathing?' — maybe no advice is necessary but if the skin is dry consider an oil water substitute such as oilatum bath oil or Alpha Keri; if infected such preparations as chlorhexidine (Hibitane) may help. A bath in the appropriate preparation can be very comforting to the patient.

5. Ask yourself, 'are oral antibiotics needed?' — they will obviously be essential in bacterial infections — but remember that patients with eczema often need oral antibiotics.

6. Ask yourself, 'do I need a dermatologist right now?'.

Appendix 1 Books for the A & E department library

A & E medicine

Emergency Medicine Evans R (ed) 1981 Butterworths, London

Current Emergency Diagnosis & Treatment, 2nd edn. Mills J, Ho M T, Salber P R 1985 Lange, Los Altos, California

Emergency Medicine: Concepts and Clinical Practice Rosen F, Baker F J, Braen R G, Dailey R H, Levy R C 1983 C V Mosby, St. Louis

Accident and Emergency Handbook Wilson D H, Flowers M W 1985 Butterworths, London

Lecture Notes on Accident and Emergency Medicine Yates D W, Redmond A D 1985 Blackwell Scientific Publications, Oxford

Medicine

Cardiac Arrhythmias: Practical Notes on Interpretation and Treatment, 2nd edn. Bennett D H 1985 Wright, Bristol

ABC of Resuscitation Evans T R (ed) 1986 British Medical Journal, London

Emergencies in Clinical Medicine Kennedy H J (ed) 1985 Blackwell Scientific Publications, Oxford

Environmental Emergencies Nelson R N, Rund D A, Keller M D 1985 Saunders, Philadelphia

Birch's Emergencies in Medical Practice 11th edn. Ogilvie C (ed) 1981 Churchill Livingstone, Edinburgh

Oxford Textbook of Medicine, 2nd edn. Weatherall D J, Ledingham J G G, Warrell D A (eds) 1987 Oxford University Press, Oxford

Drugs

ABPI Data Sheet Compendium (Annual) Datapharm Publications, London

British National Formulary (Twice yearly) British Medical Association and The Pharmaceutical Society of Great Britain, London

MIMS (Monthly) Medical Publications, London

Practical Prescribing Brodie M J, Harrison P I 1986 Churchill Livingstone, Edinburgh

Martindale: The Extra Pharmacopoeia, 28th edn. Reynold J E F (ed) 1982 Pharmaceutical Press, London

Poisons

Poisonous Plants in Britain and their Effects on Animals and Man Cooper M R, Johnson A W 1984 HMSO, London

Dangerous Chemicals: Emergency First Aid Guide Houston A (ed) 1983 Wolters Samsom, New Malden, Surrey

Diagnosis and Management of Acute Poisoning Proudfoot A T 1982 Blackwell Scientific Publications, Oxford

Poisoning: Diagnosis and Treatment Vale J A, Meredith T J (eds) 1981 Update Books, London

Infectious diseases and dermatology

ABC of AIDS Adler M W (ed) 1987 British Medical Journal, London

A Colour Atlas of Infectious Diseases, 2nd edn. Emond R T D, Rowland H A K 1987 Wolfe Medical Publications, London

A Colour Atlas of AIDS, Acquired Immune Deficiency Syndrome Farthing C F, Brown S E, Staughton R C D, Cream J J, Muhlemann M 1986 Wolfe Medical Publications, London

Dermatology: an Illustrated Guide, 3rd edn. Fry L 1984 Butterworths, London

Paediatrics

Paediatric Emergencies, 2nd edn. Black J A (ed) 1987 Butterworths, London

The Diagnosis and Primary Care of Accidents and Emergencies in Children, 2nd edn. Illingworth CM 1982 Blackwell Scientific Publications, Oxford

Common Symptoms of Disease in Children, 9th edn. Illingworth R S 1987 Blackwell Scientific Publications, Oxford

Paediatric Emergencies: A Practical Guide to Acute Paediatrics Lissauer T 1982 MTP Press, Lancaster

The Battered Child: Recognition in Primary Care O'Doherty N 1982 Baillière Tindall, London

Trauma

Shock Trauma/Critical Care Manual: Initial Assessment and Management Cowley R A, Dunham C M 1982 University Park Press, Baltimore

ABC of Spinal Cord Injury Grundy D, Russell J, Swain A 1986 British Medical Journal, London

Management of Head Injuries Jennett B, Teasdale G 1981 Davis, Philadelphia

Field Surgery Pocket Book Kirby N G, Blackburn G (ed) 1981 HMSO, London

Advances in Trauma, vol 1 Maull K 1986 Year Book Medical Publications, Chicago

Trauma Care Odling-Smee W, Crockard A (eds) 1981 Academic Press, London

Orthopaedics and fractures

A Colour Atlas of Hand Conditions Conolly W B 1980 Wolfe Medical Publications, London

Musculoskeletal Disease Dickson R A, Wright V (eds) 1984 Heinemann Medical Books, London

Clinical Orthopaedic Examination, 2nd edn. McRae R 1983 Churchill Livingstone, Edinburgh

Practical Fracture Treatment McRae R 1981 Churchill Livingstone, Edinburgh

Sports Injuries: Their Prevention and Treatment Peterson L, Renstrom P 1986 Martin Dunitz, London

Children's Fractures, 2nd edn. Rang M 1983 Lippincott, Philadelphia

The Primary Management of Hand Injuries Semple C 1979 Pitman Medical, Tunbridge Wells

Burns

Burns and Their Treatment, 3rd edn. Muir L F K, Barclay T L, Settle J A D 1987 Butterworths, London

Burns, the First Five Days Settle J A D 1987 Smith & Nephew Pharmaceuticals, Romford

Surgery

Diagnosis of Acute Abdominal Pain de Dombal F T 1980 Churchill Livingstone, Edinburgh

Hamilton Bailey's Emergency Surgery, 11th edn. Dudley H A F (ed) 1986 Wright, Bristol

Plain X-ray Diagnosis of the Acute Abdomen, 2nd edn. Gough M H, Gear M W L, Daar A S 1986 Blackwell Scientific Publications, Oxford

Abdominal Pain in Children O'Donnell B 1985 Blackwell Scientific Publications, Oxford

Eyes, ENT

Atlas of Ophthalmology Glasspool M G 1982 MTP Press, Lancaster

ABC of Ear, Nose and Throat, 2nd edn. Ludman H 1987 British Medical Journal, London

Obstetrics

Essential Management of Obstetric Emergencies Baskett T F 1985 Wiley, Chichester

Anaesthesia

Emergency Anaesthesia Adams A P, Hewitt P B, Rogers M C (eds) 1986 Edward Arnold, London

A Synopsis of Anaesthesia, 10th edn. Atkinson R S, Rushman G B, Lee J A 1987 Wright, Bristol

Illustrated Handbook in Local Anaesthesia, 2nd edn. Eriksson E 1979 Lloyd-Luke, London

Anatomy

A Colour Atlas of Surface Anatomy, Clinical and Applied Backhouse K M, Hutchings R T 1986 Wolfe Medical Publications, London

Aids to Investigating the Peripheral Nervous System Guarantors of 'Brain' 1986 Baillière Tindall, London

A Colour Atlas of Human Anatomy McMinn R M H, Hutchings R T 1977 Wolfe Medical Publications, London

Practical Procedures

Practical Procedures in Accident and Emergency Medicine Ferguson D G, Lord S M 1986 Butterworths, London

Handbook of Percutaneous Central Venous Catheterisation Rosen M, Latto I P, Ng W S 1981 Saunders, London

Radiology

Casualty Radiology: A Practical Guide for Radiological Diagnosis Grech P 1981 Chapman and Hall, London

An Atlas of Normal Roentgen Variants that may Simulate Disease, 3rd edn. Keats T E 1984 Year Book Medical Publishers, Chicago

Nursing and first aid

A Colour Atlas of Nursing Procedures in Accidents and Emergencies Bache J B, Armitt C R, Tobiss J R 1985 Wolfe Medical Publications, London

Emergency Nursing: Principles and Practice Budassi S A, Barber J M 1981 C V Mosby, St Louis

A Colour Atlas of Plastering Techniques Mills K, Page G, Morton R 1986 Wolfe Medical Publications, London

First Aid Manual, 5th edn. St John Ambulance, St Andrew's Ambulance Association, British Red Cross Society 1987 Dorling Kindersley, London

Miscellaneous

How To Do It: 1, 2nd edn. Anonymous 1985 British Medical Journal, London

How To Do It: 2 Anonymous 1987 British Medical Journal, London

Legal Aspects of Medical Practice, 3rd edn. Knight K 1982 Churchill Livingstone, Edinburgh

A Handbook for Clinical Teachers Newble D, Cannon R 1983 MTP Press, Lancaster

Index